THE WASHINGTON MANUAL™
OF CRITICAL CARE

THE WASHINGTON MANUAL™ OF CRITICAL CARE

Marin H. Kollef, MD
Professor of Medicine
Director, Medical Intensive Care Unit
Director, Respiratory Care Unit
Division of Pulmonary and Critical Care Medicine
Washington University School of Medicine
Barnes-Jewish Hospital
St. Louis, Missouri

Timothy J. Bedient, MD
Resident Physician
Department of Internal Medicine
Washington University School of Medicine
Barnes-Jewish Hospital
St. Louis, Missouri

Warren Isakow, MD
Assistant Professor of Medicine
Division of Pulmonary and Critical Care Medicine
Washington University School of Medicine
Barnes-Jewish Hospital
St. Louis, Missouri

Chad A. Witt, MD
Resident Physician
Department of Internal Medicine
Washington University School of Medicine
Barnes-Jewish Hospital
St. Louis, Missouri

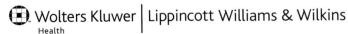
Wolters Kluwer | Lippincott Williams & Wilkins
Health
Philadelphia · Baltimore · New York · London
Buenos Aires · Hong Kong · Sydney · Tokyo

Acquisitions Editor: Brian Brown
Managing Editor: Nicole T. Dernoski
Developmental Editor: Heidi Pongrantz
Marketing Manager: Angela Panetta
Project Manager: Nicole Walz
Manufacturing Coordinator: Kathy Brown
Design Coordinator: Terry Mallon
Production Services: Aptara—India

© 2008 by LIPPINCOTT WILLIAMS & WILKINS, a Wolters Kluwer business
© 2001 by LIPPINCOTT WILLIAMS & WILKINS, © 1997, 1990 by Williams & Wilkins
530 Walnut Street
Philadelphia, PA 19106

Printed in the United States of America

Library of Congress Cataloging-in-Publication Data

The Washington manual of critical care / [edited by] Marin H. Kollef . . . [et al.].
    p. ; cm.
    Includes bibliographical references and index.
    ISBN-13: 978-0-7817-7054-5 (alk. paper)
    ISBN-10: 0-7817-7054-8 (alk. paper)
  1. Critical care medicine—Handbooks, manuals, etc. I. Kollef, Marin H.
II. Washington University (Saint Louis, Mo.). School of Medicine. III.
Title: Manual of critical care.
    [DNLM: 1. Critical Care—methods—Handbooks. 2. Critical
Illness—therapy—Handbooks. WX 39 W319 2008]
  RC86.8.W38 2008
  616.02′8—dc22

                  2007031356

---

2 3 4 5 6 7 8 9 10

We dedicate this manual to all health care providers involved in the care of critically ill patients and their families. We acknowledge their efforts and sacrifices and hope this manual can assist them in some meaningful way.
To our families for their support and to the critical care community of Washington University and Barnes-Jewish Hospital for their commitment to the education and well-being of medical students and house staff physicians.

Finally, we would like to dedicate this manual to Daniel Schuster, MD. Dan was a mentor to all of us and one of the founders of critical care at Washington University and Barnes-Jewish Hospital. He was one of the leaders in the investigation of the acute respiratory distress syndrome performing many landmark studies in this and other areas of critical care medicine. Dan will be remembered as an outstanding teacher, expert clinician, meticulous clinical researcher, close friend, and a loving husband and father.

CONTENTS

III: CARDIAC DISORDERS

IV: ELECTROLYTE ABNORMALITIES

V: ACID-BASE DISORDERS

VI: ENDOCRINE DISORDERS

XV: HEMATOPOIETIC DISORDERS

XVI: PREGNANCY

XVII: SURGICAL PROBLEMS

XVIII: NUTRITION IN THE INTENSIVE CARE UNIT

XIX: PROCEDURES

XX: END-OF-LIFE ISSUES

XXI: APPENDICES

This is the first edition of *The Washington Manual™ of Critical Care*, building on the long tradition of *The Washington Manual™ of Medical Therapeutics*, which is now in its 32nd edition and has given rise to numerous medical and surgical subspecialty manuals. This project was inspired by the expanding literature in critical care medicine and the demands this places on health care professionals treating critically ill patients. Our goal in preparing this manual is to provide clinicians and students with comprehensive and current treatment algorithms for the bedside diagnosis and management of the most frequently encountered illnesses in the intensive care unit (ICU). Many chapters begin with brief discussions of epidemiology, pathophysiology, and clinical findings. The chapters include annotated bibliographies of select references to guide more in-depth reading when time permits. Also included are sections covering common ICU procedures and equations, nutrition, and pharmacology. The chapters were written by Washington University faculty physicians and experts in their fields from the Departments of Internal Medicine, Neurology, Surgery, Obstetrics and Gynecology, and Anesthesiology, often with the assistance of subspecialty fellows and residents. In keeping with the tradition of *The Washington Manual™*, we hope that the *Manual of Critical Care* will be updated regularly and become a staple in managing critically ill patients.

Medicine is a constantly changing field and the most up-to-date treatment recommendations may outpace this manual's revisions. The tables and algorithms that accompany each chapter are meant as guides and may not be appropriate for all patients. Further reading of the literature is always encouraged and this manual is expected to be used in conjunction with trained critical care clinicians.

We would especially like to give our sincerest thanks to Becky Light for her tireless efforts in preparing chapters and for acting as the liaison between the Pulmonary and Critical Care Department, the chapter's authors, and Lippincott Williams & Wilkins. We would also like to thank Jennifer Ceccotti, Nidhi Waddon, Brian Brown, Nicole Dernoski, Nicole Walz, and the production and editorial staff at Lippincott Williams & Wilkins and Wolters Kluwer for their hard work in making this manual come to fruition.

C.W. would like to thank his wife, Jen, and his parents for their love and support. M.K. would like to thank his loving family for all of their support. T.B. would like to thank his family for believing in him, especially his mother, Laura, who is his inspiration; Alison, for her love; and Curtis J. Gravis, for wisdom. W.I. thanks his wife for her tireless support and understanding.

C.W.
M.K.
T.B.
W.I.

Sumeet Asrani, MD
Resident Physician
Department of Internal Medicine
Washington University School of Medicine
Barnes-Jewish Hospital
St. Louis, Missouri

Yekaterina Axelrod, MD
Assistant Professor
Department of Neurology
Washington University School of Medicine
Barnes-Jewish Hospital
St. Louis, Missouri

Ravi Aysola, MD
Fellow
Division of Pulmonary and Critical Care
  Medicine
Washington University School
  of Medicine
Barnes-Jewish Hospital
St. Louis, Missouri

Richard G. Bach, MD
Associate Professor of Medicine
Cardiovascular Division
Director, Cardiac Intensive Care Unit
Washington University School
  of Medicine
Barnes-Jewish Hospital
St. Louis, Missouri

Timothy J. Bedient, MD
Resident Physician
Department of Internal Medicine
Washington University School
  of Medicine
Barnes-Jewish Hospital
St. Louis, Missouri

Morey A. Blinder, MD
Associate Professor of Medicine and
  Pathology and Immunology
Division of Hematology
Washington University School
  of Medicine
Barnes-Jewish Hospital
St. Louis, Missouri

Alan C. Braverman, MD
Professor of Medicine
Cardiovascular Divison
Chief of Service, Inpatient
  Cardiology Firm
Director, Marfan Syndrome Clinic
Washington University School
  of Medicine
Barnes-Jewish Hospital
St. Louis, Missouri

Steven L. Brody, MD
Associate Professor of Medicine
Division of Pulmonary and Critical Care
  Medicine
Washington University School
  of Medicine
Barnes-Jewish Hospital
St. Louis, Missouri

Derek E. Byers, MD, PhD
Fellow
Division of Pulmonary and Critical Care
  Medicine
Washington University School
  of Medicine
Barnes-Jewish Hospital
St. Louis, Missouri

Bernard C. Camins, MD, MSCR
Assistant Professor of Medicine
Division of Infectious Diseases
Associate Hospital Epidemiologist
Washington University School
  of Medicine
Barnes-Jewish Hospital
St. Louis, Missouri

Mario Castro, MD, MPH
Associate Professor of Medicine and
  Pediatrics
Division of Pulmonary and Critical Care
  Medicine
Washington University School
  of Medicine
Barnes-Jewish Hospital
St. Louis, Missouri

Murali M. Chakinala, MD
Assistant Professor of Medicine
Division of Pulmonary and Critical Care
  Medicine
Washington University School
  of Medicine
Barnes-Jewish Hospital
St. Louis, Missouri

Namrata Chawla, MD
Fellow
Renal Division
Washington University School of Medicine
Barnes-Jewish Hospital
St. Louis, Missouri

William E. Clutter, MD
Associate Professor of Medicine
Division of Endocrinology, Metabolism,
  and Lipid Research
Washington University School
  of Medicine
Barnes-Jewish Hospital
St. Louis, Missouri

G. Lee Collins, MD
Assistant Professor of Anesthesiology
Department of Anesthesiology
Washington University School
  of Medicine
Barnes-Jewish Hospital
St. Louis, Missouri

Daniel H. Cooper, MD
Fellow
Cardiovascular Division
Washington University School of Medicine
Barnes-Jewish Hospital
St. Louis, Missouri

Craig M. Coopersmith, MD
Assistant Professor of Surgery and
  Anesthesiology
Division of General Surgery
Co-Director, Surgical Intensive
  Care Unit
Washington University School
  of Medicine
Barnes-Jewish Hospital
St. Louis, Missouri

Jeffrey S. Crippin, MD
Professor of Medicine
Division of Gastroenterology
Medical Director, Liver Transplantation
Washington University School of Medicine
Barnes-Jewish Hospital
St. Louis, Missouri

Phillip S. Cuculich, MD
Fellow
Cardiovascular Division
Washington University School
  of Medicine
Barnes-Jewish Hospital
St. Louis, Missouri

Alex E. Denes, MD
Associate Professor
Division of Oncology
Director, Inpatient Oncology
Washington University School
  of Medicine
Barnes-Jewish Hospital
St. Louis, Missouri

James A. Driscoll, MD
Fellow
Division of Pulmonary and Critical Care
  Medicine
Washington University School
  of Medicine
Barnes-Jewish Hospital
St. Louis, Missouri

Gregory A. Ewald, MD
Associate Professor
Cardiovascular Division
Medical Director, Cardiac Transplant
  Program
Washington University School
  of Medicine
Barnes-Jewish Hospital
St. Louis, Missouri

Ryan C. Fields, MD
Resident Physician
Division of General Surgery
Washington University School
  of Medicine
Barnes-Jewish Hospital
St. Louis, Missouri

Joseph M. Fritz, MD
Fellow
Division of Infectious Diseases
Washington University School of Medicine
Barnes-Jewish Hospital
St. Louis, Missouri

Clare N. Gentry, MD, MS
Fellow
Division of Infectious Diseases
Washington University School
  of Medicine
Barnes-Jewish Hospital
St. Louis, Missouri

Jennifer Gnerlich, MD
Fellow
Division of General Surgery
Washington University School
    of Medicine
Barnes-Jewish Hospital
St. Louis, Missouri

Seth Goldberg, MD
Fellow
Renal Division
Washington University School
    of Medicine
Barnes-Jewish Hospital
St. Louis, Missouri

Manu S. Goyal, MD, MSc
Resident Physician
Department of Neurology
Washington University School
    of Medicine
Barnes-Jewish Hospital
St. Louis, Missouri

Jonathan M. Green, MD
Associate Professor of Medicine
Division of Pulmonary and Critical Care
    Medicine
Washington University School
    of Medicine
Barnes-Jewish Hospital
St. Louis, Missouri

Brian Hamburg, MD
Resident Physician
Department of Internal Medicine
Washington University School
    of Medicine
Barnes-Jewish Hospital
St. Louis, Missouri

Anthony J. Hart, MD
Resident Physician
Department of Internal Medicine
Washington University School
    of Medicine
Barnes-Jewish Hospital
St. Louis, Missouri

Michael J. Hersh, MD
Fellow
Division of Gastroenterology
Washington University School
    of Medicine
Barnes-Jewish Hospital
St. Louis, Missouri

Christopher L. Holley, MD, PhD
Chief Resident, Cardiology and
    Karl-Flance Firms
Department of Internal Medicine
Washington University School
    of Medicine
Barnes-Jewish Hospital
St. Louis, Missouri

Runhua Hou, MD
Fellow
Division of Endocrinology, Metabolism,
    and Lipid Research
Washington University School
    of Medicine
Barnes-Jewish Hospital
St. Louis, Missouri

Howard J. Huang, MD
Fellow
Division of Pulmonary and Critical Care
    Medicine
Washington University School
    of Medicine
Barnes-Jewish Hospital
St. Louis, Missouri

Amy M. Hueffmeier, RN, BSN
Manager, Hospital Epidemiology and
    Infection Prevention
Washington University School
    of Medicine
Barnes-Jewish Hospital
St. Louis, Missouri

Warren Isakow, MD
Assistant Professor of Medicine
Division of Pulmonary and Critical Care
    Medicine
Washington University School
    of Medicine
Barnes-Jewish Hospital
St. Louis, Missouri

Jeffrey C. Jones, MD
Fellow
Division of Infectious Diseases
Washington University School
    of Medicine
Barnes-Jewish Hospital
St. Louis, Missouri

Sreenivasa S. Jonnalagadda, MD
Associate Professor of Medicine
Division of Gastroenterology
Washington University School of Medicine
Barnes-Jewish Hospital
St. Louis, Missouri

Yo-El Ju, MD
Resident Physician
Department of Neurology
Washington University School
  of Medicine
Barnes-Jewish Hospital
St. Louis, Missouri

Andrew M. Kates, MD
Assistant Professor of Medicine
Cardiovascular Division
Washington University School
  of Medicine
Barnes-Jewish Hospital
St. Louis, Missouri

John P. Kirby, MD, FCCWS, FACS
Assistant Professor of Surgery
Division of General Surgery
Director, Wound Healing Program
Washington University School
  of Medicine
Barnes-Jewish Hospital
St. Louis, Missouri

Matthew J. Koch, MD
Assistant Professor of Medicine
Renal Division
Washington University School
  of Medicine
Barnes-Jewish Hospital
St. Louis, Missouri

Marin H. Kollef, MD
Professor of Medicine
Division of Pulmonary and Critical Care
  Medicine
Director, Medical Intensive Care Unit
Director, Respiratory Care Unit
Washington University School
  of Medicine
Barnes-Jewish Hospital
St. Louis, Missouri

Kevin M. Korenblat, MD
Assistant Professor of Medicine
Division of Gastroenterology
Washington University School
  of Medicine
Barnes-Jewish Hospital
St. Louis, Missouri

Andrew Labelle, MD
Resident Physician
Department of Internal Medicine
Washington University School
  of Medicine
Barnes-Jewish Hospital
St. Louis, Missouri

Steven J. Lawrence, MD, MSc
Assistant Professor of Medicine
Division of Infectious Diseases
Washington University School
  of Medicine
Barnes-Jewish Hospital
St. Louis, Missouri

Christopher Leach, MD
Fellow
Cardiovascular Division
Washington University School
  of Medicine
Barnes-Jewish Hospital
St. Louis, Missouri

Michael Lippmann, MD
Associate Professor
Division of Pulmonary and Critical Care
  Medicine
Washington University School
  of Medicine
St. Louis Veterans Affairs Hospital
St. Louis, Missouri

Martin L. Mayse, MD
Assistant Professor of Medicine and
  Surgery
Division of Pulmonary and Critical Care
  Medicine
Washington University School
  of Medicine
Barnes-Jewish Hospital
St. Louis, Missouri

Kevin W. McConnell, MD
Resident Physician
Division of General Surgery
Washington University School
  of Medicine
Barnes-Jewish Hospital
St. Louis, Missouri

Bryan F. Meyers, MD, MPH
Associate Professor of Surgery
Division of Cardiothoracic Surgery
Washington University School
  of Medicine
Barnes-Jewish Hospital
St. Louis, Missouri

Scott T. Micek, PharmD
Clinical Pharmacist
Department of Pharmacy
Washington University School
  of Medicine
Barnes-Jewish Hospital
St. Louis, Missouri

James C. Mosley, III, MD
Fellow
Divisions of Hematology and Oncology
Washington University School
    of Medicine
Barnes-Jewish Hospital
St. Louis, Missouri

Chandra Prakash, MD, MRCP
Associate Professor of Medicine
Division of Gastroenterology
Washington University School
    of Medicine
Barnes-Jewish Hospital
St. Louis, Missouri

Jamie M. Rosini, PharmD
Fellow
Department of Pharmacy
Washington University School of Medicine
Barnes-Jewish Hospital
St. Louis, Missouri

Nareg Roubinian, MD
Resident Physician
Department of Internal Medicine
Washington University School
    of Medicine
Barnes-Jewish Hospital
St. Louis, Missouri

Tonya D. Russell, MD
Assistant Professor of Medicine
Division of Pulmonary and Critical Care
    Medicine
Washington University School
    of Medicine
Barnes-Jewish Hospital
St. Louis, Missouri

Stephen C. Ryan, MD
Fellow
Division of Pulmonary and Critical Care
    Medicine
Washington University School
    of Medicine
Barnes-Jewish Hospital
St. Louis, Missouri

Yoel Sadovsky, MD
Professor of Obstetrics and Gynecology
    and Cell Biology and Physiology
Department of Obstetrics and Gynecology
Director, Division of Maternal-Fetal
    Medicine and Ultrasound
Washington University School of Medicine
Barnes-Jewish Hospital
St. Louis, Missouri

Kamalanathan K. Sambandam, MD
Fellow
Renal Division
Washington University School
    of Medicine
Barnes-Jewish Hospital
St. Louis, Missouri

Mark A. Schroeder, MD
Fellow
Divisions of Hematology and Oncology
Washington University School
    of Medicine
Barnes-Jewish Hospital
St. Louis, Missouri

Douglas J.E. Schuerer, MD
Assistant Professor of Surgery
Division of General Surgery
Washington University School
    of Medicine
Barnes-Jewish Hospital
St. Louis, Missouri

Daniel P. Schuster, MD
Professor of Medicine and Radiology
Division of Pulmonary and Critical Care
    Medicine
Washington University School
    of Medicine
Barnes-Jewish Hospital
St. Louis, Missouri

Lee P. Skrupky, PharmD
Fellow
Department of Pharmacy
Washington University School
    of Medicine
Barnes-Jewish Hospital
St. Louis, Missouri

Timothy W. Smith, DPhil, MD
Associate Professor of Medicine
Cardiovascular Division
Washington University School
    of Medicine
Barnes-Jewish Hospital
St. Louis, Missouri

R. Brian Sommerville, MD
Resident Physician
Department of Neurology
Washington University School
    of Medicine
Barnes-Jewish Hospital
St. Louis, Missouri

Rael Sundy, MD
Fellow
Division of Pulmonary and Critical Care
   Medicine
Washington University School
   of Medicine
Barnes-Jewish Hospital
St. Louis, Missouri

Beth E. Taylor, MS, RD, CNSD, FCCM
Nutrition Support Specialist
Department of Food and Nutrition
Washington University School
   of Medicine
Barnes-Jewish Hospital
St. Louis, Missouri

Garry S. Tobin, MD
Associate Professor
Division of Endocrinology
Director, Diabetes Center
Washington University School
   of Medicine
Barnes-Jewish Hospital
St. Louis, Missouri

Tracy M. Tomlinson, MD
Fellow
Division of Maternal-Fetal Medicine and
   Ultrasound
Washington University School
   of Medicine
Barnes-Jewish Hospital
St. Louis, Missouri

Anitha Vijayan, MD
Associate Professor of Medicine
Renal Division
Medical Director, Acute Dialysis Unit
Washington University School
   of Medicine
Barnes-Jewish Hospital
St. Louis, Missouri

David K. Warren, MD, MPH
Assistant Professor of Medicine
Division of Infectious Diseases
Hospital Epidemiologist
Washington University School
   of Medicine
Barnes-Jewish Hospital
St. Louis, Missouri

John Welch, MD, PhD
Fellow
Divisions of Hematology and Oncology
Washington University School
   of Medicine
Barnes-Jewish Hospital
St. Louis, Missouri

Robb R. Whinney, DO, FACOS
Assistant Professor of Surgery
Division of General Surgery
Washington University School
   of Medicine
Barnes-Jewish Hospital
St. Louis, Missouri

Chad A. Witt, MD
Resident Physician
Department of Internal Medicine
Washington University School
   of Medicine
Barnes-Jewish Hospital
St. Louis, Missouri

Keith F. Woeltje, MD, PhD
Associate Professor of Medicine
Division of Infectious Diseases
Medical Director, Infection Control and
   Healthcare Epidemiology
Washington University School
   of Medicine
Barnes-Jewish Hospital
St. Louis, Missouri

ACKNOWLEDGMENTS

The editors would like to thank Becky Light who coordinated all of the communications and manuscript preparation for this manual.

Management of Shock

INTRODUCTION TO SHOCK

Marin H. Kollef

Shock is a common problem in the intensive care unit, requiring immediate diagnosis and treatment. It is usually defined by a combination of hemodynamic parameters (mean blood pressure <60 mm Hg, systolic blood pressure <90 mm Hg), clinical findings (altered mentation, decreased urine output), and abnormal laboratory values (elevated serum lactate, metabolic acidosis). The first step is to identify the cause of shock, as each condition will require different interventions. The overall goal of therapy is to reverse tissue hypoperfusion as quickly as possible in order to preserve organ function. Table 1.1 and Algorithms 1.1 and 1.2 offer an approach for determining the main cause of shock. Specific management of the various shock states is presented in the following chapters. Early evaluation with echocardiography, intraesophageal aortic waveform assessment, or right heart catheterization will allow determination of the cause of shock and will assist in management.

TABLE 1.1	Hemodynamic Patterns Associated with Specific Shock States[a]

Type of shock	CI	SVR	PVR	Svo$_2$	RAP	RVP	PAP	PAOP
Cardiogenic (e.g., myocardial infarction or cardiac tamponade)	↓	↑	N	↓	↑	↑	↑	↑
Hypovolemic (e.g., hemorrhage, intravascular volume depletion)	↓	↑	N	↓	↓	↓	↓	↓
Distributive shock (e.g., septic, anaphylaxis)	N-↑	↓	N	N-↑	N-↓	N-↓	N-↓	N-↓
Obstructive (e.g., pulmonary embolism)	↓	N-↑	↑	N-↓	↑	↑	↑	N-↓

CI, cardiac index; SVR, systemic vascular resistance; PVR, pulmonary vascular resistance; Svo$_2$, mixed venous oxygen saturation; RAP, right arterial pressure; RVP, right ventricular pressure; PAP, pulmonary artery pressure; PAOP, pulmonary artery occlusion pressure; ↑, increased; ↓, decreased; N, normal.
[a]Equalization of RAP, PAOP, diastolic PAP, and diastolic RVP indicates cardiac tamponade.

ALGORITHM 1.1   **Main Causes of Shock**

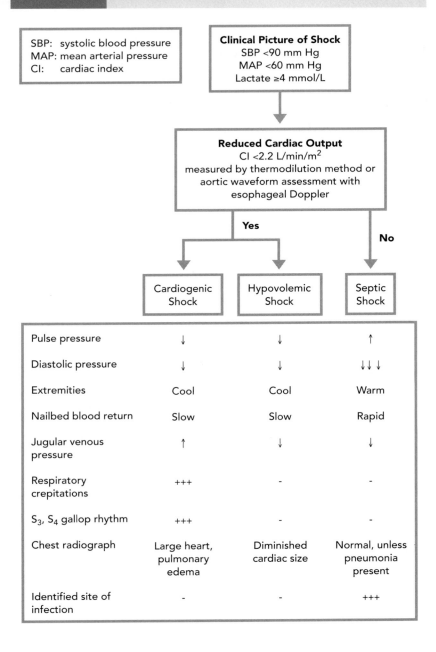

	Cardiogenic Shock	Hypovolemic Shock	Septic Shock
Pulse pressure	↓	↓	↑
Diastolic pressure	↓	↓	↓ ↓ ↓
Extremities	Cool	Cool	Warm
Nailbed blood return	Slow	Slow	Rapid
Jugular venous pressure	↑	↓	↓
Respiratory crepitations	+++	-	-
S_3, S_4 gallop rhythm	+++	-	-
Chest radiograph	Large heart, pulmonary edema	Diminished cardiac size	Normal, unless pneumonia present
Identified site of infection	-	-	+++

Text within the algorithm figure:

SBP: systolic blood pressure
MAP: mean arterial pressure
CI: cardiac index

Clinical Picture of Shock
SBP <90 mm Hg
MAP <60 mm Hg
Lactate ≥4 mmol/L

Reduced Cardiac Output
CI <2.2 L/min/m^2
measured by thermodilution method or
aortic waveform assessment with
esophageal Doppler

Yes   No

ALGORITHM 1.2	Miscellaneous Causes of Shock

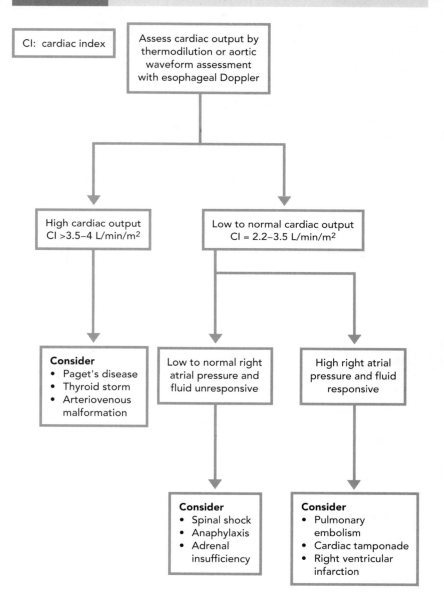

HYPOVOLEMIC SHOCK

Marin H. Kollef

2

Hypovolemic shock occurs as a result of decreased circulating blood volume, most commonly from acute hemorrhage. It may also result from heat-related intravascular volume depletion or fluid sequestration within the abdomen. Table 2.1 provides a classification of hypovolemic shock based on the amount of whole blood volume lost. In general, the greater the loss of whole blood, the greater the resultant risk of mortality. However, it is important to note that other factors can influence the outcome of hypovolemic shock including age, underlying comorbidities (e.g., cardiovascular disease), and the rapidity and adequacy of the fluid resuscitation.

Lactic acidosis occurs during hypovolemic shock because of inadequate tissue perfusion. The magnitude of the serum lactate elevation is correlated with mortality in hypovolemic shock and may be an early indicator of tissue hypoperfusion, despite near-normal-appearing vital signs. The treatment of lactic acidosis depends on reversing organ hypoperfusion. This is reflected in the equation for tissue oxygen delivery shown here. Optimizing oxygen delivery to tissues requires a sufficient hemoglobin concentration to carry oxygen to tissues. Additionally, ventricular preload is an important determinant of cardiac output. Providing adequate intravascular volume will ensure that stroke volume and cardiac output are optimized to meet tissue demands for oxygen and other nutrients. If, despite adequate preload, cardiac output is not sufficient for the demands of tissues, then dobutamine can be employed to further increase cardiac output and oxygen delivery.

$$\dot{D}o_2 = Cao_2 \times CO$$
$$Cao_2 = (Hb \times 1.34 \times Sao_2) + 0.0031\ Pao_2$$
$$CO = SV \times HR$$

where $\dot{D}o_2$ = oxygen delivery, Cao_2 = arterial oxygen content, CO = cardiac output, Hb = hemoglobin concentration, Sao_2 = arterial hemoglobin oxygen saturation, Pao_2 = arterial oxygen tension, SV = stroke volume, and HR = heart rate.

The treatment goals in hypovolemic shock are to control the source of hemorrhage and to administer adequate intravascular volume replacement. Control of the source of hemorrhage may be as simple as placing a pressure dressing on an open bleeding wound, or it may require urgent operative exploration to identify and control the bleeding source from an intra-abdominal or intrathoracic injury. Angiographic embolization of a bleeding vessel may also be helpful for bleeding injuries that are not amenable to surgical intervention (e.g., multiple pelvic fractures with ongoing hemorrhage). Therefore, most episodes of hypovolemic shock are managed by trauma specialists, usually in the emergency department setting. However, all clinicians caring for critically ill patients should be able to recognize the early clinical manifestations of hypovolemic shock and to initiate appropriate fluid management.

An algorithm for the fluid management of hypovolemic shock is provided in Algorithm 2.1. At least two large-bore (14 to 16 gauge or larger) peripheral vein catheters and/or an 8.5 French central vein catheter should be placed to allow rapid blood product and crystalloid administration. A mechanical rapid transfusion device should also be used to decrease the time required for each unit of blood or liter of crystalloid to be infused. In a patient with ongoing hemorrhage, initial administration of 2 to 4 liters of crystalloid (0.9 NaCl or lactated Ringer solution) and group O blood should be given. Most hospitals will employ four units of Rh-positive O blood for men and women who are not in childbearing age and

ALGORITHM 2.1   Management of Hypovolemic Shock

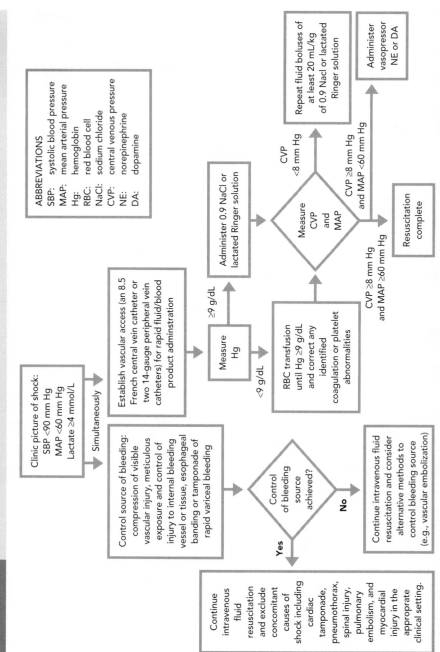

ABBREVIATIONS

SBP:	systolic blood pressure
MAP:	mean arterial pressure
Hg:	hemoglobin
RBC:	red blood cell
NaCl:	sodium chloride
CVP:	central venous pressure
NE:	norepinephrine
DA:	dopamine

Clinic picture of shock:
SBP <90 mm Hg
MAP <60 mm Hg
Lactate ≥4 mmol/L

Simultaneously

Establish vascular access (an 8.5 French central vein catheter or two 14-gauge peripheral vein catheters) for rapid fluid/blood product adminstration

Control source of bleeding: compression of visible vascular injury, meticulous exposure and control of injury to internal bleeding vessel or tissue, esophageal banding or tamponade of rapid variceal bleeding

Measure Hg

≥9 g/dL → Administer 0.9 NaCl or lactated Ringer solution

<9 g/dL → RBC transfusion until Hg ≥9 g/dL and correct any identified coagulation or platelet abnormalities

Measure CVP and MAP

CVP <8 mm Hg → Repeat fluid boluses of at least 20 mL/kg of 0.9 Nacl or lactated Ringer solution

CVP ≥8 mm Hg and MAP <60 mm Hg → Administer vasopressor NE or DA

CVP ≥8 mm Hg and MAP ≥60 mm Hg → Resuscitation complete

Control of bleeding source achieved?

Yes → Continue intravenous fluid resuscitation and exclude concomitant causes of shock including cardiac tamponade, pneumothorax, spinal injury, pulmonary embolism, and myocardial injury in the appropriate clinical setting.

No → Continue intravenous fluid resuscitation and consider alternative methods to control bleeding source (e.g., vascular embolization)

TABLE 2.1	Classification of Hypovolemic Shock

Category	Whole blood volume loss (%)	Pathophysiology
Mild (compensated)	<20	Peripheral vasoconstriction to preserve blood flow to critical organs (brain and heart)
Moderate	20–40	Decreased perfusion of organs such as the kidneys, intestine, and pancreas
Severe (uncompensated)	>40	Decreased perfusion to brain and heart

TABLE 2.2	Adjunctive Therapies for Hypovolemic Shock

Therapy	Rationale
Airway control	To provide appropriate gas exchange in the lungs and to prevent aspiration
Cardiac/hemodynamic monitoring	To identify dysrhythmias and inadequate fluid resuscitation (Fig. 2.1)
Platelet/fresh-frozen plasma administration	Required because of dilutional effects of crystalloid and blood administration as well as consumption from ongoing bleeding. The prothrombin time and partial thromboplastin time should be corrected and the platelet count should be kept >50,000/mm^3 with ongoing bleeding
Activated Factor VII	Should be considered in the presence of diffuse or nonoperative ongoing hemorrhage when clotting abnormalities have been corrected
Calcium chloride, magnesium chloride	To reverse ionized hypocalcemia and hypomagnesemia resulting from the administration of citrate with transfused blood, which binds ionized calcium and magnesium
Rewarming techniques (e.g., warm fluids, blankets, radiant lamps, head covers, warmed humidified air, heated body cavity lavage)	Hypothermia is a common consequence of massive blood transfusion that can contribute to cardiac dysfunction and coagulation abnormalities
Monitor for and treat for transfusion-related complications including transfusion-related acute lung injury (TRALI) and transfusion reactions	These are immunologically mediated, requiring appropriate use of mechanical ventilation with positive end-expiratory pressure for TRALI and bronchodilators and corticosteroids for severe bronchoconstriction, subglottic edema, and anaphylaxis
Antibiotics	When open dirty or contaminated wounds are present to prevent and treat bacterial infections
Corticosteroids	For patients presumed to have adrenal injury and patients unable to mount an appropriate stress response

Rh-negative O blood for women who are in childbearing age. Type-specific blood is usually administered after the first four units of nontyped blood are given. The goal of blood transfusion therapy during ongoing hemorrhage is to maintain the hemoglobin value above 8 g/dL.

In addition to the initial administration of crystalloid and red blood cells, other therapies will be required in patients with hypovolemic shock. These are summarized in Table 2.2, and are especially important for patients requiring massive transfusions or those with ongoing blood loss.

Suggested Reading

Bilkovski RN, Rivers EP, Horst HM. Targeted resuscitation strategies after injury. *Curr Opin Crit Care*. 2004;10:529–538.

Provides end points for the management of hypovolemic shock in patients with blunt or penetrating injury.

Kelley DM. Hypovolemic shock: an overview. *Crit Care Nurs Q*. 2005;28:2–19.

A concise review of hypovolemic shock including initial evaluation and management.

Stein DM, Dutton RP. Use of recombinant factor VIIa in trauma. *Curr Opin Crit Care*. 2004;10:520–528.

Summarizes potential uses of recombinant factor VIIa in patients with trauma and ongoing hemorrhage.

Uses of recombinant factor VIIa in trauma.

SEVERE SEPSIS AND SEPTIC SHOCK

3

Marin H. Kollef and Scott T. Micek

Severe sepsis is an infection-induced syndrome resulting in a systemic inflammatory response that is complicated by dysfunction of at least one organ system. In the United States, approximately 750,000 cases of sepsis occur each year. The mortality associated with severe sepsis ranges from 30% to 50%, with mortality increasing with advancing age. Although complex, the pathophysiology of sepsis involves a series of interacting pathways involving immune stimulation, immune suppression, hypercoagulation, and hypofibrinolysis. Cardiovascular management plays an important role in the treatment of septic shock. Hypotension occurs because of failure of vasoconstriction by vascular smooth muscle resulting in peripheral vasodilation. Goal-directed cardiovascular resuscitation has been demonstrated to be an important determinant of survival in patients with septic shock. In addition to cardiovascular management, appropriate initial antimicrobial treatment of patients with severe sepsis also appears to be an important determinant of patient outcome.

The unscrambling of the complex pathophysiology associated with severe sepsis and septic shock has made much progress, and current understanding of this process is no longer rudimentary. Novel drug entities and new therapeutic strategies targeting these pathways have demonstrated efficacy in reducing patient mortality (Table 3.1). The challenge for clinicians is the integration of these pharmacotherapies to confer the recognized survival benefit into critical care practice. The Surviving Sepsis Campaign has teamed with the Institute for Healthcare Improvement to create the Severe Sepsis Bundles, which are designed in an effort to optimize the timing, sequence, and goals of the individual elements of care as delineated in the Surviving Sepsis Guidelines. The benefits associated with the use of comprehensive treatment protocols integrating goal-directed hemodynamic stabilization, early appropriate antimicrobial therapy, and associated adjunctive severe sepsis therapies initiated in the emergency department and continued in the intensive care unit have been reported in several prospective trials (Algorithms 3.1 through 3.3).

The significance of early, aggressive, volume resuscitation and hemodynamic stabilization was demonstrated in a randomized, controlled, single-center trial in patients who presented to the emergency department with signs of the systemic inflammatory response syndrome and hypotension, as published by Rivers et al. Administration of crystalloids, red blood cell transfusions, vasopressors, and inotropes based on aggressive monitoring of intravascular volume and a tissue oxygen marker within 6 hours of presentation to the emergency department resulted in a 16% decrease in absolute 28-day mortality. The major differences in treatment between the intervention and control groups were in the volume of intravenous fluids received, the number of patients transfused packed red blood, the use of dobutamine, and the presence of a dedicated study team for the first 6 hours of care.

The implementation of treatment pathways mimicking the interventions of the well-scripted, carefully performed procedures employed by Rivers et al. have been put into practice in the clinical setting. Micek et al. employed standardized order sets that focused on intravenous fluid administration and the appropriateness of initial antimicrobial therapy for severe sepsis and septic shock. Patients managed in this manner were more likely to receive intravenous fluids >20 mL/kg of body weight prior to vasopressor administration, and consequently were less likely to require vasopressor administration at the time of transfer to the intensive care unit. Patients managed with this approach were also more likely to be treated with an appropriate initial antimicrobial regimen. As a result of the aggressive

TABLE 3.1	Medications Commonly Used in Septic Shock			

		CO	MAP	SVR
I. Vasopressors				
Norepinephrine	0.05–0.5 mcg/kg/min	−/+	++	+++
Dopamine	5–20 mcg/kg/min	++	+	++
Epinephrine	0.05–2 mcg/kg/min	++	++	+++
Phenylephrine	2–10 mcg/kg/min	0	++	+++
Vasopressin	0.04 units/min	0	+++	+++
II. Inotrope				
Dobutamine	2.5–10 mcg/kg/min	+++	−/+	−/0
III. Drotrecogin alfa (activated)	24 mcg/kg/hr for 96 hr			
IV. Corticosteroids				
Hydrocortisone	50 mg every 6 hr			
(+/− fludrocortisone 50 mcg daily)				
V. Antibiotic management				
(See Algorithm 3.3)				

CO, cardiac output; MAP, mean arterial blood pressure; SVR, systemic vascular resistance.

management initiated in the emergency department and continued in the intensive care unit, patients managed via the severe sepsis order sets had statistically shorter hospital lengths of stay and a lower risk for 28-day mortality.

In summary, the initial management of patients with septic shock appears to be critical in terms of determining outcome. Institution of standardized physician order sets, or some other systematic approach, for the management of patients with severe infections appears to consistently improve the delivery of recommended therapies and, as a result, may improve patient outcomes. Given that evidence-based treatment pathways typically have no additional risks and are associated with little to no acquisition costs, their implementation should become the standard of care for the management of septic shock.

ALGORITHM 3.1   Fluid Management of Septic Shock

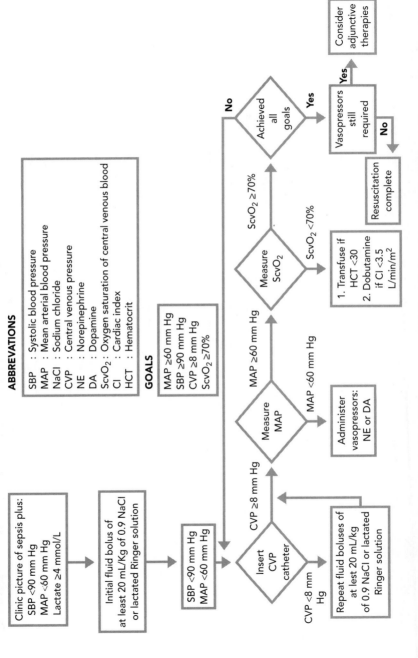

ABBREVATIONS

SBP   : Systolic blood pressure
MAP : Mean arterial blood pressure
NaCl : Sodium chloride
CVP : Central venous pressure
NE   : Norepinephrine
DA   : Dopamine
$ScvO_2$: Oxygen saturation of central venous blood
CI   : Cardiac index
HCT : Hematocrit

GOALS

MAP $\geq$60 mm Hg
SBP $\geq$90 mm Hg
CVP $\geq$8 mm Hg
$ScvO_2$ $\geq$70%

Clinic picture of sepsis plus:
SBP <90 mm Hg
MAP <60 mm Hg
Lactate $\geq$4 mmol/L

Initial fluid bolus of at least 20 mL/Kg of 0.9 NaCl or lactated Ringer solution

SBP <90 mm Hg
MAP <60 mm Hg

Insert CVP catheter

CVP <8 mm Hg

Repeat fluid boluses of at lest 20 mL/kg of 0.9 NaCl or lactated Ringer solution

CVP $\geq$8 mm Hg

Measure MAP

MAP <60 mm Hg

Administer vasopressors: NE or DA

MAP $\geq$60 mm Hg

Measure $ScvO_2$

$ScvO_2$ <70%

1. Transfuse if HCT <30
2. Dobutamine if CI <3.5 L/min/m²

$ScvO_2$ $\geq$70%

Achieved all goals

No

Yes

Vasopressors still required

Yes

Consider adjunctive therapies

No

Resuscitation complete

11

ALGORITHM 3.2   Adjunctive Therapies for Septic Shock

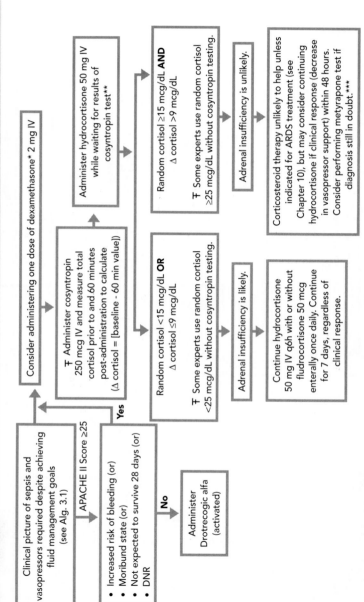

APACHE, acute physiology and chronic health evaluation; ARDS, acute respiratory distress syndrome; DNR, do not resuscitate; IV, intravenously; Δ Cortisol, change in cortisol level in mcg/dL.
*Dexamethasone does not interfere with the cosyntropin test and 2 mg IV is equivalent to approximately 50 mg of hydrocortisone.
**Administer only if dexamethasone was not given initially.
***Metyrapone blocks the conversion of 11-deoxycortisol to cortisol by CYP11B1 and causes a rapid fall in cortisol. To test, give metyrapone PO at 30 mg/kg at 12 AM and measure 11-deoxycortisol and cortisol 8 hours later. A normal response is an 8 AM serum 11-deoxycortisol level of 7 to 22 mcg/dL, and serum cortisol <5 mcg/dL. Serum 11-deoxycortisol <7 mcg/dL indicates adrenal insufficiency. Patients who undergo metyrapone testing should receive at least 24 hours of corticosteroid replacement. *Metyrapone is not currently available for routine clinical use in the United States.*

ALGORITHM 3.3   **Antibiotic Management of Severe Sepsis and Septic Shock**

Is patient immunocompromised?
- HIV-positive
- Neutropenia
- Chronic corticosteroids
- Malnutrition
- Receiving chemotherapy

Yes →

Consider obtaining consultation with infectious disease expert. Patient may need antimicrobial therapy directed to opportunistic pathogens in addition to bacterial pathogens.

↓ **No**

Consider likely bacterial infection based on clinical presentation (patients with viral, fungal, or ehrlichial infections who are not immunocompromised may also present with severe sepsis or septic shock).

ABBREVIATIONS
HIV: Human immunodeficiency antibody
ESBL: Extended-spectrum beta-lactamase
MRSA: Methicillin-resistant *Staphylococcus aureus*

↓

Risk factors for health care-associated infection present:
- Recent hospitalization
- Residence in nursing home/rehabilitation facility
- Regular visits to hospital clinic and dialysis
- Home infusion or wound therapy

Yes →

Consider nosocomial bacterial pathogens that are potentially antibiotic resistant:
- MRSA
- *Pseudomonas aeruginosa*
- *Acinetobacter species*
- *Klebsiella pneumonia* (ESBL+)
- *Escherichia coli* (ESBL+)

↓ **No**

Consider community-based bacterial pathogens that are antibiotic sensitive:
- *Streptococcus pneumoniae*
- *Escherichia coli*
- *Legionella pneumophila*
- Methicillin-susceptible *Staphylococcus aureus*
- *Haemophilius Influenza*
- *Klebsiella pneumonia*

↓

Select single agent or combination therapy if *Legionella* is possible:
- Ceftriaxone
    or
- Ampicillin/sulbactam
    or
- Ertapenem
    plus
- Macrolide (azithromycin, clarithromycin)
    or
- Fluoroquinolone (levofloxacin, moxifloxacin)

Broad-spectrum cephalosporin (cefepime, ceftazidime)
    or
Carbapenem (imipenem, meropenem, doripenem)
    or
Beta-lactam/beta-lactamase inhibitor (piperacilin-tazobactam)
    plus
Fluoroquinolone (ciprofloxacin or levofloxacin)
    or
Aminoglycoside (gentamicin, tobramycin, amikacin)
    plus
MRSA-directed agent (vancomycin, linezolid, tigecycline)

↓

Modify and/or narrow antibiotic regimen based on organism identified and susceptibility testing. ←

Suggested Reading

Annane D, Sebille V, Charpentier C, et al. Effect of treatment with low doses of hydrocortisone and fludrocortisone on mortality in patients with septic shock. *JAMA*. 2002;288:862–871.
Randomized trial demonstrating survival benefit amongst patients with septic shock not responding appropriately to administration of corticotropin.

Bernard GR, Vincent JL, Laterre PF, et al. Efficacy and safety of recombinant human activated protein C for severe sepsis. *N Engl J Med*. 2001;344:699–709.
A randomized blinded trial demonstrating the mortality advantage of patients receiving activated protein C for severe sepsis and high acuity of illness.

Dellinger RP, Carlet JM, Masur H, et al. Surviving Sepsis Campaign guidelines for management of severe sepsis and septic shock. *Crit Care Med*. 2004;32:858–873.
Evidence-based recommendations for the initial resuscitation and treatment of patients with septic shock and severe sepsis.

Kollef MH, Sherman G, Ward S, et al. Inadequate antimicrobial treatment of infections: a risk factor for hospital mortality among critically ill patients. *Chest*. 1999;115:462–474.
Cohort study demonstrating greater hospital mortality among infected patients in the intensive care unit setting receiving inappropriate initial antibiotic treatment of their infections.

Kortgen A, Niederprum P, Bauer M. Implementation of an evidence-based "standard operating procedure" and outcome in septic shock. *Crit Care Med*. 2006;34:943–949.
Evaluation of an algorithm defining resuscitation according to early goal-directed therapy, glycemic control, administration of stress doses of hydrocortisone, and use of recombinant human activated protein C demonstrating improved clinical outcomes.

Micek ST, Roubinian N, Heuring T, et al. A before-after study of a standardized hospital order set for the management of septic shock. *Crit Care Med*. 2006;34:2707–2713.
A before-after study demonstrating improvements in 28-day mortality and length of stay for patients with septic shock managed with a standardized order set in the emergency department.

Rivers E, Nguyen B, Havstad S, et al. Early goal-directed therapy in the treatment of severe sepsis and septic shock. *N Engl J Med*. 2001;345:1368–1377.
Randomized trial demonstrating the survival benefit of a goal-directed approach to the initial resuscitation of patients with severe sepsis and septic shock.

CARDIOGENIC SHOCK

Christopher Leach and Richard G. Bach

4

Cardiogenic shock refers to a condition in which there is inadequate circulation and compromised organ perfusion primarily due to cardiac dysfunction. This failure of pump function results in an inability to maintain circulation to vital organs that, without treatment, will lead to multisystem failure and death. To differentiate cardiogenic from other forms of shock, it is characterized by prolonged hypotension (systolic blood pressure <90 mm Hg) in the setting of decreased cardiac output (typically <2.2 L/min/m^2) despite adequate intravascular volume (pulmonary artery occlusion pressure >15 mm Hg). This is clinically suggested when there are signs of systemic hypoperfusion manifest by cool mottled extremities, altered mentation, and/or oliguria. However, these classic signs may not always be present. Despite recent advances in management, cardiogenic shock from pump failure remains associated with a very high mortality. Among patients hospitalized with an acute myocardial infarction (AMI) that is complicated by cardiogenic shock, the rate of death within the first 30 days is in the range of 40% to 50% and within the first year it is 55% to 65%.

ETIOLOGY

Cardiogenic shock has multiple possible causes (Table 4.1), although the most common cause is AMI. Shock occurs in approximately 5% to 10% of patients with AMI. It may develop as a consequence of either left or right ventricular infarction, although hemodynamically significant right ventricular infarction occurs most commonly in combination with inferior wall, left ventricular infarction. The severity of shock from left ventricular infarction is generally related to the quantitative loss of functional myocardium, although other factors also play a role. Complications of AMI, such as arrhythmias, ventricular septal defects, papillary muscle dysfunction, or myocardial rupture causing pericardial tamponade, may also trigger the onset of shock. Less frequently, cardiogenic shock may be caused by severe cardiomyopathy (dilated or hypertrophic), acute myocarditis, or severe valvular disease.

PATHOPHYSIOLOGY

Cardiogenic shock generally occurs when myocardial dysfunction exceeds a critical threshold from a single large myocardial infarction (typically considered to involve >40% of the myocardium), a cumulative amount of damage from multiple infarctions, or from diffuse myocardial injury from other inciting factors. With shock there is increasing myocardial oxygen demand due to elevated end-diastolic ventricular pressure along with decreasing oxygen supply from hypotension and falling cardiac output. This results in a self-perpetuating spiral of progressive ischemia and cardiac dysfunction, ultimately culminating in death (Algorithm 4.1). Treatments of cardiogenic shock have sought to interrupt this spiral at various steps. The situation is further complicated by the fact that the majority of patients with cardiogenic shock secondary to AMI have significant multivessel coronary artery disease (CAD) that can limit any compensatory increase in contractility of noninfarct territories. Recent observations of the inflammatory cascade have modified traditional thinking on this syndrome. First, the average left ventricular ejection fraction among patients with AMI and cardiogenic shock is 30%, not lower as might be expected, and yet many patients with an ejection fraction significantly <30% still do not develop cardiogenic shock. In addition, the

15

TABLE 4.1	Causes of Cardiogenic Shock

Acute myocardial infarction
   Left ventricular pump failure
      Large infarction
      Smaller infarction with pre-existing LV dysfunction
   Mechanical complications
      Free wall rupture/tamponade
      Papillary muscle dysfunction/rupture
      Right ventricular infarction
      Ventricular septal defect
Severe cardiomyopathy/congestive heart failure
   Dilated cardiomyopathy
   Stress-induced or Tako-tsubo cardiomyopathy
Acute myocarditis (infectious, toxin/drug, transplant rejection)
Myocardial contusion
Acute/severe valvular insufficiency
   Acute mitral regurgitation (e.g., chordal rupture)
   Acute aortic insufficiency
Obstruction to left ventricular outflow
   Hypertrophic obstructive cardiomyopathy
   Aortic stenosis
Obstruction to ventricular filling
   Pericardial effusion/tamponade
   Mitral stenosis
   Left atrial myxoma

systemic vascular resistance in patients with cardiogenic shock is often not elevated and may be unexpectedly low. This may be the result of a systemic inflammatory response syndrome not unlike septic shock and putatively related to high levels of cytokines and systemic/vascular nitric oxide, which have both negative inotropic and vasodilatory effects.

PATIENT CHARACTERISTICS

Shock is more likely to develop in the setting of AMI among patients who are older, female, and who have significantly more comorbid conditions (diabetes, prior known CAD, history of cerebrovascular disease, and history of renal insufficiency). Cardiogenic shock can complicate ST elevation myocardial infarction (MI) or non-ST elevation MI; it is most common in patients with anterior location of MI. By angiography, the left anterior descending artery is most commonly the culprit vessel, but patients with cardiogenic shock are likely to have multivessel CAD. Signs and symptoms of cardiogenic shock usually develop after hospital admission (median, 6.2 hours after initial MI symptoms) and the majority of patients develop shock within the first 24 hours. A significant minority (~25%) of patients may develop cardiogenic shock after 24 hours, possibly due to recurrent ischemia. Note should be made of a select subset of cardiogenic shock patients who present with poor cardiac output and evidence of systemic hypoperfusion but without frank hypotension. These so-called normotensive cardiogenic shock patients have a lower mortality than their hypotensive counterparts (43% vs. 66%, respectively) but their risk of death is still much higher than AMI patients without hypoperfusion.

EVALUATION

Prompt recognition of cardiogenic shock is essential for management, as timely and appropriate treatment can significantly reduce mortality. Patients with low blood pressure

ALGORITHM 4.1   **Pathophysiology of Cardiogenic Shock**

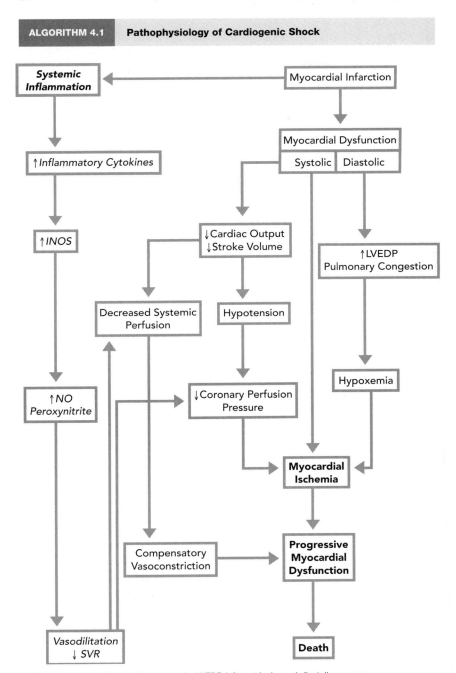

INOS, nitric oxide synthase; NO, nitric oxide; LVEDP, left ventricular end-diastolic pressure; SVR, systemic vascular resistance.

(<90 mm Hg) should be quickly assessed for the presence of pulsus paradoxus (potentially indicating cardiac tamponade), signs of congestive heart failure (elevated jugular venous pressure JVP, pulmonary edema, S3 gallop), and evidence of end-organ hypoperfusion (cool mottled extremities, weak pulses, clouded mental status, reduced urine output). A careful cardiac examination should be performed to assess for the presence of valvular disease or uncommon mechanical causes, although in the setting of AMI or low cardiac output, the murmurs of mitral regurgitation or critical aortic stenosis or insufficiency may be diminished or virtually inaudible. An electrocardiogram should be obtained without delay to look for evidence of acute ischemia or infarction, and serum cardiac biomarkers should be measured at presentation and serially to diagnose acute myocardial injury even when the electrocardiogram is nondiagnostic. A bedside echocardiogram is usually indicated as soon as possible at initial evaluation to assess left and right ventricular function, valvular function, and to exclude cardiac tamponade. When detected, certain mechanical causes of circulatory failure, such as acute mitral regurgitation or ventricular rupture, warrant emergency surgical intervention. When the etiology remains unclear, bedside pulmonary artery catheterization can be helpful in differentiating cardiogenic from other forms of shock, although in cases of shock due to suspected acute myocardial ischemia or infarction, such studies should not delay definitive evaluation by left heart catheterization and coronary angiography. In addition to assisting with diagnosis, pulmonary artery catheter monitoring can help to guide therapy with vasopressor and inotropic medications and gauge hemodynamic improvement versus deterioration prior to any clinically evident signs.

TREATMENT

Initial Medical Management

Patients with cardiogenic shock require immediate attention to the stabilization of adverse hemodynamics in order to interrupt the viscous cycle of tissue hypoperfusion and the potential for rapid development of irreversible organ damage (Algorithm 4.2). Such patients typically need central venous access and continuous monitoring of arterial pressure and urine output in a hospital environment where advanced management options are readily available. The cause must be considered when choosing therapeutic interventions because the application of certain therapies commonly used in other forms of shock can be deleterious to the acutely dysfunctional heart, especially in the setting of AMI. In the absence of overt pulmonary congestion, fluid resuscitation may help reverse hypotension but must be monitored carefully to avoid pulmonary edema and respiratory failure. Systemic hypotension may initially require treatment with a vasopressor, although it should be remembered that peripheral vasoconstrictors typically further increase afterload and oxygen demand for the failing myocardium. For this reason, the lowest dose of pressor empirically effective in achieving an adequate BP response should be employed. The first-line agent for hypotension in the setting of cardiogenic shock is usually dopamine (5 to 20 mcg/kg/min), which is preferred over other pressors because of its combined inotropic and vasopressor effects, and for theoretical preservation of renal perfusion by mesenteric vasodilation at low doses. If hypotension remains refractory, norepinephrine (1 to 20 mcg/min) can be added, but as a peripheral vasoconstrictor, it may aggravate pump failure by increasing ventricular afterload.

In patients with relatively stable blood pressure (systolic blood pressure >90 mm Hg) but low cardiac output and evidence of hypoperfusion, dobutamine (2.5 to 10 mcg/min) may provide additional benefit from its inotropic effect. Because of its potential for peripheral vasodilation, dobutamine should be avoided or used with caution in patients with hypotension. Milrinone (0.375 to 0.75 mcg/kg/min, with or without a loading dose of 50 mcg/kg), another potent inotrope, typically causes significant vasodilation and should be used with caution in the patient with low blood pressure and avoided in patients with renal insufficiency. Because of the potential adverse effects of pressor agents and the favorable effects of intra-aortic counterpulsation, patients with shock due to primary pump failure should always be considered for intra-aortic balloon pump support early in the course of shock. If, however, hypertrophic cardiomyopathy and shock due to outflow tract obstruction is suspected, drugs with positively inotropic effects and intra-aortic balloon pumping should be avoided and the peripheral vasoconstrictor phenylephrine administered as the pressor of choice.

ALGORITHM 4.2 **Management of Suspected Cardiogenic Shock**

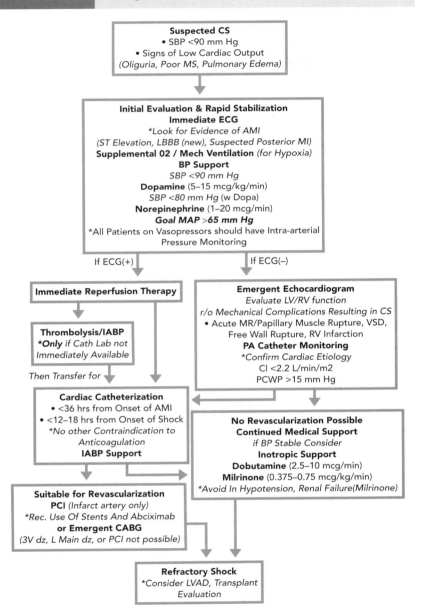

CS, cardiogenic shock; SBP, systolic blood pressure; MS, mental status; ECG, electrocardiogram; AMI, acute myocardial infarction; BP, blood pressure; MAP, mean arterial pressure; LV/RV, left ventricular/right ventricular; IABP, intra aortic balloon counterpulsation; MR, mitral regurgitation; VSD, ventricular septal defect; PA, pulmonary artery; PCI, percutaneous coronary intervention; CABG, coronary artery bypass surgery; LVAD, left ventricular assist device.

Intra-Aortic Balloon Counterpulsation

An intra-aortic balloon catheter is a device inserted via an accessible artery, usually the femoral artery, into the descending aorta and then inflated and deflated with helium gas by a computerized console in synchrony with the cardiac cycle to provide hemodynamic support for patients in shock. By balloon inflation that is timed just after aortic valve closure and deflation just prior to the next ventricular systole, balloon pump counterpulsation is the only means to augment central aortic pressure and vital organ perfusion (including coronary blood flow) while simultaneously reducing afterload and myocardial oxygen demand. Early intra-aortic balloon pump support can be beneficial as a bridge to revascularization, to recovery following transient myocardial stunning, or en route to more advanced support devices or cardiac transplantation. It should be considered as an early intervention for most patients with cardiogenic shock in whom there are no contraindications (severe aortic insufficiency, severe peripheral vascular disease, aortic dissection).

Reperfusion Therapy: Thrombolytic Therapy and Primary Percutaneous Coronary Intervention

A fundamental concept of current treatment of cardiogenic shock in patients with ischemic heart disease is the recognition that rapid reperfusion of AMI and early revascularization for patients with obstructive coronary artery disease are key interventions that have been proven in clinical trials to reduce mortality. Because randomized trials of reperfusion for ST-elevation MI have suggested that the presence of cardiogenic shock is associated with reduced efficacy of pharmacologic reperfusion by thrombolytic therapy and superior outcomes after successful percutaneous coronary intervention (PCI), timely primary PCI is the preferred mode of reperfusion when available for patients with cardiogenic shock complicating AMI. There is a significant increase in mortality for such patients even with delays to reperfusion as short as minutes to hours. However, for patients who cannot undergo timely coronary angiography there are also limited data that thrombolysis combined with intra-aortic balloon counterpulsation may have benefit as a temporizing measure to be followed by mechanical revascularization when feasible.

Coronary Revascularization

Patients with evidence of an acute coronary syndrome and cardiogenic shock should be referred for urgent left heart catheterization and revascularization if coronary anatomy is favorable. Results from the randomized SHOCK trial comparing early revascularization with conservative management showed that patients (age <75 years) with AMI and cardiogenic shock had significant mortality benefit from early PCI or coronary artery bypass surgery. Current guidelines recommend early revascularization, when feasible, for patients who are within 36 hours of the onset of AMI. Of note, reflecting the complex and extensive coronary artery disease in these high-risk patients, 36% of the patients in the SHOCK trial who underwent revascularization received coronary artery bypass surgery. Nonrandomized data show there may also be a benefit from early revascularization in those patients more than 75 years old. Current guidelines recommend that such patients should be considered for early revascularization on an individual basis.

Left Ventricular Assist Devices

When medical therapy and intra-aortic balloon pump support are inadequate to stabilize vital organ perfusion, more advanced forms of support may be necessary and should be considered before irreversible end-organ damage occurs. Left ventricular assist devices (LVADs) that are inserted surgically or, more recently, percutaneously, can provide significant improvements in cardiac output, blood pressure, pulmonary artery wedge pressure, and end-organ perfusion that can be lifesaving. In a suitable patient with cardiogenic shock, an LVAD is most commonly used as a means of temporary support or as a "bridge" to definitive treatment such as orthotopic heart transplantation. However, there are ongoing clinical trials investigating use of LVADs as definitive therapy for patients with end-stage cardiac failure refractory to more conservative management who may not be candidates for heart transplantation.

CARDIAC TAMPONADE

Cardiac tamponade represents a unique cause of shock in which external compression of the heart significantly restricts filling and limits output. Because it represents a not uncommon and rapidly reversible form of shock, prompt recognition is essential. An important clinical sign on examination is the presence of pulsus paradoxus, where the inspiratory fall in systolic blood pressure exceeds ~10 mm Hg. Distended jugular veins are also usually present. The most common cause is a significant pericardial effusion, although more unusual causes of impaired filling—such as a localized thrombus compressing the left atrium of a patient following cardiac surgery—are possible. Echocardiography may demonstrate the classic findings of a significant pericardial effusion with evidence of diastolic compression of the right side of the heart and exaggerated respiratory variation in Doppler-measured mitral inflow velocities. When hypotension is present, rapid infusion of intravenous fluids may help maintain blood pressure, but removal of the offending pericardial fluid by percutaneous subxiphoid pericardiocentesis or surgical drainage may be needed without delay. If the diagnosis is in question, pulmonary artery catheterization may be useful to confirm hemodynamic evidence of tamponade, suggested by equalization of elevated right atrial, right ventricular diastolic, pulmonary artery diastolic, and pulmonary artery wedge pressures.

CONCLUSION

Cardiogenic shock is a condition associated with profound cardiac dysfunction from several potential causes, but is seen most commonly in the setting of acute MI. It is associated with a high rate of death. Optimal management requires early recognition and aggressive medical and potentially mechanical intervention. When anatomically feasible for patients with acute coronary syndromes and shock, early revascularization has been shown to be effective for improving both short- and long-term survival.

Suggested Reading

Hochman JS. Cardiogenic shock complicating acute myocardial infarction: expanding the paradigm. *Circulation*. 2003;107:2998–3002.
   A review of cardiogenic shock including newer information regarding pathophysiology and management.
Hochman JS. Early revascularization in acute myocardial infarction complicated by cardiogenic shock. *N Engl J Med*. 1999;341:625–634.
   Published results of the landmark SHOCK trial showing reduced mortality for patients (less than age 75) randomized to a strategy of early revascularization vs. conservative management.
Hollenberg SM, et al. Cardiogenic shock. *Ann Intern Med*. 1999;131:47–59.
   A general review of cardiogenic shock and evidence-based management.
Various Authors. *J Am Coll Cardiol*. 2000;36(3, Suppl 1).
   JACC supplement with several publications on clinically relevant sub-studies from the SHOCK trial and Registry.

5

ANAPHYLACTIC SHOCK
Timothy J. Bedient

Anaphylaxis refers to the characteristic and often life-threatening clinical manifestations of the immunoglobulin E (IgE)-mediated immediate hypersensitivity reaction involving mast cell and basophil degranulation and release of histamine, tryptase, prostaglandins, and leukotrienes that occurs following exposure to various substances. Anaphylactoid reactions are clinically indistinguishable from anaphylaxis, but are not IgE-mediated. They are thought to result from direct mast cell degranulation independent of IgE, or alterations in arachidonic acid metabolism. The substances that trigger anaphylaxis and anaphylactoid reactions differ, and are outlined in Table 5.1.

Reactions can develop within minutes, but usually <1 hour, after exposure to a triggering substance. More rapid reactions occur with parenteral exposure. Initial symptoms include flushing, pruritis, and a sense of doom. Characteristic clinical manifestations of varying severity develop involving the skin, eyes, respiratory and gastrointestinal tracts, and cardiovascular and central nervous systems, as listed in Table 5.2. Cardiovascular collapse (shock) occurs in approximately 30% of cases and results from (a) hypovolemia induced by increased vascular permeability and loss of intravascular volume, (b) hypotension from peripheral vasodilation, (c) myocardial depression, and (d) bradycardia. Up to 50% of patients describe respiratory symptoms, which can progress to respiratory failure from severe upper airway edema, bronchospasm, and cardiogenic and noncardiogenic pulmonary edema. Biphasic reactions occur in up to 20% of patients, characterized by a second round of symptoms 1 to 8 hours after the initial reaction (although up to 72 hours has been reported).

Diagnosis is clinical and involves a broad differential diagnosis including urticaria, status asthmaticus, "red man" syndrome (vancomycin), scromboidosis (histaminelike compound in spoiled fish such as tuna, mackerel, mahi-mahi, and blue fish), carcinoid, pheochromocytoma, mastocytosis, monosodium glutamate ingestion, and panic attacks. Serum levels of tryptase (especially the beta subtype) and histamine, when elevated, support the diagnosis. Tryptase levels are elevated for 1-6 hours after the event, but serum histamine levels fall within 30–60 minutes. A 24 hour urine n-methyl histamine level compared to a later baseline can be a helpful alternative. Patients should be questioned about exposure to potential triggers, but no substance is identified in up to 60% of cases.

Treatment is outlined in Algorithm 5.1 and is based on the joint recommendations of the American Academy of Allergy, Asthma, and Immunology and the American College of Allergy, Asthma and Immunology. Pharmacologic therapy involves epinephrine to reverse the respiratory and cardiovascular effects, and blocking the effects of histamine with histamine 1 and 2 receptor blockers. There are no contraindications to the use of epinephrine, and numerous studies have shown that it is underused in emergency treatment, with delay resulting in shock and respiratory failure. In a study by Korenblat et al., 70% of patients with severe symptoms required at least two epinephrine injections. Intravenous steroids have no role in the acute treatment of anaphylaxis but may prevent phase 2 reactions that can occur up to 72 hours after initial presentation. Steroids are given as an initial dose of 1 to 2 mg/kg of intravenous methylprednisolone, or equivalent, and continued for up to 4 days (intravenously or orally). On discharge, patients should be referred to an allergist for testing and monitoring, and provided with home epinephrine self-injectors (EpiPen).

TABLE 5.1	Causes of Anaphylaxis and Anaphylactoid Reactions (Substances Are Paired with the Most Common Associated Mechanism)

Anaphylaxis (IgE-mediated)
   Foods (especially nuts, eggs, fish, shellfish, and cow's milk)
   Antibiotics (especially penicillin; 4% positive by allergy testing also test positive to
      cephalosporins)
   Vaccines
   Anesthetics
   Insulin and other hormones
   Antitoxins
   Blood and blood products
   Insect stings and bites (bee, wasp, and ant)
   Snake bites
   Latex
   Allergy immunotherapy
Anaphylactoid reactions (direct mast cell degranulation, altered AA metabolism)
   Nonsteroidal anti-inflammatory drugs (especially aspirin)
   Opiates
   Sulfites
   Radiocontrast media
   Neuromuscular blocking agents (curoniums and succinylcholine)
   Gamma globulin
   Antisera
   Exercise

IgE, immunoglobulin E; AA, arachidonic acid.

TABLE 5.2	Clinical Manifestations of Anaphylaxis and Anaphylactoid Reactions

Eyes
   Pruritis
   Lacrimation
   Conjunctival erythema
   Periorbital edema
Cardiovascular
   Hypotension
   Tachycardia (bradycardia when severe)
   Arrhythmias
   Cardiac arrest
Gastrointestinal
   Nausea/vomiting
   Diarrhea
   Abdominal pain

Skin
   Pruritis
   Flushing
   Urticaria
   Angioedema
Respiratory
   Dyspnea
   Stridor/wheezing/hoarseness
   Difficulty swallowing
   Pulmonary edema
Neurologic
   Anxiety and "sense of doom"
   Presyncope and syncope
   Seizures

ALGORITHM 5.1	Acute Treatment of Patients with Anaphylaxis and Anaphylactoid Reactions

Immediate treatment is indicated for all patients with significant respiratory, cardiac, or gastrointestinal symptoms as symptoms can progress rapidly to shock, respiratory failure, and death, and there are **NO absolute contraindications to epinephrine.**

Suspected impending respiratory collapse (stridor, wheezing, tachypnea, dyspnea, difficulty swallowing)

No   **Yes**

Place patient in recumbent position. Obtain large-bore IV access (but do not delay epinephrine) Continuous monitoring of blood pressure, heart rate, oxygen saturation, and respiratory symptoms.

Immediate intubation as delay may increase difficulty of endotracheal intubation. Cricothyroidotomy may be necessary if severe airway edema.

IM epinephrine 0.3–0.5 mg 1:1,000 to anterior or lateral thigh, preferably. Repeat after 5 minutes as needed (up to 70% can require second dose) **FOR SEVERE SYMPTOMS OR POOR RESPONSE TO IM GIVE** IV epinephrine 0.1–0.2 mg (1 mL 1:1,000 in 10 mL 0.9% NaCl [0.1 mg/mL]) 1–2 min until response **IF HYPOTENSIVE GIVE** 1–2 L IV 0.9% NaCl rapid infusion.

Treat all patients with histamine 1 and 2 (H1, H2) blockers.
1) Diphenhydramine (H1) 25–50 mg IV
And
1) Ranitidine (H2) 50 mg IV
or
2) Famotidine (H2) 20 mg IV

Clinical Response?   **Yes**

No

If patient taking home beta-blocker;
1) Glucagon 1– 2 mg IV/IM q5min to effect
For continued hypotension;
1) Start continuous IV epinephrine infusion at 0.1–1 mcg/kg/min titrated to effect.
2) Continued aggressive fluid resuscitation (via rapid transfuser if available).
For continued respiratory symptoms, if not intubated
1) Inhaled beta-agonists (albuterol) 0.5 mL 0.5% soln in 2.5 mL 0.9% NaCl nebulized q15min.

IV, intravenous; IM, intramuscular.

Suggested Reading

Joint Task Force on Practice Parameters; American Academy of Allergy, Asthma and Immunology; American College of Allergy, Asthma and Immunology; Joint Council of Allergy, Asthma and Immunology. The diagnosis and management of anaphylaxis: an updated practice parameters. *J Allergy Clin Immunol.* 2005;115:S483–S523.

Joint recommendations on the definition, causes, manifestations, diagnosis, and treatment for patients with anaphylaxis and anaphylactoid reactions.

Korenblat P, Lundie MJ, Dankner RE, et al. A retrospective study of epinephrine administration for anaphylaxis: how many doses are needed? *Allergy Asthma Proc.* 1999;20: 383–386.

Retrospective review of 105 anaphylactic episodes to determine the level of severity and corresponding number of epinephrine injections required for symptom reversal.

6

MECHANICAL CAUSES OF SHOCK
Howard J. Huang

The mechanical causes of shock encompass a heterogeneous group of syndromes that produce an acute elevation in pulmonary vascular resistance, either through direct obstruction of the pulmonary vasculature or via vasoactive mediators that cause pulmonary vasoconstriction. These events precipitate acute cor pulmonale and right ventricular (RV) strain, eventually resulting in shock due to RV failure. *Mechanical shock* has also been described as *obstructive shock*, and these terms have been used interchangeably in the literature. Among the mechanical shock syndromes, massive acute pulmonary embolism (PE) is the prototypical and most commonly encountered syndrome. However, the pathogenesis of shock and clinical findings in air, fat, and amniotic fluid embolism syndromes shares many similar features. The specific diagnosis depends on the clinical context in which the syndrome occurs.

Cardiac tamponade has also been described as a mechanical cause of shock. However, its pathophysiology is distinct from that of obstructive shock. A concise discussion on the pathogenesis, diagnosis, and treatment of cardiac tamponade is included in the chapter on cardiogenic shock. Although the various causes of shock are discussed in isolation in this manual, it is important to recognize that multiple forms of shock may be present simultaneously in the same patient.

The severity of hemodynamic derangements seen in obstructive shock is determined by (a) the magnitude of pulmonary arterial vascular obstruction and/or vasoconstriction, (b) RV performance, and (c) pre-existing cardiopulmonary disease (CPD). As an example, a segmental PE that is normally survivable in an otherwise healthy patient may produce hemodynamic compromise in a patient with pre-existing pulmonary arterial hypertension and marginal RV function.

Because the pulmonary circulation is typically a low-resistance circuit, a normal right ventricle is incapable of sustaining a mean pulmonary arterial pressure (mPAP) >40 mm Hg. The finding of mPAP values >40 mm Hg in the absence of RV failure suggests a subacute or chronic cause for pulmonary arterial hypertension. Without pre-existing CPD, the rise in RV afterload and mPAP is directly related to the magnitude of pulmonary vascular obstruction and/or pulmonary vasoconstriction. Evidence of acute RV dysfunction typically can be detected by echocardiography after a 25% to 30% loss of pulmonary vascular cross-sectional area. However, in the setting of pre-existing CPD, the amount of obstruction necessary to cause hemodynamic compromise may be much smaller and difficult to predict.

Without prompt intervention, an acute elevation of pulmonary arterial (PA) pressure and RV afterload beyond the capacity for RV compensation will precipitate a deleterious sequence of events that ends in refractory shock and circulatory collapse. Algorithm 6.1 illustrates the interdependent nature of the multiple contributing factors and events that lead to obstructive shock. Successful management of mechanical shock syndromes requires early recognition and rapid initiation of supportive measures to restore and maintain hemodynamic stability. Common clinical findings of mechanical shock states include tachycardia, hypotension, and signs of end-organ hypoperfusion (i.e., decreased urine output, cool extremities, and altered mental status). Hypoxemia and tachypnea are frequently present because of abnormalities in ventilation-perfusion matching. In catastrophic cases, ventricular fibrillation, asystole, or pulseless electrical activity may be the initial presentation. Physical examination may reveal signs of RV failure, including jugular venous distention, tricuspid regurgitation murmur, accentuated P2, hepatojugular reflux, and the Kussmaul sign.

ALGORITHM 6.1   Pathophysiology of Mechanical Shock

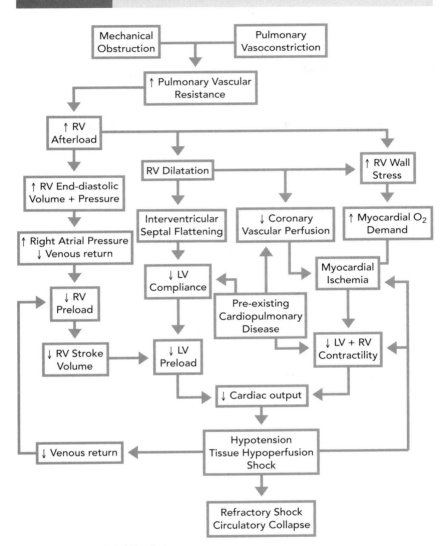

RV, Right Ventricular; LV, Left Ventricular.

Sinus tachycardia is frequently observed on electrocardiogram, with or without changes consistent with RV strain and myocardial ischemia. Transthoracic echocardiography usually reveals evidence of RV dysfunction, including RV distention and hypokinesis, tricuspid regurgitation, and flattening of the interventricular septum. McConnell sign, characterized by global RV hypokinesis with relative sparing of the apical segments on echo, may be observed. Common hemodynamic findings on right heart catheterization and transesophageal Doppler are described at the beginning of this chapter.

The mainstay of treatment in mechanical shock is restoration and maintenance of hemodynamic stability to reverse end-organ hypoperfusion. It is important to recognize that excessive fluid administration may be counterproductive by exacerbating RV distention and impairing left ventricular (LV) filling. Vasopressor and inotropic agents should be initiated early, and additional fluid administration may be guided by clinical assessment and diagnostic measurements of hemodynamic status using bedside echocardiography, transesophageal Doppler, or pulmonary arterial catheter.

The following sections review the pathophysiology, unique features, and management algorithms for four common mechanical shock syndromes. Table 6.1 contains a list of common risk factors and presenting signs and symptoms for each of these syndromes.

PULMONARY EMBOLISM

Venous thromboembolism (VTE) is a frequent complication in critically ill medical and surgical patients. Most intensive care unit patients have multiple major risk factors for VTE, including prolonged immobilization, trauma, malignancy, advanced age, cardiopulmonary disease, and indwelling vascular access devices. Clinical studies in medical intensive care unit patients have shown that up to one third of patients not receiving deep venous thrombosis prophylaxis develop VTE at some point during their hospital course. Approximately 5% to 10% of patients with VTE will develop PE, with approximately 10% of these cases causing hemodynamically significant or massive PE. The presence of shock in the setting of PE is associated with a five- to sevenfold increase in mortality. Patients presenting with cardiopulmonary arrest have mortality rates exceeding 65%.

Bedside echocardiography offers a readily accessible modality for evaluating hemodynamic status in patients with suspected massive PE. Alternative diagnoses, such as cardiomyopathy, valvular disease, cardiac tamponade, pericardial effusion, and aortic dissection, can be quickly excluded. Occasionally, a large thrombus in transit may be directly visualized by echocardiogram. Initiation of therapy should not be delayed for confirmatory diagnostic testing. Management should be focused on (a) restoring and maintaining hemodynamic stability, (b) maintaining adequate oxygenation, and (c) preventing thrombus propagation and recurrent PE. A management algorithm for massive PE is shown in Algorithm 6.2.

Multiple clinical trials have been conducted to address the role of thrombolytic (fibrinolytic) therapy in massive PE. Yet, no single trial to date has demonstrated a clear mortality benefit for thrombolytics over high-dose anticoagulation with unfractionated or low-molecular-weight heparin. However, there is some evidence that thrombolytic administration results in faster improvement in RV function and hemodynamic status. Most experts recommend use of thrombolytics in the setting of massive acute PE when supportive measures are ineffective at restoring hemodynamic stability, and no absolute contraindications to thrombolytic use (Algorithm 6.2) can be identified. In patients with strong contraindications to thrombolytics, catheter thrombectomy or open surgical thrombectomy may be attempted as salvage therapy.

Unfortunately, mortality in such patients frequently exceeds 90%. If hemodynamic stability is restored, definitive diagnosis with computed tomographic angiography or pulmonary angiography may be conducted. An evaluation for deep venous thrombosis should be conducted with consideration of inferior vena cava filter placement in patients with marginal cardiac function and significant clot burden.

AIR EMBOLISM

Air embolism syndrome (AES) occurs when gas enters the venous or arterial circulation driven by a pressure gradient favoring entrainment of gas, or through inadvertent injection,

TABLE 6.1	Risk Factors and Common Manifestations of Mechanical Shock States	

State	Risk factors	Common signs and symptoms
Massive pulmonary embolism	■ Immobilization ■ Surgery within last 3 months ■ Prior history of VTE ■ Malignancy ■ Chronic cardiopulmonary disease ■ Trauma ■ Obesity ■ Central venous catheters ■ Hypercoagulable state	■ Pleuritic chest pain ■ Respiratory distress ■ Cough ■ Wheezing ■ Hemoptysis ■ Hypoxemia ■ Cyanosis ■ Fever
Air embolism syndrome	■ Open surgical site above RA (craniotomy, cesarean section) ■ Use of medical gases in laparoscopic or endoscopic procedures ■ Volume depletion ■ Barotrauma ■ Pulmonary vasodilators ■ Biopsy of airway or lung parenchyma ■ Venous access devices ■ Contrast injection ■ Trauma	■ Anxiety ■ Sense of impending doom ■ Chest pain ■ Respiratory distress ■ Wheezing ■ Cyanosis ■ Hypoxemia ■ Gasp reflex ■ Mill-wheel murmur ■ Agitation, delirium, seizure activity (systemic gas embolization)
Fat embolism syndrome	■ Blunt-force trauma resulting in long-bone and pelvic fractures ■ Orthopaedic procedures ■ Extensive rib fractures ■ Burn injury ■ Acute pancreatitis ■ Diabetes mellitus ■ Sickle cell anemia ■ Liposuction ■ Parenteral lipid infusion	■ Agitation ■ Delirium ■ Seizure activity ■ Fevers and chills ■ Chest pain ■ Respiratory distress ■ Wheezing ■ Cyanosis ■ Hypoxemia ■ Petechial rash involving axilla and upper trunk
Amniotic fluid embolism syndrome	■ Pregnancy ■ Peripartum ■ Postpartum (up to 48 hours) ■ Difficult labor ■ Use of labor induction agents ■ Amniocentesis ■ First or second trimester abortion ■ Trauma	■ Agitation and delirium ■ Seizure activity ■ Fevers and chills ■ Nausea and vomiting ■ Respiratory distress ■ Wheezing ■ Chest pain ■ Cyanosis ■ Hypoxemia ■ Profuse hemorrhage with no obvious structural cause ■ Fetal bradycardia or late decelerations

VTE, Venous thromboembolism; RA, right atrium.

ALGORITHM 6.2 Management Algorithm for Massive Pulmonary Embolism (PE)

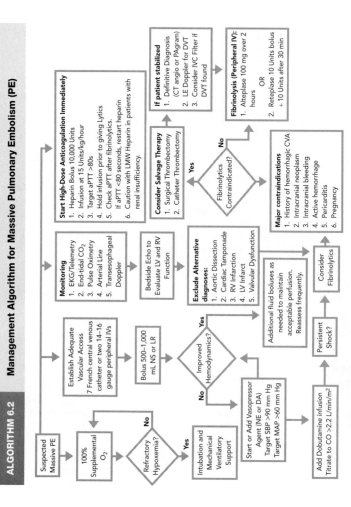

IVs, intravenous catheters; EKG, electrocardiogram; aPTT, activated partial thromboplastin time; LMW, low-molecular-weight; NS, normal saline; LR, lactated ringers; CT, computed tomography; PA, pulmonary arterial; DVT, deep venous thrombosis; IVC, inferior vena cava; NE, norepinephrine; DA, dopamine; SBP, systolic blood pressure; MAP, mean arterial pressure; CVA, cerebral vascular accident.

producing hemodynamic and gas exchange abnormalities and end-organ dysfunction. Air enters the venous circulation when there is transient negative intrathoracic pressure in the presence of an open central or peripheral vein, or if the open vein is elevated above the right atrium. A negative pressure gradient as small as 5 cm H_2O through a 14-gauge peripheral IV is sufficient to allow air to enter the venous circulation at up to 100 mL/sec. In the setting of volume depletion and decreased central venous pressure, or if the extravascular environment is under positive pressure (e.g., CO_2 insufflation during laparoscopic surgery), the rate of gas entry is increased. Gas can enter the arterial circulation via anatomic shunts, pulmonary vasodilator administration, or if the filtration capacity of the pulmonary circulation is overwhelmed by large volumes of gas. Consequently, every case of venous air embolism is a potential case of arterial air embolism. The severity of hemodynamic and gas exchange abnormalities caused by venous air embolism depends on (a) total volume of gas entrained, (b) the rate at which gas enters the pulmonary arterial circulation, (c) pre-existing cardiopulmonary disease, and (d) severity of the inflammatory response triggered by gas deposited in the pulmonary circulation.

The cause of shock in the setting of AES is mainly obstructive in nature. However, arterial air embolism can result in cardiogenic shock if gas enters the coronary circulation. A sufficiently large venous air embolus can completely obstruct the RV outflow tract. Animal studies have shown that acute, large-volume gas embolism is lethal, whereas slow, continuous small-volume gas embolism is survivable, even if the total volume of gas embolized is much greater. In humans, the estimated lethal dose in venous AES is approximately 300 to 500 mL if gas is entrained slowly. However, acute embolism of as little as 50 mL of air may be sufficient to cause hemodynamic compromise. Unlike embolism of solid materials such as thrombus or fat, gas entering the pulmonary arterial circulation is eliminated continuously via diffusion across alveolar capillaries. Thus, as long as RV performance is capable of compensating for the acute rise in PA pressure and the portal of air entry is eliminated, shock due to AES will resolve over time as the embolized gas is cleared.

In the correct clinical setting, AES should be included in the differential diagnosis for patients presenting acutely with hemodynamic instability and gas-exchange abnormalities. The cardiopulmonary manifestations of AES may be indistinguishable from acute massive PE, fat embolism, hypovolemic shock, and anaphylaxis or septic shock. If paradoxic embolism occurs and air enters the coronary arterial circulation, cardiogenic shock is added to the picture. Early assessment of cardiac function using transthoracic echocardiography, transesophageal Doppler, or PA catheter will help determine the predominant cause of shock.

Therapy for AES is supportive and should focus on (a) eliminating the portal of air entry, (b) restoring and maintaining hemodynamic stability, and (c) promoting clearance of entrained air. A management algorithm for AES is shown in Algorithm 6.3. Air aspiration from the RV has been described, and can remove up to 50% of the embolized air in some patients, producing rapid hemodynamic improvement. The patient is placed in the left lateral decubitus position, elevating the RV above its outflow tract and promoting migration of entrained air back into the RV. A central venous catheter is then placed with the tip approximately 2 cm below the superior vena cava/right atrial junction, and air is aspirated through the distal port. In the setting of refractory cardiopulmonary arrest, emergency thoracotomy, closed-chest cardiac massage, and direct aspiration of air through the right ventricle may be attempted as a last resort.

Emphasis should be placed on prevention of gas embolization during medical procedures through adequate hydration, proper patient positioning, avoidance of barotrauma, and observing proper procedures for central venous catheter placement and removal. Patients at high risk for AES should be closely monitored via capnography or precordial Doppler ultrasound to detect gas embolization during surgical procedures. Early detection and prompt supportive treatment of AES can lead to dramatic improvement in outcomes.

FAT EMBOLISM

Fat embolism syndrome (FES) occurs when fat from necrotic bone marrow or adipocytes is released into the venous circulation following trauma or tissue injury, resulting in mechanical obstruction of the pulmonary vascular bed and triggering a systemic inflammatory

ALGORITHM 6.3   Management Algorithm for Air Embolism Syndrome

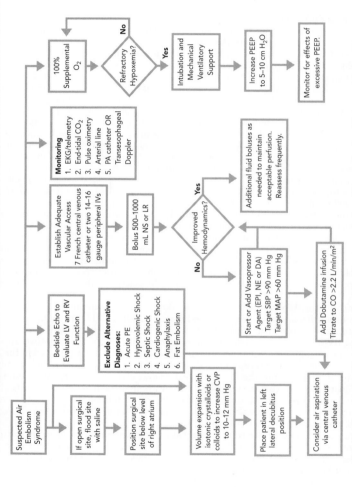

CVP, LV, left ventricular; RV, right ventricular; PE, pulmonary embolism; NS, normal saline; LR, lactated ringers; EPI, epinephrine; NE, norepinephrine; DA, dopamine; SBP, systolic blood pressure; MAP, mean arterial pressure; IVs, intravenous catheters; EKG, electrocardiogram; PA, pulmonary arterial.; PEEP, positive end-expiratory pressure.

response. Approximately 90% of cases of FES occur following blunt trauma resulting in pelvic and long-bone fractures. The risk of developing FES rises with the severity of the injury and the number of large marrow-containing bones involved.

The pathophysiologic changes precipitated by FES appear to be the result of mechanical obstruction and a severe vasoconstrictive, inflammatory response triggered by the deposition of free fatty acids in the pulmonary arterial vasculature. However, the precise mechanisms underlying this syndrome remain incompletely understood. Studies have shown circulating fat in blood specimens collected from patients undergoing orthopaedic surgery. This observation suggests the presence of fat in the circulation is necessary but not sufficient to precipitate FES. Development of FES likely depends on multiple factors, including (a) the total volume and rate of fat embolization, (b) immunogenicity of the embolized material, (c) intensity of the host inflammatory response, and (d) pre-existing CPD.

Shock in the early phase of FES is mainly due to mechanical obstruction of the pulmonary vasculature causing acute RV failure. Within 24 to 72 hours of the initial insult, toxic free fatty acid metabolites cause systemic inflammation, acute lung injury, and end-organ dysfunction with hemodynamic derangements similar to those found in septic or distributive shock. The classic triad of clinical findings described in FES includes hypoxemia, neurologic dysfunction, and petechial rash involving the upper trunk and axilla may be found in some patients.

No specific diagnostic test is available for FES. Treatment for FES is supportive and should be focused on (a) restoring and maintaining hemodynamic stability and (b) maintaining adequate oxygenation to avoid end-organ dysfunction. There is some evidence for prophylactic administration of corticosteroids in patients at high risk for FES. However, no prospective data are available to support corticosteroid use after the FES has occurred. A management algorithm for FES is shown in Algorithm 6.4. A high index of suspicion and early institution of supportive care is necessary to improve outcomes for patients with FES.

AMNIOTIC FLUID EMBOLISM

Amniotic Fluid Embolism Syndrome (AFES) is a relatively uncommon but devastating syndrome that occurs when amniotic fluid enters the maternal circulation during labor and delivery or in the postpartum period due to cervical, uterine wall, or placental membrane disruption. Classic findings include the acute onset of shock, hypoxemia, encephalopathy, coagulopathy, and disseminated intravascular coagulation. Many patients deteriorate rapidly and die of circulatory collapse within the first hour of presentation. Survivors are frequently left with severe neurologic impairment.

The pathogenesis of AFES remains incompletely understood. Amniotic fluid is a heterogeneous mixture of water, electrolytes, hormones, and fetal components. It is unclear which are the principle agents responsible for AFES. Amniotic fluid components are routinely isolated in blood specimens from pregnant women who are asymptomatic, suggesting that the presence of amniotic fluid in the maternal circulation is necessary but not sufficient to cause AFES. The development of AFES may depend on multiple factors, including (a) absolute volume of amniotic fluid and its rate of entry into the maternal circulation, (b) amniotic fluid composition, which affects its immunogenicity and vasoactive properties, (c) maternal immune response, and (d) pre-existing maternal cardiopulmonary disease.

The cause of shock in AFES is frequently multifactorial and temporally heterogeneous. In humans, the early phase of AFES is frequently dominated by severe acute LV systolic dysfunction and cardiogenic shock. This may be accompanied by bradycardia, ventricular fibrillation, pulseless electrical activity, or asystole. Deposition of amniotic fluid in the pulmonary circulation triggers intense pulmonary vasoconstriction, RV strain, and obstructive shock. The late phase of AFES, typically occurring 1 to 2 hours after presentation, is frequently complicated by the onset of distributive shock likely due to a systemic inflammatory response syndrome triggered by immunogenic amniotic fluid components. Cardiogenic and obstructive shock may persist into the late phase of AFES, but typically improve over time. Finally, with the onset of disseminated intravascular coagulation and coagulopathy, severe hemorrhaging may occur, adding hypovolemic shock to the picture.

The acute onset of agitation, altered mental status, dyspnea, and hemodynamic instability in a pregnant or peripartum woman should immediately raise clinical suspicion for

| ALGORITHM 6.4 | Management Algorithm for Fat Embolism Syndrome |

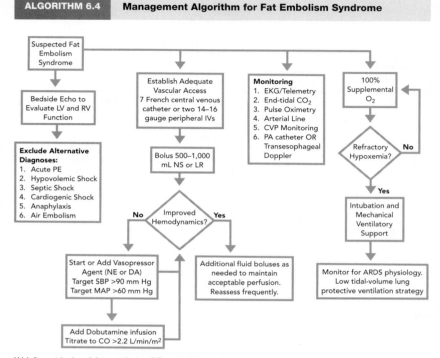

LV, left ventricular; right ventricular; PE, pulmonary embolism; IVs, intravenous catheters; NS, normal saline; LR, lactated ringers; NE, norepinephrine; DA, dopamine; SBP, systolic blood pressure; MAP, mean arterial pressure; EKG, electrocardiogram; CVP, central venous pressure; PA, pulmonary arterial; ARDS, acute respiratory distress syndrome.

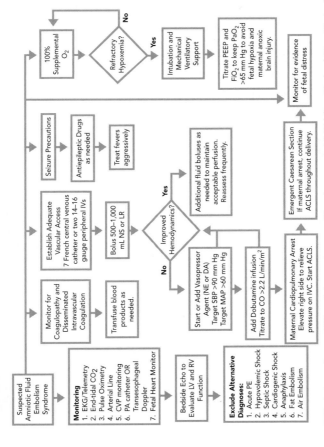

EKG, electrocardiogram; CVP, central venous pressure; PA, pulmonary arterial; LV, left ventricular; RV, right ventricular; PE, pulmonary embolism; IVs, intravenous catheters; NS, normal saline; LR, lactated ringers; NE, norepinephrine; DA, dopamine; SBP, systolic blood pressure; MAP, mean arterial pressure; IVC, inferior vena cava; ACLS, advanced cardiac life support; PEEP, positive end-expiratory pressure.

AFES. Because there are no diagnostic laboratory tests specific for AFES, it is a clinical diagnosis made by exclusion. Management of AFES is supportive and consists of the following objectives: (a) restoring and maintaining maternal hemodynamic stability, (b) maintaining adequate oxygenation to prevent maternal and fetal hypoxia, (c) correcting anemia and coagulopathy, (d) treating neurologic manifestations, and (e) expediting delivery of the fetus. A management algorithm for AFES is shown in Algorithm 6.5. Overly aggressive volume resuscitation may be counterproductive because LV systolic dysfunction is a common feature in AFES. Bedside echocardiography is a useful modality for rapid assessment of LV and RV function. Because multiple causes of shock are frequently encountered during the course of AFES, a transesophageal Doppler or PA catheter is useful for monitoring changing hemodynamic parameters and guiding fluid resuscitation and titration of vasopressors and inotropes. Successful management of this catastrophic syndrome requires early recognition, prompt initiation of supportive measures, and close cooperation between the intensivist, obstetrician, and anesthesiologist.

Suggested Reading

Claus MM, Shank ES. Gas embolism. *N Engl J Med.* 2000;342;476–482.
   A concise review of venous and arterial gas embolism syndromes.
Goldhaber SZ. Echocardiography in the management of pulmonary embolism. *Ann Intern Med.* 2002;136:691–700.
   Review of common echocardiographic findings in pulmonary embolism.
Mellor A, Soni N. Fat embolism. *Anaesthesia.* 2001;56:145–154. A review of etiology, diagnosis, and treatment of fat embolism syndrome.
Moore J, Baldisseri MR. Amniotic fluid embolism. *Crit Care Med.* 2005;33[Suppl]: S279–S285.
   Thorough discussion of pathogenesis, diagnosis, and treatment of the amniotic fluid embolism syndrome.
Piazza G, Golhaber SZ. The acutely decompensated right ventricle: pathways for diagnosis and management. *Chest.* 2005;128:1836–1852.
   Thorough review of signs, symptoms and management strategy for acute right ventricular decompensation.
Wood KE. Major pulmonary embolism: review of a pathophysiologic approach to the golden hour of hemodynamically significant pulmonary embolism. *Chest.* 2002;121:877–905.
   Comprehensive review of the pathogenesis, diagnosis, and management of hemodynamically significant pulmonary embolism.

Management of Respiratory Disorders

II

AN APPROACH TO RESPIRATORY FAILURE

Warren Isakow

7

Respiratory failure is a common reason for intensive care unit admission and is the final pathway for a number of diseases of differing pathophysiology. A mechanism-based approach enables the clinician to identify the most likely cause for the respiratory failure and to treat appropriately. In general, patients with respiratory failure may be classified into two groups, depending on the component of the respiratory system that is involved.

- Hypercapnic respiratory failure is a consequence of ventilatory failure and is recognized by an elevated $PaCO_2$ above normal (>45 mm Hg at sea level). This denotes failure of the respiratory pump and can occur with normal lungs.
- Hypoxemic respiratory failure is a consequence of gas exchange failure and is recognized by hypoxemia (PaO_2 <60 mm Hg) with or without widening of the alveolar arterial O_2 gradient.

HYPERCAPNIC RESPIRATORY FAILURE

The hallmark of hypercapnic respiratory failure is an elevated $PaCO_2$ above 45 mm Hg.

$$\blacksquare \; PaCO_2 = K \times \frac{VCO_2}{(1 - Vd/Vt) \times VA}$$

where $PaCO_2$ = the partial pressure of carbon dioxide in the blood, K = constant, VCO_2 = carbon dioxide production, Vd/Vt = dead space ratio of each tidal volume breath, VA = minute ventilation.

Analysis of the previous equation shows that hypercapnea can occur from three processes: (a) an increase in CO_2 production, (b) a decrease in minute ventilation, and (c) an increase in dead-space ventilation. Understanding of the "respiratory pump" enables the clinician to systematically consider the cause of hypercapnic respiratory failure in different patients, as depicted in Algorithm 7.1.

The acuity of onset of the hypercapnea is also an important determinant of management. An acute change in $PaCO_2$ of 10 mm Hg will change the blood pH by 0.08 in the

ALGORITHM 7.1   **Causes of Hypercapnic Respiratory Failure Based on Components of the Respiratory Pump**

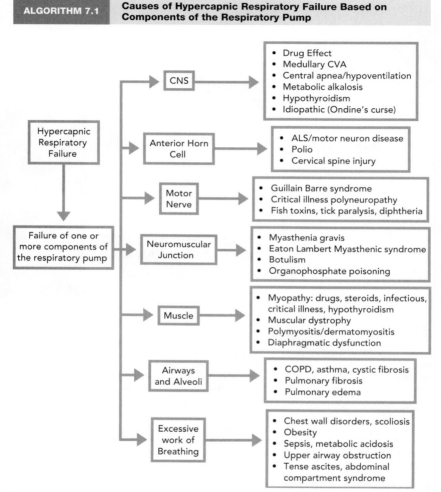

CVA, cerebrovascular accident; ALS, amyotrophic lateral sclerosis; COPD, chronic obstructive pulmonary disease.

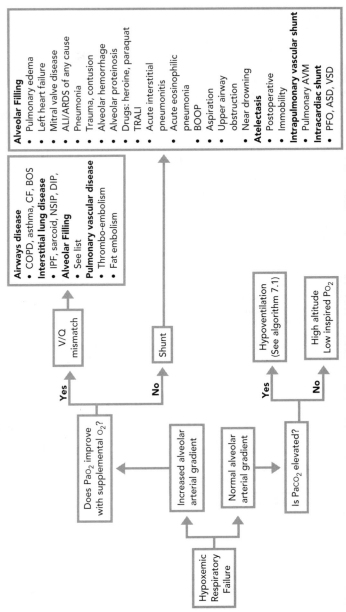

Airways disease
- COPD, asthma, CF, BOS

Interstitial lung disease
- IPF, sarcoid, NSIP, DIP,

Alveolar Filling
- See list

Pulmonary vascular disease
- Thrombo-embolism
- Fat embolism

Alveolar Filling
- Pulmonary edema
- Left heart failure
- Mitral valve disease
- ALI/ARDS of any cause
- Pneumonia
- Trauma, contusion
- Alveolar hemorrhage
- Alveolar proteinosis
- Drugs: heroine, paraquat
- TRALI
- Acute interstitial pneumonitis
- Acute eosinophilic pneumonia
- BOOP
- Aspiration
- Upper airway obstruction
- Near drowning

Atelectasis
- Postoperative
- Immobility

Intrapulmonary vascular shunt
- Pulmonary AVM

Intracardiac shunt
- PFO, ASD, VSD

V/Q mismatch

Shunt

Hypoventilation
(See algorithm 7.1)

High altitude
Low inspired Po_2

Yes

No

Does Pao_2 improve with supplemental o_2?

Increased alveolar arterial gradient

Normal alveolar arterial gradient

Is $Paco_2$ elevated?

Yes

No

Hypoxemic Respiratory Failure

COPD, chronic obstructive pulmonary disease; CF, cystic fibrosis; BOS, bronchiolitis obliterans syndrome; IPF, interstitial pulmonary fibrosis; NSIP, non-specific interstitial pneumonitis; DIP, desquamative interstitial pneumonia; ALI/ARDS, acute lung injury/acute respiratory distress syndrome; TRALI, transfusion-related acute lung injury; BOOP, bronchiolitis obliterans-organizing pneumonia; AVM, arteriovenous malformation; PFO, patent foramen ovale; ASD, atrial septal defect; VSD, ventricular septal defect.

opposite direction. In patients with chronic hypercapnea, renal compensation occurs by bicarbonate retention and tends to correct the pH toward normal. In these cases, a change in $PaCO_2$ of 10 mm Hg is reflected by a change of 0.03 in the blood pH in the opposite direction. Recognition of acute hypercapnea or acute on chronic hypercapnea is vitally important as it is a harbinger of an imminent respiratory arrest and potential development of severe hypoxemia.

Important principles in managing patients with hypercapnea are:

- Never sedate a patient with hypercapnea or a patient who has neuromuscular weakness.
- Cautious use of supplemental oxygen is necessary as oxygen can worsen hypercapnea by a number of mechanisms: worsening of V/Q matching, the Haldane effect, and suppression of central hypoxemic drive. Enough oxygen should be given to keep the hemoglobin molecules >90% saturated with oxygen.
- Rapidly institute adequate ventilation: in carefully selected patients, noninvasive ventilation can be tried prior to intubation and mechanical ventilation.

HYPOXEMIC RESPIRATORY FAILURE

Hypoxemic respiratory failure occurs because of impaired gas exchange or hypoventilation and is defined by a PaO_2 of <60 mm Hg. The first step in ascertaining a cause is looking for concomitant hypercapnea as would occur with hypoventilation or severe intrinsic lung disease with increased dead-space ventilation, and calculating the alveolar-arterial oxygen gradient by using the alveolar gas equation. The approach to hypoxemic respiratory failure is summarized in Algorithm 7.2.

The alveolar gas equation follows:

$$PAO_2 = FIO_2 (PB - PH_2O) - \frac{PaCO_2}{R}$$

where PAO_2 = alveolar partial pressure of oxygen, FIO_2 = fraction of inspired oxygen, PB = barometric pressure (760 mm Hg at sea level), PH_2O = water vapor pressure (47 mm Hg), $PaCO_2$ = partial pressure of carbon dioxide in the blood, and R = respiratory quotient, assumed to be 0.8.

The alveolar-arterial oxygen gradient = $PAO_2 - PaO_2$. The normal value is between 10 and 15 mm Hg and is influenced by age, increasing by 3 mm Hg every decade after the age of 30 years. For an FIO_2 = 21%, it should be 5 to 25 mm Hg and for an FIO_2 = 100%, it should be <150 mm Hg. Hypoxemic respiratory failure with a widened alveolar-arterial oxygen gradient is caused by V/Q mismatching or shunt pathophysiology. These two processes can be differentiated by improvement of the hypoxemia with supplemental oxygen, in the case of V/Q mismatch, and no improvement in cases with shunt. Diseases that cause airspace flooding, atelectasis, airway disease, or pulmonary vascular problems are common causes of hypoxemic respiratory failure.

Management principles for patients with hypoxemic respiratory failure include:

- Rapid restoration of an adequate arterial saturation, which often requires intubation and mechanical ventilation. Patients with hypoxemia as a group respond less well to noninvasive ventilation.
- Use of adequate amounts of positive end-expiratory pressure to reduce FIO_2 to nontoxic levels (FIO_2 <60%).
- A low tidal volume strategy with permissive hypercapnea in patients with acute lung injury/acute respiratory distress syndrome.
- General supportive care in the intensive care unit while the patient's pulmonary process resolves.

It is worthwhile to note that hypoxia refers to an oxygen deficit at a tissue level and depends on oxygen delivery. Therefore, hypoxia can be a result of any process that affects oxygen delivery to the tissues, and includes:

- Hypoxic hypoxia (low arterial oxygen saturation and a low PaO_2)
- Anemic hypoxia (low circulating hemoglobin with impaired oxygen delivery)

- Circulatory hypoxia (low cardiac output states)
- Histotoxic hypoxia (poisoning with cyanide where oxygen is delivered to the tissues but cannot be used).

Oxygen delivery $=$ Cardiac Output $\times$ Arterial Oxygen Content

$$Do_2 = CO \times Cao_2$$

$$Do_2 = CO \times (1.39 \times [Hb\ (g/dL)] \times Sao_2) + 0.003 \times Pao_2$$

Suggested Reading

Lanken PN. Approach to acute respiratory failure. In: Lanken PN, ed. *The Intensive Care Unit Manual.* Philadelphia: Saunders; 2001;1–12.

A superb concise chapter focusing on developing a pathophysiological approach to all patients with respiratory failure.

Wood LDH. The pathophysiology and differential diagnosis of acute respiratory failure. In: Hall JB, Schmidt GA, Wood LDH, eds. *Principles of Critical Care.* New York: McGraw Hill 2005;417–426.

Another superb textbook chapter focusing on pathophysiology.

8 INITIAL VENTILATOR SETUP
Warren Isakow

The initiation of mechanical ventilation is a critical period during the course of a patient's stay in the intensive care unit. The clinician is encouraged to monitor the patient closely during initiation of mechanical ventilation as this period often provides important answers regarding a patient's underlying pathophysiologic abnormality. This simple bedside process allows for verification of the underlying cause of the decompensation requiring ventilatory support, assessment of severity of the disease process, the likely response to standard therapies, and it helps with planning of care during the next few days to weeks.

Table 8.1 provides a general guideline to the initial ventilator settings in different clinical circumstances. The table is simply a guide, and the reader should understand that every patient is unique and should have the ventilator adjusted according to the individual's clinical status.

Algorithm 8.1 is a management algorithm for troubleshooting the situation of a patient with persistent high peak airway pressures, a common ventilator-related problem in the intensive care unit. Table 8.2 provides potential causes for an alarm resulting from a low exhaled tidal volume/low minute ventilation.

TABLE 8.1 Guidelines for Initial Ventilator Settings in Different Clinical Scenarios

Indication for mechanical ventilation	Mode of choice	Respiratory rate (breaths/min)	Tidal volume (mL/kg)	Fio₂	PEEP	Additional ventilator issues	Adjunctive therapies	Additional comments
Airway protection, spontaneously breathing patient. (e.g., hepatic encephalopathy, upper airway obstruction)	AC (volume) SIMV PSV	10–14	8–10	100%, Obtain ABG and wean for sats >92% to goal Fio₂ of 40%	5	Peak flow 60 L/min Trigger sensitivity −2 cm H_2O	DVT GI	Maintain on MV until upper airway issues resolved. Patients with hepatic encephalopathy are prone to develop a respiratory alkalosis, so TV may need to be reduced.
Asthma exacerbation	AC (volume)	Set rate low, 8–12	6–8	100%, obtain ABG and wean for sats >92% to goal Fio₂ of 40%	0–5	Set peak flows high, allow adequate expiratory time. Consider square wave ventilation. Use flow-by for easier triggering	BD ST AB SDN DVT GI	Tolerate hypercarbia, higher peak airway pressures. Monitor for auto-PEEP and barotrauma Do not ventilate for a "normal" ABG Apply external PEEP to overcome intrinsic PEEP when triggering Often need heavy sedation initially Once bronchospasm and acute issues adequately resolved, do not do prolonged weaning trials, consider trial of extubation.

(continued)

TABLE 8.1 Guidelines for Initial Ventilator Settings in Different Clinical Scenarios *(Continued)*

Indication for mechanical ventilation	Mode of choice	Respiratory rate (breaths/min)	Tidal volume (mL/kg)	FiO_2	PEEP	Additional ventilator issues	Adjunctive therapies	Additional comments
COPD exacerbation	AC (volume)	Set rate low, 8–12	6–8	100%, obtain ABG and wean for sats >92% to goal FiO_2 of 40%	0–5	Set peak flows high, allow adequate E time. Use flow by for easier triggering	BD ST AB DVT GI NUTR	Monitor for autoPEEP. Avoid posthypercapnic alkalosis. Tolerate hypercarbia; do not ventilate for a "normal" ABG Monitor for barotrauma Apply external PEEP to overcome intrinsic PEEP when triggering. Consider extubation to NIPPV
Hypoxemic respiratory failure with pneumonia or pulmonary edema	AC (volume)	Often need high rates, 16–24 because of high V_E requirements	6–8	100%, obtain ABG and wean for sats >92% to goal FiO_2 of 40%	5–10	Often have high V_E requirements	BD AB DVT GI NUTR	Secretion management is important. In septic patients, allow full MVS to divert CO from the respiratory muscles to other vital organs. Follow improvement clinically as improved pulmonary compliance

Condition	Mode	Rate		FiO2	PEEP		Prophylaxis	Comments
ALI/ARDS	AC (volume) PCV, high frequency oscillator	6	Often need high rates, up to 30, because of high V_E requirements	100%, obtain ABG and wean for sats >92% to "safe" FiO_2 of <60%	5–15	May need I:E of 1:1 or 1.5:1 (IRV) Need higher mean airway pressures Allow permissive hypercarbia to a pH of 7.20	BD DVT GI NUTR SDN	Consider nebulized prostacyclin, nitric oxide or oscillator Monitor for barotrauma Often require heavy sedation Try to avoid neuromuscular blockade if possible. Consider adjunctive steroids after 7 days. Monitor for septic complications
Postoperative respiratory failure	AC (volume)	8–10	Set rate at 10–16	100%, wean rapidly for sats. >92% to goal FiO_2 of 30%	5	Verify placement of all lines, tubes placed in OR. Peak flow 60 L/min	DVT GI	Await sedatives, paralytics to be cleared and perform weaning rapidly. Prone to hypoventilation after extubation. Prone to atelectasis and splinting due to pain which can cause hypoxemia
Hypoventilation from CNS depression, neuromuscular weakness	AC (volume)	8–10	Set rate at 10–16	100%, obtain ABG and wean rapidly for sats of <92% to goal FiO_2 of 30%	5	Peak flow 60 L/min	GI DVT NUTR	Avoid sedatives Prone to atelectasis Follow NIF in patients with weakness

PEEP, positive end-expiratory pressure; AC, assist control; SIMV, synchronized intermittent mandatory ventilation; PSV, pressure support ventilation; ABG, arterial blood gas; sats, saturation; DVT, deep venous thrombosis prophylaxis; GI, gastrointestinal prophylaxis; MV, mechanical ventilation; TV, tidal volume; BD, bronchodilator regimen; ST, steroids; AB, antibiotics; SDN, sedation; COPD, chronic obstructive pulmonary disease; NIPPV, noninvasive positive pressure ventilation; V_E, minute ventilation; MVS, mechanical ventilator support; CO, cardiac output; PCV, pressure control ventilation; I:E, expiratory time ratio; IRV, inverse ratio ventilation; NUTR, nutritional support; OR, operating room; NIF, negative inspiratory force.

ALGORITHM 8.1   **Management Algorithm for High Peak Airway Pressures**

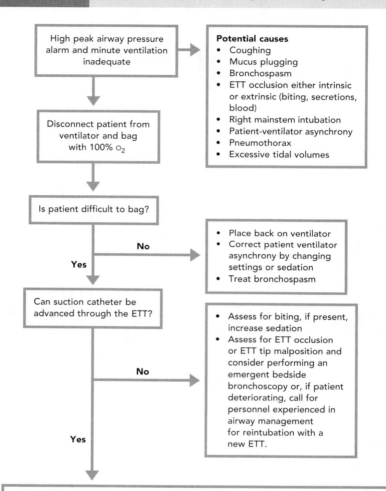

ETT, endotracheal tube; ICS, intercostal space.

TABLE 8.2	Potential Causes for a Low Exhaled Tidal Volume/Low Minute Ventilation Alarm

Leak in the circuit
- Tracheal cuff leak
- Patient inadvertently extubated or endotracheal tube tip high, causing a leak
- Ventilator circuit disconnected at any point from the patient to the ventilator
- Large bronchopleural fistula with leak through a chest tube

In patients on pressure support ventilation
- Worsening respiratory system compliance
- Decreased patient effort
- Decreased patient respiratory rate
- Inadequate pressure support being provided

In patients on pressure control ventilation
- Worsening respiratory system compliance

Suggested Reading

Reily DJ, Lanken PN. Ventilator Alarm Situations. In: Lanken PN, ed. *The Intensive Care Unit Manual.* Philadelphia: Saunders; 2001;553–561.
A practical chapter with clinical information on how to deal with common ventilator alarms.

9

UPPER AIRWAY OBSTRUCTION
Warren Isakow

Upper airway obstruction is a medical emergency that requires rapid evaluation of the patient with simultaneous therapy to ensure adequate oxygenation and ventilation of the patient. Prompt recognition of premonitory symptoms and signs may enable the physician to buy precious time for evaluation and planning patient care. The common causes of upper airway obstruction are presented in Table 9.1 and an algorithm for the rapid assessment and management of the patient is presented in Algorithm 9.1. It is important to note that with most patients, upper airway obstruction is a clinical diagnosis that does not allow for laboratory testing, arterial blood gas analysis, or even imaging in the acute setting, and all resources should be directed to preventing cardiorespiratory arrest and securing the airway. Figures 9.1 through 9.5 review the anatomy of the upper airway, intubation technique, and illustrate practical aspects of performing emergent airway access.

Some common etiologies and their management will be briefly reviewed.

INFECTIOUS EPIGLOTTITIS AND LARYNGITIS

Routine pediatric vaccination against *Haemophilus influenzae* has now made epiglottitis more common in adults than in children. The potential pathogens include *Haemophilus influenzae* and *Haemophilus parainfluenzae, Streptococcus pneumoniae, Streptococcus pyogenes, Staphylococcus aureus,* and occasionally anaerobes, while laryngitis is often caused by viruses and rarely *Corynebacterium diphtheriae,* which is more common in unvaccinated individuals.

The classic presentation is of an adult who is drooling, appears toxic, and is sitting upright in the tripod position. These patients have a high potential for complete occlusion of the airway and should be treated with empiric intravenous (IV) antibiotics (ceftriaxone, 2 g IV every 24 hours, or TMP-SMX, 10 mg/kg per day divided every 6 hours if allergic to penicillin). Personnel with experience in handling difficult airways should be called in to evaluate the patient, and a tracheostomy set should be brought into the examining room. If an examination is to be performed fiberoptically, preferentially this should be done in the operating room with a tracheostomy set available. The examination needs to be performed cautiously so as not to precipitate further narrowing of the airway.

In cases of epiglottitis, the epiglottis appears swollen and beefy. Diphtheria is characterized by a gray membrane. Blood cultures may occasionally be positive for bacteria, and a lateral radiograph of the neck may show the swollen epiglottis. The patient should not be sent out of the intensive care unit for any studies and should not be left alone. Most patients improve rapidly with antibiotics; patients with diphtheria should also receive equine antitoxin and a macrolide antibiotic.

ANGIOEDEMA

Angioedema can occur through a variety of mechanisms and results in painless swelling of the soft tissues of the face. The common precipitants are angiotensin-converting enzyme inhibitors, immunoglobulin E-mediated allergic reactions to foods or medications, and complement activation through an inherited or acquired C1 esterase inhibitor deficiency/ impairment.

Patients are treated with antihistamines, steroids, and epinephrine, with airway management as noted in the algorithm. Patients with hereditary deficiency of C1 esterase inhibitor respond to therapy with androgens (danazol) and antifibrinolytic agents.

TABLE 9.1	Etiology and Specific Therapy of Upper Airway Obstruction by Site	

Site of obstruction	Etiology	Specific therapy
Nasopharynx	■ Nasal polyps ■ Nasal tumors, lymphoma ■ Adenoidal hypertrophy ■ Trauma ■ Nasal packing	■ Nasal steroids, surgery ■ Radiation, surgery, chemotherapy ■ Adenoidectomy ■ Fracture reduction, incise hematomas ■ Prophylactic antibiotics for sinusitis, humidified oxygen
Oropharynx	■ Ludwig's angina ■ Odontogenic abscess ■ Retropharyngeal abscess ■ Peritonsillar abscess ■ Tonsillar enlargement ■ Macroglossia ■ Angioedema ■ Stevens-Johnson syndrome ■ Burkitt lymphoma ■ Salivary tumors ■ LeFort fractures 2 and 3 ■ Obstructive sleep apnea	■ Antibiotics, drainage, may need tracheotomy ■ Antibiotics and drainage ■ Antibiotics and drainage ■ Tonsillectomy ■ Supportive, tracheotomy ■ Antihistamines, steroids, epinephrine (see text) ■ Supportive care, tracheotomy ■ Chemoradiation ■ Resection ■ Tracheotomy, fixation ■ CPAP, UPPP, tracheotomy
Laryngopharynx	■ Epiglottitis ■ Acute bacterial laryngotracheitis (diphtheria) ■ Neoplasms: SCC, papillomatosis ■ Angioedema ■ Rheumatoid arthritis ■ Relapsing polychondritis ■ Wegener's granulomatosis ■ Midline granuloma ■ ETT injury: subglottic stenosis ■ Trauma, burns, inhalation injury ■ Hemangiomas ■ Foreign body aspiration, dislodged tooth ■ Iatrogenic: laryngospasm, epistaxis	■ Antibiotics ■ Antibiotics ■ Resection, laser removal ■ Antihistamines, steroids, epinephrine (see text) ■ Corticosteroids, tracheotomy ■ Corticosteroids, tracheotomy ■ Corticosteroids, cyclophosphamide, tracheotomy ■ Radiation ■ Resection, dilation, cryotherapy ■ Tracheotomy ■ Laser, intralesional steroids, tracheotomy ■ Endoscopy ■ Supportive

CPAP, continuous positive airway pressure; UPPP, uvulopalatopharyngoplasty; SCC, squamous cell carcinoma; ETT, endotracheal tube.

POSTEXTUBATION STRIDOR

Stridor occurs in up to 15% of patients after extubation, and most cases are caused by laryngeal edema. Laryngospasm and secretions in the airway are less common causes of stridor in this situation. Immediate management should consist of nebulized racemic epinephrine, which

ALGORITHM 9.1	Algorithm for the Management of a Patient with Airway Obstruction

Airway obstruction suspected by history and physical examination:
- Inspiratory stridor: lesion at or above glottis
- Biphasic stridor and wheeze: subglottic lesion or below the glottis
- Impaired phonation
- Poor air entry
- Suprasternal retractions
- Universal choking sign
- Respiratory distress
- Tachycardia
- Agitation
- Angioedema
- Wheezing
- Neck swelling

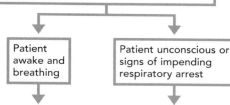

Patient awake and breathing

Patient unconscious or signs of impending respiratory arrest

- Attempt to localize cause by history and examination
- Assemble help with personnel experienced in difficult airways (anesthesia, ENT)
- Assemble intubation equipment and a tracheostomy tray
- Consider transfer to the operating room to optimize available equipment and personnel
- Careful performance of indirect laryngoscopy or fiberoptic nasopharyngolaryngoscopy

- Call for help to assemble personnel experienced in difficult airways (anesthesia and/or ENT)
- Head tilt-chin lift
- Jaw thrust (if C-spine unstable)
- Insert an oral or nasal airway
- Ventilate with a bag-valvemask
- Attempt direct laryngoscopy and endotracheal intubation
- Surgical airway (bedside tracheostomy)
- Cricothyroidotomy or needle cricothyrotomy if personnel not available to perform a bedside surgical airway

- Management based on diagnosis
- Can use heliox or BiPAP if etiology not progressive.
- Close monitoring

- Additional management based on etiology

ENT, ear, nose, and throat specialist.

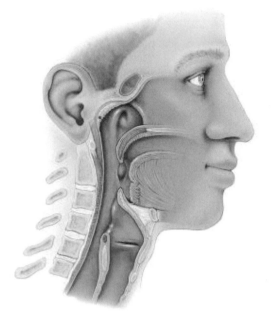

Figure 9.1. Anatomy of the pharynx and larynx—sagittal section. (From ACC Systems and Structures Chart Images, Anatomical Chart Company, with permission.)

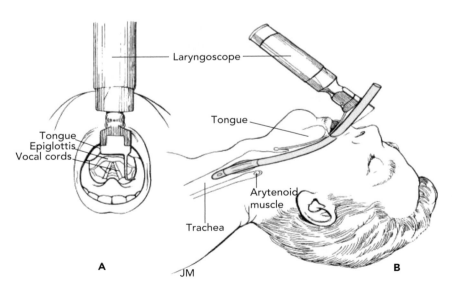

Laryngoscope

Tongue

Tongue
Epiglottis
Vocal cords

Arytenoid muscle

Trachea

A

JM

B

Figure 9.2. Endotracheal intubation in a patient without a cervical spine injury. **A:** The primary glottic landmarks for tracheal intubation as visualized with proper placement of the laryngoscope. **B:** Positioning the endotracheal tube. (From Smeltzer SC, Bare BG. *Textbook of Medical-Surgical Nursing.* 9th ed. Philadelphia: Lippincott Williams & Wilkins, 2000.)

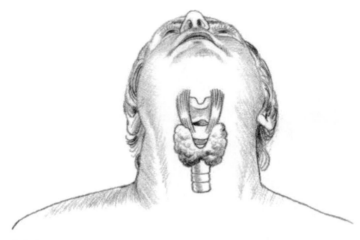

Figure 9.3. Landmarks for performing a cricothyrotomy. (From *Nursing Procedures.* 4th ed. Philadelphia: Lippincott Williams & Wilkins; 2004.)

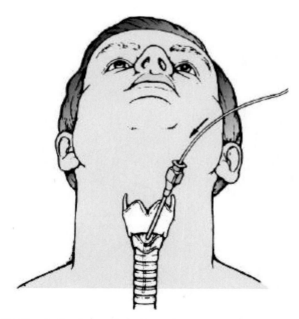

Figure 9.4. Needle cricothyrotomy with a 12- or 14- gauge needle. The catheter should be attached to high-flow oxygen from a wall source (15 L/min). (From Nettina SM. *The Lippincott Manual of Nursing Practice.* 7th ed. Philadelphia: Lippincott, Williams & Wilkins; 2001.)

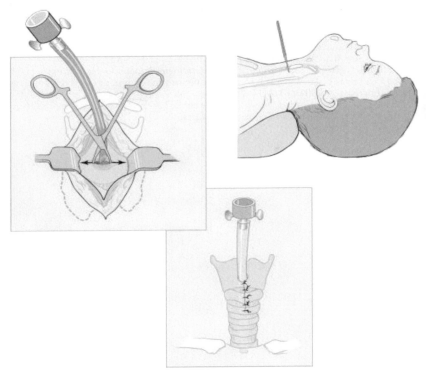

Figure 9.5. Cricothyrotomy. Illustrations showing scalpel in position to perform horizontal incision through cricothyroid membrane; hemostats maintain opening for insertion of tracheal tube, and tracheal tube is secured in place. (From LifeART image. Philadelphia: Lippincott Williams & Wilkins. All rights reserved.)

will cause local vasoconstriction and reduce edema. Most physicians also use short courses of IV corticosteroids; however, there are no randomized data to support this treatment. These patients need to be monitored in the ICU with all airway precautions fulfilled, as noted in the algorithm. Prevention of this problem by doing a cuff-leak test prior to all extubations is controversial because failing a cuff-leak test is not an accurate predictor of postextubation stridor.

Suggested Reading
Aboussouan LS, Stoller JK. Diagnosis and management of upper airway obstruction. *Clin Chest Med.* 1994;15:1:35–53.
   An excellent review article on the topic.
Gehlbach B, Kress JP. Upper airway obstruction. In: Hall JB, Schmidt GA, Wood LDH, eds. *Principles of Critical Care.* 3rd ed. New York: McGraw Hill, 2005;455–464.
   An excellent review article on the topic.
Goodenberger D. Medical emergencies. In: Carey CF, Lee HH, Woeltje KF, eds. *The Washington Manual of Medical Therapeutics.* 29th ed. Philadelphia: Lippincott, Williams & Wilkins, 1998; 494–526.
   An excellent concise chapter on the management of common emergencies in the ICU.
Jaber S, Chanques G, Matecki S, et al. Post extubation stridor in intensive care unit patients: risk factors, evaluation and importance of the cuff leak test. *Intensive Care Med.* 2003;29:69–74.

Risks for stridor include increased severity of illness, medical cause for intubation, traumatic and difficult intubations, a history of self extubation, overdistended endotracheal tube cuffs and a prolonged period of intubation.

Khosh MM, Lebovics RS. Upper airway obstruction. In: Parillo JE, Dellinger RP, eds. *Critical Care Medicine.* 2nd ed., St Louis: Mosby, 2001:808–825.

A thorough textbook chapter which divides etiologies into anatomic location.

Nzeako UC, Frigas E, Tremaine WJ. Hereditary angioedema. A broad review for clinicians. *Arch Intern Med.* 2001;161:2417–2429.

Reviews the genetic forms of the disease, the clinical presentation, diagnosis and therapeutic options as well as options for prophylaxis.

10

ACUTE LUNG INJURY AND THE ACUTE RESPIRATORY DISTRESS SYNDROME
Timothy J. Bedient and Daniel P. Schuster

Acute lung injury (ALI) and the acute respiratory distress syndrome (ARDS) are life-threatening examples of acute pulmonary edema. Although a distinction between ALI and ARDS was originally conceived as representing a spectrum of severity (ALI less severe than ARDS), overlap between the two entities is sufficiently great so that most experts no longer believe the distinction is clinically important.

The incidence of ALI/ARDS in the United States is estimated to be 200,000 cases per year, with a mortality rate of 35% to 40%, which has significantly decreased from a rate of 65% to 70% in the early 1980s. The major physiologic consequence of ALI/ARDS is hypoxia, but most patients ultimately die from the underlying cause (e.g., sepsis) or associated complications (e.g., multiorgan failure) rather than from refractory hypoxemia per se. Current therapy for ALI/ARDS centers around treatment of the underlying cause, a pressure-targeted strategy of low tidal volume ventilation aimed at preventing further lung injury, and appropriate fluid management.

In 1994, the American-European Consensus Conference on ARDS convened to develop a set of diagnostic criteria for ALI and ARDS. With these criteria, in conjunction with the more recent view that there is little importance in the distinction between ALI and ARDS, along with evolving changes in the use of hemodynamic monitoring (see later discussion), the diagnosis of ALI/ARDS should be considered whenever the following criteria are met (Algorithm 10.1): (a) an appropriate clinical setting (i.e., a likely underlying cause), (b) the development of bilateral alveolar and/or interstitial infiltrates of acute onset (<72 hours) on frontal chest radiograph, (c) a ratio of the pulmonary arterial oxygen pressure in millimeters of mercury (PaO_2) divided by the fraction of inspired oxygen (FiO_2) of <300, and (d) no clinical evidence that left ventricular failure or intravascular volume overload are the principle cause for the acute radiographic pulmonary infiltrates.

ALI/ARDS can arise from direct injury to the lung parenchyma or from indirect systemic insults transmitted to the lung by the pulmonary circulation (Table 10.1). Direct causes of ALI/ARDS include pneumonia, gastric aspiration, blunt chest trauma, near drowning, and toxic inhalations. Common indirect causes include sepsis, large-volume blood transfusions (typically >15 units), massive tissue trauma, lung transplantation, reperfusion after cardiopulmonary bypass, drug overdoses, and pancreatitis. Although more than 60 conditions have been associated with ARDS, the most frequent cause is sepsis, followed by pneumonia and aspiration.

The pathogenesis of ARDS starts with a pulmonary or systemic insult that triggers an inflammatory response within the lungs. The resulting "noncardiogenic, increased permeability" form of pulmonary edema follows a predictable clinical and pathologic course that has been separated into three clinically meaningful phases. The exudative phase occurs immediately and lasts approximately 3 to 7 days. Pathologically, it is characterized by "diffuse alveolar damage," the cardinal features of which are (a) the accumulation of extravascular lung water, protein, and inflammatory cells (primarily neutrophils) in the interstitial and alveolar spaces, precipitates of which result in the characteristic intra-alveolar "hyaline membranes," (b) type 1 alveolar cell necrosis, and (c) intra-alveolar hemorrhage. The physiologic consequences of filling alveoli with edema and cellular debris are reduced alveolar ventilation, intrapulmonary shunting, and reduced lung compliance with increased work of breathing. The clinical consequences are a need for mechanical ventilatory support to reduce the work of breathing, a high FiO_2 to achieve an acceptable PaO_2, and positive airway pressure throughout the respiratory cycle to improve alveolar ventilation.

| ALGORITHM 10.1 | Ventilator Management in Acute Lung Injury/Acute Respiratory Distress Syndrome |

Acute Hypoxic Respiratory Failure with the Following
- Appropriate clinical setting
- Bilateral patchy, diffuse, or homogenous pulmonary infiltrates on frontal radiograph
- PaO_2/FiO_2 ≤300
- Suspicion of left heart failure?

ABBREVIATIONS
PaO_2 arterial partial pressure of oxygen in mm Hg
FiO_2 fraction inspired oxygen e.g., room air = 0.21
PBW   predicted body weight
VT   tidal volume
PEEP   positive end expiratory pressure in cm H_2O
RR   respiratory rate
PP   plateau pressure in cm H_2O
A/C   assist/control mode of mechanical ventilation

No ↓   **Yes** →

Calculate PBW in kg
- Men = 50 + 2.3 (height in inches - 60)
- Women = 45.5 + 2.3 (height in inches - 60)

Cardiogenic Pulmonary Edema Supported by
- Clinical signs
- Pulmonary capillary wedge pressure >18 mm Hg
- Esophageal doppler ultrasonography with decreased cardiac index and increased corrected flow time
- Echocardiographic evidence of left heart failure

Start Mechanical Ventilation in A/C Mode with the Following Initial Parameters
- VT 6 mL/kg PBW
- PEEP 5 cm H_2O
- RR ≤35

Mechanical Ventilation Goals
- PaO_2 55–80 mm Hg or SaO_2 ≥88%
- PP ≤30 cm H_2O
- FiO_2 <0.6
- pH 7.30–7.45
*Obtain PP at least every 4 hours with 0.5 second end inspiratory pause

GOALS MET?
No ← | → **Yes**

Go To Algorithm 10.2

- If PP >30 cm H_2O, decrease VT 1 mL/kg PBW to as low as 4 mL/kg to achieve PP ≤30 cm H_2O
- If PP <25 cm H_2O and TV <6 mL/kg PBW, increase TV by 1 mL/kg until PP >25 cm H_2O or TV = 6 mL/kg
- Increase PEEP using minimal amount necessary to maintain FiO_2 <0.7 (see **Table 10.3**)*
- If pH 7.15–7.30 increase RR until pH >7.30 or $PaCO_2$ <25 (consider $NaHCO_3$ if RR = 35 and $PaCO_2$ <25)
- If pH <7.15 increase RR to 35; if pH remains <7.15 and $NaHCO_3$ used or considered, increase TV by 1 mL/kg until pH >7.15 (may exceed PP of 30 cm H_2O)

* Some experts prefer PEEP of 10–15 cm H_2O during the first 48–96 hr of ALI/ARDS if other parameters, like PP, remain within acceptable limits

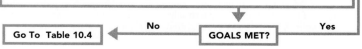

Go To Table 10.4 ← **No** — **GOALS MET?** — **Yes** →

TABLE 10.1	Common Causes of Acute Lung Injury and Acute Respiratory Distress Syndrome	
Direct causes	**Indirect causes**	
Pneumonia	Sepsis	
Aspiration	Severe traumatic shock	
Inhalation injuries	Large-volume blood transfusions (>15 units)	
Blunt pulmonary trauma	Pancreatitis	
Near drowning	Reperfusion after cardiopulmonary bypass	

Overlapping with the late exudative phase is a proliferative phase, which usually lasts another 2 to 3 weeks, and is characterized by increased numbers of type 2 pneumocytes, clearing of alveolar edema and debris, improving gas exchange, and, eventually, liberation from the ventilator.

Finally, some patients may progress after 2 to 3 weeks to a clinically obvious fibrotic phase. These patients develop progressive interstitial and alveolar fibrosis, occasionally with large emphysematous bullae prone to rupture, and prolonged ventilator dependency with increased morbidity and mortality.

ARDS must be distinguished from cardiogenic pulmonary edema and other less common causes of diffuse pulmonary infiltrates because these different diagnoses could lead to differences in treatment. If the underlying cause of the acute pulmonary infiltrates is not certain, then x-ray computed tomography, bronchoalveolar lavage, or other diagnostic tests should be performed to exclude such entities as diffuse alveolar hemorrhage, acute interstitial pneumonia, disseminated cancer, acute eosinophilic pneumonia, miliary tuberculosis, and cryptogenic organizing pneumonia (Table 10.2). Although radiographically and physiologically similar, diffuse alveolar damage is not a prominent pathologic feature of these disease entities.

The evidence base for a particular strategy of mechanical ventilatory support for ALI/ARDS was greatly strengthened in 2000 by the landmark ARMA clinical trial, conducted by the National Institutes of Health ARDS Network. This trial demonstrated a 22% relative reduction in mortality when tidal volumes of 6 mL/kg of predicted body weight were used rather than more traditional volumes of 12 mL/kg. The lower tidal volumes are thought to prevent microscopic barotrauma to relatively normal alveoli, which can worsen the extent and/or severity of inflammatory pulmonary edema, an outcome sometimes described as *ventilator-induced lung injury*.

The other major, and still controversial, aspect of mechanical ventilatory support concerns the use of positive end-expiratory pressure (PEEP). PEEP increases the amount of aerated lung, thereby improving oxygenation by decreasing the shunt fraction, allowing a lower fraction of inspired oxygen to be used. However, it can also be associated with barotrauma and depressed cardiovascular function. Because of these potentially conflicting effects, another major clinical trial (ALVEOLI) was conducted by the ARDS Network to determine the relative benefit of high versus low PEEP. The results of this study showed no difference in outcomes between higher PEEP (mean, 13.2 cm H_2O) and lower PEEP (mean, 8.3 cm H_2O) levels. Thus, some recommend that the lowest level of PEEP be used

TABLE 10.2	Conditions Mimicking Acute Lung Injury/Acute Respiratory Distress Syndrome	
Cardiogenic pulmonary edema	Acute eosinophilic pneumonia	
Diffuse alveolar hemorrhage	Miliary tuberculosis	
Acute interstitial pneumonia- (Hamman-Rich syndrome)	Cryptogenic organizing pneumonia Disseminated cancer	

TABLE 10.3	Suggested combinations of Fio_2 and PEEP in ARDS		
Fio_2	0.3	0.4	0.5	0.6
PEEP	5	5–8	8–10	10
Fio_2	0.7	0.8	0.9	1.0
PEEP	10–14	14	14–18	18–23

PEEP, positive end-expiratory pressure.

to support oxygenation and to maintain an Fio_2 at or below 0.7. However, the algorithm for administering PEEP changed during the trial, and a favorable trend toward improved survival was possibly missed because of inadequate statistical power. Therefore, some experts still favor higher (10 to 15 cm H_2O) rather than lower (5 to 10 cm H_2O) PEEP during the early phase of ALI/ARDS (Table 10.3).

Other ventilation strategies can be used as "rescue" therapies when oxygenation is inadequate despite the previously mentioned approach to ventilatory support, or when patients require unacceptable levels of Fio_2 or airway pressure. These include prone ventilation, inverse ratio ventilation, high-frequency ventilation, extracorporeal membrane oxygenation, or inhalational prostacyclin or nitric oxide (Table 10.4).

With the exception of glucocorticoids, no pharmacologic therapy has yet been shown to decrease the mortality of ALI/ARDS independent of treating the underlying cause. The benefit or harm of using glucocorticoids, however, appears to depend on dose, duration, and timing. In a prospective, randomized, double-blind, placebo-controlled clinical trial by Bone et al. in 1987 of very high-dose methylprednisolone (30 mg/kg every 6 hours for four doses) in 308 patients with sepsis, 88 developed ARDS. Of the patients who developed ARDS, significantly fewer reversed their ARDS within 14 days of onset in the treatment group than in the placebo group (31% vs. 61%, respectively); mortality was also significantly higher in the methylprednisolone-treated group than in the placebo group (52% vs. 22%, respectively). Another prospective, randomized, double-blind, placebo-controlled clinical trial by Bernard et al. in 1987, using the same methylprednisolone dose in 99 patients with early ARDS, showed no difference in mortality or in the reversal of ARDS between the two groups after 45 days.

In contrast, a more recent prospective, randomized, double-blind, placebo-controlled clinical trial in 2007 by Meduri et al. of moderate-dose methylprednisolone (1 mg/kg for 2 weeks followed by a taper during 2 weeks) reported significantly reduced duration of mechanical ventilation (5 vs. 9.5 days; $p = 0.002$), length of intensive care unit (ICU) stay (7 vs. 14.5 days; $p = 0.007$), and pulmonary and extrapulmonary organ dysfunction in the methylprednisolone-treated group. There was also significantly reduced ICU mortality with a strong trend ($p = 0.07$) toward reduced hospital mortality. Finally, the corticosteroid treatment group also had a significantly lower rate of infections ($p = 0.0002$).

Two prospective, randomized, double-blind, placebo-controlled clinical trials of corticosteroid administration have also been conducted in patients with unresolving (>7 days) ARDS (one by the Meduri et al. group with 24 patients and conducted at four medical centers, and the other by the multicenter National Institutes of Health-sponsored ARDS Network with 180 patients). Both studies showed significant improvements in ventilator-free days, shock-free days, and ICU-free days. The study by Meduri et al. reported improved ICU ($p = 0.002$) and in-hospital ($p = 0.03$) mortality, but the ARDS Network study did not. Indeed, in the latter study, there was a trend toward increased mortality in patients administered glucocorticoids >2 weeks after the onset of ARDS. Possible confounding factors in the latter study, however, include a greater use of paralytic agents in the treated group and a shortened course of therapy compared with the Meduri et al. protocol.

Overall, we believe data from these various studies support the use of moderate-dose steroids for all ARDS patients of duration <2 weeks (Table 10.4). Steroids should be withheld until it is certain that paralytic agents are not required concomitantly. Because physiologic and radiologic parameters appear to improve substantially within 3 to 5 days after beginning

TABLE 10.4	Rescue Therapies and Steroids in Acute Lung Injury/Acute Respiratory Distress Syndrome[a]

Rescue therapies indicated when Pao$_2$ <55 mm Hg or Sao$_2$ <88% with
- Fio$_2$ ≥0.7 **or**
- PP >30 cm H$_2$O

Inhaled pharmacologic agents[b] (see Common Drug Dosages and Side Effects)
- Inhaled epoprostenol
- Inhaled nitric oxide
- Inhaled iloprost (prostaglandin I$_2$)

Prone ventilation
- Contraindications:
  - ☐ Open wounds/burns on the ventral body surface
  - ☐ Unstable fractures
  - ☐ Spinal instability
  - ☐ Increased intracranial pressure
  - ☐ Hemodynamic instability
- Caution if tracheostomy, chest tubes, obesity, ascites.
- Maintain in prone position for 18–20 hr of every 24

Other adjunctive/salvage ventilator strategies
- Inverse ratio ventilation (inspiratory time > expiratory time)
- High-frequency ventilation
- Extracorporeal membrane oxygenation

Steroids
- 1–7 days but ideally ≤72 hr;
  - ☐ Give methylprednisolone (or equivalent) 1 mg/kg IV bolus, then 1 mg/kg/day continuous IV infusion for 14 days.
  - ☐ If receiving paralytics, delay use until concomitant use of paralytic agents is not required.
  - ☐ If no clear physiologic or radiologic benefit in 3–5 days, discontinue.
  - ☐ After 14 days or successful patient extubation, decrease to 0.5 mg/kg/day IV and continue for 7 days, then decrease to 0.25 mg/kg/day IV and continue for 7 days, then stop.
- 7–14 days, if steroids were not started earlier;
  - ☐ Benefit less certain, but in select cases may try the same protocol as above. If no clear physiologic or radiologic benefit in 3–5 days, discontinue.
- 14 days
  - ☐ Probably no role for steroid use in these cases (may cause increased mortality if used routinely in this time course). However, a trial may still be considered in select cases.

IV, intravenously.
[a]Pao$_2$, arterial oxygen pressure in millimeters of mercury; Sao$_2$, oxygen saturation in percent; Fio$_2$, fraction inspired oxygen; PP, plateau pressure in centimeters of H$_2$O.
[b]These agents should not be given IV as they may worsen shunting by vasodilating capillaries in nonaerated alveoli.

steroid use, it may be reasonable to discontinue steroids after this time in those patients who fail to show any significant response. In those who do respond, however, steroids should be continued for up to 4 weeks (Table 10.4).

Corticosteroids should not be *routinely* started in patients with unresolving ARDS more than 2 weeks after onset. However, they may be considered in selected cases; here again, a 3- to 5-day course should at least establish whether there will be physiologic or radiologic improvement before longer trials are considered.

The injured lung during ALI/ARDS is also highly vulnerable to worsening pulmonary edema by high pulmonary capillary pressures. However, until recently, fluid management during ALI/ARDS often emphasized the need to maintain intravascular volume to optimize hemodynamic performance, even at the risk of worsening pulmonary edema. Even though

ALGORITHM 10.2 — Fluid Management in Acute Lung Injury/Acute Respiratory Distress Syndrome

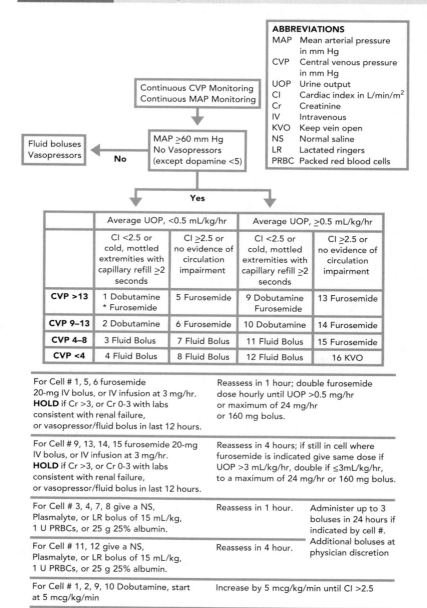

ABBREVIATIONS

MAP	Mean arterial pressure in mm Hg
CVP	Central venous pressure in mm Hg
UOP	Urine output
CI	Cardiac index in L/min/m²
Cr	Creatinine
IV	Intravenous
KVO	Keep vein open
NS	Normal saline
LR	Lactated ringers
PRBC	Packed red blood cells

Continuous CVP Monitoring
Continuous MAP Monitoring

MAP ≥60 mm Hg
No Vasopressors
(except dopamine <5)

No → Fluid boluses / Vasopressors

Yes

	Average UOP, <0.5 mL/kg/hr		Average UOP, ≥0.5 mL/kg/hr	
	CI <2.5 or cold, mottled extremities with capillary refill ≥2 seconds	CI ≥2.5 or no evidence of circulation impairment	CI <2.5 or cold, mottled extremities with capillary refill ≥2 seconds	CI ≥2.5 or no evidence of circulation impairment
CVP >13	1 Dobutamine * Furosemide	5 Furosemide	9 Dobutamine Furosemide	13 Furosemide
CVP 9–13	2 Dobutamine	6 Furosemide	10 Dobutamine	14 Furosemide
CVP 4–8	3 Fluid Bolus	7 Fluid Bolus	11 Fluid Bolus	15 Furosemide
CVP <4	4 Fluid Bolus	8 Fluid Bolus	12 Fluid Bolus	16 KVO

For Cell # 1, 5, 6 furosemide 20-mg IV bolus, or IV infusion at 3 mg/hr. **HOLD** if Cr >3, or Cr 0-3 with labs consistent with renal failure, or vasopressor/fluid bolus in last 12 hours.
Reassess in 1 hour; double furosemide dose hourly until UOP >0.5 mg/hr or maximum of 24 mg/hr or 160 mg bolus.

For Cell # 9, 13, 14, 15 furosemide 20-mg IV bolus, or IV infusion at 3 mg/hr. **HOLD** if Cr >3, or Cr 0-3 with labs consistent with renal failure, or vasopressor/fluid bolus in last 12 hours.
Reassess in 4 hours; if still in cell where furosemide is indicated give same dose if UOP >3 mL/kg/hr, double if ≤3mL/kg/hr, to a maximum of 24 mg/hr or 160 mg bolus.

For Cell # 3, 4, 7, 8 give a NS, Plasmalyte, or LR bolus of 15 mL/kg, 1 U PRBCs, or 25 g 25% albumin.
Reassess in 1 hour.
Administer up to 3 boluses in 24 hours if indicated by cell #. Additional boluses at physician discretion

For Cell # 11, 12 give a NS, Plasmalyte, or LR bolus of 15 mL/kg, 1 U PRBCs, or 25 g 25% albumin.
Reassess in 4 hour.

For Cell # 1, 2, 9, 10 Dobutamine, start at 5 mcg/kg/min
Increase by 5 mcg/kg/min until CI >2.5

* If furosemide not available can use bumetanide with a dose equivalency of 40:1 (lasix 40 mg = bumetanide 1 mg).

From the 2006 FACTT trial, this complex algorithm may not be appropriate for all patients and in all clinical settings, and should be used with physician discretion and judgment.

hemodynamic stability and organ perfusion need to be maintained, another trial by the ARDS Network from 2006 (FACTT) showed that minimizing pulmonary capillary pressures without compromising systemic organ perfusion could be accomplished, with a decreased duration of mechanical ventilation and ICU stay as the result (Algorithm 10.2). However, no mortality benefit was shown.

The FACTT study also showed no improvement in survival or organ function if hemodynamic management was guided with pulmonary artery catheters (PACs) instead of with simple central venous pressure monitoring in patients with established ALI/ARDS, and PACs were associated with increased complications. Thus, the routine use of PACs for hemodynamic management of ALI/ARDS can no longer be recommended.

Numerous studies have examined the long-term outcome of patients who survive ALI/ARDS. In one study, the average stay in the ICU from ALI/ARDS was 25 days. At discharge, patients had lost 18% of their body weight, and had significant functional limitations. At 1 year, patients had persistent functional limitations due to muscle wasting and weakness. Lung volume and spirometric measurements in survivors were normal or near normal by 6 months to 1 year (defined as >80% of predicted amounts), and most patients did not require supplemental oxygen.

In summary, ALI/ARDS is a severe life-threatening form of pulmonary edema with characteristic clinical, radiologic, and physiologic consequences. Beyond treating the inciting event, current ALI/ARDS management centers on volume and pressure-limited lung protective ventilation, conservative fluid management, and the early use of moderate-dose corticosteroids. Rescue therapies are reserved for those patients who remain hypoxic despite steroids and optimal ventilator and fluid management. At 1 year, survivors often must endure some degree of functional disability from muscle weakness and wasting, but lung function measurements can be expected to approach normal values.

Suggested Reading

Bernard GR, Artigas A, Bringham KL, et al. The American-European Consensus Conference on ARDS: definitions, mechanism, relevant outcomes and clinical trial coordination. *Am J Respir Crit Care Med.* 1994;149:818–824.
The American-European Consensus Conference on ARDS was established in 1992 between the American Thoracic Society and the European Society of Intensive Care Medicine. The goals of the Committee were to form a uniform definition of ALI and ARDS, better define the mechanism of acute lung injury, identify risk factors, prevalence, and outcomes, and to promote clinical study coordination. The Committee's results are published in this landmark paper.

Bernard GR, Luce JM, Sprung CL, et al. High-dose corticosteroids in patients with the adult respiratory distress syndrome. *N Engl J Med.* 1987;317:1565–1570.
A prospective, randomized, double-blind, placebo-controlled trial of methylprednisolone therapy (30 mg per kilogram body weight every six hours for 24 hours) in 99 patients with ARDS. There were no differences in mortality or infectious complications between the groups.

Bone RC, Fisher CJ Jr. Clemmer TP, et al. Early methylprednisolone treatment for septic syndrome and the adult respiratory distress syndrome. *Chest.* 1987;92(6):1032–1036.
A prospective, randomized, double-blind, placebo-controlled study to determine if early treatment with methylprednisolone (MPSS) would decrease the incidence of ARDS in septic patients. Early treatment of septic patients with MPSS did not prevent the development of ARDS. Additionally, MPSS treatment impeded the reversal of ARDS and increased the mortality rate in patients with ARDS.

Herridge MS, Cheung AM, Tansey CM, et al. One-year outcomes in survivors of the acute respiratory distress syndrome. *N Engl J Med.* 2003;348:683–693.
This longitudinal study was conducted at four medical-surgical intensive care units in Toronto, Canada. At the time of discharge, patients had lost 18% of their body weight, with 71% returning to their baseline body weight by one year. Lung volume and spirometric measurements were normal by six months, defined as being within 80% predicted.

Meduri GU, Golden E, Freire AX, et al. Methylprednisolone infusion in early severe ARDS. Results of a randomized controlled trial. *Chest.* 2007;131:954–963.
Randomized, double blinded, placebo controlled trial of moderate dose methylprednisolone in early ARDS conducted in the surgical and medical intensive care units at

5 medical centers in Memphis, TN, randomizing patients 2:1 to methylprednisolone versus placebo (n = 63 vs. 28) and treating patients for up to 28 days, showing a significant reduction in duration of mechanical ventilation, length of ICU stay, and organ dysfunction in the treatment group.

Meduri GU, Headley AS, Golden E, et al. Effect of prolonged methylprednisolone therapy in unresolving acute respiratory distress syndrome. JAMA. 1998;280:159–165.

Randomized, double blinded, placebo controlled clinical trail conducted at 4 medical centers in Memphis, TN of 24 patients with ARDS that did not show improved lung injury scores by day 7 assigned 2:1 to receive methylprednisolone (initially 2mg/kg/day and continued for 32 days) versus placebo. The study showed significant improvement in the primary outcomes of lung injury, MODS scores, and ICU and in-hospital mortality in the methylprednisolone treated patients.

The Acute Respiratory Distress Syndrome Network. Ventilation with lower tidal volumes as compared with traditional tidal volumes for acute lung injury and the acute respiratory distress syndrome. N Engl J Med. 2000;342:1301–1308.

The "ARMA" trial was conducted at 10 university centers in the ARDS Network. The trial enrolled patients with ALI/ARDS and compared ventilation with traditional tidal volumes (mean 11.8±0.8 ml/kg PBW) versus low tidal volumes (mean 6.2±0.8 ml/kg PBW). The trial was stopped after enrolling 861 patients after the lower tidal volume group had significantly lower mortality (31% vs. 39%).

The National Heart, Lung, and Blood Institute ARDS Clinical Trials Network. Higher versus lower positive end-expiratory pressures in patients with the acute respiratory distress syndrome. N Engl J Med. 2004;351:327–336.

The "ALVEOLI" trial was conducted by the ARDS Network at 23 affiliated centers. The trial compared mechanical ventilation with higher PEEP (mean 13.2±3.5cm H2O) versus lower PEEP (mean 8.3±3.2) when tidal volumes of 6ml/kg PBW were used. The trial was stopped after 549 patients were enrolled when no significant difference was found between the two groups for death.

The National Heart, Lung, and Blood Institute Acute Respiratory Distress Syndrome Clinical Trials Network. Efficacy and safety of corticosteroids for persistent acute respiratory distress syndrome. N Engl J Med. 2006;354:1671–1684.

The "LaSRS" trial was a double-blind randomized controlled clinical trial conducted by the ARDS Network at 25 affiliated centers. The study enrolled 180 patients with ALI/ARDS of at least 7–28 days duration and randomly assigned them to receive either methylprednisolone (2mg/kg bolus then 0.5mg/kg every 6 hours for 14 days, 0.5mg/kg every 12 hours for 7 days, then tapered over four days), or placebo. The study found no difference in 60 day mortality between those treated with corticosteroids versus placebo (29.2% vs. 28.6%) but did identify significant physiologic and radiologic improvements favoring corticosteroids. Some have criticized the trial for too rapid withdrawal of steroids and for significant differences in use of paralytics between groups.

The National Heart, Lung, and Blood Institute Acute Respiratory Distress Syndrome (ARDS) Clinical Trials Network. Comparison of two fluid-management strategies in acute lung injury. N Engl J Med. 2006;354:2564–2575.

The "FACTT" trial was a randomized controlled clinical trial conducted by the ARDS Network at 20 affiliated centers. The study enrolled 1000 patients with ALI/ARDS of less than 48 hours duration and randomly assigned them to a conservative vs. liberal fluid management strategy for seven days. Patients were also randomly assigned to treatment guided by PAC vs. CVP monitoring (see the following citation). The study found no difference in 60 day mortality (25.5% vs. 28.4%) but did identify significant differences in ventilator time and ICU stay favoring the conservative fluid management strategy.

The National Heart, Lung, and Blood Institute Acute Respiratory Distress Syndrome (ARDS) Clinical Trials Network. Pulmonary artery versus central venous catheter to guide treatment of acute lung injury. N Engl J Med. 2006;354:2213–2224.

The "FACTT" study also yielded this paper based on outcome among the 1000 patients with ALI/ARDS who were randomly assigned to conservative versus liberal fluid management for seven days. Patients were randomly assigned to treatment guided by pulmonary vs. central venous catheter monitoring. The study found no difference between the PAC and CVP groups in 60-day mortality (27.4% vs. 26.3%).

STATUS ASTHMATICUS

Ravi Aysola and Mario Castro

11

Asthma is a common disorder affecting approximately 30 million Americans. It is a chronic inflammatory disease of the airways characterized by airway hyperreactivity and inflammation, bronchoconstriction, and mucus hypersecretion. In 2002, asthma exacerbations resulted in nearly 2 million emergency department visits, 484,000 hospitalizations, and 4,200 deaths in the United States. In school-aged children, asthma accounts for nearly 15 million missed-school days per year. In adults, nearly 12 million days of work are missed because of asthma. The economic impact of asthma is estimated to be $13 billion annually.

Approximately 10% of patients hospitalized with asthma are admitted to the intensive care unit, and 2% are intubated. Mortality rates range from 0.5% to 3% in hospitalized patients. Morbidity and mortality from asthma disproportionately affect the economically disadvantaged, women, and minorities, especially African Americans and Hispanics from Puerto Rico. A recent study, the Nationwide Inpatient Sample from >80,000 U.S. hospital admissions for asthma, reported a hospital mortality rate of 0.5%. The majority of asthma-related deaths occurred in patients older than 35 years. The study found no significant differences in hospitalized mortality rates in regard to race, suggesting that the disproportionate affect on minorities may be the result of prehospital factors such as access to health care, inadequate preventive therapy, or delay in seeking medical treatment. Risk factors for death from asthma are listed in Table 11.1.

Clinically, patients present with dyspnea, cough, chest tightness, and wheezing. In severe asthma episodes, airway obstruction, respiratory muscle fatigue, and altered V/Q relationships can lead to hypercapnia and hypoxemic respiratory failure. This chapter will focus on the initial hospital and intensive care unit management, as well as ventilatory strategies for patients with status asthmaticus.

Status asthmaticus is defined as a prolonged severe episode of asthma that is unresponsive to initial standard therapy that may lead to respiratory failure. The episodes may be rapid onset (in a matter of hours) or, more typically, progress during several hours to days. The former is often referred to as *asphyxic* asthma and occurs in a minority of cases. Rapid-onset status asthmaticus is more common in men, and is oftentimes triggered by exposure to allergens, irritants, exercise, psychosocial stress, and inhaled illicit drugs. It may also develop after exposure to aspirin, nonsteroidal anti-inflammatory drugs, or β-blockers in susceptible individuals. This form of status asthmaticus represents a more "bronchospastic" pathophysiology, and is associated with rapid resolution with treatment. More commonly, asthma episodes develop during several hours to days, and may be triggered by viral or atypical infection. Airway obstruction in these cases is due to airway inflammation, bronchoconstriction, and mucus plugging.

In both forms, the pathologic processes result in airway obstruction and expiratory airflow limitation. Insufficient expiratory time results in air trapping, dynamic hyperinflation (DHI), and persistent positive end-expiratory alveolar pressure, also referred to as *intrinsic positive end-expiratory pressure* (iPEEP). This alters lung mechanics by increasing work of breathing while simultaneously placing the diaphragm at a mechanical disadvantage. The increased work load placed on the respiratory muscles results in increased O_2 consumption and CO_2 production, setting up a vicious cycle.

DHI adversely affects cardiovascular function because of the dramatic fluctuations in intrathoracic pressure during inspiration and expiration (evident on physical examination as pulsus paradoxus). During inspiration, there can be exaggerated right ventricular filling and paradoxic interventricular septal motion, resulting in impaired left ventricular filling.

TABLE 11.1	Risk Factors for Death from Asthma

Lower socioeconomic status
Female gender
African American or Puerto Rican race
Smoking
"Labile asthma," high degree of variability in peak expiratory flow
Blood eosinophilia
Poor perception of dyspnea: alexithymia, a psychological trait characterized by difficulty in perceiving and expressing emotions and body sensations.
History of sudden severe exacerbations (asphyxic asthma)
History of intubation for asthma
History of ICU admission for asthma
Two or more hospitalizations for asthma within the past year
Three or more ED visits for asthma in the past year
Hospitalization or ED visit for asthma within past month
Use of more than two canisters per month of inhaled short-acting β_2-agonists
Current use or recent withdrawal of oral corticosteroids
Poor perception of airflow obstruction
Comorbid cardiovascular disease
Sensitivity to Alternaria

ICU, intensive care unit; ED, emergency department.

During expiration, the increased intrathoracic pressure impairs ventricular diastolic filling, resulting in decreased cardiac output and compromised diaphragmatic blood flow, exacerbating metabolic acidosis and respiratory muscle fatigue. This downward spiral from the multiple pathophysiologic processes results in hypoxemic and hypercapnic respiratory failure (Algorithm 11.1).

Rapid evaluation of the patient presenting with status asthmaticus is essential, focusing on key points of the history such as duration of symptoms, potential inciting exposures, medication use, and previous history of severe attacks. Patients should be questioned regarding the presence of symptoms suggestive of comorbid, complicating, or similarly presenting conditions (Table 11.2). Key historical and physical examination findings are listed in Table 11.3.

TREATMENTS

Standard Treatment for All Patients

Oxygen
Supplemental oxygen to maintain SaO_2 >92%.

Inhaled Bronchodilators

- β_2-agonists administered via metered dose inhalers (MDIs) with a spacer are as effective as nebulized bronchodilators. Albuterol (2.5 to 5 mg) nebulization every 20 minutes (or four to eight puffs of MDI with spacer) within first hour. Alternatively, albuterol may be given as a continuous nebulization at a dose of 10 to 15 mg during 1 hour with telemetry monitoring.
- Levalbuterol (1.25 mg) every 20 minutes within the first hour, then every 40 minutes times three doses.
- Initial treatment should include ipratropium 0.5 mg nebulized every 20 minutes, given concomitantly with albuterol (shown to improve airflow limitation in acute asthma exacerbations in first 36 hours).

ALGORITHM 11.1   Status Asthmaticus Pathophysiology

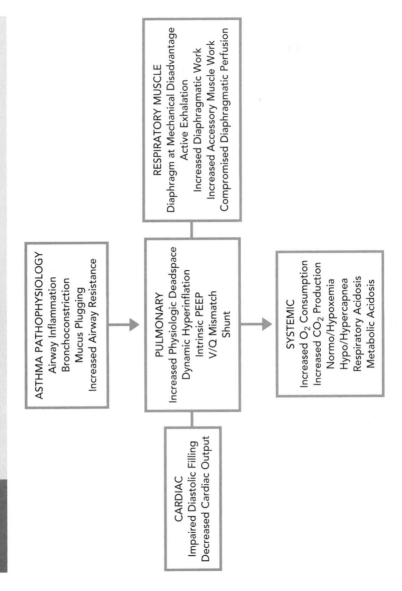

ASTHMA PATHOPHYSIOLOGY
Airway Inflammation
Bronchoconstriction
Mucus Plugging
Increased Airway Resistance

RESPIRATORY MUSCLE
Diaphragm at Mechanical Disadvantage
Active Exhalation
Increased Diaphragmatic Work
Increased Accessory Muscle Work
Compromised Diaphragmatic Perfusion

PULMONARY
Increased Physiologic Deadspace
Dynamic Hyperinflation
Intrinsic PEEP
V/Q Mismatch
Shunt

CARDIAC
Impaired Diastolic Filling
Decreased Cardiac Output

SYSTEMIC
Increased O_2 Consumption
Increased CO_2 Production
Normo/Hypoxemia
Hypo/Hypercapnea
Respiratory Acidosis
Metabolic Acidosis

TABLE 11.2	Differential Diagnoses to Consider

Upper airway obstruction
Tumor
Epiglottitis
Vocal cord dysfunction
Foreign body aspiration
Endobronchial lesion
Congestive heart failure
Gastroesophageal reflux
Obstructive sleep apnea
Tracheomalacia
Herpetic tracheobronchitis
Mitral stenosis
Adverse drug reaction
    Aspirin sensitivity
    Angiotensin converting enzyme inhibitor
    β_2-adrenergic antagonist
    Inhaled pentamidine

TABLE 11.3	Typical Physical Examination and Laboratory Findings in Asthma by Severity

Finding	Mild	Moderate	Severe	Respiratory arrest imminent
Breathless	Walking Can lie down	Talking Prefers sitting	At rest Hunched forward	
Speaks in	Sentences	Phrases	Words	
Alertness	May be agitated	Usually agitated	Usually agitated	Drowsy or confused
Respiratory rate	Increased	Increased	>30 breaths/min	
Accessory muscle use and retractions	Usually not	Usually	Usually	
Wheeze	Moderate, often end-expiratory	Loud	Usually loud	Absent
Pulse (beats/min)	<100	100–120	>120	Bradycardia (<60)
Pulsus paradoxus	Absent (<10 mm Hg)	May be present (10–25 mm Hg)	Often present (>25 mm Hg)	Absence suggests respiratory muscle fatigue
PEF	>80%	60%–80%	<60%	
Pao_2	Normal	>60 mm Hg	<60 mm Hg	
$Paco_2$	<45 mm Hg	<45 mm Hg	>45 mm Hg	
Sao_2	>95%	91%–95%	<90%	

PEF, peak expiratory flow.

- In the case of intubated patients, bronchodilators should be given via MDI (e.g., albuterol along the inspiratory circuit or between a Y-piece and the endotracheal tube).
- Long-acting β_2-agonists, salmeterol and formoterol, are not indicated for treatment of acute asthma. Long-acting β_2-agonists may be continued as add-on therapy in the hospitalized patient and in the outpatient setting.
- The administration of intravenous β_2-agonists is no more effective and potentially more toxic than delivery via aerosol and is therefore not recommended.

Corticosteroids

- Initial dose of methylprednisolone, 125 mg intravenously once, or equivalent oral dose if the patient is able to tolerate oral administration.
- Subsequently, methylprednisolone, 40 to 60 mg intravenously every 6 hours or equivalent dose given orally if there is no suspected impairment in gastrointestinal absorption.
- Consider tapering dose after 36 to 48 hours, depending on clinical response.

Additional Therapeutic Considerations
Antibiotics

- Not recommended routinely for uncomplicated asthma exacerbation.
- Justified if patients have fever, purulent sputum, or if there is evidence of pneumonia or bacterial sinusitis complicating the asthma exacerbation.

Magnesium

- IV magnesium (2 g infused during 20 minutes) is relatively safe but does not appear to be more effective than standard therapy.
- Less data available regarding use of inhaled magnesium but may be added to inhaled bronchodilators.

Methylxanthines

- Not recommended for initial treatment in acute asthma.
- Equivalent bronchodilator properties as β_2-agonists but with increased potential of toxicity (tachyarrhythmia).

Epinephrine

- No proven advantage over inhaled bronchodilator therapy, but with added potential for toxicity, especially in hypoxemic patients.
- Consider in patients who do not respond or are unable to cooperate with intensive inhaled bronchodilator treatment.
- Dosing: 0.5 mg of a 1:1000 dilution given subcutaneously every 20 minutes times three if needed.

Heliox

- The use of helium-oxygen (HeO_2) mixtures in severe obstructive airway disease is based on the decreased density of heliox compared with air, resulting in more laminar rather than turbulent airflow.
- Use either 60%:40% or 70%:30% heliox (helium: O_2) mixtures.
- Limited data suggest improved delivery of aerosolized bronchodilators when given with heliox rather than oxygen.
- The use of heliox in the mechanically ventilated patient should only be considered in those institutions that have significant experience and familiarity with its use because of potential technical complications regarding volume and pressure monitoring with standard ventilators.

Ventilator Strategies

The goal of management in status asthmaticus is to unload the respiratory muscles, correct hypoxemia, provide adequate ventilation, and minimize lung injury, particularly from DHI, while treating the underlying airway inflammation and bronchoconstriction.

Noninvasive Ventilation

- Data regarding the use of noninvasive positive pressure ventilation (NIPPV) in severe asthma are limited.
- NIPPV with either continuous positive airway pressure or bilevel positive airway pressure may be considered as initial treatment of patients presenting to the emergency department with status asthmaticus who are alert, cooperative, and able to protect their airways while tolerating a full face mask.
- Initial bilevel positive airway pressure settings, IPAP (inspiratory positive airway pressure) of 8 and EPAP (expiratory positive airway pressure) of 5, and adjusted promptly to achieve patient comfort and compliance and decrease work of breathing (decreased respiratory rate, increased tidal volume) without exceeding IPAP of 15 and EPAP of 5.
- Aerophagia with subsequent vomiting and aspiration are potential complications of NIPPV, and patients should be closely monitored and kept in nothing by mouth status.
- Clinical improvement after initiation of NIPPV (decreased respiratory rate, improved air movement, decreased $PaCO_2$) should be documented shortly after initiation of NIPPV and pharmacologic treatment (within 30 minutes).
- Lack of improvement should prompt the clinician to the need for intubation and mechanical ventilation. Once deemed necessary, intubation should not be delayed.
- NIPPV is contraindicated in patients with decreased mental status and hemodynamic instability.

Ventilator strategies should concentrate on allowing adequate expiratory time to avoid DHI and barotrauma. Mechanical ventilation with volume-controlled ventilation is preferable. Suggested initial settings are listed in Table 11.4. A lung protective and permissive hypercapnia strategy should be employed, targeting a plateau pressure <30 cm H_2O. iPEEP should be monitored by performing an end-expiratory hold maneuver. The iPEEP is equal to total PEEP minus set PEEP (set on ventilator) (Fig. 11.1). The goal should be to maintain iPEEP <20 cm H_2O.

ADDITIONAL CONSIDERATIONS

Postintubation hypotension is common in status asthmaticus because of multiple factors, including the application of positive pressure throughout the respiratory cycle in patients with pre-existing DHI and iPEEP, hypovolemia, and sedation. It should be managed with

TABLE 11.4	Initial Ventilator Settings in Status Asthmaticus
Parameter	**Setting**
Mode	Volume controlled
Minute ventilation	<10 L
Tidal volume	7–8 mL/kg
Respiratory rate	12–14 breaths/min
Inspiratory flow rate	60–80 LPM
PEEP	0–5 cmH$_2$O
Fio$_2$	Titrate to keep Spo$_2$ >90%

LPM, liters per minute, PEEP, positive end-expiratory pressure.

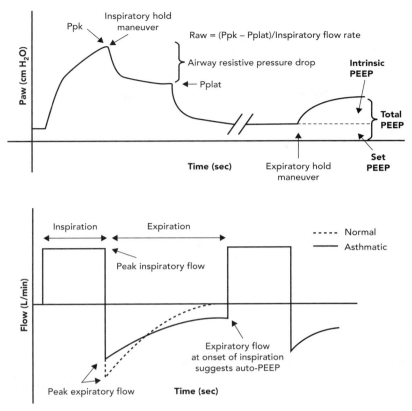

Figure 11.1. Intrinsic positive end-expiratory pressure (PEEP). Ppk, peak pressure; Pplat, plateau pressure.

sedatives and liberal IVF (intravenous fluids) as well as the aforementioned ventilatory strategies to minimize DHI. If needed, with close monitoring of SpO_2, the patient can be disconnected from the ventilator circuit to allow adequate exhalation of trapped gas and decrease intrathoracic pressure.

Neuromuscular blockade should be considered in patients with status asthmaticus on mechanical ventilation who demonstrate considerable patient-ventilator dyssynchrony with unacceptably high plateau pressures and iPEEP despite adequate sedation and analgesia. Neuromuscular blocking agents should be given as intermittent boluses with neuromuscular (train of four) monitoring. Administration of neuromuscular blocking agents as continuous infusions should be avoided because of the increased risk of myopathy associated with concurrent corticosteroid use.

Suggested Reading

Barr RG, Woodruff PG, Clark S, et al. Sudden-onset asthma exacerbations: clinical features, response to therapy, and a 2-week follow-up. Multicenter Airway Research Collaboration (MARC) investigators. *Eur Respir J*. 2000;15:266–273.

Brandstetter RD, Gotz VP, Mar DD. Optimal dosing of epinephrine in acute asthma. *Am J Hosp Pharm*. 1980;37:1326–1329.

British Guideline on the Management of Asthma. British Thoracic Society & Scottish Intercollegiate Guidelines Network. April 2004. Thorax 2003;58: Supplement I.

Calverley PMA, Koulouris NG. Flow limitation and dynamic hyperinflation: key concepts in modern respiratory physiology. *Eur Respir J.* 2005;25:186–199.

Castro M. Near-fatal asthma what have we learned? *Chest.* 2002;121:1394–1395.

Cates CJ, Crilly JA, Rowe BH. Holding chambers (spacers) versus nebulisers for beta-agonist treatment of acute asthma. *Cochrane Database Syst Rev.* 2006.

Dolan CM, Fraher KE, Bleecker ER, et al. Design and baseline characteristics of The Epidemiology and Natural History of Asthma: Outcomes and Treatment Regimens (TENOR) study: a large cohort of patients with severe or difficult-to-treat asthma. *Ann Allergy Asthma Immunol.* 2004;92:32–39.

Global Strategy for Asthma Management and Prevention. Global Initiative for Asthma (GINA). 2006. www. ginasthma.com. Accessed 7/12/2007.

Guidelines for the Diagnosis and Management of Asthma—expert panel report 2. National Asthma Education and Prevention Program, National Institutes of Health, National Heart, Lung and Blood Institute. www.nhlbi.nih.gov/guidelines/asthma/index.htm. Accessed 7/12/2007.

Gupta D, Keogh B, Chung KF, et al. Characteristics and outcome for admissions to adult, general critical care units with acute severe asthma: a secondary analysis of the ICNARC case mix programme database. *Crit Care.* 2004;9:112–121.

Krishnan V, Diette GB, Rand CS, et al. Mortality in patients hospitalized for asthma exacerbations in the United States. *Am J Respir Crit Care Med.* 2006;174:633–638.

Levy BD, Kitch B, Fanta CH. Medical and ventilatory management of status asthmaticus. *Intensive Care Med.* 1998;24:105–117.

MacIntyre NR. Current issues in mechanical ventilation for respiratory failure. *Chest.* 2005;128:561–567.

McFadden ER. Acute severe asthma. *Am J Respir Crit Care Med.* 2003;168:740–759.

Oddo M, Feihl F, Schaller MO, et al. Management of mechanical ventilation in acute severe asthma: practical aspects. *Intensive Care Med.* 2006;32:501–510.

Pendergraft TB, Stanford RH, Beasley R, et al. Rates and characteristics of intensive care unit admissions and intubations among asthma-related hospitalizations. *Ann Allergy Asthma Immunol.* 2004;93:29–35.

Ram FSF, Wellington SR, Rowe B, Wedzicha JA. Non-invasive positive pressure ventilation for treatment of respiratory failure due to severe acute exacerbations of asthma (review). *Cochrane Database Syst Rev.* 2005.

Rodrigo GJ, Castro-Rodriguez JA. Anticholinergics in the treatment of children and adults with acute asthma: a systematic review with meta-analysis. *Thorax.* 2005;60:740–746.

Rodrigo GJ, Rodrigo C, Pollack CV, et al. Use of helium-oxygen mixtures in the treatment of acute asthma: a systematic review. *Chest.* 2003;123:891–896.

Rodrigo GJ, Rodrigo C. First-line therapy for adult patients with acute severe asthma receiving a multiple-dose protocol of ipratropium bromide plus albuterol in the emergency department. *Am J Resp Crit Care Med.* 200l;161:1862–1868.

Rodrigo GJ, Rodrigo C. Rapid-onset asthma attack: a prospective cohort study about characteristics and response to emergency department treatments. *Chest.* 2000;118: 1547–1552.

Rodrigo GJ, Rodrigo C. The role of anticholinergics in acute asthma treatment: an evidence-based evaluation. *Chest.* 2002;121:1977–1987.

Serrano J, Plaza V, Sureda B, et al. Alexithymia: a relevant psychological variable in near-fatal asthma. *Eur Respir J.* 2006;28:296–302.

Soroksky A, Stav D, Shpirer I, et al. A pilot prospective, randomized, placebo-controlled trial of bilevel positive airway pressure in acute asthmatic attack. *Chest.* 2003:123; 1018–1025.

Turner MO, Noertjojo K, Vedal S, et al. Risk factors for near-fatal asthma. *Am J Respir Crit Care Med.* 1998;157:1804–1809.

Weiss KB, Sullivan SD. The health economics of asthma and rhinitis. *J Allergy Clin Immunol.* 2001;107:3–8.

Wenzel, S. Severe asthma in adults. *Am J Respir Crit Care Med.* 2005;172:140–160.

ACUTE EXACERBATIONS OF CHRONIC OBSTRUCTIVE PULMONARY DISEASE

Chad A. Witt and Marin H. Kollef

In the United States, more than 16 million adults have chronic obstructive pulmonary disease (COPD). COPD can manifest as predominantly chronic bronchitis or predominantly emphysema. In 2001, COPD accounted for more than 16 million office visits, 500,000 hospitalizations, and 110,000 deaths, making COPD the fourth leading cause of death in the United States, behind heart disease, cancer, and cerebrovascular disease. The number of patients with COPD is expected to rise with the aging of the population.

There are many definitions for what represents an acute exacerbation of COPD. One of the most widely used definitions evaluates the severity of exacerbation based on three symptoms: (a) worsening dyspnea, (b) an increase in sputum purulence, and (c) an increase in sputum volume. Type 1 exacerbations (severe) have all three symptoms and type 2 exacerbations (moderate) exhibit two of the three symptoms. Type 3 exacerbations (mild) include one of the symptoms and at least one of the following: upper respiratory tract infection within the past 5 days, fever without apparent cause, increased wheezing, increased cough, or a 20% increase in respiratory rate or heart rate over baseline. Acute exacerbations can be triggered by infections or environmental exposures; however, given that many patients have associated clinical conditions, such as congestive heart failure or extrapulmonary infections, defining which symptoms are secondary to acute exacerbations and which symptoms are secondary to other medical conditions is a clinical diagnosis. All patients who present with symptoms consistent with an acute exacerbation of COPD should undergo chest radiography to evaluate for evidence of pneumonia or pulmonary edema and measurement of arterial oxygen content by arterial blood glass analysis (Algorithm 12.1). Routine spirometric evaluation has not been shown to be beneficial in the setting of acute exacerbations of COPD, and therefore is not recommended. Further evaluation should be dictated by the clinical scenario.

The medical management of acute exacerbations of COPD has been studied extensively. The treatment includes bronchodilator therapy, oxygen therapy, systemic corticosteroids, and antibiotics (Table 12.1). Although the exact duration of treatment with systemic corticosteroids and antibiotics has not been defined, the benefit of the use of these agents has been shown repeatedly.

Studies on bronchodilator therapy have shown that inhaled bronchodilators are superior to systemic bronchodilators, and that there is no advantage of nebulized treatment over metered-dose inhaler treatment. Bronchodilator therapy includes treatment with short acting β_2-adrenergic receptor agonists and short-acting anticholinergic agents. Overall, the side effect profile of anticholinergic agents is favorable compared with β_2-adrenergic receptor agonists; thus, anticholinergic agents should be the first option. Additionally, if the patient is not improving with maximum doses of anticholinergic treatment, the addition of a short-acting β_2-agonist has been shown to be beneficial.

Oxygen therapy has not been as rigorously studied because the benefit has been inferred. Oxygen should be administered by nasal canula or face mask to improve PaO_2 to >60 mm Hg or SaO_2 to 90% to 92%, with care not to increase oxygen tension to a high enough level to precipitate hypercapnia.

Corticosteroid treatment has been studied extensively, and the benefit of treating patients with acute exacerbations of COPD with systemic corticosteroids is clear. In the largest study comparing a 2-week course of corticosteroids to an 8-week course, there was no benefit to treating patients for 8 weeks compared with 2 weeks. Most patients will respond to treatment with corticosteroids for 5 to 10 days.

ALGORITHM 12.1	Initial Evaluation and Medical Management of Acute Exacerbations of Chronic Obstructive Pulmonary Disease (COPD)

Initial Evaluation:
- Initial clinical evaluation, including history and physical examination
- Basic laboratory studies, including complete blood cell count and basic metabolic panel
- Chest radiography
- Arterial blood gas analysis

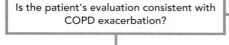

Is the patient's evaluation consistent with COPD exacerbation? — **No** → Treat underlying medical condition

Yes

Treat acute exacerbation of COPD:
- Oxygen therapy by nasal cannula or face mask. Titrate PaO_2 to >60 mm Hg or SaO_2 >90%, with care not to over correct hypoxemia and decrease respiratory drive.
- Bronchodilator therapy (Table 12.1)
- Corticosteroid therapy (Table 12.1)
- Antibiotic therapy (Table 12.1)
- Proceed with mechanical ventilatory support if needed (Algorithm 12.2).

TABLE 12.1	Medications Commonly Used for Acute Exacerbations of Chronic Obstructive Pulmonary Disease	

Medication	Dose and route	Frequency
Bronchodilators		
Anticholinergic agent		
Ipratropium bromide	0.5 mg nebulized or 18–36 mcg metered-dose inhaler	Every 4–6 hr
β_2-adrenergic receptor agonists		
Albuterol	2.5–5 mg nebulized 180 mcg metered-dose inhaler	Every 4–6 hours
Corticosteroids		
Methylprednisolone	125 mg intravenously	Every 6 hr for 3 days then
	60 mg by mouth	Every day for 4 days then
	40 mg by mouth	Every day for 4 days then
	20 mg by mouth	Every day for 4 days
Prednisone	30–60 mg by mouth	For example: every day for 5–7 days or longer course with taper
Antibiotics		
Trimethoprim-sulfamethoxazole	160 mg/800 mg by mouth	Every 12 hr for 5–10 days
Amoxicillin	250 mg by mouth	Every 6 hr for 5–10 days
Doxycycline	200 mg by mouth	First day followed by
	100 mg by mouth	Every 12 hr for 5–10 days
Azithromycin	500 mg by mouth	First day followed by
	250 mg by mouth	Every day for 4 days or
	500 mg by mouth	Every day for 3 days

Treatment of acute exacerbations of COPD with antibiotics has been shown to be beneficial, especially in patients with moderate-to-severe exacerbations. The most commonly identified organisms from sputum in patients with acute exacerbations of COPD include *Streptococcus pneumoniae, Moraxella catarrhalis,* and *Haemophilus influenzae.* In patients with more severe disease, other Gram-negative bacteria, such as *Pseudomonas aeruginosa,* are identified with increasing frequency. Many antibiotics have been studied, including, but not limited to, amoxicillin, trimethoprim-sulfamethoxazole, tetracycline, clarithromycin, azithromycin, levofloxacin, and moxifloxacin. There have been no studies that demonstrate the superiority of the newer, broader spectrum antibiotics over the older, narrower spectrum antibiotics. However because of concern of antibiotic resistance, broader spectrum agents are frequently used now, such as clarithromycin, azithromycin, levofloxacin, and moxifloxacin. Given the lack of evidence to dictate exact duration of treatment, patients are most commonly treated with antibiotics for 5 to 10 days.

There are other medical therapies that have been used to treat acute exacerbations of COPD, including mucolytic medications, chest physiotherapy, and methylxanthine bronchodilators. There is no evidence to support the use of these therapies, and, in fact, the latter two may be detrimental. No study has ever shown benefit of chest physiotherapy for acute exacerbations of COPD, and there are studies that have shown a transient decrease in forced expiratory volume in 1 second after treatment, thus raising the possibility that chest physiotherapy is harmful. Given the frequent and significant side effect profile of methylxanthines, and the lack of evidence demonstrating improved outcomes with these agents, the routine use of methylxanthines for acute exacerbations of COPD is not recommended.

In addition to the therapies already discussed, mechanical ventilatory support is an important treatment modality in patients with severe acute exacerbations of COPD (Algorithm 12.2). In patients with increasing respiratory distress, demonstrated by clinical

ALGORITHM 12.2   **Mechanical Ventilation in Acute Exacerbations of Chronic Obstructive Pulmonary Disease**

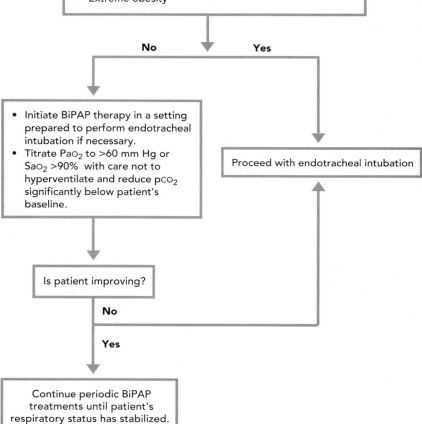

Are there reasons why patient cannot tolerate noninvasive ventilation?
- Acute respiratory failure
- Agitation or decreased mental status
- Hemodynamic instability
- Excessive secretions
- Structural abnormality precluding mask fitting
- Extreme obesity

No — **Yes**

- Initiate BiPAP therapy in a setting prepared to perform endotracheal intubation if necessary.
- Titrate PaO_2 to >60 mm Hg or SaO_2 >90% with care not to hyperventilate and reduce pCO_2 significantly below patient's baseline.

Proceed with endotracheal intubation

Is patient improving?

No

Yes

Continue periodic BiPAP treatments until patient's respiratory status has stabilized.

BiPAP, bilevel positive airway pressure.

evaluation, worsening hypercapnia and respiratory acidosis, worsening hypoxemia, and worsening dyspnea, mechanical ventilatory support may be temporarily necessary. Multiple studies have shown that noninvasive positive-pressure ventilation is beneficial in patients with acute exacerbations of COPD. This strategy decreases the likelihood of needing endotracheal intubation, as well as possibly improving survival. In patients with altered mental status, acute respiratory failure, hemodynamic compromise, and those with extreme obesity, proceeding directly to endotracheal intubation and mechanical ventilation may be necessary.

Initial ventilator settings in patients with COPD should take into account the patients' need for a long expiratory phase. Appropriate initial ventilator settings would be volume assist control, rate 10 to 12 beats/min; tidal volume, 8mL/kg; positive end-expiratory pressure (PEEP) of 0 to 5 cm H_2O; and an adequate FIO_2 to keep the hemoglobin saturation around 92%. These patients require high flows (peak flow in the 75 to 90 L/min range) to allow for an inspiratory to expiratory ratio of 1:4 if possible. The initial settings should be adjusted by assessing the patient's comfort level and synchrony with the ventilator and by arterial blood gas analysis. The patient should not be ventilated for a "normal" arterial blood gas and hypercapnia close to the patient's baseline level should be allowed.

It is also important to monitor the patient for the development of auto-PEEP while receiving mechanical ventilation. This can be detected by monitoring ventilator waveforms and the capnograph tracing. Auto-PEEP can occur with inadequate flows, excessive tidal volume, and high respiratory rates, and can result in a reduction of venous return and systemic hypotension. Auto-PEEP also makes it more difficult for the patient to trigger the ventilator, and extrinsic PEEP can be added to offset this. Additionally, patients with COPD on mechanical ventilator support should receive adequate deep venous thrombosis and stress ulcer prophylaxis. Nutritional support is vitally important in these patients, but should not contain excessive carbohydrates as this will increase CO_2 production.

Suggested Reading

Bach PB, Brown C, Gelfand SE, et al. Management of acute exacerbations of chronic obstructive pulmonary disease: a summary and appraisal of published evidence. *Ann Intern Med.* 2001;134;600–620.
  Review of studies guiding management of acute exacerbations of COPD including evidence for or against oxygen therapy, bronchodilators, corticosteroids, antibiotics, and non-invasive ventilation.
Brochard L, Mancebo J, Wysocki M, et al. Noninvasive ventilation for acute exacerbations of chronic obstructive pulmonary disease. *N Eng J Med.* 1995;333;817–822.
  Randomized study showing that noninvasive ventilation for acute exacerbations of COPD reduced the need for endotracheal intubation, reduced hospital stay, and reduced in-hospital mortality.
Lightowler JV, Wedzicha JA, Elliot MW, et al. Non-invasive positive pressure ventilation to treat respiratory failure resulting from exacerbations of chronic obstructive pulmonary disease: Cochrane systematic review and meta-analysis. *BMJ.* 2003;326;185–189.
  Systematic review of randomized controlled trials showing that the use of non-invasive positive pressure ventilation should be first line therapy to decrease the need for endotracheal intubation and decrease mortality in patients with acute exacerbations of COPD.
McCrory DC, Brown C, Gelfand SE, et al. Management of acute exacerbations of COPD: a summary and appraisal of published evidence. *Chest.* 2001;119;1190–1209.
  Review of available data on the evaluation, risk stratification, and management of patients with acute exacerbation of COPD.
Niewoehner D, Erbland M, Deupree RH, et al. Effect of systemic glucocorticoids on exacerbations of chronic obstructive pulmonary disease. *N Eng J Med.* 1999;340;1941–1947.
  Randomized controlled trial showing clinical benefit of systemic glucocorticoids for acute exacerbations of COPD, as well as showing that there was no benefit to an 8 week course of corticosteroids over a 2 week course.
Saginer A, Aytemur ZA, Cirit M, et al. Systemic glucocorticoids in severe exacerbations of COPD. *Chest.* 2001;119;726–730.
  Randomized trial showing that patients receiving 10 days of glucocorticoid treatment instead of 3 days had significant improvements in arterial oxygen tension, FEV_1, and dyspnea on exertion.

Snow V, Lascher S, Mottur-Pilson C, et al. Evidence base for management of acute exacerbations of chronic obstructive pulmonary disease. *Ann Intern Med.* 2001;134;595–599.
Review of evidence concerning risk stratification, diagnostic testing, and therapeutic interventions for management of acute exacerbation of COPD.
Stoller J. Acute exacerbations of chronic obstructive pulmonary disease. *N Engl J Med.* 2002;346;988–994.
Review of treatment of acute exacerbations of COPD, including medical management and ventilatory support.

SLEEP-DISORDERED BREATHING IN THE INTENSIVE CARE UNIT

13

Tonya D. Russell

Sleep has a range of effects on respiratory physiology in healthy patients, as outlined in Table 13.1. In patients with underlying comorbidities, such as severe chronic obstructive pulmonary disease or neuromuscular disease, these changes in respiratory physiology can lead to compromise of the cardiopulmonary status. In addition, there are sleep-related breathing disorders that can lead to respiratory failure in which the main pathophysiology occurs during sleep, such as obstructive sleep apnea and sleep-related obesity hypoventilation.

Obstructive sleep apnea occurs when there is upper airway obstruction due to excess soft tissue, resulting in limitation or cessation of airflow during sleep, which can be associated with arousals or oxygen desaturations. Obstructive sleep apnea has been associated with increased risk of excessive daytime somnolence, hypertension, stroke, and heart failure. The prevalence of obstructive sleep apnea-hypopnea syndrome (OSAHS) has been estimated to be 4% of men and 2% of women. The severity of obstructive sleep apnea can be quantified by the number of events per hour (apnea-hypopnea index) or by the severity of sleepiness, as shown in Table 13.2.

Obesity hypoventilation syndrome (OHS) is frequently used to describe hypoventilation during sleep occurring in obese patients, which results in daytime hypercapnia. The prevalence of obesity hypoventilation syndrome is not clear, and the definition of OHS in the literature is variable. However, the American Academy of Sleep Medicine Task Force has made recommendations for diagnostic criteria for sleep hypoventilation syndrome, of which OHS is a part, as shown in Table 13.3. It is apparent that hypercapnia can occur in the setting of severe OSAHS alone, sleep-related hypoventilation without apneic or hypopneic events (OHS), or in combination.

Obstructive sleep apnea and obesity hypoventilation should be considered in patients with hypercapnic respiratory failure who have signs and symptoms as listed in Table 13.4. In patients with hypercapnia related to obstructive sleep apnea alone, continuous positive airway pressure (CPAP), at a pressure that resolves the obstructive events, should correct the hypercapnia. However, in patients in whom there is a component of sleep-related hypoventilation, bilevel positive airway pressure (BiPAP) is usually required.

Unfortunately, there is not much guidance in the literature for empirically picking pressures for CPAP or BiPAP in the setting of OSAHS or OHS. In the outpatient setting, typically a split sleep study is performed, in which the first part of the study allows for the diagnosis of the sleep-disordered breathing, and the second part of the study allows for the titration of CPAP or BiPAP. If an inpatient sleep study is available, this would be the best way to establish a diagnosis of OSAHS or OHS, and the best way to determine the necessary pressures required to treat the disorder. However, if a patient requires initiation of therapy without the benefit of a sleep study, it should be initiated in a closely monitored setting such as an intensive care unit or step-down unit.

Patients who are morbidly obese or have very severe obstructive sleep apnea will frequently require high pressures to resolve the sleep-disordered breathing. If the pressure is underestimated, then the apnea events or hypoventilation may not be fully resolved, leading to prolonged hypoxemia. Severe hypoxemia has been reported to occur during the empiric use of CPAP. If the pressure is overestimated, then the patient may experience other complications related to CPAP, as outlined in Table 13.5, which may decrease the patient's ability to comply with CPAP or BiPAP.

TABLE 13.1	Effects of Sleep on Respiratory Physiology

Decreased hypoxic ventilatory response
Decreased hypercapnic ventilatory response
Increased muscle hypotonia
Increased airway resistance
Increased arousal threshold from events related to increased airway resistance
  (NREM > REM)

NREM, nonrapid eye movement; REM, rapid eye movement.

TABLE 13.2	Severity of Obstructive Sleep Apnea

Severity	AHI[a]	Level of impairment[b]
Mild	5–15	Sedentary activities requiring minimal attention (i.e., watching television, reading, passenger in a car)
Moderate	15–30	Activities requiring some attention (i.e., meetings, concerts)
Severe	>30	Activities requiring active attention (i.e., conversation, eating, driving)

[a]AHI (apnea-hypopnea index), number of apneas and hypopneas per hour; apnea is defined as cessation of airflow; hypopnea is defined as $\geq$30% reduction in airflow associated with 4% oxygen desaturation; all events must be at least 10 seconds.
[b]Extent of daytime somnolence.

TABLE 13.3	Diagnostic Criteria for Sleep Hypoventilation Syndrome[a]

Signs and symptoms	Monitoring
Cor pulmonale	Increase in $Paco_2$ during sleep >10 mm Hg from awake supine values
Pulmonary hypertension	
Unexplained excessive daytime somnolence	Oxygen desaturations during sleep not associated with apneas or hypopneas
Erythrocytosis	
Waking hypercapnia ($Paco_2$ >45 mm Hg)	

[a]Must meet at least one criterion from each column.

TABLE 13.4	Signs and Symptoms of Obstructive Sleep Apnea-Hypopnea Syndrome and Obesity Hypoventilation Syndrome

Obesity
Snoring
Awakening snorting or gasping
Witnessed apneas
Excessive daytime somnolence
Morning headaches
Large neck circumference
Unrefreshing sleep
Poorly controlled hypertension
Craniofacial abnormalities (micrognathia, retrognathia, macroglossia)
Nocturnal oxygen desaturations
Hypercapnia not explained by other etiology
Hypothyroidism

TABLE 13.5	Common Complications and Side Effects of Continuous Positive Airway Pressure or Bilevel Positive Airway Pressure

Nasal/oral dryness
Eye dryness
Mask leak
Aerophagia/gastric distention
Skin irritation

In patients who cannot tolerate CPAP or BiPAP, tracheotomy is the gold standard treatment for obstructive sleep apnea because it allows for the area of upper airway obstruction to be bypassed. However, some morbidly obese patients may require custom tracheotomy tubes in order to fully resolve the obstruction. In addition, if there is a component of sleep-related hypoventilation, not solely due to OSAHS, then nocturnal ventilation through the tracheotomy tube is required. Algorithm 13.1 demonstrates a proposed algorithm for the evaluation and treatment of patients in the intensive care unit who are suspected of having severe obstructive sleep apnea or sleep-related hypoventilation.

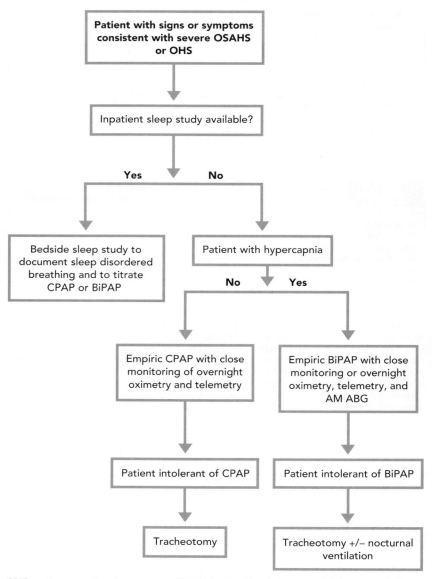

ALGORITHM 13.1	Proposed Evaluation and Treatment Guideline for Intensive Care Unit Patients Suspected of Having Severe Obstructive Sleep Apnea-Hypopnea Syndrome (OSAHS) or Obesity Hypoventilation Syndrome (OHS)

CPAP, continuous positive airway pressure; BiPAP, bilevel positive airway pressure; AM, morning; ABG, arterial blood gas.

Suggested Reading

American Academy of Sleep Medicine Task Force. Sleep related breathing disorders in adults: recommendations for syndrome definitions and measurement techniques in clinical research. *Sleep.* 1999;22:667–689.
Reviews recommended definitions for sleep disordered breathing.

Berger KI, Ayappa I, Chatr-Amontri B, et al. Obesity hypoventilation syndrome as a spectrum of respiratory disturbances during sleep. *Chest.* 2001;120:1231–1238.
Retrospective review of 23 patients with daytime hypercapnia and excessive daytime somnolence.

Douglas NJ. Respiratory physiology: control of ventilation. In: Kryger MH, Roth T, Dement WC, eds. *Principles and Practices of Sleep Medicine.* Philadelphia: WB Saunders; 2000:221–228.
Review of respiratory physiology in sleep.

Kreiger J, Weitzenblum E, Monassier JP, et al. Dangerous hypoxaemia during continuous positive airway pressure treatment of obstructive sleep apnoea. *Lancet.* 1983;322:1429–1430.
Report of a patient with severe hypoxemia occurring with empiric CPAP use for obstructive sleep apnea.

Krieger J. Respiratory physiology: breathing in normal subjects. In: Kryger MH, Roth T, Dement WC, eds. *Principles and Practices of Sleep Medicine.* Philadelphia: WB Saunders; 2000:229–241.
Review of respiratory physiology in sleep.

Meoli AL, Casey KR, Clark RW, et al. Hypopnea in sleep disordered breathing in adults. *Sleep.* 2001;24:469–470.
Reviews recommended definitions of apnea and hypopnea.

Shamsuzzaman AS, Gersh BJ, Somers VK. Obstructive sleep apnea—implications for cardiac and vascular disease. *JAMA.* 2003;290:1906–1914.
Report of MEDLINE review of 154 peer reviewed studies assessing cardiovascular complications associated with obstructive sleep apnea.

Thorpy M, Chesson A, Sarkis D, et al. Practice parameters for the treatment of obstructive sleep apnea in adults: the efficacy of surgical modification of the upper airway. *Sleep.* 1996;19:152–155.
Reviews indications and efficacy of surgical treatment of obstructive sleep apnea.

Young T, Palta M, Dempsey J, et al. The occurrence of sleep disordered breathing among middle-aged adults. *N Engl J Med.* 1993;328:1230–1235.
A random sample of state employees of Wisconsin who underwent polysomnograms to evaluate the prevalence of sleep disordered breathing.

14

PULMONARY HYPERTENSION AND RIGHT VENTRICULAR FAILURE IN THE INTENSIVE CARE UNIT

Rael Sundy and Murali M. Chakinala

Decompensated right ventricular failure (DRVF) is a less common cause of shock, which is frequently underdiagnosed, and recognizing its presence requires vigilance for a constellation of symptoms and signs. The treatment of this condition also differs somewhat from the routine shock management guidelines as elucidated elsewhere in this book. Most often, DRVF occurs in the setting of chronic pulmonary hypertension (i.e., mean pulmonary artery pressure ≥25 mm Hg) with an inciting acute illness that converts a compensated right ventricle (RV) into DRVF and a hemodynamically unstable emergency.

PATHOPHYSIOLOGY OF RV FAILURE

The RV is a thin-walled chamber that empties by sequential contraction into a low-resistance, high-capacitance pulmonary vascular circuit over the entire period of RV systole. Despite a three to fourfold increase in cardiac output, there is no increase in pulmonary pressure and RV workload, thanks to pulmonary vasodilation and recruitment of pulmonary vasculature. When faced with acutely elevated afterload (e.g., massive pulmonary embolism), the RV can decompensate rapidly, leading to shock (Algorithm 14.1). But in the setting of chronic pulmonary hypertension, the RV has an innate but limited ability to adapt through myocardial hypertrophy, thus maintaining contractility for a finite period of time. Even then, a hypertrophied and compensated RV can deteriorate rapidly in the setting of acute volume or pressure overload (Algorithm 14.1).

CAUSES OF DRVF

Table 14.1 lists causes of acute RV failure. Table 14.2 lists the etiology of acute on chronic decompensation in patients with known pulmonary hypertension.

DIAGNOSIS OF DRVF

Clinical Presentation

DRVF typically manifests as shock due to a low flow state. A history of pulmonary hypertension raises the possibility for an acute on chronic decompensation due to any of the causes listed in Table 14.2. Signs and symptoms of DRVRF are shown in Table 14.3.

Diagnostic Testing

Radiology
Plain radiographs may show enlarged central pulmonary arteries with peripheral pruning if chronic pulmonary hypertension is present. RV enlargement manifests with filling of the retrosternal space. Right-sided pleural effusions rarely may be present. If an acute pulmonary embolism is suspected, lower extremity Doppler examinations and either VQ scan or pulmonary embolism protocol computed tomography should be obtained.

ALGORITHM 14.1 **Pathophysiology of Decompensated Right Ventricular Failure**

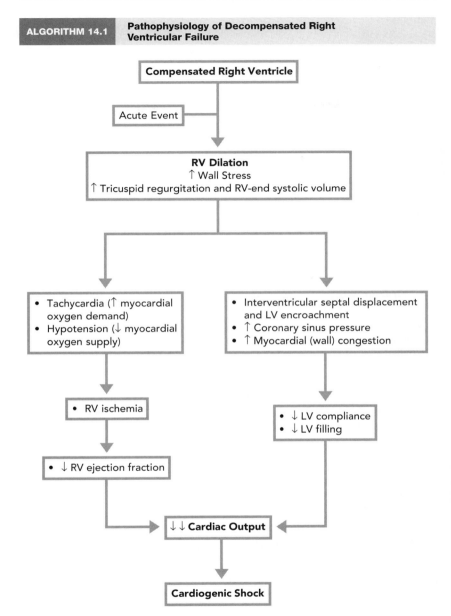

RV, right ventricular; LV, left ventricular.

TABLE 14.1	Etiology of Right Ventricular (RV) Failure

RV infarct or perioperative injury
Cardiac tamponade (mimicker of RV failure)
Tricuspid incompetence
Acute massive pulmonary embolus (thrombus, fat, air or amniotic fluid)
Acute lung injury/adult respiratory distress syndrome
Sickle cell chest syndrome
Acute decompensation of chronic pulmonary arterial hypertension (Table 14.2)

Electrocardiogram
Table 14.4 shows the RV changes that can be seen by electrocardiography.

Laboratory Data
In keeping with a low-output state, typical laboratory values include an anion gap acidosis, elevated lactate, prerenal blood urea nitrogen to creatinine ratio, low urine sodium. Hepatic congestion results in elevated liver enzymes and hyperbilirubinemia. RV strain can result in elevated B-type natriuretic peptide, and an elevated troponin I level would be consistent with RV infarction.

Echocardiography
Cardiac echocardiography is arguably the most useful examination in this scenario. Table 14.5 lists echocardiographic findings in DRVF. It provides rapid and important data for diagnosing RV failure, elucidating precipitating causes, and triaging patients into three groups: RV failure with elevated pulmonary artery (PA) pressures, RV failure without elevated pressures, and pericardial disease (Algorithm 14.2).

Pulmonary Artery Catheter
A complementary diagnostic tool in the management of DRVF is the pulmonary artery catheter (PAC). Indications for use of a PAC include differentiating pump failure from other causes of shock or assistance with the management of DRVF (i.e., regulation of volume status, use of inotropes, and assessing response to pulmonary vasodilators). Challenges to using PAC in DRVF include difficulty introducing the catheter, increased risk of PA rupture from "overwedging" the distal balloon tip, and poor tolerance of arrhythmias. The characteristic pattern of DRVF includes elevated central venous, RV, and PA pressures with reduced cardiac output, stroke volume, and mixed-venous oxygen saturation. With end-stage RV failure or in the setting of RV infarction, the PA pressure may not be elevated as the RV is unable to generate enough force to eject blood into the pulmonary vasculature. The PA occlusion pressure is variable and may actually be elevated as left ventricular (LV) compliance worsens.

TABLE 14.2	Causes of Acute Hemodynamic Instability in Chronic Pulmonary Arterial Hypertension

Acute medication failure (e.g., noncompliance, interruption of therapy)
Dietary or fluid indiscretion
Increased metabolic demands (e.g., infection, fever, environmental heat, pregnancy)
Venous thromboembolism (submassive)
Induction of general anesthesia
Surgery (left-sided valvular repair, pulmonary thromboendarterectomy, lung transplantation, lobectomy, or pneumonectomy)
Dysrhythmias
Endocrinopathies (e.g., thyroid disorders, adrenal insufficiency)

TABLE 14.3	Signs and Symptoms

Symptoms	Signs
Syncope, dizziness	Decreased pulses
RUQ pain	Cool extremities
Abdominal distention	Lower extremity edema
Weight gain	Elevated jugular venous pulsation
Early satiety	Right-sided S3
	Hepatojugular reflux
	Ascites

RUQ, right upper quadrant.

Cardiac output should be measured by the Fick method as tricuspid regurgitation or intracardiac shunts make the thermodilution method unreliable. Lastly, one should place more emphasis on trends gleaned from PAC readings rather than on absolute values.

TREATMENT OF ACUTE DECOMPENSATED RV FAILURE

The treatment of acute DRVF (Algorithm 14.3) includes:

- Identify and correct precipitating factors
- Correct hypoxemia
- Reverse hypotension and restore circulation
- Treat volume overload and RV encroachment

Identify and Correct Precipitating Factors

In patients with known pulmonary hypertension (PH) and chronic RV dysfunction, identification of precipitating factors (Table 14.2) must be sought and corrected. Maintain a high index of suspicion for occult infection in patients with chronic indwelling venous catheters; empiric therapy to treat bacteremia is appropriate. Atrial tachyarrhythmias should be slowed with digoxin, amiodarone, or cardioversion. Beta blockers or verapamil should not be used because of their negative inotropic effects. Bradycardias may require temporary pacing as the situation demands.

Correct Hypoxemia

Oxygen is the most potent pulmonary vasodilator, and liberal oxygen administration will reduce pulmonary vascular resistance (PVR) and improve cardiac output. Patients may

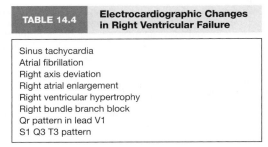

TABLE 14.4	Electrocardiographic Changes in Right Ventricular Failure

Sinus tachycardia
Atrial fibrillation
Right axis deviation
Right atrial enlargement
Right ventricular hypertrophy
Right bundle branch block
Qr pattern in lead V1
S1 Q3 T3 pattern

TABLE 14.5	Echocardiographic Findings in Right Ventricular (RV) Failure

RV hypertrophy (in chronic pulmonary hypertension)
RV dilation and hypokinesis
Paradoxic septal motion due to RV pressure overload
Right atrial enlargement
D-shaped left ventricle and late systolic left ventricular filling
Pericardial effusion
Tricuspid regurgitation
Elevated pulmonary arterial systolic pressure
Pulmonary artery dilatation
Lack of inspiratory collapse of the inferior vena cava

require mechanical ventilation to maintain oxygenation; however, the lowest possible positive end-expiratory pressure should be used to limit increases in RV afterload (from intra-alveolar vessel compression) and decreases in venous return. Permissive hypercapnia should be avoided as hypoxic pulmonary vasoconstriction is augmented in hypercarbic conditions.

Lastly, bronchospasm and agitation are frequently overlooked causes of elevated PVR in ventilated patients and should be managed aggressively.

Reverse Hypotension and Restore Circulation

Factors governing RV stroke volume are the same as those for the LV: preload, afterload, and myocardial contractility. Treatment of the unstable patient with severe PH encompasses all three parameters, and the PAC may assist.

Preload
Insufficient preload is generally not an issue in DRVF. If shock is due to decreased preload (i.e., central venous pressure <5 mm Hg) cautious volume challenges of 250 mL crystalloid should be employed until a central venous pressure of 10 to 12 mm Hg is reached. Overexuberant volume administration can worsen RV distention and encroach on the LV, further reducing cardiac output and worsening hypotension.

Systemic Hypotension
Vasopressors have an important role in restoring systemic blood pressure to maintain myocardial perfusion and minimize RV ischemia. No agent is clearly superior, but norepinephrine has both inotropic and peripheral vasopressor properties without major pulmonary vascular constriction. Dopamine, which may result in marked tachycardia, is a reasonable alternative. The lowest doses of inotropes and pressors should be used to minimize tachycardia, dysrhythmias, myocardial oxygen consumption, and pulmonary vasoconstriction.

Afterload Reduction
Selective pulmonary arterial dilation is a critical therapeutic step in breaking the spiral of RV decompensation. Inhaled agents preferentially lower PVR with minimal decreases in systemic vascular resistance and also minimize ventilation-perfusion mismatching and hypoxemia. The two available agents are inhaled nitric oxide and inhaled epoprostenol. Inhaled nitric oxide up to 40 ppm is administered via face mask or endotracheal tube, measuring methemoglobin levels every 6 hours. Inhaled epoprostenol at 5,000 to 20,000 ng/mL via continuous nebulization is a cheaper and efficacious alternative. Once cardiac output and blood pressure have improved, the patient can be transitioned to continuous intravenous epoprostenol, which is titrated by side effects and systemic blood pressure. Nonselective vasodilators such as nitroprusside, nitrates, hydralazine, and calcium channel antagonists should not be used as they preferentially cause peripheral vasodilation and aggravate hypotension.

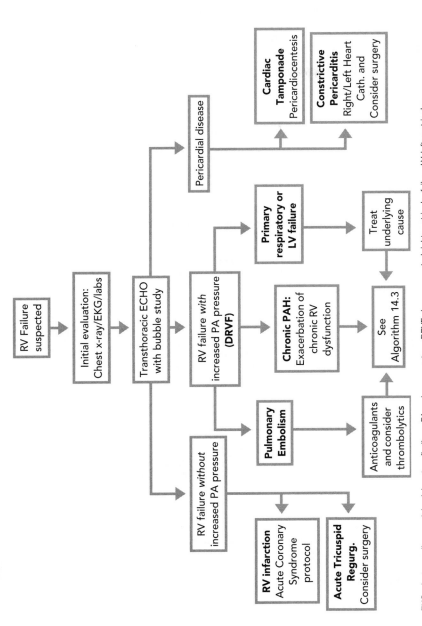

ALGORITHM 14.2   Diagnostic Pathway in Suspected Right Ventricular (RV) Failure

RV Failure suspected

↓

Initial evaluation: Chest x-ray/EKG/labs

↓

Transthoracic ECHO with bubble study

Pericardial disease

Cardiac Tamponade Pericardiocentesis

Constrictive Pericarditis Right/Left Heart Cath. and Consider surgery

RV failure with increased PA pressure **(DRVF)**

Primary respiratory or LV failure

Treat underlying cause

Chronic PAH: Exacerbation of chronic RV dysfunction

See Algorithm 14.3

Pulmonary Embolism

Anticoagulants and consider thrombolytics

RV failure without increased PA pressure

RV infarction Acute Coronary Syndrome protocol

Acute Tricuspid Regurg. Consider surgery

EKG, electrocardiogram; labs, laboratory findings; PA, pulmonary artery; DRVF, decompensated right ventricular failure; LV, left ventricular; PAH, pulmonary arterial hypertension; Cath., catheterization.

ALGORITHM 14.3   **Management of Decompensated Right Ventricular (RV) Failure**

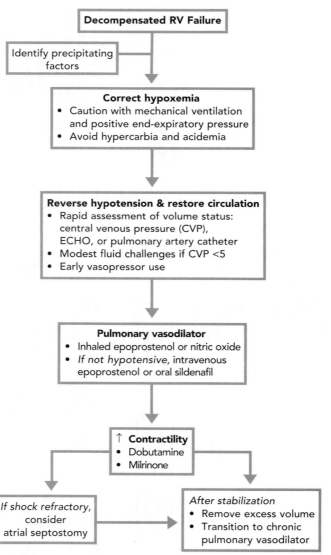

ECHO, echocardiography.

Contractility

In normotensive patients with persistently unmet peripheral metabolic needs, the next step is addition of an inotrope. There is no ideal inotrope that increases RV contractility without worsening systemic blood pressure. Options include dobutamine at 1 to 5 mcg/kg/min or the longer-acting milrinone, which requires dosage reduction in renal insufficiency. Digoxin is a much weaker alternative.

Treat Volume Overload and RV Encroachment

Once adequate circulation is restored and the patient has stabilized, excess volume can be removed. Severe right heart failure can be associated with diuretic resistance, due to poor intestinal absorption, decreased glomerular filtration rate with poor renal arterial perfusion, renal venous congestion from elevated central venous pressures, and intense neurohormonal activation. A suggested stepwise approach is:

1. Loop diuretic by intravenous bolus or continuous infusion. The latter maintains a continuous renal threshold of drug with constant diuresis and less ototoxicity.
2. If loop diuretic is insufficient, intravenous chlorthalidone or oral metolazone can be added.
3. Spironolactone is effective to counter the intense neurohormonal pathway and can be added unless hyperkalemia is present.
4. Finally, mechanical fluid removal with continuous veno-venous hemodialysis (CVVHD) may be appropriate.

SURGICAL INTERVENTIONS

Atrial septostomy, which is the creation of an intracardiac, right-to-left shunt at the atrial level, allows for right-sided decompression. Although right-to-left shunting results in oxygen desaturation, this is counterbalanced by improved left-sided filling, cardiac output, and total oxygen delivery. Septostomy is a risky procedure with high mortality and should be performed only at centers with expertise.

GENERAL MEASURES

1. Control agitation
2. Suppress fevers
3. Place filters on intravenous catheters to prevent air embolization through intracardiac shunts
4. Deep venous thrombosis prophylaxis
5. Minimize Valsalva maneuvers (e.g., constipation)
6. Practice caution with colloid infusions.

Suggested Reading

DeMarco T, McGlothin D. Managing right ventricular failure in PAH. Adv Pulm Hypertens 2005;14(4):16–26.
A review article with excellent flowcharts, algorithms & detailed pathophysiology & therapeutic discussion.

Mebazaa A, Karpati P. Acute right ventricular failure—from pathophysiology to new treatments. *Intensive Care Med.* 2004;30:185–196.
A clinical case based review.

Piazza G, Goldhaber S. The acutely decompensated right ventricle: Pathways for diagnosis & management. *Chest* 2005;128:1836–1852.
A detailed review article focusing on pathophysiology, diagnosis & treatment of this increasingly common condition.

Taichman DB, Jeffery ME. Management of the acutely ill patient with pulmonary arterial hypertension. In: Mandel J, Taichman D, eds. *Pulmonary Vascular Disease.* Philadelphia: Saunders Elsevier; 2006:254–265.
A textbook chapter which discusses issues to consider when caring for patients with PAH in the ICU.

15

PLEURAL DISORDERS IN THE INTENSIVE CARE UNIT

Brian Hamburg and Martin L. Mayse

Disorders of the pleura are found often in the intensive care unit (ICU). The management of these problems can be crucial in the patient's outcome. This chapter will review the pathophysiology of these disorders and provide guidelines for managing these conditions in the ICU.

PLEURAL EFFUSIONS

The pleural space is a potential space between the visceral pleura, which covers the outer surface of the lung, and the parietal pleura, which lines the inside of the chest wall. In this space, there is a small amount of fluid present that functions to mechanically couple the lung to the chest wall and lubricate the interface of the visceral and parietal pleura. Pleural fluid normally results from the filtration of blood through high-pressure systemic blood vessels, and is drained from the pleural space, through lymphatic openings in the parietal pleura, which drain into parietal lymphatic vessels. In different disease states, fluid may originate from the interstitial spaces of the lungs, the intrathoracic lymphatics, the intrathoracic blood vessels, or the peritoneal cavity.

A pleural effusion is defined as an abnormal collection of fluid in the pleural space. Effusions occur when the rate of fluid formation exceeds the rate of fluid absorption. The most common causes of pleural effusions are shown in Table 15.1. Pleural effusions are commonly classified as being either exudative or transudative. An exudative pleural effusion implies that there is a disease process that is affecting the pleura directly, causing the pleura and/or its vasculature to be damaged. A transudative pleural effusion results when the pleura itself is healthy, but a remote disease process affects hydrostatic and/or oncotic factors that either increase the formation of pleural fluid or decrease the absorption of pleural fluid. Deciding if the pleura is injured, or intact, helps in formulating a concise differential diagnosis for potential causes (Table 15.2).

There are certain nonspecific signs and symptoms that may indicate the presence of a pleural effusion, but these are often difficult to ascertain in the ICU. Chest pain, particularly when sharp and made worse with breathing, can result from an inflamed pleura in the presence of an effusion. Dyspnea is also common as the effusion can affect the mechanics of the diaphragm, cause a restrictive ventilatory defect, and/or cause compressive atelectasis leading to hypoxemia. The history can also help to reveal the cause of the effusion. For example, a patient with a fever and cough productive of sputum might have a pneumonia causing the effusion. On physical examination, signs that an effusion is present include dullness to percussion over the effusion, loss of fremitus, decreased breath sounds, and crackles/egophony immediately above the effusion.

The majority of ICU patients will have their pleural effusion detected first by chest x-ray. Although a posterior-anterior (PA) and lateral chest x-ray is the preferred image, ICU patients typically have portable x-rays. Blunting of the costophrenic angle and a meniscus sign are the most common findings when an effusion is present. On the lateral chest x-ray, as little as 175 mL of fluid can be detected, while on the PA film it takes approximately 500 mL of fluid. Portable films are less sensitive, and often do not show the meniscus sign. Signs on the portable chest x-ray include loss of the diaphragm silhouette and increased basilar opacity with gradation over the entire hemithorax (more opaque at the base than the apex). Once a pleural effusion is detected radiographically, a lateral decubitus chest x-ray (where the dependent side is the side of the effusion) can

TABLE 15.1	Common Causes of Pleural Effusions

1. CHF, 36%
2. Pneumonia, 22%
3. Malignancy, 14%
4. Pulmonary embolism, 11%
5. Other infections, 7%
6. Other causes, 10%

CHF, congestive heart failure.

quantitate the volume of fluid present and determine if the effusion is free-flowing or loculated. If the fluid is free-flowing, fluid can be detected as a straight line between the chest wall and lower border of the lung. Measurement of the distance between the chest wall and the lower border of the lung can give an idea of how much fluid is present. It is generally accepted that if this distance is >1 cm, then the amount of fluid is significant. Diagnostic evaluation of the effusion from this point is discussed in Algorithms 15.1 and 15.2.

Other imaging modalities can also detect, quantify, and sometimes even characterize the pleural effusion. Chest computed tomography (CT) is a useful imaging tool in assessing pleural effusions and can help the clinician diagnose not only the presence of the effusion, but also delineate possible causes. Different techniques yield different information, so it is important to select the appropriate technique:

■ Noncontrast CT scans can give a better idea of the amount of fluid within the pleural space, whether the fluid is loculated, and can detect abnormalities in the lungs that can be obscured by the effusion on standard chest x-ray.
■ Standard contrast CT scans also assess the pleural surface for abnormalities that might suggest empyema or pleural malignancy.
■ CT scans with contrast given by pulmonary embolism protocol can detect a pulmonary embolism as the cause of the effusion, but do not provide information about the pleural surface beyond that of a noncontrast CT.

CT scans cannot be done at bedside, a big disadvantage when dealing with a patient who is not stable enough to travel out of the ICU.

Ultrasound is beneficial for multiple reasons. It gives a real-time image that can be done at the bedside and used not only for diagnosis that an effusion is present, but also

TABLE 15.2	Pathophysiological Causes of Pleural Effusions	
How pleura are affected	Example	Exudate/transudate
Pleura damaged ■ Local disease in pleural space ■ Local disease adjacent to pleural space	■ Malignancy ■ Pneumonia, PE, subdiaphragmatic abscess	■ Exudate ■ Exudate
■ Systemic diseases that affect the pleural surface	■ Autoimmune disease (lupus, rheumatoid arthritis)	■ Exudate
Pleura intact ■ Systemic disease that does not directly affect the pleural surface	■ CHF, myxedema	■ Transudate

PE, pulmonary embolism; CHF, congestive heart failure.

ALGORITHM 15.1 Evaluation of the Unknown Effusion

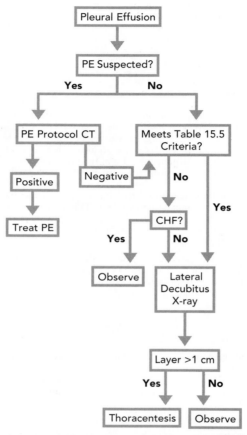

PE, pulmonary embolism; CT, computed tomography; CHF, congestive heart failure. Note: 90% of pleural effusions are caused by five processes shown in Table 15.1.

ALGORITHM 15.2   **Evaluation and Management of Pleural Fluid after Thoracentesis**

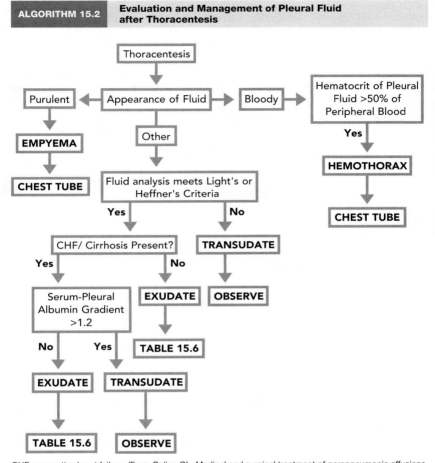

CHF, congestive heart failure. (From Colice GL. Medical and surgical treatment of parapneumonic effusions. Chest. 2000;118:1161, with permission.)

guide diagnostic and therapeutic interventions (i.e., thoracentesis, tube thoracostomy). Ultrasound can detect whether the fluid is loculated or free-flowing, and can give clues as to whether the fluid is transudative, exudative, or even whether it is an empyema.

Once a pleural effusion is identified, it is important to attempt to diagnose the etiology of the effusion by obtaining a sample of the fluid for analysis. This is most often done by a thoracentesis. Thoracenteses can be safely performed as long as there is >1 cm of layered fluid on the lateral decubitus chest x-ray, even in patients receiving mechanical ventilation. One can remove a small amount of fluid for analysis or as much as 1,500 mL per drainage of fluid for both diagnostic and therapeutic goals (Algorithms 15.2 through 15.4). The most common criteria used to separate exudates from transudates are known as Light's criteria (Table 15.3). Heffner's criteria (Table 15.4) can also differentiate exudate from transudate. Heffner's criteria has a similar sensitivity (98.4%) as Light's criteria (97.9%) and does not require simultaneous blood work to be drawn.

Other specific tests (Table 15.6) can help determine a specific diagnosis.

TABLE 15.3	**Light's Criteria**

- Pleural fluid to serum protein ratio >0.5
- Pleural fluid to serum LDH ratio >0.6
- Pleural fluid LDH >2/3 upper limit of normal for serum LDH

LDH, lactate dehydrogenase.

TABLE 15.4	**Heffner's Criteria**

- Pleural fluid protein >2.9 g/dL
- Pleural fluid LDH >0.45 upper limit of normal

LDH, lactate dehydrogenase.

TABLE 15.5	**Indications for Thoracentesis**

1. Pleural effusion of unknown etiology
2. Fever in setting of long-standing pleural effusion
3. Air-fluid level in the pleural space
4. Rapid change in size of effusion
5. Concern that empyema is developing

TABLE 15.6	**Diagnostic Tests to Consider in Evaluation of Pleural Effusions**

Diagnostic test	Type of effusion
1. Cytology	1. Malignant effusion
2. Gram stain or culture positive	2. Infectious effusion (i.e., bacterial, fungal)
3. AFB positive; pleural fluid ADA >70 U/L	3. Tuberculous effusion
4. Rheumatoid arthritis cells	4. Rheumatoid effusion
5. Chylomicrons present; pleural fluid triglycerides >110 mg/dL	5. Chylothorax
6. Salivary amylase present in pleural fluid	6. Esophageal rupture
7. Pleural creatinine/serum creatinine >1	7. Urinothorax

AFB, acid-fast bacillus; ADA, adenosine deaminase

ALGORITHM 15.3   Management of Parapneumonic Effusions

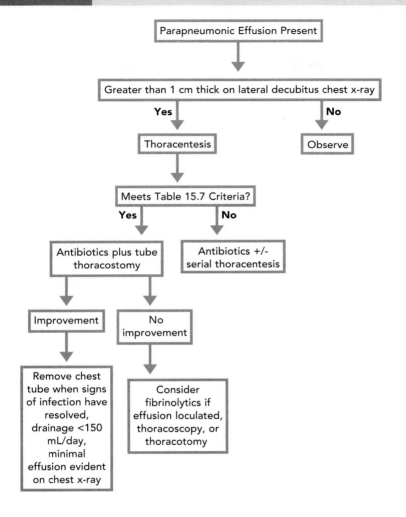

ALGORITHM 15.4   **Management of Recurrent Malignant Effusions**

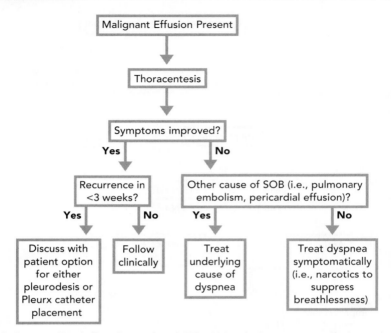

SOB, shortness of breath; (From Antunes G, et al. BTS guidelines for the management of malignant pleural effusions. *Thorax*. 2003;58[Suppl II]: ii30, with permission.)

As many as 20% of pleural effusions remain undiagnosed even after extensive investigation, and it is often unclear as to what the appropriate management of these effusions is in these situations. These idiopathic effusions with no clinical or radiologic evidence of malignancy will often resolve spontaneously without further therapy. In the ICU setting, as long as the patient does not clinically deteriorate, there is benefit in a conservative approach to the pleural effusion when a diagnosis cannot be made after initial evaluation. If the patient continues to deteriorate despite serial thoracenteses, thoracoscopy can be considered as the next step to assess the pleural effusion.

SPECIAL SITUATIONS

Parapneumonic Effusion

A parapneumonic effusion is defined as any pleural effusion associated with bacterial pneumonia, lung abscess, or bronchiectasis. Parapneumonic effusions progress through different stages and, depending on when the patient presents, the treatment of the effusion will be different. The main distinction is whether the effusion is uncomplicated or complicated. Complicated effusions and empyemas will not resolve on their own and will require tube thoracostomy. As shown in Algorithm 15.3 and Table 15.7, radiographic, microbiologic, and chemical characteristics of the effusion will dictate whether thoracentesis with antibiotics alone will be sufficient to treat the effusion, or whether a chest tube must be inserted to effectively treat the effusion. If the chest tube is not effective in draining the fluid, intrapleural fibrinolytics might be required to break up the loculations and allow effective drainage of the infected fluid. If fibrinolytics are unsuccessful, the patient may require more invasive therapy, including thoracoscopy with breakdown of adhesions or thoracotomy with decortication.

Malignant Effusion

Malignant pleural effusions occur from a number of causes. Pleural metastases occur causing increased permeability of the pleura, and lymphatic obstruction can occur, which impairs drainage of pleural fluid through regional lymphatics. Table 15.8 shows the most common malignancies associated with pleural effusions. When these effusions occur, they are often large and lead to significant symptoms in the patient. Often, drainage of the effusion with thoracentesis alone is not sufficient as the effusion frequently recurs. Other management options include insertion of a chest tube followed by pleurodesis, which can obliterate the pleural space and prevent the effusion from recurring. Alternatively, insertion of a long-term indwelling catheter will allow the patient to drain the effusion at home and is a viable option that decreases hospitalizations and increases the quality of life of the patient. Management of this type of effusion is outlined in Algorithm 15.4.

Hemothorax

A hemothorax is the presence of blood in the pleural space such that the ratio of pleural fluid hematocrit to blood hematocrit is >0.5. This can be a serious condition and may result in ICU admission for treatment. Hemothoraces can be due to traumatic, nontraumatic, or rarely from iatrogenic causes (Table 15.9). Diagnosis is made after a thoracentesis returns bloody fluid (Algorithm 15.2). It should be noted that even a small amount of blood can make pleural fluid appear bloody; therefore, the fluid's hematocrit needs to be compared with peripheral blood hematocrit to confirm the presence of a hemothorax. Initial treatment for hemothoraces of all causes is tube thoracostomy. If bleeding is voluminous and persists, transfusion and surgical intervention may be required.

TABLE 15.7	Indication for Tube Thoracostomy in Parapneumonic Effusions

1. Radiographic
   - ☐ Pleural fluid loculation
   - ☐ Effusion filling more than half of hemithorax
   - ☐ Air-fluid level present
2. Microbiologic
   - ☐ Pus in pleural space
   - ☐ Positive Gram stain for microorganisms
   - ☐ Positive pleural fluid cultures
3. Chemical:
   - ☐ Pleural Fluid pH <7.2
   - ☐ Pleural Fluid glucose <60

Pneumothorax

A pneumothorax is the presence of air in the pleural space. When this occurs, it can be an acute emergency that requires immediate attention. A pneumothorax can be spontaneous or traumatic. Spontaneous pneumothoraces are either primary, if no other disease process is present, or secondary, if there is an underlying disease process such as chronic obstructive pulmonary disease. Traumatic pneumothoraces include iatrogenic causes that may occur following a procedure (i.e., central line placement) or barotrauma. Primary spontaneous and traumatic pneumothoraces can often be treated effectively with observation or tube thoracostomy. Secondary spontaneous pneumothoraces typically require tube thoracostomy and may also require pleurodesis for definitive treatment.

Tension pneumothorax is the most serious consequence of a pneumothorax. This occurs when a one-way valve process develops, which allows air to enter the pleural space during inspiration but not leave during expiration. As the air builds up in the pleural space, the lung and intrathoracic vasculature become compressed, leading to dyspnea, hypoxemia, and hemodynamic compromise. Physical examination may reveal absent breath sounds on the side of the pneumothorax and/or shift of the trachea to the contralateral side of the pneumothorax. Tension pneumothorax should be suspected in unstable patients with absent breath sounds over one hemithorax, in mechanically ventilated patients who suddenly decompensate, in patients with known previously stable/improving pneumothorax who suddenly decompensate, or in patients who become unstable during or after a procedure known to cause a pneumothorax. Algorithm 15.5 give further information on the evaluation and management of pneumothoraces. Table 15.10 covers the indications for removal of the chest tube.

TABLE 15.8	Most Common Primary Tumors of Malignant Effusions	
Primary malignancy		**Rate (%)**
Lung		38
Breast		17
Lymphoma		12
Unknown primary		11
GU tract		9
GI tract		7
GU, genitourinary; GI, gastrointestinal.		

ALGORITHM 15.5   **Management of Pneumothorax**

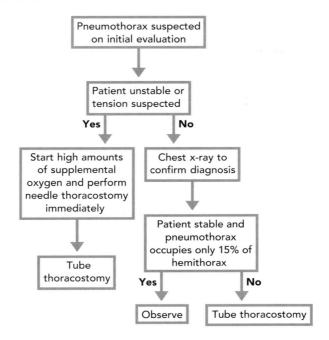

TABLE 15.9	Causes of Hemothoraces

Causes	Examples
Traumatic	Penetrating trauma (gunshot wound), blunt trauma (usually with displaced rib fracture)
Nontraumatic	Metastatic malignant pleural disease, complication of anticoagulant therapy for pulmonary emboli
Iatrogenic	Perforation of a central vein from percutaneous catheter placement, following thoracentesis, following pleural biopsy

TABLE 15.10	Indications for Removal of Chest Tube

1. Pneumothorax resolved
2. No air leak present in chest tube
3. Lung remains expanded after chest tube placed on water seal for 24 hours

If concern remains, chest tube can be clamped for 4–8 hours followed by chest radiograph; if lung expanded, then it is safe to remove the chest tube.

Suggested Reading

Abrahamian FM. Pleural effusions. Available at: http://www.emedicine.com/emerg/topic 462.htm. Accessed October 24, 2006.

Antunes G, Neville E, Duffy J, et al. BTS guidelines for the management of malignant pleural effusions. *Thorax.* 2003;58[Suppl II]:ii29–ii38.

Colice GL, Curtis A, Deslauriers J, et al. Medical and surgical treatment of parapneumonic effusions: an evidence-based guideline. *Chest.* 2000;118:1158–1171.

Fartoukh M, Azoulay E, Galliot R, et al. Clinically documented pleural effusions in medical ICU Patients: how useful is routine thoracentesis. *Chest.* 2002;121:178–184.

Ferrer JS, Munoz XG, Orriols RM, et al. Evolution of idiopathic pleural effusion: a prospective, long-term follow-up study. *Chest.* 1996;109:1508–1513.

Heffner JE, Brown LK, Barbieri CA. Diagnostic value of tests that discriminate between exudative and transudative pleural effusions. *Chest. 1997;*111: 970–980.

Lichtenstein DA, Meziere G, Lascols N, et al. Ultrasound diagnosis of occult pneumothorax. *Crit Care Med.* 2005;33:1231–1238.

Light RW. *Pleural Diseases.* 4th ed. Philadelphia: Lippincott Willams & Wilkins; 2001.

Mattison LE, Coppage L, Alderman DF, et al. Pleural effusions in the medical ICU: prevalence, causes, and clinical implications. *Chest.* 1997;111:1018–1023.

Tu C-Y, Hsu W-H, Hsia T-C, et al. Pleural effusions in febrile medical ICU patients: chest ultrasound study. *Chest.* 2004;126:1274–1280.

Vives M, Porcel JM, Vicente de Vera M, et al. A study of Light's criteria and possible modifications for distinguishing exudative from transudative pleural effusions. *Chest.* 1996;109: 1503–1507.

WEANING OF MECHANICAL VENTILATION

Chad A. Witt

16

The gradual withdrawal of mechanical ventilation is termed *weaning*. Weaning can be divided into two components: (a) *liberation* refers to no longer requiring mechanical ventilatory support, and (b) *extubation/decannulation* refers to the removal of the endotracheal or tracheostomy tube. Because of well-described complications of mechanical ventilation, such as infection and airway trauma, it is important to proceed with liberation and extubation as quickly as the patient will tolerate.

The first step in weaning a patient off mechanical ventilation is to determine whether the patient is ready for a spontaneous breathing trial. For patients to tolerate a spontaneous breathing trial, several requirements must be met. Most importantly, the cause of the patient's initial respiratory failure must be significantly improved or resolved. Additionally, the patient must be awake and able to cooperate, hemodynamically stable, and able to cough and protect the airway. Patients who are intubated on mechanical ventilation should be evaluated for readiness to undergo a spontaneous breathing trial on a daily basis (Algorithm 16.1). Protocols driven by nurses and respiratory therapists have been shown to improve the efficiency of the weaning process.

There are multiple weaning strategies and spontaneous breathing trial protocols. Spontaneous breathing trials can be performed using pressure support ventilation, continuous positive airway pressure (CPAP), or the T-tube technique. Using pressure support ventilation, a pressure support of 5 to 7 cm of H_2O is delivered to help the patient overcome the resistance of the endotracheal tube. During a CPAP trial, 5 cm of H_2O of CPAP is provided to the patient during the spontaneous breathing trial. Lastly, the T-tube technique provides oxygen flow without any pressure support or CPAP during the trial. Determining success or failure of spontaneous breathing trials performed using the T-tube technique has been studied rigorously, and the most useful measure is the rapid shallow breathing index, defined as the respiratory rate/tidal volume (breaths/minute/liter). A rapid shallow breathing index of <100 breaths/min/L during a spontaneous breathing trial indicates that a patient is more likely to be successfully extubated. It should be kept in mind that there will be extubation failures in patients who are deemed ready by all objective evaluation, and it is these patients who may benefit most from early tracheostomy.

Difficult-to-wean patients are those who do not wean from mechanical ventilation within 48 to 72 hours of resolution of their underlying disease process. In such patients, the acronym "WEANS NOW" has been developed as a set of factors to be considered in difficult-to-wean patients (Table 16.1).

ALGORITHM 16.1	Readiness to Liberate and Wean from Mechanical Ventilation

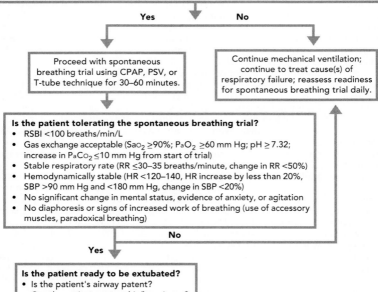

Is the patient ready for a spontaneous breathing trial?
- Evidence for reversal of the underlying cause of respiratory failure
- Patient is awake, alert, and cooperative
- Adequate oxygenation (e.g., PEEP $\leq$5 cm H_2O; Pao_2 >60 mm Hg with Fio_2 <0.50)
- Hemodynamically stable: on no vasopressor or inotropic agents or stable minimal doses of vasopressors or inotropes; no evidence of myocardial ischemia; HR <140 beats per minute.
- Afebrile (T <38.0°C)
- pH and $PaCO_2$ appropriate for patient's baseline respiratory status

Yes   **No**

Proceed with spontaneous breathing trial using CPAP, PSV, or T-tube technique for 30–60 minutes.

Continue mechanical ventilation; continue to treat cause(s) of respiratory failure; reassess readiness for spontaneous breathing trial daily.

Is the patient tolerating the spontaneous breathing trial?
- RSBI <100 breaths/min/L
- Gas exchange acceptable (Sao_2 $\geq$90%; PaO_2 $\geq$60 mm Hg; pH $\geq$ 7.32; increase in $PaCo_2$ $\leq$10 mm Hg from start of trial)
- Stable respiratory rate (RR $\leq$30–35 breaths/minute, change in RR <50%)
- Hemodynamically stable (HR <120–140, HR increase by less than 20%, SBP >90 mm Hg and <180 mm Hg, change in SBP <20%)
- No significant change in mental status, evidence of anxiety, or agitation
- No diaphoresis or signs of increased work of breathing (use of accessory muscles, paradoxical breathing)

No

Yes

Is the patient ready to be extubated?
- Is the patient's airway patent?
- Can the patient protect his/her airway?
- Can the patient clear his/her secretions?

No   **Yes**

Continue mechanical ventilation, consider causes for weaning failure (Table 16.1), and consider evaluation for tracheostomy.

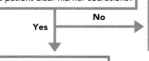

Proceed with extubation

Abbreviations:
Pao_2:	arterial partial pressure of oxygen
Fio_2:	fraction of inspired oxygen
PEEP:	positive end expiratory pressure
HR:	heart rate
T:	temperature
$PaCo_2$:	arterial partial pressure of carbon dioxide
CPAP:	continuous positive airway pressure
PSV:	pressure support ventilation
RSBI:	rapid shallow breathing index
Sao_2:	arterial oxygen saturation
RR:	respiratory rate
SBP:	systolic blood pressure

TABLE 16.1	Issues to Be Considered When Weaning Efforts Fail

Weaning parameters   (see Algorithm 16.1)
   Endotracheal tube
      Use the largest tube possible.
      Consider use of supplemental pressure-support ventilation during spontaneous
         breathing
      Suction secretions
   Arterial blood gases
      Avoid or treat metabolic alkalosis
      Maintain Pao_2 at 60–65 mm Hg to avoid blunting of respiratory drive
      For patients with CO_2 retention, keep $Paco_2$ at or above the baseline level
Nutrition
   Ensure adequate nutritional support
   Avoid electrolyte deficiencies
   Avoid excessive calories
Secretions
   Clear regularly
   Avoid excessive dehydration
Neuromuscular factors
Avoid neuromuscular-depressing drugs (neuromuscular blockers, aminoglycosides,
   clindamycin) in patients with muscle weakness
   Avoid unnecessary corticosteroids
Obstruction of airways
   Use bronchodilators when appropriate
   Exclude foreign bodies within the airway
Wakefulness
   Avoid oversedation
   Wean in morning or when patient is most awake

From *The Washington Manual of Medical Therapeutics.* 31st ed. Philadelphia: Lippincott Williams & Wilkins; 2004:192.

Suggested Reading

Calfee C, Matthay M. Recent advances in mechanical ventilation. *Am J Med.* 2005;118: 584–591.
   Review of mechanical ventilation, including noninvasive ventilation, ventilating patients with acute respiratory distress syndrome, and weaning of mechanical ventilation.

Kollef MH. Critical Care. Green GB, Harris IS, Lin GA, Moylan KC, eds. The Washington Manual of Medical Therapeutics. 31st ed. Philadelphia: Lippincott Williams & Wilkins, 2004:192.
   "WEANS NOW" acronym for the difficult to wean patient.

Kollef MH, Shapiro SD, Silver P, et al. A randomized, controlled trial of protocol-directed versus physician-directed weaning from mechanical ventilation. *Crit Care Med.* 1997; 25;4:567–574.
   Randomized, controlled trial showing that protocol-guided weaning of mechanical ventilation performed by nurses and respiratory therapists is effective, and resulted in earlier extubation than physician-directed weaning.

MacIntyre N. Evidence-based guidelines for weaning and discontinuing ventilatory support: a collective task force facilitated by the American College of Chest Physicians; the American Association for Respiratory Care; and the American College of Critical Care Medicine. *Chest.* 2001;120:375–396.
   Evidence-based review and guidelines for weaning, including spontaneous breathing trials, weaning protocols, and the use of tracheostomy for failure to wean.

Manthous CA, Schmidt GA, Hall JB. Liberation from mechanical ventilation: a decade of progress. *Chest.* 1998;114:886–901.
Review of current practices and advances in assessment of readiness for liberation, weaning strategies, and extubation.

Meade M, Guyatt G, Cook D, et al. Predicting success in weaning from mechanical ventilation. *Chest.* 2001;120:400–424.
Meta-analysis of sixty three studies evaluating predictors of successful weaning, including the rapid-shallow breathing index.

Rumbak MJ, Newton M, Truncale T, et al. A prospective, randomized, study comparing early percutaneous dilational tracheotomy to prolonged translaryngeal intubation (delayed tracheotomy) in critically ill medical patients. *Crit Care Med.* 2004;32:8; 1689–1694.
Prospective, randomized trial showing the benefit of early tracheotomy over prolonged translaryngeal intubation.

Tobin M. Advances in mechanical ventilation. *N Engl J Med.* 2001;334:1986–1996.
Review of mechanical ventilation strategies, including modes of ventilation, use of positive end expiratory pressure, and discontinuation of mechanical ventilation.

NONINVASIVE POSITIVE PRESSURE VENTILATION

17

Michael Lippmann

Noninvasive positive pressure ventilation (NPPV) delivers mechanically assisted breaths using tight-fitting nasal or facial masks, obviating the need for endotracheal intubation. The assisted ventilation is usually pressure-cycled either via pressure support ventilation or bilevel positive airway pressure. Although NPPV can be used successfully in a number of clinical situations, there are specific contraindications to its use (Table 17.1) and it should not delay clinically indicated tracheal intubation and invasive ventilation. Additionally, NPPV is a supportive therapy, and patients require prompt treatment of the underlying medical conditions leading to the respiratory failure.

Thorough patient assessment is critical prior to initiation of NPPV. NPPV is not indicated in patients with cardiac or respiratory arrest; nonrespiratory organ failure, impaired consciousness, unstable cardiac rhythm, hemodynamic instability, severe upper gastrointestinal bleeding, inability to protect upper airway or clear secretions, facial surgery, trauma, or deformity.

Clinical trials and subsequent meta-analyses demonstrate that NPPV is beneficial in the management of chronic obstructive pulmonary disease (COPD) exacerbations, cardiogenic pulmonary edema, immunocompromised patients with acute respiratory failure, and in selected patients with hypoxemic respiratory failure (Table 17.2). Patients with these conditions should receive a trial of NPPV if emergent intubation is not indicated, there are no contraindications, and qualified personnel are available to initiate the trial. Patients whose pH and PCO_2 improve after a short trial have better outcomes. Worsening gas exchange, increasing tachypnea, hemodynamic instability, or mental status changes necessitate tracheal intubation and invasive mechanical ventilation. Algorithm 17.1 provides an algorithmic approach to initiating NPPV in a patient with an exacerbation of COPD.

The American Association for Respiratory Care recommends that patients with COPD exacerbations be started on NPPV if they have no contraindications and meet two or more of the following criteria: respiratory distress with moderate-to-severe dyspnea; arterial pH <7.35 with $PaCO_2$ >45; and respiratory rate ≥25 breaths/minute. In these patients, NPPV decreases intubation, mortality, complications, treatment failure, and length of stay. Patients with less severe derangements in function do not benefit from NPPV and tend to tolerate it poorly. Patients with a Glasgow coma scale <11, pH <7.25, and respiratory rate >30 breaths/minute are more likely to fail trials of NPPV.

In cardiogenic pulmonary edema, NPPV decreases preload by increasing thoracic pressure with consequent decrease in venous return, and decreases afterload by decreasing intrathoracic transaortic pressure. The diminished work of breathing also lowers myocardial oxygen demands. A meta-analysis of 15 randomized, controlled trials showed NPPV decreased mortality and decreased the need for intubation. Early concerns that use of bilevel positive airway pressure is associated with an increased risk of myocardial infarction were not confirmed in larger, more recent trials.

A randomized study of immunocompromised patients with acute respiratory failure demonstrated that patients receiving NPPV had lower rates of endotracheal intubation, serious complications, and all-cause mortality when compared with patients randomized to receive usual care.

NPPV appears beneficial in selected patients with hypoxemic respiratory failure. Randomized studies demonstrate reductions in mortality, need for intubation, intensive care unit stay and serious complications including sepsis and nosocomial pneumonias. The benefit appears to be greatest in patients whose arterial PCO_2 are >45 mm Hg.

TABLE 17.1	Contraindications to Noninvasive Positive Pressure Ventilation
Cardiac or respiratory arrest Nonrespiratory organ failure Severe encephalopathy Severe UGI bleeding Hemodynamic instability High risk for aspiration	Unstable cardiac rhythm Facial surgery, trauma, or deformity Upper airway obstruction Inability to protect airway Inability to clear secretions
UGI, upper gastrointestinal.	

NPPV appears to decrease the incidence of respiratory failure when applied immediately after extubation, especially in patients with COPD and hypercapnia during spontaneous breathing trials preextubation. NPPV does not prevent reintubation when applied after a recently extubated patient develops respiratory failure. In this population, patients randomized to receive a trial of NPPV demonstrated an increase in all-cause mortality when compared with patients receiving standard medical therapy.

Physicians initiating NPPV must select the mode of ventilation, the patient interface, and ventilator settings. Most studies have applied NPPV using pressure-controlled ventilators, which supply variable levels of inspiratory positive pressure to assist inspiration, and a lower level of expiratory positive pressure to unload inspiratory muscles and potentially recruit closed airways. This bilevel ventilation is generally well tolerated and decreases the work of breathing and improves gas exchange more effectively than pressure support ventilation, which applies only positive inspiratory pressure.

Full facial masks are associated with improved physiologic parameters when compared with nasal masks, likely because of decreased air leak through the mouth and bypass of the high-resistance nasal passages that decrease airflow for any given inspiratory pressure. Patients tend to tolerate nasal masks better, however, and they tend to be associated with less abdominal distention. Regardless of the interface, appropriate fit is key to assuring patient comfort and effective ventilatory support. Air leaks due to poorly fitting masks impair detection of inspiratory effort and end-expiration, leading to failure to trigger or patient-ventilator dyssynchrony. Patients also receive less inspiratory volume and are at risk for excessive drying of the corneas. Overly tight masks lead to skin necrosis. Careful adjustment of the ventilator settings and mask fit improves patient tolerance.

Patients receiving NPPV require close monitoring with frequent clinical assessment. Most patients will be admitted to intensive care units, although studies have shown that carefully selected patients can be treated in less-acute settings. Patients must be assessed for mental status, respiratory rate, use of accessory muscles, chest wall movement, coordination of respiratory effort with the ventilator, and overall comfort. Pulse oximetry monitors oxygen saturation but does not measure $PaCO_2$ and does not replace arterial blood gas analysis in evaluating a patient's response to NPPV.

TABLE 17.2	Indications for Noninvasive Positive Pressure Ventilation (Supported by Randomized Controlled Trial Data)
COPD exacerbations Cardiogenic pulmonary edema Hypoxemic respiratory failure in immunocompromised hosts with pulmonary infiltrates Weaning adjunct in COPD	
COPD, chronic obstructive pulmonary disease.	

ALGORITHM 17.1   **Algorithm for the Initiation of Noninvasive Positive Pressure Ventilation (NPPV) in a Patient with a Chronic Obstructive Pulmonary Disease (COPD) Exacerbation**

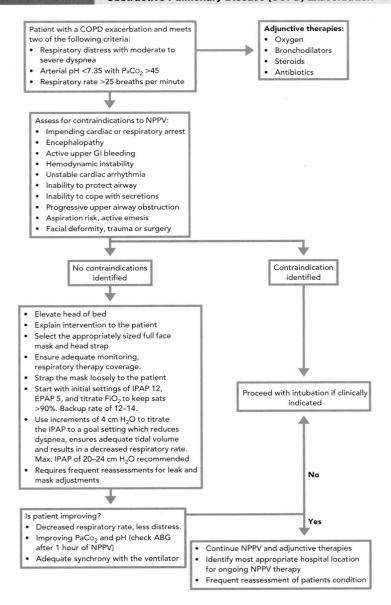

Patient with a COPD exacerbation and meets two of the following criteria:
- Respiratory distress with moderate to severe dyspnea
- Arterial pH <7.35 with P_aCO_2 >45
- Respiratory rate >25 breaths per minute

Adjunctive therapies:
- Oxygen
- Bronchodilators
- Steroids
- Antibiotics

Assess for contraindications to NPPV:
- Impending cardiac or respiratory arrest
- Encephalopathy
- Active upper GI bleeding
- Hemodynamic instability
- Unstable cardiac arrhythmia
- Inability to protect airway
- Inability to cope with secretions
- Progressive upper airway obstruction
- Aspiration risk, active emesis
- Facial deformity, trauma or surgery

No contraindications identified

Contraindication identified

- Elevate head of bed
- Explain intervention to the patient
- Select the appropriately sized full face mask and head strap
- Ensure adequate monitoring, respiratory therapy coverage.
- Strap the mask loosely to the patient
- Start with initial settings of IPAP 12, EPAP 5, and titrate FiO_2 to keep sats >90%. Backup rate of 12–14.
- Use increments of 4 cm H_2O to titrate the IPAP to a goal setting which reduces dyspnea, ensures adequate tidal volume and results in a decreased respiratory rate. Max. IPAP of 20–24 cm H_2O recommended
- Requires frequent reassessments for leak and mask adjustments

Proceed with intubation if clinically indicated

No

Is patient improving?
- Decreased respiratory rate, less distress.
- Improving $PaCO_2$ and pH (check ABG after 1 hour of NPPV)
- Adequate synchrony with the ventilator

Yes

- Continue NPPV and adjunctive therapies
- Identify most appropriate hospital location for ongoing NPPV therapy
- Frequent reassessment of patients condition

GI, gastrointestinal; IPAP, inspiratory positive pressure; EPAP, expiratory positive pressure; ABG, arterial blood gas.

Suggested Reading

Antonelli M, Conti G, Rocco M, et al. A comparison of non-invasive positive pressure ventilation and conventional ventilation in patients with acute respiratory failure. *N Engl J Med*. 1998;339:429–435.

In a prospective, randomized trial of noninvasive positive-pressure ventilation versus endotracheal intubation with conventional mechanical ventilation in patients with hypoxemic acute respiratory failure who required mechanical ventilation, noninvasive ventilation was as effective as conventional ventilation in improving gas exchange and was associated with fewer serious complications and shorter stays in the intensive care unit.

Baudouin S, Blumenthal S, Cooper B, et al. Non-invasive ventilation in acute respiratory failure. *Thorax*. 2002;57:192–211.

Recommendations of the British Society Standard of Care Committee regarding use of non-invasive ventilation.

Brochard L, Mancebo J, Wysocki M, et al. Noninvasive ventilation for acute exacerbations of chronic obstructive pulmonary disease. *N Engl J Med*. 1995;333:817–822.

A prospective, randomized study comparing noninvasive pressure-support ventilation delivered through a face mask with standard treatment in 85 patients admitted to five intensive care units over a 15-month period. In selected patients with acute exacerbations of chronic obstructive pulmonary disease, noninvasive ventilation can reduce the need for endotracheal intubation, the length of the hospital stay, and the in-hospital mortality rate.

Esteban A, Frutos-Vivar F, Ferguson ND, et al. Noninvasive positive-pressure ventilation for respiratory failure after extubation. *N Engl J Med*. 2004;350:2452–2460.

Multicenter, randomized trial in 221 patients who developed recurrent respiratory failure after extubation. The trial was stopped early after an interim analysis. The rate of death in the intensive care unit was higher in the noninvasive-ventilation group than in the standard-therapy group (25 percent vs. 14 percent; relative risk, 1.78; 95 percent confidence interval, 1.03 to 3.20; P = 0.048), and the median time from respiratory failure to reintubation was longer in the noninvasive-ventilation group (12 hours vs. 2 hours 30 minutes, P = 0.02).

Ferrer M, Esquinas A, Leon M, et al. Non-invasive ventilation in severe hypoxemic respiratory failure: a randomized clinical trial. *Am J Respir Crit Care Med*. 2003;168: 1438–1444.

The use of noninvasive ventilation in patients with hypoxemic respiratory failure prevented intubation, reduced the incidence of septic shock, and improved survival in these patients compared with high-concentration oxygen therapy.

Nava S, Ambrosino N, Clini E, et al. Noninvasive mechanical ventilation in the weaning of patients with respiratory failure due to chronic obstructive pulmonary disease: a randomized, controlled trial. *Ann Intern Med*. 1998;128:721–728.

Multicenter, randomized trial in 50 patients with COPD who failed an initial SBT. These patients were then randomized to two methods of weaning: 1) extubation and application of noninvasive pressure support ventilation by face mask and 2) invasive pressure support ventilation by an endotracheal tube. Noninvasive pressure support ventilation during weaning reduced weaning time, shortens the time in the intensive care unit, decreases the incidence of nosocomial pneumonia, and improves 60-day survival rates.

Cardiac Disorders   III

ACUTE MYOCARDIAL INFARCTION   18
Phillip S. Cuculich and Andrew M. Kates

Acute myocardial infarction (AMI) is a common diagnosis among hospitalized and critically ill patients. Each year there are approximately 650,000 new cases of AMI and 450,000 recurrent AMIs in the United States. Despite improved in-hospital survival during several decades, roughly 1 in 25 patients admitted with AMI who survive initial hospitalization will die within 1 year of discharge.

On presentation, the working diagnosis of patients with ischemic chest pain is acute coronary syndrome (ACS; Alg. 18.1). A prompt electrocardiogram (ECG) is essential to distinguish between ST segment elevation ACS (STE-ACS) and non–ST segment elevation ACS (NSTE-ACS). The diagnosis of *myocardial infarction* is supported by evidence of cardiac myocyte death; namely, elevated cardiac-specific serum biomarkers (troponin, myoglobin, creatine kinase-MB isoenzyme). Because most patients who present with ACS and STEs have actively infarcting myocardium, the term *ST-elevation myocardial infarction* (STEMI) is often used synonymously for STE-ACS. Patients without STEs are further stratified into unstable angina or non–STEMI (NSTEMI) based on the negative or positive results of serum cardiac biomarker tests respectively.

Patients with ACS typically present with moderate-to-severe chest discomfort that lasts >15 minutes. Atypical presentations are more common in patients with diabetes, advanced age, and in female patients. The goal for any ACS patient is prompt cardiac risk-stratification between STEMI, NSTEMI, and unstable angina, and appropriate treatment of ischemia.

ST-ELEVATION ACUTE CORONARY SYNDROME

STE-ACS results from sudden occlusion of a coronary artery, which almost exclusively is the product of coronary atherosclerosis with superimposed thrombus. Despite modern multimodality treatment pathways, one in three patients with ACS and STEs do not survive, with nearly half of the deaths occurring in the first hour from ventricular arrhythmias. The extent of cardiac myocyte death worsens with ischemic time and correlates strongly with

ALGORITHM 18.1   Nomenclature of Acute Coronary Syndromes

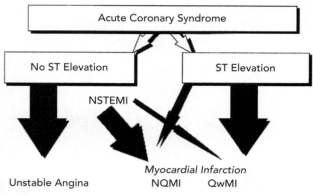

Adapted from Antman EM, Braunwald E. Acute myocardial infarction. In: Braunwald EB, ed. *Heart Disease: A Textbook of Cardiovascular Medicine*. Philadelphia, PA: WB Saunders, 1997.

cardiac morbidity and mortality, leading to the oft-quoted phrase, "time is muscle." As such, mechanical and medical therapies listed here are designed to re-establish blood flow in the shortest time possible.

Algorithm 18.2 is our recommended management pathway that combines established benchmark goals and treatment options for treating STE-ACS/STEMI.

NON–ST-ELEVATION ACUTE CORONARY SYNDROME

The common finding in most patients with NSTE-ACS is a myocardial oxygen supply-demand mismatch. For some, an unstable coronary plaque forms a thrombus (similar to STE-ACS), but does not completely occlude blood flow. Other patients have fixed coronary artery atheromas that do not cause ischemia at rest, but can induce ischemia at times of increased oxygen utilization (tachycardia, surgery, severe hypertension) or decreased oxygen delivery (anemia, hypoxia, hypotension). Cardiac ischemia is also a common intraoperative complication, often as a combination of increased oxygen demand and decreased oxygen delivery. It often manifests postoperatively as elevated cardiac biomarkers.

The initial goal in evaluating patients with NSTE-ACS is risk-stratification aimed at preventing major adverse cardiac events, defined as death, nonfatal myocardial infarction (MI), and the need for urgent revascularization. A useful and well-validated method is the thrombolysis in myocardial ischemia (TIMI) risk score. Patients with a higher score are more likely to suffer from major adverse cardiac events than those with a lower score. High-risk patients benefit more from early, aggressive medical and revascularization therapies. Our recommended algorithm for the treatment of patients with NSTE-ACS is shown in Algorithm 18.3.

HOSPITAL CARE OF THE ACS PATIENT

Patients with ACS are at an increased risk for recurrent MI and death, both in the hospital and after discharge. Each hospitalization provides a venue to work with patients to aggressively reduce the risk of these events. One thoughtful way to organize the various in-hospital and postdischarge treatments is the "ABCDE" list (Table 18.1). These 12 items should be considered an acute treatment guide as well as a discharge checklist for any patient presenting with ACS.

TABLE 18.1	ABCDE's as an Inpatient Treatment Guide and Discharge Checklist for Patients with Acute Coronary Syndrome	
A	Antiplatelet	Aspirin indefinitely. Consider clopidogrel if appropriate.
	Antithrombin	Heparin or enoxaparin during hospitalization.
	ACE-inhibitor	Particularly beneficial if reduced EF ($<$40%) or high-risk features.
	AT2-receptor blocker	For ACE-inhibitor intolerance.
B	Beta-blocker	All patients.
	Blood pressure	Goal $<$130/80 for CRI, DM. Otherwise, goal $<$140/90.
C	Cigarette cessation	Complete cessation. Nicotine replacement, oral medications, counseling.
	Cholesterol	Goal: LDL, $<$70 mg/dL; HDL, $>$40 mg/dL. Statin preferred.
D	Diet	If overweight, reduce daily diet by $>$500 calories.
	Diabetes	Goal Hgb A1C $<$7.0%.
E	Exercise	30 minutes of activity at least 4 days/week. Supervised cardiac rehab can be beneficial.
	Ejection fraction	Measurement of ejection fraction prior to discharge. Consider aldosterone antagonist, digitalis, and ICD if indicated.

EF, ejection fraction; CRI, chronic renal insufficiency; DM, diabetes mellitus; LDL, low-density lipoprotein; HDL, high-density lipoprotein; Hgb, hemoglobin; ICD, implantable cardioverter-defibrillator.

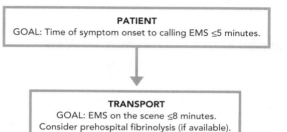

ALGORITHM 18.2 — Goals and Treatment of ST-Segment Elevation Myocardial Infarction

PATIENT
GOAL: Time of symptom onset to calling EMS ≤5 minutes.

TRANSPORT
GOAL: EMS on the scene ≤8 minutes.
Consider prehospital fibrinolysis (if available).

MEDICAL FACILITY- 3Ds-DATA, DECISION, DRUGS
DATA- Focused history and physical exam. GOAL: ECG ≤10 minutes
STEMI = ischemic symptoms <u>with</u>;
1) ≥1 mm ST elevation in two contiguous leads **OR**
2) New LBBB
- If inferior MI (leads II, III, avF)→ <u>right-sided ECG</u> (rV4) for right ventricular MI
- If ST-depression in precordial leads→ <u>posterior ECG</u> (V7, V8, V9) for posterior MI

DECISION—PRIMARY PCI
GOAL: Door-to-balloon time ≤90 minutes
<u>Preferred over fibrinolytics</u> if available
Also preferred when:
- Cardiogenic shock
- Contraindication to fibrinolytic therapy
- Late presentation (>3 hours of symptoms)
- The diagnosis of STEMI is in doubt

Continued on next page

DECISION—FIBRINOLYTIC THERAPY
GOAL: Door-to-needle time ≤30 minutes
Preferred when:
- Lack of available PCI facility
- Delay in transport to PCI facility
<u>Absolute</u> contraindications to fibrinolytics:
  Prior hemorrhagic stroke
  Any stroke <1 year
  Known intracranial neoplasm
  Active internal bleeding
  Known or suspected aortic dissection
<u>Relative</u> contraindications to fibrinolytics:
  BP >180/110
  CPR >10 minutes
  Remote history of stroke
  INR >2.0
  Recent trauma, major surgery, or
    internal bleeding within 4 weeks
  Noncompressible vascular puncture

Continued on next page

ALGORITHM 18.2 | **Goals and Treatment of ST-Segment Elevation Myocardial Infarction (Continued)**

DRUGS-UNLESS CONTRAINDICATED, ALL PATIENTS RECEIVE:

- Aspirin 160–325 mg chewed
- Metoprolol 5 mg IV × 3 doses- caution if SBP <100, HR <50 or early signs of shock.
- IV nitroglycerin, started at 10 mcg/min & titrated for symptoms-caution if suspected inferior MI, SBP <90 mm Hg, HR <50 bpm or >100 bpm, or phosphodiesterase inhibitors for erectile dysfunction in past 24 hours.
- Consider morphine sulfate 2–4 mg IV for chest pain unresponsive to nitrates
- Antithrombin therapy:
  Unfractionated heparin 60 U/kg IV bolus, max 4,000 U; then 14 U/kg/hr, max 1,000 U /hr **OR**, Enoxaparin (Lovenox) 1 mg/kg SQ- *avoid Lovenox if renal insufficiency.*
- Clopidogrel (Plavix) 300–600 mg PO for one dose-**unless high suspicion for surgical CAD** (i.e., advanced age, diabetes, known multivessel CAD)

DRUGS-PRIMARY PCI
Consider an "upstream" GP-IIb/ IIIa inhibitor:
Abciximab (Reopro) 0.25 mg/kg IV bolus then 0.125 mcg/kg/min (max 10 mcg/min)

DRUGS-FIBRINOLYTIC
1. Regimens include:
   Reteplase (Retavase) + UFH (**Preferred for age ≥75 years**)
   Retaplase 10 U IV bolus over 2 min and repeat 10 U IV bolus 30 min later.
   UFH IV as listed above.
2. Tenecteplase (TNKase) + Enoxaparin (**Preferred for age <75 years and/or >4 hours of symptoms if no PCI available**)
   TNKase dose is based on weight and given as a single IV bolus*.
   Enoxaparin 30 mg IV push followed by 1 mg/kg SQ.
3. $^1/_2$ dose Reteplase + Abciximab + $^1/_2$ dose UFH (**Preferred for age <75 years or those with large anterior MIs**)
   Retaplase 5 U IV bolus over 2 min and repeat 5 U IV bolus 30 min later.
   Abciximab 0.25 mg/kg IV bolus then 0.125 mcg/kg/min (max 10 mcg/min).
   UFH 60 U/kg IV bolus, max 4,000 U; then 7 U/kg/hr infusion, max 1,000 U/hr).

REPERFUSION-PRIMARY PCI
GOAL: Restoration of TIMI 3 flow
Advantages of PCI over fibrinolytics:
1) Superior restoration of coronary flow
2) Defines anatomy & risk stratification
3) Fewer complications
4) Treatment of thrombus AND plaque

*TNKase Dosing	
Weight (kg)	**TNKase (mg)**
<60	30
60–69	35
70–79	40
80–89	45
≥90	50

REPERFUSION-THROMBOLYSIS
Considered successful if:
1) Complete resolution of chest pain
2) ST segment elevation improvement >50%
3) Accelerated idioventricular rhythm (AIVR)

EMS, emergency medical services; STEMI, ST-elevation myocardial infarction; ECG, electrocardiogram; LBBB, left bundle branch block; MI, myocardial infarction; PCI, percutaneous coronary intervention; BP, blood pressure; CPR, cardiopulmonary resuscitation; INR, international normalized ratio; IV, intravenous; SBP, systolic blood pressure; HR, heart rate; bpm, beats per minute; SQ, subcutaneous; CAD, coronary artery disease; GP, glycoprotein; TIMI, thrombolysis in myocardial ischemia; UFH, unfractionated heparin.

ALGORITHM 18.3   **Risk-Stratification and Treatment Algorithm for Non-ST-Segment Elevation Acute Coronary Syndrome**

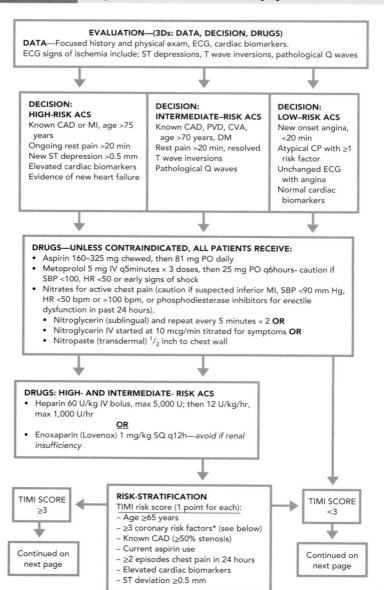

EVALUATION—(3Ds: DATA, DECISION, DRUGS)
DATA—Focused history and physical exam, ECG, cardiac biomarkers.
ECG signs of ischemia include; ST depressions, T wave inversions, pathological Q waves

DECISION:
HIGH-RISK ACS
Known CAD or MI, age >75 years
Ongoing rest pain >20 min
New ST depression >0.5 mm
Elevated cardiac biomarkers
Evidence of new heart failure

DECISION:
INTERMEDIATE–RISK ACS
Known CAD, PVD, CVA, age >70 years, DM
Rest pain >20 min, resolved
T wave inversions
Pathological Q waves

DECISION:
LOW–RISK ACS
New onset angina, <20 min
Atypical CP with ≥1 risk factor
Unchanged ECG with angina
Normal cardiac biomarkers

DRUGS—UNLESS CONTRAINDICATED, ALL PATIENTS RECEIVE:
• Aspirin 160–325 mg chewed, then 81 mg PO daily
• Metoprolol 5 mg IV q5minutes × 3 doses, then 25 mg PO q6hours- caution if SBP <100, HR <50 or early signs of shock
• Nitrates for active chest pain (caution if suspected inferior MI, SBP <90 mm Hg, HR <50 bpm or >100 bpm, or phosphodiesterase inhibitors for erectile dysfunction in past 24 hours).
  • Nitroglycerin (sublingual) and repeat every 5 minutes × 2 **OR**
  • Nitroglycerin IV started at 10 mcg/min titrated for symptoms **OR**
  • Nitropaste (transdermal) $^1/_2$ inch to chest wall

DRUGS: HIGH- AND INTERMEDIATE- RISK ACS
• Heparin 60 U/kg IV bolus, max 5,000 U; then 12 U/kg/hr, max 1,000 U/hr
                    OR
• Enoxaparin (Lovenox) 1 mg/kg SQ q12h—*avoid if renal insufficiency*

TIMI SCORE
≥3

RISK-STRATIFICATION
TIMI risk score (1 point for each):
– Age ≥65 years
– ≥3 coronary risk factors* (see below)
– Known CAD (≥50% stenosis)
– Current aspirin use
– ≥2 episodes chest pain in 24 hours
– Elevated cardiac biomarkers
– ST deviation ≥0.5 mm

TIMI SCORE
<3

Continued on next page

Continued on next page

*Coronary risk factors include diabetes, cigarette smoking, HTN (BP 140/90 mm Hg or on antihypertensive medication), low HDL cholesterol (<40 mg/dL), family history of premature CAD (CAD in male first-degree relative 55 or younger, CAD in female first-degree relative 65 or younger), and age (men 45 years and older; women 55 years and older).

ALGORITHM 18.3	Risk-Stratification and Treatment Algorithm for Non-ST-Segment Elevation Acute Coronary Syndrome (*Continued*)

Calculated TIMI score	14-day Risk of MACE
0 or 1	5 %
2	8 %
3	13 %
4	20 %
5	28 %
6 or 7	41 %

TIMI score ≥3

TIMI score <3

EARLY INVASIVE STRATEGY
GP-IIb/IIIa inhibitor:
Eptifibitide (Integrillin) 180 mcg/kg
   bolus (max 22.6 mg), then 2 mcg/
   kg/min (max 15 mg/hr) infusion.
   Can reduce infusion to
   1 mcg/kg/min if CrCl <50 mL/min
OR
Tirofiban (Aggrastat) 0.4 mcg/kg/min
   for 30 min, then 0.1 mcg/kg/min
   infusion. Can reduce bolus and
   infusion to half-dose for
   CrCl <30 mL/min

Consider Clopidogrel (Plavix)
   300–600 mg PO loading dose
   (unless high suspicion for
   surgical CAD (i.e., advanced age,
   diabetes, known multi-vessel CAD))

CONSERVATIVE STRATEGY
Noninvasive cardiac stress test
Exercise is preferred for prognostic
   information

Avoid adenosine if bronchospasm
Avoid dobutamine if
   tachyarrhythmias, severe
   AS, uncontrolled HTN, AAA.

Exercise Treadmill (men)–
   68% sensitive, 77% specific
Exercise Treadmill (women)–
   61% sensitive, 70% specific
Exercise, Adenosine Thallium–
   88% sensitive, 77% specific
Exercise or Dobutamine Echo–
   76% sensitive, 88% specific

High-risk result

Low-risk result

EARLY INVASIVE MANAGEMENT PLAN
Cardiac catheterization within 4-48 hours
If chest pain is not controlled,
   consider emergent catheterization
Medical management (ABCDE*)

CONSERVATIVE MANAGEMENT PLAN
Medical management (ABCDE*)
Cardiac risk factor modification
Consider other causes of
   chest pain

*See Table 18.1.
ECG, electrocardiogram; ACS, acute coronary syndrome; CAD, coronary artery disease; MI, myocardial infarction; PVD, peripheral vascular disease; CVA, cerebrovascular accident; DM, diabete mellitus; CP, chest pain; PO, by mouth; SBP, systolic blood pressure; HR, heart rate; MI, myocardial infarction; bpm, beats per minute; IV, intravenous; SQ, subcutaneous; TIMI, thrombolysis in myocardial ischemia; MACE, major adverse cardiac events; CrCl, creatinine clearance; HTN, hypertension; AAA abdominal aortic aneurysm; GP, glycoprotein.

COMPLICATIONS AFTER MYOCARDIAL INFARCTION

Postinfarction complication rates have fallen dramatically since the advent of early reperfusion strategies. Nevertheless, many patients (those with large infarction, silent infarction, late presentation, delayed or incomplete reperfusion) remain at high risk for severe complications. The mnemonic FEAR AMI is a logical way to remember and respect these potential life-threatening complications while caring for patients in the intensive care unit. The following sections elucidate the individual letters of this mnemonic.

Failure

Left ventricular dysfunction is the single most powerful predictor of survival following an MI. Hypotension, tachycardia, and hypoxia predict a particularly poor outcome. Clinical symptoms of heart failure are more likely in patients with large infarcts, advanced age, and/or diabetes. Treatment for post-MI heart failure includes supplemental oxygen, diuretic therapy, afterload reduction with vasodilators and/or inhibition of the renin-angiotensin system, and digitalis. Severe heart failure may require vasopressor therapy. Beta-agonists dobutamine and dopamine and/or phosphodiesterase inhibitor, milrinone, have theoretical mechanistic benefits over epinephrine, norepinepherine, and isoproterenol (see Chapter 21).

Effusion and Pericarditis

Post-MI effusions are rarely life-threatening. However, if tamponade physiology is present, consider hemorrhagic effusion from a ventricular rupture. Generally, the presence of an effusion on echocardiogram is a reason to withhold anticoagulation in the post-MI period to avoid contributing to a hemopericardium. If anticoagulation cannot be stopped, heightened vigilance for this complication is warranted.

Post-MI pericarditis can present in the first days to 6 weeks after the infarct. This complication is due to local pericardial irritation, usually by a transmural infarct. It is essential to distinguish pericarditis from recurrent ischemia. Pericarditis pain is often worse with deep inspiration, improved with sitting forward, radiates to the scapulae, and can be associated with characteristic ECG findings.

Dressler syndrome is a type of postinfarction pericarditis that occurs 1 to 8 weeks after the infarct. It is thought to be immune-mediated and is best treated with high-dose aspirin. Glucocorticosteroids and other nonsteroidal anti-inflammatory agents are avoided in the first month after infarction because of the potential to impair ventricular healing, leading to increased rates of ventricular rupture.

Arrhythmia

The management of many common arrhythmias is discussed elsewhere (see Chapter 19). Several infarction-specific arrhythmias are presented here.

Accelerated idioventricular rhythm is considered a "reperfusion rhythm," as it is often seen immediately after a successful reperfusion. No treatment is warranted for this arrhythmia when it is combined with a clinical scenario of reperfusion.

Ventricular tachycardia is often the terminal rhythm in the peri-infarct period and is associated with increased mortality when occurring in the first 48 hours of hospitalization. Aggressive restoration of sinus rhythm is achieved through the use of antiarrhythmic medications (amiodarone, lidocaine) and/or synchronized direct current cardioversion. Because hypokalemia and hypomagnesemia have been associated with development of sustained ventricular tachycardia (NSVT), it is reasonable to correct potassium (K) and magnesium (Mg) levels in the setting of an infarction (K >4meq/L and Mg >2meq/L). In contrast, nonsustained ventricular tachycardia is not associated with an increased risk of death during the index hospitalization or during the first year after infarction and suppressive treatment of asymptomatic NSVT is not routinely recommended in the post-MI patient.

MI can cause block at any level of the conduction system. The location of the infarct has a large influence on the prognosis and treatment of conduction disease. In general, proximal (atrioventricular [AV] nodal) conduction disease is associated with a right coronary artery infarct. This causes a transient AV block and often does not warrant immediate temporary pacemaker placement in the absence of symptoms. One exception is symptomatic AV

TABLE 18.2	Features of Ischemia-Related Atrioventricular (AV) Conduction Disease	
	Proximal Conduction Disease	**Distal Conduction Disease**
Compromised artery	Right coronary/posterior descending (90%)	Septal perforators of left anterior descending
Site of block	Intranodal*	Infranodal*
Site of infarction	Inferoposterior	Anteroseptal
Type of AV block	1st degree or Mobitz I	Mobitz II or 3rd degree
Duration of AV block	Transient (2–3 days)	Variable
Mortality rate	Low, unless CHF or hypotension	High, because of extensive infarct
Temporary pacemaker	Rare	Early consideration, especially for anterior infarct and bifascicular block
Permanent pacemaker	Almost never	Indicated if high-grade block in His-Purkinje system or associated bundle branch block

CHF, congestive heart failure.
*The right coronary artery (RCA) typically supplies the sinoatrial node, AV node, and distal right bundle, while the left coronary artery supplies the Bundle of His, proximal right bundle, and left anterior fascicle. The left posterior fascicle is supplied by the posterior descending artery, typically off the RCA, as well as the distal LAD.

block in the setting of right ventricular infarction, where restoration of AV synchrony can improve right ventricular filling and thus, cardiac output. Distal (infranodal) conduction disease is frequently associated with a left anterior descending/septal infarct and is more lasting and life-threatening. Immediate pacing efforts should be pursued. Additional features of AV conduction disease are shown in Table 18.2 and acute treatment is discussed in Chapter 19.

Rupture

The clinical presentation of a ventricular rupture is often striking and life-threatening. The rupture can be in the ventricular free wall, ventricular septum, or papillary muscle (Table 18.3). A clinical suspicion and the timely use of echocardiography and pulmonary artery catheter are essential for prompt diagnosis of this serious complication.

Aneurysm

True left ventricular (LV) aneurysms complicate <5% of acute infarctions. They are thought to be a consequence of a complete occlusion of the supplying coronary artery without significant collateral blood flow. As such, anteroapical aneurysms (due to left anterior descending artery occlusion) are four times more common than inferoposterior aneurysms.

LV aneurysms are associated with a considerably lower survival rate. When compared with patients with similar ejection fractions, patients with LV aneurysms have a sixfold increase in mortality, mainly resulting from ventricular arrhythmias. LV aneurysms are often supported by fibrous tissue and, thus, rarely rupture. The characteristic ECG findings of LV aneurysms are Q waves with persistent ST elevations, although the diagnosis is best made by a noninvasive imaging study. Because of the risk of mural thrombus formation and systemic embolization, patients with an LV aneurysm are generally treated with long-term anticoagulation with warfarin. Additionally, as ST segments may remain elevated for some time after successful reperfusion, persistent ST elevations (>4 weeks after AMI) is generally required for the ECG diagnosis of LV aneurysm.

TABLE 18.3	Clinical Profile of Mechanical Complications of Myocardial Infarction (MI)		
	Ventricular Septal Defect	Free Wall Rupture	Papillary Muscle Rupture
Days post-MI	3–5	3–6	3–5
Anterior MI	66%	50%	25%
New murmur	90%	25%	50%
Palpable thrill	Yes	No	Rare
Previous MI	25%	25%	30%
2D echo findings	Visualize defect	May have pericardial effusion	Flail or prolapsing leaflet
Doppler echo findings	Detect shunt		Regurgitant jet in LA
PA catheterization	Oxygen step-up in RV	Equalization of diastolic pressure	Prominent c-v wave in PCW tracing
Medical mortality	90%	90%	90%
Surgical mortality	50%	Case reports	40%–90%

2D, two-dimensional; echo, echocardiogram; LA, left atrium; PA, pulmonary artery; RV, right ventricle; PCW, pulmonary capillary wedge.
Modified from Labovitz AJ, Miller LW and Kennedy HL. Mechanical complications of acute myocardial infarction. *Cardiovasc Rev Rep.* 1984;5:948, with permission.

Distinct from an aneurysm is a pseudoaneurysm. Rather than involving layers of muscle, the myocardium perforates and, as such, this clinical entity can be thought of as a "contained rupture." It is most often seen with inferior infarctions, and treatment is emergent surgery. Both surgical and medical treatments carry a very high mortality.

Myocardial Infarction

The complaint of chest pain after an MI may represent recurrent ischemia from incomplete revascularization. Ischemia recurs in 20% to 30% of patients receiving thrombolytic therapy and up to 10% of patients after percutaneous revascularization. Serial cardiac biomarkers and ECGs can help identify at-risk patients. Normally, antianginal medications (heparin, nitrates, beta-blockers) can control symptoms.

New postinfarct ST elevations can be caused by reinfarction, pericarditis, or dyskinetic/aneurysmal ventricular segments. Reinfarction due to stent thrombosis usually has a dramatic presentation with severe anginal pain refractory to medical therapy and evolving ST elevations on ECG. These findings warrant additional prompt revascularization efforts.

Suggested Reading

2005 American Heart Association Guidelines for Cardiopulmonary Resuscitation and Emergency Cardiovascular Care, Part 8: Stabilization of the patient with acute coronary syndromes. *Circulation.* 2005;112[Suppl I]: IV-89–110.
A thorough and easy-to-read review of the studies that form the foundation for the management of ACS patients. Available online at www.circulationaha.org
Antman EM, Cohen M, Bernink PJ, et al. The TIMI risk score for unstable angina/non-ST elevation MI: a method for prognostication and therapeutic decision making. *JAMA.* 2000;284:835–842.
One of several validations of the popular TIMI risk score for NSTE-ACS.
Antman EM, Anbe DT, Armstrong PW, et al. Management of patients with STEMI: executive summary. *J Am Coll Cardiol.* 2004;44:671–719.
Invaluable consensus guidelines detailing the state-of-the-art for management of patients with STEMI. Available online at www.acc.org

Braunwald E, Antman EM, Beasley JW, et al. Management of patients with unstable angina and non-ST-segment elevation myocardial infarction update. *J Am Coll Cardiol.* 2002;40:1366–1374.
Equally invaluable consensus guidelines for patients with NSTE-ACS. Several years older than its STEMI counterpart this document is awaiting an update. Available online at www.acc.org
Gluckman TJ, Baranowski B, Ashen MD, et al. A practical and evidence-based approach to cardiovascular disease risk reduction. *Arch Intern Med.* 2004;164:1490–1500.
A clever, organized approach to improve health-care providers' adherence to guidelines for proven, though often overlooked, therapies for ACS patients.

19

CARDIAC ARRHYTHMIAS AND CONDUCTION ABNORMALITIES
Timothy J. Bedient and Timothy W. Smith

This chapter addresses the causes, recognition, and treatment of cardiac arrhythmias occurring in hospitalized and critically ill patients. Cardiac arrhythmias can disrupt cardiac output (CO) by impairing the heart rate (HR) and/or stroke volume (SV) according to the equation $CO = HR \times SV$. The clinical presentation of cardiac arrhythmias varies widely, and they may present as (a) asymptomatic findings on an electrocardiogram (ECG) or cardiac monitor, (b) symptoms without hemodynamic instability (e.g., palpitations), (c) hemodynamic instability in conscious patients, or (d) cardiac arrest. Initial patient evaluation in hospitalized patients includes ensuring (a) adequate airway and breathing support; (b) continuous monitoring of cardiac rhythm, blood pressure, and oxyhemoglobin saturation; and (c) adequate intravenous (IV) access. The cardiac rhythm should be analyzed by 12-lead ECG when possible, but initial treatment may be based on the rhythm seen on the intensive care unit bedside monitor or defibrillator. If time permits, the specific underlying rhythm should be identified, the cause sought, and therapy tailored accordingly. However, *cardiac arrest and severely symptomatic tachycardia and bradycardia require immediate treatment based on the advanced cardiac life support (ACLS) algorithms* shown later in this chapter in Algorithms 19.4, 19.5, and 19.6.

TACHARRHYTHMIAS

Tachycardia, defined as a heart rate >100 beats per minute, can be separated into (a) those that arise above the ventricles, termed *supraventricular tachycardias,* and (b) those that arise within the ventricles, termed *ventricular tachycardias*. Tachycardias can generally be distinguished on the basis of the heart rate, the width and morphology of the QRS complex, and the length of the PR interval. The approach to differentiating narrow and wide QRS complex tachycardias is outlined in Algorithms 19.1 and 19.2, respectively.

Supraventricular Tachycardias

Sinus tachycardia originates from the sinus node, and is not considered a primary arrhythmia. The ECG shows a normal P wave preceding each QRS complex. Sinus tachycardia in the intensive care unit can be a physiologic response to volume depletion, fever, pain, anxiety, shock, hypoxia, or in patients on vasopressor or inotropic support. Humans maximum heart rate is age-dependent and roughly limited to 220 – age in years (e.g., 150 in a 70 year old man).

   Treatment of sinus tachycardia is directed at the underlying cause, which includes treating infections and fever, volume repletion, anxiolytics, and pain control. Rate-controlling agents are generally not indicated unless the rapid heart rate causes symptoms of low cardiac output, such as in severe anxiety and pain. Reflex sinus tachycardia may be important to maintain adequate cardiac output. Direct treatment of the tachycardia without treatment of the underlying cause may be deleterious.

Atrial fibrillation is a chaotic rhythm within the atria of 350 to 600 beats per minute without an appreciable P wave on ECG. All atrial beats are not conducted because of the refractory period in the atrioventricular (AV) node, and conduction is variably timed, resulting in an irregular ventricular rate. If the ventricular rate is greater than 100 beats per minute, a rapid ventricular response is said to be present. The associated rapid heart rate and the lack of atrial contribution to pumping blood can compromise cardiac output, requiring immediate

ALGORITHM 19.1 **Approach to Differentiating Narrow QRS Complex Tachycardias**

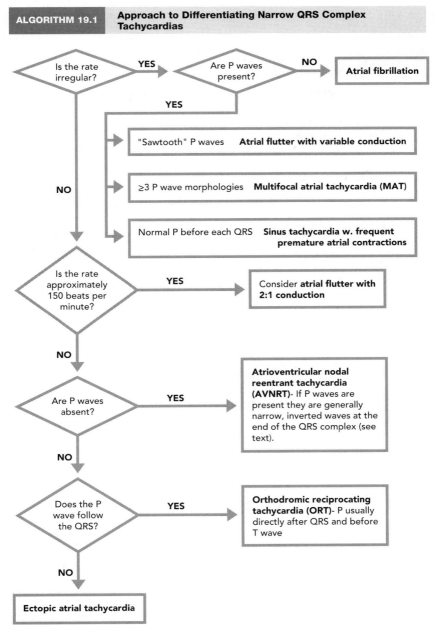

RBBB, right bundle branch block; LBBB, left bundle branch block; MAT, multifocal atrial tachycardia; PAC, premature atrial contraction; SVT, supraventricular tachycardia; ART, antidromic re-entrant tachycardia; DC, direct current; IV, intravenous.

ALGORITHM 19.2

**Approach to Differentiating Wide QRS Complex Tachycardias.
Wide complex tachycardias (except clear sinus tachycardia
with aberrancy) should initially be assumed to be ventricular
tachycardia (VT) and treatment urgency based on
assessment of patient condition and hemodynamics
(see text for details)**

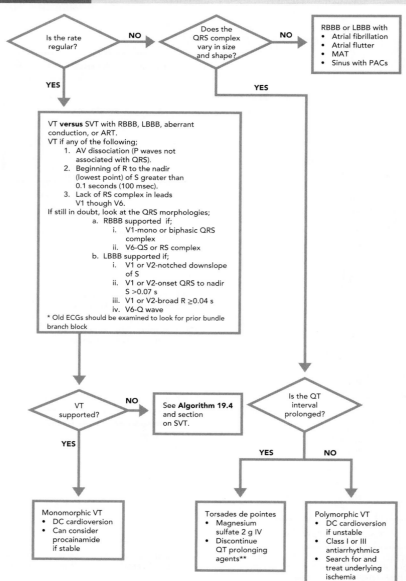

** Agents that prolong the QT interval can be found on-line at http://www.arizonacert.org/medical-pros/drug-lists/drug-lists.htm

treatment. Loss of organized atrial contraction creates stasis of the blood pool within the atria, which may facilitate intracardiac thrombus formation and thromboembolism.

Atrial fibrillation is seen in patients with chronic cardiopulmonary disease. It can also be the presenting finding of thyrotoxicosis, infection, pulmonary embolization, acute alcohol intoxication, pericarditis, and stress, and is common postoperatively. It is a rare presentation of acute myocardial infarction.

Typical *atrial flutter* is caused by a re-entrant rhythm localized to the right atrium, which generates impulses at a rate of approximately 300 beats per minute. The ventricular rate is frequently 150 beats per minute (half the atrial rate) due to 2:1 block within the AV node. In 3:1 block, every third beat is conducted, and the ventricular rate is approximately 100 beats per minute. A large portion of the atria is depolarized at once, causing a classic "sawtooth" appearance on the baseline of the ECG, with fairly narrow, negative flutter waves in the inferior leads (II, III, aVF). The ventricular rate may be regular, but can be irregular if conduction is variable (i.e., 2:1 alternating with 3:1). It is seen in patients with underlying heart disease and is also commonly seen in patients after open heart surgery. If left untreated, it may degrade to atrial fibrillation.

Treatment of atrial fibrillation and atrial flutter is outlined in Algorithm 19.3. Precipitating factors listed here should be sought and treated. Preoperative beta-blockers can reduce the incidence of postoperative atrial fibrillation/flutter. Thromboembolic risk management typically involves anticoagulation with warfarin overlapping with IV heparin until the international normalized ratio (INR) is >2. Patients with contraindications to anticoagulation should be treated with aspirin if possible. Long-term anticoagulation therapy is beyond the scope of this chapter.

Paroxysmal supraventricular tachycardias (PSVT) are characterized by sudden onset and termination (hence, the name). The most common PSVT in adults is *atrioventricular nodal re-entrant tachycardia* (AVNRT). It is caused by a re-entrant electrical loop within the AV node. The rate generally varies from 120 to 250 beats per minute and is associated with a narrow QRS complex in the absence of aberrancy or an underlying bundle branch block. The atria and ventricles typically depolarize at virtually the same time, and thus the P waves are frequently not visible, obscured by the QRS complexes. If visible, they generally present as narrow inverted P waves at the end of the QRS complex, commonly described as a "pseudo R" in V1 and/or "a pseudo S" in lead II. AV nodal re-entrant tachycardia is not associated with any specific diseases, can occur at any age, and is more common in women.

PSVT may also be mediated by an accessory pathway between the atria and ventricles that bypasses the AV node. *Manifest* accessory pathways are seen on the sinus rhythm ECG as a delta wave of pre-excitation. The pre-excitation also causes a short PR interval because the accessory pathway does not have the delayed conduction of the AV node. Accessory pathways may conduct antegrade (forming the delta wave) or retrograde. *Concealed* accessory AV pathways only conduct retrograde, and are invisible in sinus rhythm. Either of these pathways may mediate an *orthodromic re-entrant tachycardia* in which the electrical impulse propagates antegrade through the AV node and retrograde (from ventricle to atrium) through the accessory pathway. The result is a narrow QRS complex tachycardia, typically with inverted retrograde P waves between the QRS and T wave (although the QRS may be wide because of aberrancy, e.g., bundle branch block or fascicular block).

The patient with visible pre-excitation (delta wave and short PR interval) in sinus rhythm and with palpitations (usually from paroxysmal orthodromic re-entrant tachycardia) is said to have *Wolff-Parkinson-White syndrome* (WPW). Patients with WPW are also prone to arrhythmias with antegrade conduction through the accessory pathway. These include *antidromic re-entrant tachycardia*, in which the excitation propagates antegrade through the accessory pathway and retrograde through the AV node. Atrial arrhythmias (including atrial fibrillation) may also conduct antegrade through the accessory pathway. The short refractory period of the accessory pathway may allow very rapid conduction of impulses to the ventricles, resulting in rapid "pre-excited atrial fibrillation" with ventricular rates up to 300 beats per minute, often resulting in hemodynamic instability requiring urgent intervention. Rapid conduction of atrial fibrillation through an accessory pathway may also induce ventricular fibrillation. This is thought to be the pathogenesis of the rare sudden death that is associated with WPW.

Treatment of PSVT aims at aborting the re-entrant rhythm by blocking conduction through the AV node with vagal maneuvers (valsalva, carotid massage, face immersion in

ALGORITHM 19.3   Treatment of Atrial Fibrillation and Atrial Flutter (see Chapter 83 Common Drug Dosages and Side Effects)

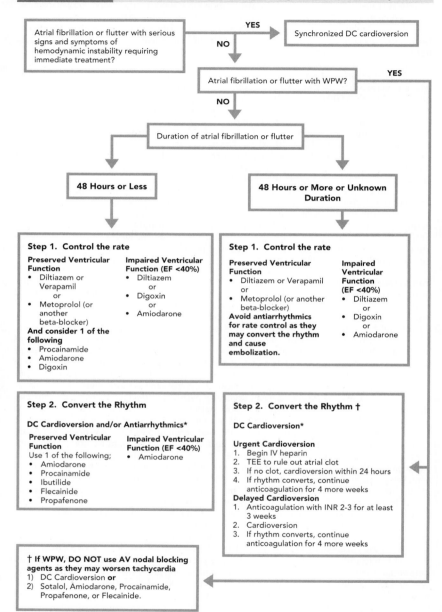

*Premedicate when possible with a sedative (e.g., diazepam, midazolam, ketamine, etomidate) and analgesic (e.g., fentanyl, morphine). Perform synchronized cardioversion with 100 J, 200 J, 300 J, 360 J, biphasic energy or monophasic equivalent, starting with lowest energy level and increasing if needed. Perform asynchronous cardioversion if delays in synchronized cardioversion with worsening clinical status.

DC, direct current; WPW, Wolff-Parkinson-White; EF, ejection fraction; IV, intravenous; TEE, transesophageal echocardiogram; INR, international normalized ratio.

cold water [diving reflex]) or adenosine given as a 6 mg IV bolus ($t_{1/2}$ approximately 10 seconds). A second 12-mg dose can be given after 1 to 2 minutes if the first was ineffective, and a third dose of 12 or 18 mg can be given if needed. If these treatments fail, the AV nodal blocking agents beta-blockers, calcium channel blockers, or digoxin should be used. Patients with WPW and pre-excited atrial fibrillation or flutter must be rapidly treated with direct current cardioversion or class IA, IC, or III drugs (e.g., procainamide, flecainide, and amiodarone), which slow myocardial conduction and prolong the refractory period, and not AV nodal blocking agents as they can increase conduction down the accessory pathway (Alg. 19.3).

Ectopic atrial tachycardia occurs when there is automaticity at a single focus outside the sinoatrial (SA) node. A P wave precedes each QRS as in sinus tachycardia, but the P wave axis is altered. When increased automaticity occurs at three or more different atrial sites, which may include the SA node, it is termed *multifocal atrial tachycardia*, with the alternating foci causing at least three P wave morphologies on ECG. Both can be seen in cases of digitalis toxicity (which causes increased automaticity), severe cardiopulmonary disease, hypokalemia, hyperadrenergic states, and as a side effect of theophylline.

Treatment includes AV nodal blocking agents and removal of inciting agents/factors.

Ventricular Tachycardias

The two main tachyarrhythmias arising from the ventricles are *ventricular fibrillation* (VF) and *ventricular tachycardia* (VT). VT may be monomorphic, if the QRS morphology is fixed, or polymorphic, if the QRS complex is variable. Polymorphic VT is more like VF than monomorphic VT in that it results in chaotic ventricular activation, often with hemodynamic instability, possibly leading to cardiac arrest and sudden death. Also like VF, it is more likely to occur in the setting of acute ischemia, infarct, or acute heart failure.

Monomorphic VT results from re-entrant electrical impulses within the ventricles or from a focal ventricular site with frequent spontaneous action potentials that propagate to the remainder of the ventricles. VT is characterized on ECG by a wide QRS complex (>0.12 seconds), and a rate usually between 100 and 200 beats per minute (although it may be higher). VT that lasts <30 seconds is termed *nonsustained VT* (NSVT), and sustained VT (just termed *VT*) if it lasts >30 seconds. The most common setting for monomorphic VT is in healed myocardial infarction. It occurs less commonly in acute ischemia and infarct. Importantly, monomorphic VT may occur in the absence of structural heart disease. The "idiopathic VTs" do not have a poor prognosis and may not cause hemodynamic instability, emphasizing the need to assess and treat the patient's condition, and not solely the ECG.

An important specific type of polymorphic VT is *torsades de pointes*, which is polymorphic VT associated with prolongation of the QT interval (in sinus rhythm) from numerous causes, including (a) drugs (especially tricyclic antidepressants, certain antiarrhythmics, macrolides, and fluoroquinolone; see website in Algorithm 19.2), (b) electrolyte abnormalities (hypokalemia, hypomagnesemia, and hypocalcemia), and (c) congenital long QT syndromes. Torsades de pointes appears on ECG as a characteristic pattern of oscillating amplitude of the QRS, or "twisting," around the baseline. Torsades de pointes is generally symptomatic but may be nonsustained. If prolonged, hemodynamic instability, syncope, and/sudden death may result.

Wide complex tachycardias (except clear sinus tachycardia with aberrancy) should initially be assumed to be VT and the urgency of treatment should depend on assessment of the patient and the hemodynamic situation. Distinguishing VT from SVT with a wide QRS is therefore of secondary importance. Mistaken diagnosis of "SVT with aberrancy" can result in mistreatment. The differential diagnosis of wide complex tachycardia is threefold: (a) VT, (b) SVT with aberrancy (typical bundle branch or fascicular blocks or atypical aberrancy), and (c) pre-excited supraventricular rhythm (including atrial fibrillation) in which case the ECG in sinus rhythm will typically feature a delta wave.

Algorithm 19.2 shows the ECG criteria that favor VT. Also, old ECGs should be examined for bundle branch blocks or ventricular pre-excitation syndromes. As previously mentioned, if the diagnosis of the wide complex rhythm is uncertain, it should be assumed to be VT, and treatment should proceed according to the patient's condition.

NSVT may occur in the setting of acute ischemia, and evaluation and treatment should be focused on the ischemia. Direct pharmacologic treatment (e.g., lidocaine, amiodarone) of NSVT in ischemia/infarct is not advisable. In the patient not suffering from active ischemia, NSVT is frequently asymptomatic and has little prognostic utility for malignant arrhythmia, especially in the absence of structural heart disease and ventricular dysfunction. Symptomatic NSVT may be treated pharmacologically, primarily to relieve symptoms.

Sustained VT generally causes symptoms by impairing cardiac output, resulting in hypotension, loss of consciousness, and possibly cardiac arrest. It may also deteriorate into ventricular fibrillation.

Treatment of symptomatic VT with a detectable pulse is synchronous direct current cardioversion (with sedation or anesthesia in the awake patient) or, if the VT is well tolerated, with an antiarrhythmic drug (such as procainamide, amiodarone, or lidocaine). Patients with hemodynamically compromising, pulseless monomorphic or polymorphic VT usually require immediate treatment with asynchronous defibrillation (see section "Cardiac Arrest"), followed by antiarrhythmic drugs if necessary.

Sustained torsades de pointes with hemodynamic collapse also requires asynchronous cardioversion. Treatment of torsades de pointes aims at correcting any underlying electrolyte abnormalities and stopping any drugs known to prolong the QT interval. Torsades de pointes is likely to recur if the inciting factors cannot be eliminated immediately. Magnesium sulfate given at 1 to 2 mg IV may have utility, particularly in hypomagnesemic patients. Lidocaine or phenytoin may also be suppressive. Torsades de pointes is frequently *bradycardia-dependent*, and temporary pacing or isoproterenol infusion may be used to increase the heart rate and prevent recurrences.

Ventricular fibrillation is the result of chaotic electrical currents within the ventricles, preventing coordinated contractions. VF on ECG has a chaotic appearance without any discernable QRS complex. Untreated VF rapidly results in death. VF may be preceded by VT and is most commonly seen in patients with acute myocardial infarction.

Treatment is immediate asynchronous electrical defibrillation, followed by antiarrhythmic drugs when a stable rhythm returns (see "Cardiac Arrest"). Also see treatment Algorithm 19.6.

BRADYARRHYTHMIAS

Bradycardia, defined as a heart rate of less than 60 beats per minute, occurs from (a) SA node dysfunction or (b) disturbances of the AV conduction system. Clinically significant bradycardia occurs when there is inadequate cardiac output, generally associated with hypotension, and which may manifest as any or all of presyncope, syncope, fatigue, confusion, depressed level of consciousness, chest pain, shock, or congestive heat failure. Acute treatment aims at restoring adequate cardiac output and identifying the underlying rhythm and its cause.

SA node dysfunction occurs in a number of pathophysiologic states seen in the intensive care unit including increased intracranial pressure, prolonged apneic periods in patients with the obstructive sleep apnea/hypopnea syndrome, myocardial infarction (especially of the right coronary artery, which normally supplies the SA node), advanced liver disease, hypothyroidism, hypothermia, hypercapnia, acidemia, hypervagotonia, and certain infections. It may also be due to depression of the sinus node by drugs, including sympatholytics such as beta-blockers and clonidine, the cardioselective calcium channel blockers verapamil and diltiazem, parasympathomimetics, and antiarrhythmic drugs such as amiodarone. Sick sinus syndrome refers to intrinsic sinus node dysfunction with any of the previously mentioned clinical symptoms associated with the decrease in cardiac output. An important variant of sick sinus syndrome is sinus bradycardia or prolonged sinus pause occurring after termination of atrial fibrillation or other atrial arrhythmias due to depression of SA node automaticity during the tachyarrhythmia, which may be slow to recover. Syncope is a common presentation of this variant, termed the *tachy-brady syndrome*.

Disturbances of the AV conduction system can occur in the atria, AV node, or His-Purkinje system. When there is complete block in any part of the AV conduction system (termed *third-degree AV block*) an escape pacemaker generally develops. When complete blockage occurs in the AV node, the His bundle escape pacemaker generally takes over at a

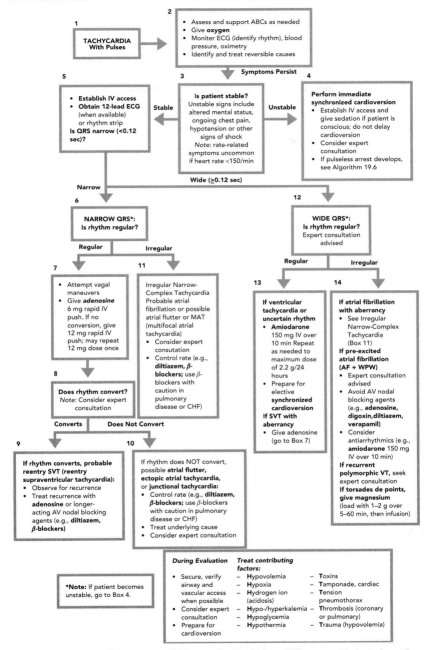

ALGORITHM 19.4 — Advanced Cardiac Life Support Tachycardia Treatment Algorithm

1
TACHYCARDIA With Pulses

2
- Assess and support ABCs as needed
- Give **oxygen**
- Moniter ECG (identify rhythm), blood pressure, oximetry
- Identify and treat reversible causes

Symptoms Persist

3
Is patient stable?
Unstable signs include altered mental status, ongoing chest pain, hypotension or other signs of shock
Note: rate-related symptoms uncommon if heart rate <150/min

Stable → **5**
Unstable → **4**

5
- Establish IV access
- Obtain 12-lead ECG (when available) or rhythm strip
Is QRS narrow (<0.12 sec)?

4
Perform immediate synchronized cardioversion
- Establish IV access and give sedation if patient is conscious; do not delay cardioversion
- Consider expert consultation
- If pulseless arrest develops, see Algorithm 19.6

Narrow

Wide (≥0.12 sec)

6
NARROW QRS*:
Is rhythm regular?

12
WIDE QRS*:
Is rhythm regular?
Expert consultation advised

Regular / Irregular

Regular / Irregular

7
- Attempt vagal maneuvers
- Give **adenosine** 6 mg rapid IV push. If no conversion, give 12 mg rapid IV push; may repeat 12 mg dose once

11
Irregular Narrow-Complex Tachycardia
Probable atrial fibrillation or possible atrial flutter or MAT (multifocal atrial tachycardia)
- Consider expert consutation
- Control rate (e.g., **diltiazem, β-blockers;** use β-blockers with caution in pulmonary disease or CHF)

13
If ventricular tachycardia or uncertain rhythm
- **Amiodarone** 150 mg IV over 10 min Repeat as needed to maximum dose of 2.2 g/24 hours
- Prepare for elective **synchronized cardioversion**
If SVT with aberrancy
- Give adenosine (go to Box 7)

14
If atrial fibrillation with aberrancy
- See Irregular Narrow-Complex Tachycardia (Box 11)
If pre-excited atrial fibrillation (AF + WPW)
- Expert consultation advised
- Avoid AV nodal blocking agents (e.g., **adenosine, digoxin, diltiazem, verapamil**)
- Consider antiarrhythmics (e.g., **amiodarone** 150 mg IV over 10 min)
If recurrent polymorphic VT, seek expert consultation
If torsades de points, **give magnesium** (load with 1–2 g over 5–60 min, then infusion)

8
Does rhythm convert?
Note: Consider expert consultation

Converts / Does Not Convert

9
If rhythm converts, probable reentry SVT (reentry supraventricular tachycardia):
- Observe for recurrence
- Treat recurrence with **adenosine** or longer-acting AV nodal blocking agents (e.g., **diltiazem, β-blockers**)

10
If rhythm does NOT convert, possible **atrial flutter, ectopic atrial tachycardia,** or **junctional tachycardia:**
- Control rate (e.g., **diltiazem, β-blockers;** use β-blockers with caution in pulmonary disease or CHF)
- Treat underlying cause
- Consider expert consultation

*Note: If patient becomes unstable, go to Box 4.

During Evaluation
- Secure, verify airway and vascular access when possible
- Consider expert consultation
- Prepare for cardioversion

Treat contributing factors:
- Hypovolemia
- Hypoxia
- Hydrogen ion (acidosis)
- Hypo-/hyperkalemia
- Hypoglycemia
- Hypothermia
- Toxins
- Tamponade, cardiac
- Tension pneumothorax
- Thrombosis (coronary or pulmonary)
- Trauma (hypovolemia)

ECG, electrocardiogram; IV, intravenous; CHF, congestive heart failure; SVT, supraventricular tachycardia; AF, atrial fibrillation; WPW, Wolff-Parkinson-White; VT, ventricular tachycardia. (From 2005 American Heart Association Guidelines for Cardiopulmonary Resuscitation and Emergency Cardiovascular Care, Part 7.3: Management of Symptomatic Bradycardia and Tachycardia. *Circulation.* 2005;112[suppl IV]:IV-70, with permission.)

rate of 40 to 60 beats per minute, and is associated with a narrow QRS complex (in the absence of an underlying bundle branch block or other aberrant conduction). Complete heart block distal to the AV node often results in an escape pacemaker originating from the more distal conduction system, usually with a rate between 25 and 45 beats per minute. These fascicular escape rhythms generate a QRS complex consistent with their origin (e.g., if the origin is in the right bundle, the QRS has a left bundle branch block pattern). If the conduction system fails, a rhythm from the ventricular myocardium may generate a heart beat, with a wide complex of ventricular origin. Thus, in general, the more distal the escape rhythm, the slower and less reliable it tends to be. Heart block with irregular fascicular escapes may require urgent temporary pacing. The ECG shows AV dissociation with non-conducted P waves that "march" out independently of the ventricular escape rhythm. There are many causes of third-degree heart block including acute myocardial infarction, drug toxicity (e.g., digitalis, beta-blockers, cardioselective calcium channel blockers), chronic cardiopulmonary disease, idiopathic fibrosis, congenital heart disease, infiltrative diseases (sarcoidosis), infections/inflammatory diseases, collagen vascular diseases, trauma, and tumors.

First-degree AV block is not truly *block*, but is a PR interval >200 ms. It is in itself generally benign, but may result in symptoms if the degree of AV dyssynchrony is severe.

Second-degree AV block occurs when some atrial impulses fail to conduct to the ventricles. **Mobitz type I second-degree AV block** (AV Wenckebach block) is characterized on ECG by a variable (usually progressively prolonging) PR interval culminating in a nonconducted atrial beat. Mobitz I uncommonly progresses to complete heart block. When it does, the escape pacemaker of 40 to 60 beats per minute in the His bundle usually provides an adequate backup rate to maintain cardiac output. Mobitz I block can be caused by drugs such as digoxin, beta-blockers, certain calcium channel blockers, ischemia (especially of the inferior wall), or in healthy individuals from hypervagotonia.

Mobitz type II second-degree AV block generally is due to disease in the His-Purkinje system and is characterized on ECG by a fixed PR interval with one or more non-conducting atrial impulses. It is more likely to progress to complete heart block than Mobitz 1, sometimes precipitously. The typical escape pacemaker rate of 25 to 45 arises in the more distal His-Purkinje system and has a wide QRS. The escape rhythm may not be sufficient to maintain cardiac output and can progress rapidly to cardiac arrest and death. Mobitz II can occur from ischemia (especially anteroseptal infarcts), endocarditis, valvular or congenital heart disease, drugs such as procainamide, disopyramide, and quinidine, or idiopathic progressive cardiac conduction system diseases.

Treatment of clinically significant bradycardia follows the ACLS algorithm outlined in Algorithm 19.5, and aims at maintaining adequate cardiac output. Atropine is first-line pharmacologic therapy, and is more successful in patients with sinus bradycardia or block within the AV node, rather than block in the more distal His-Purkinje system. Patients who remain clinically unstable require immediate transcutaneous or transvenous pacing. Reversible causes should be identified. In patients with sinus node dysfunction in which the cause is not reversible, permanent pacing can relieve symptoms. Permanent pacing is typically indicated in Mobitz II or third-degree AV block. If symptoms of bradycardia are present in Mobitz I AV block, permanent pacing is indicated.

CARDIAC ARREST

Cardiac arrest refers to the cessation of a detectable noninvasive blood pressure and pulse. Cardiac arrest can be separated into three main types: (a) pulseless electrical activity (PEA), (b) VT and VF, and (c) asystole. All three fall under the overall heading of pulseless arrest outlined in Algorithm 19.6. Treatment of PEA and asystole are similar and center on identifying reversible causes and pharmacologic intervention. VT and VF are treated with immediate electrical defibrillation.

Treatment of cardiac arrest in an intensive care unit setting requires a team of nurses and physicians trained in advanced cardiac life support. Ideally there should be an established and easily identifiable team leader responsible for continuously evaluating the patient's condition and the ECG, assimilating incoming data, and giving all orders. In addition, there should be a scribe, recording changes in condition, ECG and laboratory data,

ALGORITHM 19.5   **Advanced Cardiac Life Support Bradycardia Treatment Algorithm**

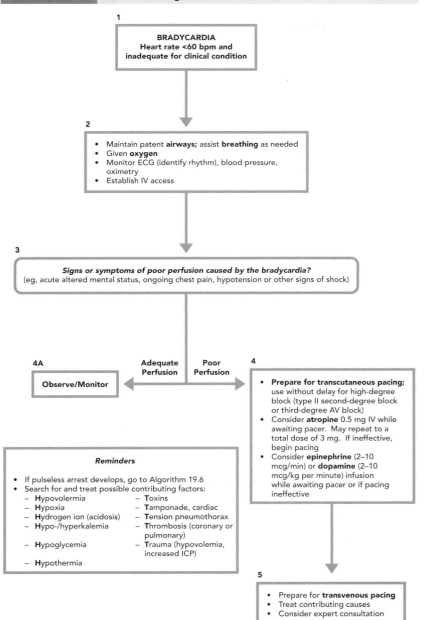

1

BRADYCARDIA
Heart rate <60 bpm and
inadequate for clinical condition

2

- Maintain patent **airways;** assist **breathing** as needed
- Given **oxygen**
- Monitor ECG (identify rhythm), blood pressure, oximetry
- Establish IV access

3

Signs or symptoms of poor perfusion caused by the bradycardia?
(eg, acute altered mental status, ongoing chest pain, hypotension or other signs of shock)

Adequate Perfusion   Poor Perfusion

4A

Observe/Monitor

4

- **Prepare for transcutaneous pacing;** use without delay for high-degree block (type II second-degree block or third-degree AV block)
- Consider **atropine** 0.5 mg IV while awaiting pacer. May repeat to a total dose of 3 mg. If ineffective, begin pacing
- Consider **epinephrine** (2–10 mcg/min) or **dopamine** (2–10 mcg/kg per minute) infusion while awaiting pacer or if pacing ineffective

Reminders

- If pulseless arrest develops, go to Algorithm 19.6
- Search for and treat possible contributing factors:
  - **H**ypovolermia
  - **H**ypoxia
  - **H**ydrogen ion (acidosis)
  - **H**ypo-/hyperkalemia
  - **H**ypoglycemia
  - **H**ypothermia
  - **T**oxins
  - **T**amponade, cardiac
  - **T**ension pneumothorax
  - **T**hrombosis (coronary or pulmonary)
  - **T**rauma (hypovolemia, increased ICP)

5

- Prepare for **transvenous pacing**
- Treat contributing causes
- Consider expert consultation

bpm, beats per minute; ECG, electrocardiogram; AV, atrioventricular; IV, intravenous; ICP, intracranial pressure. (From 2005 American Heart Association Guidelines for Cardiopulmonary Resuscitation and Emergency Cardiovascular Care, Part 7.3: Management of Symptomatic Bradycardia and Tachycardia. *Circulation*. 2005;112[suppl IV]:IV-68, with permission.)

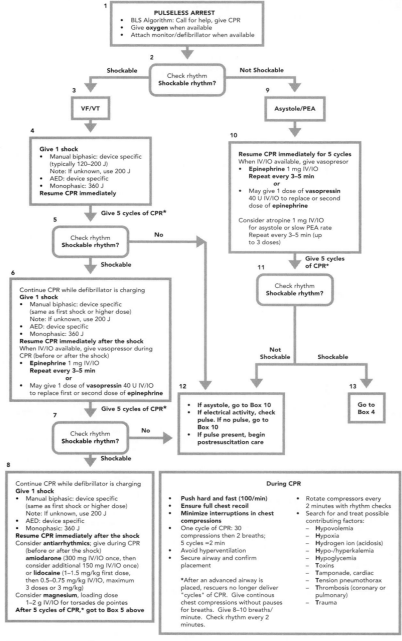

ALGORITHM 19.6 **Advanced Cardiac Life Support Pulseless Arrest Algorithm**

1
PULSELESS ARREST
- BLS Algorithm: Call for help, give CPR
- Give **oxygen** when available
- Attach monitor/defibrillator when available

2
Check rhythm
Shockable rhythm?

Shockable ← → Not Shockable

3
VF/VT

9
Asystole/PEA

4
Give 1 shock
- Manual biphasic: device specific (typically 120–200 J)
  Note: If unknown, use 200 J
- AED: device specific
- Monophasic: 360 J
Resume CPR immediately

Give 5 cycles of CPR*

10
Resume CPR immediately for 5 cycles
When IV/IO available, give vasopressor
- **Epinephrine** 1 mg IV/IO
  Repeat every 3–5 min
  or
- May give 1 dose of **vasopressin** 40 U IV/IO to replace or second dose of **epinephrine**

Consider atropine 1 mg IV/IO for asystole or slow PEA rate
Repeat every 3–5 min (up to 3 doses)

5
Check rhythm
Shockable rhythm? — No →

Shockable ↓

6
Continue CPR while defibrillator is charging
Give 1 shock
- Manual biphasic: device specific (same as first shock or higher dose)
  Note: If unknown, use 200 J
- AED: device specific
- Monophasic: 360 J
Resume CPR immediately after the shock
When IV/IO available, give vasopressor during CPR (before or after the shock)
- **Epinephrine** 1 mg IV/IO
  Repeat every 3–5 min
  or
- May give 1 dose of **vasopressin** 40 U IV/IO to replace first or second dose of **epinephrine**

Give 5 cycles of CPR*

11
Check rhythm
Shockable rhythm?

Not Shockable ↓   Shockable →

7
Check rhythm
Shockable rhythm? — No →

Shockable ↓

12
- **If asystole, go to Box 10**
- **If electrical activity, check pulse. If no pulse, go to Box 10**
- **If pulse present, begin postresuscitation care**

13
Go to Box 4

8
Continue CPR while defibrillator is charging
Give 1 shock
- Manual biphasic: device specific (same as first shock or higher dose)
  Note: If unknown, use 200 J
- AED: device specific
- Monophasic: 360 J
Resume CPR immediately after the shock
Consider **antiarrhythmics**; give during CPR (before or after the shock)
  amiodarone (300 mg IV/IO once, then consider additional 150 mg IV/IO once) or **lidocaine** (1–1.5 mg/kg first dose, then 0.5–0.75 mg/kg IV/IO, maximum 3 doses or 3 mg/kg)
Consider **magnesium**, loading dose 1–2 g IV/IO for torsades de pointes
After 5 cycles of CPR,* got to Box 5 above

During CPR
- **Push hard and fast (100/min)**
- **Ensure full chest recoil**
- **Minimize interruptions in chest compressions**
- One cycle of CPR: 30 compressions then 2 breaths; 5 cycles ≈2 min
- Avoid hyperventilation
- Secure airway and confirm placement

*After an advanced airway is placed, rescuers no longer deliver "cycles" of CPR. Give continous chest compressions without pauses for breaths. Give 8–10 breaths/minute. Check rhythm every 2 minutes.

- Rotate compressors every 2 minutes with rhythm checks
- Search for and treat possible contributing factors:
  - Hypovolemia
  - Hypoxia
  - Hydrogen ion (acidosis)
  - Hypo-/hyperkalemia
  - Hypoglycemia
  - Toxins
  - Tamponade, cardiac
  - Tension pneumothorax
  - Thrombosis (coronary or pulmonary)
  - Trauma

BLS, basic life support; CPR, cardiopulmonary resuscitation; VF/VT, ventricular fibrillation/ventricular tachycardia; PEA, pulseless electrical activity; AED, automated external defibrillator; IV/IO, intravenous/intraosseous. (From 2005 American Heart Association Guidelines for Cardiopulmonary Resuscitation and Emergency Cardiovascular Care, Part 7.2: Management of Cardiac Arrest. *Circulation.* 2005;112[suppl IV]:IV-59, with permission).

and therapies delivered. Initial patient evaluation follows the ABC's of cardiac arrest in a coordinated and overlapping fashion, ensuring adequate airway control, breathing (i.e., ventilation), and circulation. In non-intubated patients, an oral airway device should be placed and a bag-valve-mask should be used to deliver breaths. Intubation is performed when possible. Cardiopulmonary resuscitation (CPR) should begin immediately with chest compressions given at a rate of 100 compressions per minute at 1.5 to 2 inches depth, allowing full chest recoil between compressions. Patients should also be immediately connected to an automated external defibrillator (AED), or a manual defibrillator if an AED is not available. The defibrillator is connected to two pads or paddles placed on the chest wall, with one to the right of the sternum centered on the second intercostal space, and one on the left chest wall centered in the midaxillary line at the fifth intercostal space. IV access should be ensured for delivery of medications and fluids. Peripheral IV access is initially adequate. However, central IV access should be obtained as soon as possible via the femoral vein, subclavian vein, or internal jugular vein. Pulses are best monitored in the femoral artery, but the carotid arteries may be used. Once airway control is established and the patient is connected to an external defibrillator, the cardiac rhythm should be rapidly analyzed.

Pulseless VT and VF

Confirmed VT and VF with hemodynamic collapse should be treated with *immediate* asynchronous defibrillation. Automated AED devices typically deliver escalating biphasic shocks at 200, 300, and 360 Joules (J). Manual devices may generate monophasic or biphasic waveforms. If a manual biphasic device is used and the devices recommended dose scale is unknown, an initial dose of 200 J should be used, with subsequent shocks at the same or higher doses. If a monophasic device is used, the dose should be 360 J for all shocks. The patient's rhythm, blood pressure, and responsiveness must be continuously monitored with appropriate adjustment of therapy (e.g., continuation/discontinuation of CPR, infusion of new medications). If VT/VF persists or recurs after initial treatment, CPR should be resumed immediately after the first shock is given and continued for 2 minutes along with continuous ventilation via a mask airway or endotracheal tube. The rhythm and pulse should be reassessed 2 minutes after the shock is given. Shocks should be repeated if patients remain in pulseless VT/VF and the CPR cycle repeated. When IV access is established, patients should be concomitantly treated with 1 mg IV epinephrine every 3 to 5 minutes. Vasopressin, 40 U IV, may also be substituted for the first or second dose. Studies comparing epinephrine and vasopressin given to hospitalized patients in cardiac arrest have shown no difference in survival. After the third shock is given, patients who remain in VF/VT should be considered for amiodarone or lidocaine at the doses shown in Algorithm 19.6. If the rhythm on the monitor appears to be torsades de pointes, patients should be given IV magnesium sulfate. If a pulse becomes present at any point in treatment, the rhythm should be identified and appropriately treated according to Algorithms 19.4 and 19.5.

PEA and Asystole

PEA includes numerous pulseless rhythms such as bradyasystolic rhythms, idioventricular rhythms, and ventricular escape rhythms. PEA and asystole are not treated with electrical defibrillation. Treatment centers on well-delivered CPR and pharmacologic intervention as illustrated in Algorithm 19.6. Epinephrine should be given at 1 mg IV every 3 to 5 minutes and may be replaced with vasopressin 40 U for the first or second dose. If a slow rhythm is seen on the monitor, consider giving atropine 1mg IV. If IV access is not available, the drugs may be given endotracheally, in which case the dose is generally doubled

The five H's and five T's listed in Algorithm 19.6 are common conditions that may contribute to cardiac arrest. Airway control and ventilation can correct *hypoxemia*. IV fluids should be given at a wide open rate or via a rapid infuser to correct *hypovolemia*. If *hypoglycemia* is suspected, give 1 ampule (amp) of 50% Dextrose, or 1 mg of intramuscular glucagon if IV access is not available. If *hypokalemia* or acidosis (*hydrogen ion*) are suspected, give 1 amp of sodium bicarbonate (50 mEq NaHCO$_3$). *Hypothermia* should be treated as outlined in Chapter 31. Cases of suspected cardiac *tamponade* should be treated with immediate pericardiocentesis (see Chapter 79). Suspected *tension* pneumothorax should be treated with rapid decompression by inserting a large-bore catheter (14- or 16-gauge) into the second intercostal space in the midclavicular line, or unilateral or bilaterally inserted thoracostomy tubes. Ischemia from coronary *thrombosis* should be rapidly identified and treated when patients are stabilized (see Chapter 18). If pulmonary thrombosis is suspected, fibrinolytics may be beneficial but are not recommended for routine use.

Cycles of CPR should continue until patients have palpable pulses and a detectable blood pressure or until resuscitation efforts have failed. There is no set period for when to stop resuscitation efforts. The decision to stop CPR is made by the medical team when a full trial at resuscitation has failed and the patient's chances of regaining a pulse and neurologic function are negligible. If patients do regain a pulse, the rhythm on the monitor should be identified and the patient treated accordingly. Blood pressure should be checked and hypotension should be treated with IV vasopressors and IV fluids. An arterial blood gas and other laboratory tests should be checked and abnormalities treated.

Postresuscitation hypothermia often occurs naturally after cardiac arrest. Active induction of hypothermia has also been evaluated in numerous randomized trials of patients with VF arrest and PEA/asystolic arrest occurring both in and out of the hospital. Patients were generally hemodynamically stable but comatose. They were cooled within minutes to hours to between approximately 32°C and 34°C, generally with cooling blankets. There were improved outcomes and metabolic endpoints in patients who were actively cooled. Thus, it is a current American Heart Association Class IIb recommendation for in-hospital cardiac arrest and non-VF arrest, and Class IIa for out-of-hospital VF arrest to cool hemodynamically stable but unconscious patients to between 32°C and 34°C for 12 to 24 hours after cardiac arrest. Patients with spontaneous hypothermia should not be actively rewarmed. Complications of cooling include coagulopathies and arrhythmias.

Suggested Reading

2005 American Heart Association Guidelines for Cardiopulmonary Resuscitation and Emergency Cardiovascular Care, Part 3: Overview of CPR, Part 4: Adult Basic Life Support, Part 5: Electrical Therapies, Part 6: CPR Techniques and Devices, Part 7: Advanced Cardiovascular Life Support. *Circulation.* 2005;112[Suppl IV]:IV12–88. *Current recommendations from the AHA based on evaluation of current treatment evidence reviewed at the 2005 International Consensus Conference on Cardiopulmonary Resuscitation and Emergency Cardiovascular Care, and published in the supplement to Circulation.*

Aung K, Htay T. Vasopressin for cardiac arrest: a systematic review and meta-analysis. *Arch Intern Med.* 2005;165:17–24. *Summation of evidence from 5 randomized trials comparing vasopressin and epinephrine in cardiac arrest showing no clear advantage of vasopressin over epinephrine.*

Hypothermia After Cardiac Arrest Study Group. Mild therapeutic hypothermia to improve the neurologic outcome after cardiac arrest. *N Engl J Med.* 2002;346:549–556. *Multicenter trial of patients resuscitated after cardiac arrest due to ventricular fibrillation who were randomly assigned to undergo therapeutic hypothermia or standard treatment with normothermia. The primary end point was a favorable neurologic outcome within six months after cardiac arrest, which was achieved by 55% of patients in the hypothermia group compared to 39% in the normothermia group. Mortality was 41% versus 55%, favoring the hypothermia group.*

AORTIC DISSECTION

Anthony J. Hart and Alan C. Braverman

20

Aortic dissection is a potentially life-threatening acute aortic syndrome that accounts for a small but significant proportion of cardiovascular system disease. It carries substantial morbidity and mortality, with a mortality rate up to 1% per hour within the first 48 hours when untreated. An algorithm for the immediate approach to the patient with aortic dissection is presented in Algorithm 20.1.

Classic aortic dissection occurs in approximately 90% of cases and results from a tear in the aorta's intimal layer, which allows blood to enter the medial layer and propagate in an anterograde or retrograde direction, resulting in a second "false" lumen. Additional intimal tears can allow reconnection with the true lumen (the so-called *double-barrel aorta*). Variants of aortic dissection include penetrating atherosclerotic aortic ulcer and aortic intramural hematoma. Penetrating atherosclerotic ulceration occurs when an atherosclerotic plaque ruptures into the aorta's media with development of a dissection flap and variable propagation along the aorta. In aortic intramural hematoma, no dissection flap is visualized, but there is blood in the wall of the aorta secondary to apoplexy of the vasa vasorum. Once dissection occurs, hydrodynamic forces stemming from the rate of change in pressure (dP/dt) and mean blood pressure contribute to spread of the tear.

Several conditions predispose the aorta to dissection, mostly as a result of disruption of the normal arterial wall composition (Table 20.1). Heritable conditions such as Marfan syndrome and Ehlers-Danlos syndrome type IV are particularly prone to aortic dilatation and dissection. A congenital bicuspid aortic valve may be associated with abnormalities of the aortic root, leading to enlargement and increased risk of dissection. Acquired conditions such as hypertension, inflammation, and direct trauma can damage arterial walls. Once the intima becomes injured, it is vulnerable to shear stresses, with progression to intramural hemorrhage, rupture, or dissection.

There are several classification systems for aortic dissections, with involvement of the ascending aorta as the defining characteristic (Fig. 20.1). Type I and II, or type A, dissections occur proximal to the left subclavian artery with or without distal involvement. Distal dissection (type III or type B) involves any segment of the aorta distal to the left subclavian artery. The dissection's anatomic location is important because it guides patient management. Broadly, proximal aortic involvement requires immediate surgical repair, and dissections that begin distal to the arch (type III or type B) are often initially medically manageable.

An aortic dissection's clinical presentation is variable, requiring a high index of suspicion for diagnosis. Multiple symptoms have been ascribed to dissection, but the most common presentation is abrupt onset of severe, sharp, or "tearing" pain in the chest, neck, or interscapular areas. Limb blood pressures with a difference >20 mm Hg may be an independent predictor of dissection. However, if the patient is hypotensive, care should be taken to rule out pseudohypotension with false low blood pressures secondary to occlusion of the brachiocephalic trunk, left subclavian artery, or distal aorta. Careful examination of all the major vessels should be performed at the bedside, and differences in pulse strength and blood pressure may offer a clue to the presence of an aortic dissection. Cardiac auscultation may reveal an aortic regurgitation murmur. However, clinical examination alone is often insufficient to rule out aortic dissection. Pulse differentials and an aortic regurgitation murmur are present in a minority of patients. The anteroposterior chest radiograph may demonstrate a widened mediastinum or abnormal aortic contour, but up to 20% of aortic dissections are associated with an unremarkable radiograph.

Significant morbidity and mortality from dissection is attributed to end-organ damage and aortic rupture (Table 20.2). Organ damage occurs from ischemia secondary to

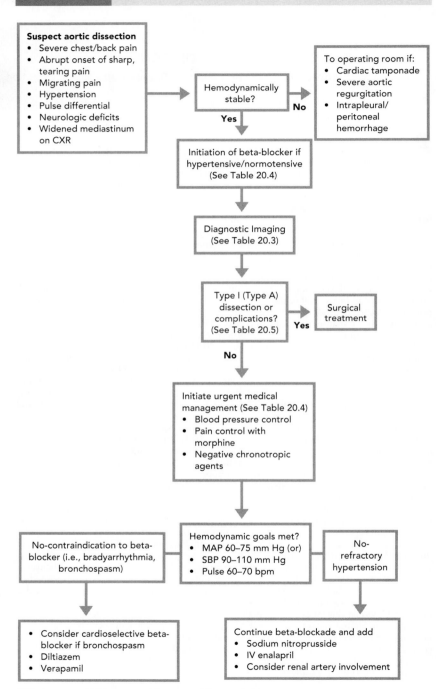

ALGORITHM 20.1 Algorithm for Aortic Dissection

Suspect aortic dissection
- Severe chest/back pain
- Abrupt onset of sharp, tearing pain
- Migrating pain
- Hypertension
- Pulse differential
- Neurologic deficits
- Widened mediastinum on CXR

Hemodynamically stable?

No → To operating room if:
- Cardiac tamponade
- Severe aortic regurgitation
- Intrapleural/peritoneal hemorrhage

Yes ↓

Initiation of beta-blocker if hypertensive/normotensive (See Table 20.4)

Diagnostic Imaging (See Table 20.3)

Type I (Type A) dissection or complications? (See Table 20.5) — **Yes** → Surgical treatment

No ↓

Initiate urgent medical management (See Table 20.4)
- Blood pressure control
- Pain control with morphine
- Negative chronotropic agents

Hemodynamic goals met?
- MAP 60–75 mm Hg (or)
- SBP 90–110 mm Hg
- Pulse 60–70 bpm

No-contraindication to beta-blocker (i.e., bradyarrhythmia, bronchospasm)

No-refractory hypertension

- Consider cardioselective beta-blocker if bronchospasm
- Diltiazem
- Verapamil

Continue beta-blockade and add
- Sodium nitroprusside
- IV enalapril
- Consider renal artery involvement

CXR, chest x-ray; MAP, mean arterial pressure; SBP, systolic blood pressure; bpm, beats per minute; IV, intravenous.

TABLE 20.1	Common Risk Factors for Aortic Dissection

- Hypertension
- Connective tissue disorders
  - Marfan syndrome
  - Vascular Ehlers-Danlos syndrome
  - Bicuspid aortic valve
  - Coarctation of the aorta
  - Loeys-Deitz syndrome
  - Hereditary thoracic aortic aneurysm/dissection
- Cocaine use
- Atherosclerosis, penetrating aortic ulcer
- Trauma, blunt or iatrogenic
  - Catheter
  - Aortic/valvular surgery
  - Coronary artery bypass grafting
  - Motor vehicle accident (lap belt)
- Inflammatory conditions
  - Giant cell arteritis
  - Takayasu's arteritis
  - Behçet disease

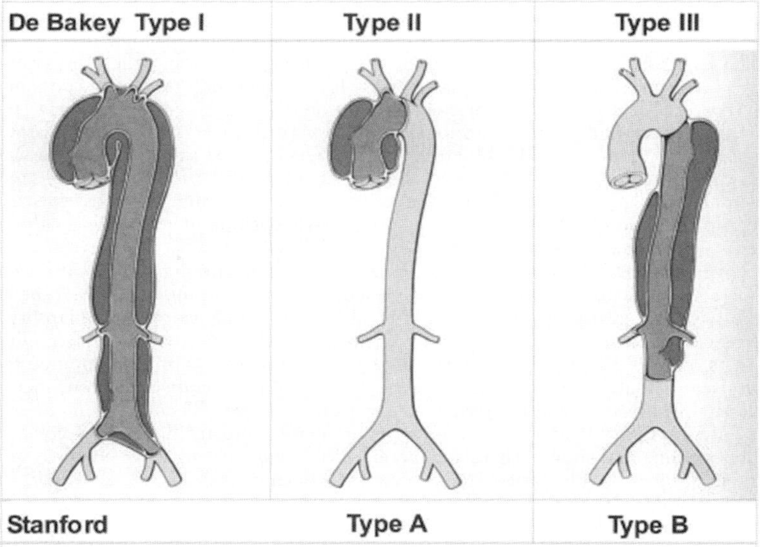

De Bakey

Type I   Originates in the ascending aorta, propagates at least to the aortic arch and often beyond it distally

Type II   Originates in and is confined to the ascending aorta

Type III Originates in the descending aorta and extends distally down the aorta or, rarely, retrograde into the aortic arch and ascending aorta

Stanford

Type A   All dissections involving the ascending aorta, regardless of the site of origin

Type B   All dissections not involving the ascending aorta

Figure 20.1. Classification systems for aortic dissection: Stanford and DeBakey. (From SP Nienaber CA, Eagle KA. Aortic dissection: new frontiers in diagnosis and management. Part I: from etiology to diagnostic strategies. *Circulation.* 2003;108:628–635, with permission.)

TABLE 20.2	Complications of Aortic Dissection

- Aortic rupture
- Neurologic deficits: coma, altered consciousness, syncope.
- Malperfusion: myocardial, mesenteric, limb, spinal cord, renal, hepatic.
- Hypotension
- Hemothorax
- Cardiac effusion ± tamponade
- Acute aortic regurgitation ± congestive heart failure
- Subsequent aneurysm formation

branch vessel obstruction from direct dissection into the arterial wall, or by compression of the vessel by an expanding false lumen. Cardiovascular and neurologic manifestations are two particularly devastating complications of aortic dissection. When the ascending aorta is involved, acute aortic regurgitation may lead to heart failure. Cardiac tamponade, aortic rupture, or myocardial infarction from coronary artery involvement, may lead to cardiogenic shock and death. Neurologic sequelae may also result from acute dissection, with cerebral hypoperfusion leading to syncope, altered mental status, and stroke. Spinal perfusion may be compromised via occlusion of the intercostal arteries, the great anterior segmental medullary artery (of Adamkiewicz), or the thoracic radicular arteries. This can present in the form of transverse myelitis, progressive myelopathy, paraplegia, or quadriplegia.

Given the critical nature of aortic dissections, immediate diagnostic confirmation is imperative once aortic dissection is suspected. The choice of imaging should be made on the basis of sensitivity, specificity, clinical stability, and operator availability and experience (Table 20.3). If the patient presents with hemodynamic instability or hypotension, rapid evaluation by transesophageal echocardiogram or computed tomography scan should be performed to assess for complications of dissection, including pericardial effusion, aortic regurgitation, or aortic rupture. When tamponade occurs, poor outcomes have been reported from percutaneous pericardiocentesis secondary to further bleeding and shock. Therefore, pericardiocentesis should be avoided in favor of emergent surgery. Stable patients with renal insufficiency may be evaluated with magnetic resonance imaging.

When aortic dissection is suspected, initiation of beta-blocker therapy to reduce shear forces is paramount while pursuing confirmation of the diagnosis (Table 20.4). Blood pressure should be reduced to as low a level as possible without compromising organ perfusion. Beta-blocker therapy is recommended to achieve a target heart rate <70 beats per minute. Cardioselective calcium channel blockers (diltiazem, verapamil) may be considered if beta-blocker therapy is contraindicated. Care should be taken to avoid direct acting vasodilators in the absence of negative chronotropic medications, as they may induce reflex tachycardia, increasing dP/dt with worsening dissection.

Surgery is indicated with type I and II (type A) dissection as medical therapy alone is associated with a high risk of morbidity and mortality. Surgery in type III (type B) dissection is reserved for life-threatening complications such as end-organ ischemia, refractory pain, uncontrolled hypertension, or a rapidly expanding aortic diameter (Table 20.5). There is growing experience managing distal aortic dissections with percutaneous interventional therapy using stent-grafting and balloon fenestration, which involve sealing the intimal tear with stents, and fenestration of a false lumen to relieve ischemia, respectively. These techniques and others continue to evolve the management of complex aortic dissections.

TABLE 20.3	Comparison of Diagnostic Imaging Modalities			
Test	Sensitivity (%)	Specificity (%)	Advantages	Disadvantages
TTE	35–80	39–96	Rapid bedside test; useful (highest sensitivity and specificity) in diagnosing proximal dissection, as well as evaluating for tamponade and aortic regurgitation	Much less accurate than other diagnostic tests for detection of dissection
TEE	98–99	94–97	Excellent evaluation of aortic root and descending thoracic aorta, aortic valve and pericardium	Requires esophageal intubation; limited to thoracic aorta
CT	96–100	96–100	Superior imaging of aortic arch vessel involvement as well as visceral and iliac arteries	Limited identification of the intimal tear/site of entry; nephrotoxic iodinated contrast required
MRI	98	98	Superior accuracy, sensitivity, and specificity for all types of dissection	Limited availability, time-consuming procedure

TTE, transthoracic echocardiogram; TEE, transesophageal echocardiogram; CT, computed tomography; MRI, magnetic resonance imaging.
Adapted from Khan, IA, Nair CK. Clinical, diagnostic, and management perspectives of aortic dissection. *Chest*. 2002;122;311–328, with permission.

TABLE 20.4	Selected Pharmacologic Therapy[a]

- Labetalol: Give 20 mg IV over 2 min, then 40 to 80 mg IV every 15min until adequate response (maximum 300 mg), then continuous IV infusion at 2–10 mg/min IV, titrated to effect. Has good alpha and beta antagonism.
- Esmolol: Give 500 mcg/kg IV bolus, then continuous IV infusion at 50–200 mcg/kg/min, titrated to effect. Short half-life allows rapid titration.
- Sodium nitroprusside: Start continuous infusion with no bolus at 20 mcg/min, maximum 800 mcg/min, titrated to effect. **Use only in presence of rate-controlling agents**.
- Enalapril: Give 0.625–1.25 mg IV, then increase by 0.625–1.25 mg every 6 hr to a maximum of 5 mg every 6 hr, titrated to effect. Ideal agent for dissection of the renal artery with concurrent hypertension.
- Diltiazem: Give 0.25 mg/kg IV during 2 min, then continuous IV infusion at 5–15 mg/hr, titrated to effect. Used for rate control if contraindications to B-blocker therapy.

[a]Goal of therapy is HR less than 70 beats per minute and blood pressure as low as possible without compromising organ perfusion.
IV, intravenously.

TABLE 20.5	Indications for Surgery[a]

- Type I (type A) dissection
- Type III (type B) with
  - □ Rupture
  - □ Branch vessel ischemia with vital organ compromise

- Refractory pain
- Refractory hypertension
- Rupture
- Aneurysmal dilation

[a]Endovascular repair may be effective in certain aortic/branch vessel complications of distal dissections.

Suggested Reading

Hagan PG, Nienaber CA, Isselbacher EM, et al. The international registry of acute aortic dissection (IRAD). New insights into an old disease. *JAMA.* 2000;283:897–903.
The largest database of acute aortic dissection with emphasis on clinical presentation.

Hirst A, Johns V, Kime W. Dissecting aneurysms of the aorta. A review of 505 cases. *Medicine* 1958;37: 217–279.
An early review of aortic dissection.

Isselbacher EM, Cigarroa JE, Eagle, KA. Cardiac tamponade complicating proximal aortic dissection: is pericardiocentesis harmful? *Circulation.* 1994; 90:2375–2379.
Small, retrospective study which reviewed outcomes of aortic dissection complicated by cardiac tamponade with and without pericardiocentesis.

Khan, IA, Nair CK. Clinical, diagnostic, and management perspectives of aortic dissection. *Chest.* 2002;122;311–328.
Broad overview of aortic dissection with concise description of secondary organ involvement.

Mehta RH, Suzuki T, Hagan PG, et al. Predicting death in patients with acute type A aortic dissection. *Circulation.* 2002;105:200–206.
IRAD study of 547 patients which develops a risk prediction tool in patients with acute type A aortic dissection.

Nienaber CA, Eagle KA. Aortic dissection: new frontiers in diagnosis and management. Part I: from etiology to diagnostic strategies. *Circulation.* 2003;108:628–635.
A broad review of aortic dissection with emphasis on etiology and diagnostic methods of detecting aortic dissection.

Nienaber CA, von Kodolitsch Y, Petersen B, et al. Intramural hematoma of the thoracic aorta: diagnostic and therapeutic implications. *Circulation.* 1995;92:1465–1472.
Describes clinical features and prognosis of a series of patients with aortic intramural hematoma.

Von Kodolitsch Y, Schwartz AG, Nienaber CA. Clinical prediction of acute aortic dissection. *Arch Intern Med.* 2000;160:2977–2982.
Proposes independent predictors of acute aortic dissection and creates a prediction model for facilitated estimation of the individual risk of dissection.

21

ACUTE DECOMPENSATED HEART FAILURE

Christopher L. Holley and Gregory A. Ewald

The combination of an increasing elderly population and the relatively recent era of successful reperfusion strategies for acute myocardial infarction (MI) have led to a nearly epidemic growth in the number of patients with left ventricular dysfunction and heart failure (HF). It is estimated that there are five million Americans living with HF, with 500,000 new cases occurring each year. In fact, HF is the leading cause of hospitalization for patients age 65 or more years and costs nearly 40 billion dollars per year in the United States and is an estimated 1% to 2% of the entire health care budget in Europe. The 1-year mortality from this condition approaches 50% for patients with advanced HF, corresponding to 300,000 deaths yearly in the United States.

The management of chronic HF has improved substantially during the past decade. Successful approaches validated by clinical trials have become well established and are documented in numerous evidence-based guidelines. These approaches will not be detailed here but involve (a) modulation of neurohormonal activation, specifically the renin-angiotensin-aldosterone system (via angiotensin converting enzyme inhibitors [ACEIs], angiotensin receptor blockers [ARBs], and aldosterone antagonists) and sympathetic nervous system (via beta-blockers); (b) fluid management (via diuretics and sodium/water restriction); and (c) reducing cardiac work and improving cardiac output (via hydralazine, nitrates, and digoxin).

In contrast to chronic HF, the management of acute decompensated HF (ADHF) is not as well studied in randomized controlled trials, and evidence-based guidelines have only recently appeared. There are now two sets of guidelines that provide the clinician with recommendations for treating ADHF, with one from the European Society of Cardiology, and another from the Heart Failure Society of America. Our approach to HF in the critical care setting is consistent with these guidelines and is summarized in this chapter.

Recognizing HF is an important first step, as previously extant HF may not have been diagnosed, or there may be acute HF in the setting of MI or acute cardiomyopathy. Typical patients have a history of coronary artery disease, MI, or HF with subjective complaints of paroxysmal nocturnal dyspnea, orthopnea, and dyspnea on exertion. Physical findings that correlate with HF include a third heart sound (S3) and signs of volume overload, such as jugular venous distention, hepatojugular reflux, pulmonary rales, and lower extremity edema. Chest radiography may show cardiomegaly or pulmonary venous congestion. Electrocardiogram findings are not specific but may show atrial fibrillation, ventricular hypertrophy, or evidence of prior MI.

It is important to remember that although HF is a clinical diagnosis, echocardiography, angiography, and invasive hemodynamic monitoring are useful to document systolic or diastolic dysfunction. The role of blood testing is limited in the diagnosis of HF, although B-type natriuretic peptide (BNP) levels can be helpful if the diagnosis is uncertain. In particular, patients with serum BNP <100 pg/mL are very unlikely to have decompensated HF, and values >500 pg/mL are consistent with the diagnosis, with the exception of patients on hemodialysis or with an estimated glomerular filtration rate <60 ml/min. In these patients, the BNP should not be used for diagnosis as it is typically elevated out of proportion to the degree of heart failure. Elevated serum creatinine and hepatic function tests may suggest poor end-organ perfusion secondary to reduced cardiac output.

It is critical to make an accurate assessment regarding the precipitating events for the patient's decompensated state. Common precipitants include acute MI, hypertensive crisis, arrhythmias, sepsis, anemia, and simple decompensation of pre-existing HF secondary to medical or dietary noncompliance. Less common precipitating factors include acute

TABLE 21.1	Precipitants of Acute Decompensated Heart Failure

Common	Less Common
Medical/dietary noncompliance	Peripartum cardiomyopathy
Acute myocardial infarction	Acute myocarditis
Hypertensive crisis	Infective endocarditis
Arrhythmias	Valvular heart disease
Sepsis	Cardiac tamponade
Anemia	Thyrotoxicosis

myocarditis, peripartum cardiomyopathy, valvular heart disease (including infective endocarditis), cardiac tamponade, and thyrotoxicosis (Table 21.1).

Once the diagnosis of ADHF is confirmed, an initial algorithmic approach should focus on stabilizing the patient and performing noninvasive assessments of heart rhythm, oxygenation, hemodynamics, and volume status (Alg. 21.1). This will guide therapies, such as digoxin or amiodarone for atrial fibrillation with rapid ventricular response, vasodilators to reduce afterload and the work of the failing heart, or inotropes for the patient with inadequate end-organ perfusion.

Two classification schemes are frequently used for ADHF: the Killip and Forrester classifications, both of which were developed for ADHF in the setting of MI. The Forrester classification is useful with both noninvasive data (clinical perfusion status and evidence of pulmonary congestion) or invasive hemodynamic data (Alg. 21.2). When an accurate clinical assessment of hemodynamic and volume status cannot be made, a pulmonary artery catheter (Swan-Ganz) can be useful to measure the cardiac index, pulmonary capillary wedge pressure (PCWP), and systemic vascular resistance (SVR), with the additional benefit of monitoring the response to therapy. However, this procedure is not without risks, should be reserved for selected cases, and should only be performed by an experienced operator (see Chapter 76).

TREATMENT

Most patients with ADHF present with volume overload and pulmonary congestion. The mainstays of therapy are diuretics and vasodilators, reserved for those patients with adequate cardiac output to maintain sufficient blood pressure (systolic blood pressure >85 to 90 mm Hg) and end-organ perfusion (Alg. 21.2, Forrester Class II) prior to their initiation. These therapies are considered Class I recommendations by the European Society of Cardiology, and their effect is to reduce the work that must be performed by the failing heart by reducing both preload and afterload. Initial therapy with intravenous (IV) diuretics has a relatively rapid effect, with reductions in right atrial pressure, PCWP, and PVR within 5 to 30 minutes. For patients requiring high doses of furosemide, a continuous drip may be more effective than boluses >1 mg/kg. Guidelines for practical diuretic use are shown in Table 21.2, and include adding thiazide diuretics for refractory cases. In selected patients with ADHF (such as MI with pulmonary edema), vasodilator therapy with IV nitroglycerin should be considered the first-line agent (Table 21.3). Nitroglycerin IV is a balanced arterial and venous vasodilator when given in appropriate doses, effectively reducing both preload and afterload without impairing tissue perfusion. At low doses, IV nitroglycerin induces venodilation (without significant coronary artery dilation), and may not effectively unload the failing heart. Therefore, IV nitroglycerin should be titrated aggressively (with careful blood pressure monitoring) in patients suffering from ADHF in the setting of MI. In other patients with pulmonary congestion in the setting of ADHF, the combination of IV nitroglycerin and IV loop diuretics provides rapid symptomatic relief and has been found to be more effective than high-dose diuretics alone.

Nesiritide is recombinant B-type natriuretic peptide that, like nitroglycerin, is a balanced arterial and venous vasodilator, but also promotes natriuresis in combination with loop diuretics. Nesiritide decreases PCWP promptly and improves dyspnea in patients with

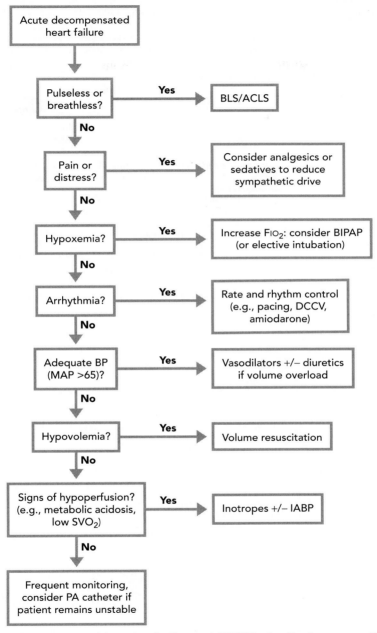

ALGORITHM 21.1 — Algorithmic Approach to Acute Decompensated Heart Failure

Acute decompensated heart failure

Pulseless or breathless? — **Yes** → BLS/ACLS

No

Pain or distress? — **Yes** → Consider analgesics or sedatives to reduce sympathetic drive

No

Hypoxemia? — **Yes** → Increase F_{IO_2}: consider BIPAP (or elective intubation)

No

Arrhythmia? — **Yes** → Rate and rhythm control (e.g., pacing, DCCV, amiodarone)

No

Adequate BP (MAP >65)? — **Yes** → Vasodilators +/− diuretics if volume overload

No

Hypovolemia? — **Yes** → Volume resuscitation

No

Signs of hypoperfusion? (e.g., metabolic acidosis, low SVO_2) — **Yes** → Inotropes +/− IABP

No

Frequent monitoring, consider PA catheter if patient remains unstable

BLS/ACLS, basic life support/advanced cardiac life support; BiPAP, bilevel positive airway pressure; DCCV, direct current cardioversion; BP, blood pressure; MAP, mean arterial pressure; IABP, intra-aortic balloon pump; PA, pulmonary artery; SVO_2, venous oxygen saturation.

ALGORITHM 21.2	Acute Decompensated Heart Failure Therapies by Clinical Presentation (Forrester Classification)

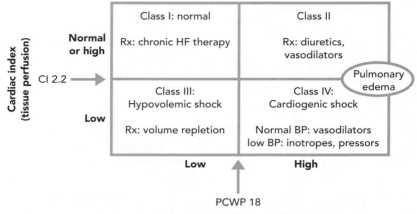

HF, heart failure; Rx, therapy; CI, cardiac index; BP, blood pressure; PCWP, pulmonary capillary wedge pressure.

TABLE 21.2	Diuretics for Acute Decompensated Heart Failure

Severity of Volume Overload	Diuretic	Dose	Comments
Mild to moderate	Furosemide	20–40 mg PO or IV	Follow Na^+ and K^+
Severe	Furosemide	40–120 mg IV, or IV drip at 2–20 mg/hr	Up to every 6 hr for bolus dosing
Refractory to loop diuretics	Add metolazone 30 min prior to each furosemide dose	2.5–5 mg PO	Most helpful when CrCl <30 mL/min
Refractory to combination of loop and thiazide diuretics	Consider inotrope (dobutamine) if renal perfusion is inadequate. Consider renal replacement therapy if renal failure (HD or CVVHDF).		

PO, by mouth; IV, intravenously; CrCl, creatinine clearance; HD, hemodialysis CVVHDF, continuous venovenous hemodiafiltration.

ADHF. Nesiritide can be initiated most safely without a bolus at 0.01 mcg/kg/min, with titration to a maximum dose of 0.03 mcg/kg/min.

ACEIs and ARBs have an important role in the management of chronic HF, but their role in the setting of ADHF is less clear. Chronic ACEI or ARB therapy promotes afterload reduction, but may require dosage reduction or discontinuation to facilitate diuresis without impairing renal function. Cautious initiation of ACEI or ARB therapy in the intensive care unit setting may be helpful with careful monitoring of renal function and electrolytes. The short-acting ACEI captopril (starting dose 6.25 to 12.5 mg every 6 to 8 hours) may be carefully titrated with each dose until a prespecified goal is met (systolic blood pressure <100 mm Hg, reduced SVR, or 300-mg daily dose). For patients with chronic HF, ACEIs or ARBs should be initiated approximately 48 hours after stabilization of an ADHF episode, most likely after transfer out of the critical care setting (Class I recommendation, Level of Evidence A).

Other medical therapies such as beta-blockers and calcium channel blockers generally have little role in the setting of ADHF. Beta-blockade is a mainstay of treatment for acute MI as well as for chronic HF, but patients presenting with MI and ADHF involving hypotension, or more than mild-to-moderate pulmonary congestion, have not been included in most of the relevant clinical trials. As such, IV metoprolol and other agents should be used with caution in this setting because of negative inotropic effects. Patients receiving chronic beta-blocker therapy should have their dosage reduced, but not abruptly discontinued to avoid rebound hypertensive effects. Milrinone should be considered for these patients if they require inotropic support as it acts downstream from the beta-adrenergic receptor. Calcium channel blockers (including diltiazem, verapamil, and amlodipine) are contraindicated in patients with ADHF, secondary to their negative inotropic effects.

TABLE 21.3	Vasodilators (all have potential for causing hypotension)

Indication	Vasodilator	Dose (mcg/min)	Comments
ADHF	Nitroglycerin	10–200	Headache, tachyphylaxis
ADHF	Nesiritide	0.01–0.03	Use bolus dosing with caution
Hypertensive crisis	Nitroprusside	0.5–5	Isocyanate toxicity

ADHF, acute decompensated heart failure.

TABLE 21.4	Inotropic Agents and Vasopressors

Drug	Class	Dose (mcg/kg/min)	Comments
Dobutamine	Inotrope	2.5–10	First line for ADHF
Milrinone	Inotrope/vasodilator	0.25–0.75	Useful with beta-blockade
Dopamine	Inotrope/vasopressor	5–50	Relatively weak agonist
Epinephrine	Inotrope/vasopressor	0.05–0.5	If refractory to dobutamine
Norepinephrine	Vasopressor	0.05–1	More appropriate for sepsis

ADHF, acute decompensated heart failure.

For patients in cardiogenic shock with hypotension and evidence of inadequate tissue perfusion (Alg. 21.2, Forrester Group IV) dobutamine and milrinone are the inotropic agents of choice. Dobutamine is predominantly a beta-1 and beta-2 adrenergic receptor agonist, which augments both inotropy and chronotropy. There is frequently a reflex decrease in sympathetic tone that leads to lowered SVR, further augmenting cardiac output. In patients receiving chronic beta-blocker therapy or in patients in whom tachycardia is problematic, milrinone is an effective alternative to dobutamine. Milrinone is a type-III phosphodiesterase inhibitor with characteristics of both an inotrope and peripheral vasodilator. Unfortunately, it has the disadvantage of renal clearance, making it contraindicated in patients with renal failure. The peripheral vasodilation of milrinone may also cause hypotension, particularly if it is given inappropriately in the setting of volume depletion (Alg. 21.2, Forrester Class III). Dobutamine and milrinone increase myocardial oxygen demand and should be reserved for cases of documented or suspected cardiogenic shock and systemic hypoperfusion. They do not have a role for mild episodes of ADHF. The use of vasopressors (e.g., dopamine or norepinephrine) may also be necessary in urgent situations to maintain blood pressure while the patient is being stabilized, but they should be weaned quickly as they increase afterload, and may further reduce end-organ perfusion. Table 21.4 shows typical dosing of inotropic agents and vasopressors.

For patients who cannot be adequately stabilized with medical therapy, consideration should be given to mechanical support, particularly if the patient is a candidate for advanced HF therapies such as cardiac transplantation or mechanical circulatory support with a left ventricular assist device. Intra-aortic balloon pump placement can provide mechanical afterload reduction, and augmented diastolic pressure to improve coronary artery filling in low-output states. Acute dialysis, especially continuous venovenous hemodiafiltration, can be used for volume control of diuretic-refractory patients with renal failure. Pursuing more advanced mechanical therapy (e.g., left ventricular assist device support) or cardiac transplantation is an increasingly viable option for patients without irreversible end-organ damage who are at centers with the appropriate resources.

Suggested Reading

Cuffe MS, Califf RM, Adams KF Jr, et al. Short-term intravenous milrinone for acute exacerbation of chronic heart failure: a randomized controlled trial. *JAMA*. 2002;287: 1541–1547.
  This RCT highlights the dangers of routine inotrope use in ADHF and demonstrates that inotropic agents should be reserved for those patients with evidence of clinically significant hypoperfusion.
Heart Failure Society of America. Executive summary: HFSA (Heart Failure Society of America) 2006 Comprehensive Heart Failure Practice Guideline. *J Card Fail*. 2006;12: 10–38.
  While the ESC guidelines above are dedicated specifically to ADHF, the 2006 HFSA guidelines represent a consensus-driven approach to establish best practices for diagnosis and treatment of HF in general, including ADHF.

Hunt SA, Abraham WT, Chin MH, et al. ACC/AHA 2005 Guideline Update for the Diagnosis and Management of Chronic Heart Failure in the Adult: a report of the American College of Cardiology/American Heart Association Task Force on Practice Guidelines (Writing Committee to Update the 2001 Guidelines for the Evaluation and Management of Heart Failure): developed in collaboration with the American College of Chest Physicians and the International Society for Heart and Lung Transplantation: endorsed by the Heart Rhythm Society. *Circulation.* 2005;112:e154–235.

The ACC/AHA practice guidelines regarding chronic heart failure provide a broad review of the data substantiating state-of-the art therapies for management of the heart failure patient.

McCullough PA, Nowak RM, McCord J, et al. B-type natriuretic peptide and clinical judgment in emergency diagnosis of heart failure: analysis from Breathing Not Properly (BNP) Multinational Study. *Circulation.* 2002;106:416–422.

This study is the most widely recognized trial validating the utility of serum BNP measurement for differentiating heart failure from other entities with similar presentations.

Nieminen MS, Bohm M, Cowie MR, et al. Executive summary of the guidelines on the diagnosis and treatment of acute heart failure: the Task Force on Acute Heart Failure of the European Society of Cardiology. *Eur Heart J.* 2005;26:384–416.

These ESC guidelines were the first to address the diagnosis and treatment of ADHF in a systematic fashion, and the Executive Summary cited here is an excellent overview of the topic and the supporting scientific literature.

Publication Committee for the VI. Intravenous nesiritide vs nitroglycerin for treatment of decompensated congestive heart failure: a randomized controlled trial. [erratum appears in *JAMA.* 2002;288:577]. *JAMA.* 2002;287:1531–1540.

This trial demonstrates the utility of nesiritide for improving the hemodynamics of patients with ADHF.

Thom T, Haase N, Rosamond W, et al. Heart Disease and Stroke Statistics—2006 Update: a report from the American Heart Association Statistics Committee and Stroke Statistics Subcommittee. *Circulation.* 2006;113ie85–e151.

This AHA update details the extensive cardiovascular disease burden in the United States.

22

HYPERTENSIVE EMERGENCIES
Daniel H. Cooper

True hypertensive emergencies have become a relatively infrequent cause for admission to the intensive care unit (ICU) in the current medical environment. The widespread availability of antihypertensive medications has drastically reduced the once-common scenario of the untreated hypertensive patient presenting to the emergency department with crisis related to elevated blood pressure. Only 1% to 2% of the hypertensive population will present with a hypertensive emergency in their lifetime. It is not an uncommon scenario, however, for our patients to present with severe hypertension. This may seem contradictory but to truly diagnose a hypertensive *emergency*, acute and progressive end-organ damage must be present, distinguishing it from other hypertensive syndromes. Terminology used in the description of hypertensive syndromes is often overlapping and confusing, which makes the following terms worth defining.

- *Hypertensive crisis:* Severe elevations in blood pressure that have the potential to cause target organ (heart, vasculature, kidneys, eyes, brain) damage. These include *emergencies* and *urgencies*.
- *Hypertensive urgency:* Severe elevation in blood pressure *without* evidence of acute and ongoing target-organ damage (TOD).
- Hypertensive emergency: Severe elevation in blood pressure with evidence of acute, ongoing TOD.
  - *Hypertensive encephalopathy*: a hypertensive emergency characterized by irritability, headaches, and mental status changes caused by significant and often rapid elevations in blood pressure.
  - *Accelerated malignant hypertension*: a hypertensive emergency characterized by fundoscopic findings of papilledema (grade 4 Keith-Wagener retinopathy) and/or acute retinal hemorrhages and exudates (grade 3 Keith-Wagener retinopathy). See Figure 22.2.

Timely differentiation between hypertensive emergencies and urgencies is imperative so that patients with severely elevated blood pressure can be triaged to the appropriate level of care and monitoring (i.e., outpatient follow-up vs. inpatient ward vs. ICU) with the appropriate antihypertensive agents initiated (parenteral vs. oral) and the establishment of blood pressure-lowering goals at the appropriate time interval (minutes-to-hours vs. days-to-weeks). In the absence of acute, progressive end-organ damage, elevated blood pressure alone does not require immediate, emergent therapy. The definitions given here intentionally are devoid of any absolute blood pressure numbers because the level at which individuals develop TOD can vary, depending on clinical substrate and the rapidity with which the blood pressure rises. For example, a patient with long-standing, poorly controlled hypertension can tolerate a blood pressure in excess of 230/120 mm Hg without evidence of acute end-organ damage, while the young healthy patient who acutely develops glomerulonephritis may become encephalopathic from hypertension at much lower pressures.

The approach to severely elevated blood pressure is outlined in Algorithm 22.1. It should be emphasized that when presented with these patients, one should perform a truncated history and physical examination that (a) quickly identifies patient characteristics that place the patient at risk for hypertensive emergencies, and (b) searches for signs and/or symptoms of underlying TOD. If rapid assessment reveals a true hypertensive emergency, then treatment should be initiated immediately, and managed in an ICU setting.

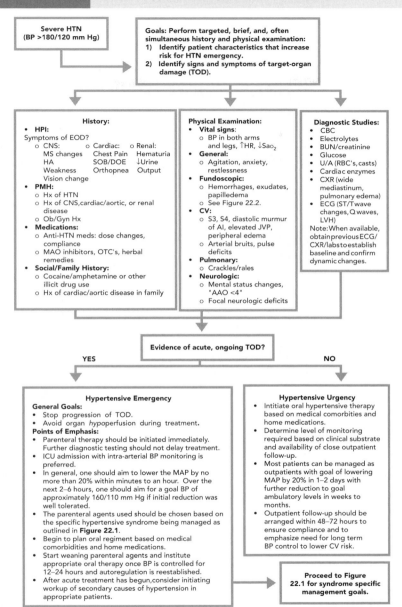

ALGORITHM 22.1   General Approach to Hypertensive Emergencies

Severe HTN
(BP >180/120 mm Hg)

Goals: Perform targeted, brief, and, often simultaneous history and physical examination:
1) Identify patient characteristics that increase risk for HTN emergency.
2) Identify signs and symptoms of target-organ damage (TOD).

History:
- **HPI:**
  Symptoms of EOD?
  - CNS:
    - MS changes
    - HA
    - Weakness
    - Vision change
  - Cardiac:
    - Chest Pain
    - SOB/DOE
    - Orthopnea
  - Renal:
    - Hematuria
    - ↓Urine Output
- **PMH:**
  - Hx of HTN
  - Hx of CNS, cardiac/aortic, or renal disease
  - Ob/Gyn Hx
- **Medications:**
  - Anti-HTN meds: dose changes, compliance
  - MAO inhibitors, OTC's, herbal remedies
- **Social/Family History:**
  - Cocaine/amphetamine or other illicit drug use
  - Hx of cardiac/aortic disease in family

Physical Examination:
- **Vital signs:**
  - BP in both arms and legs, ↑HR, ↓Sao₂
- **General:**
  - Agitation, anxiety, restlessness
- **Fundoscopic:**
  - Hemorrhages, exudates, papilledema
  - See Figure 22.2.
- **CV:**
  - S3, S4, diastolic murmur of AI, elevated JVP, peripheral edema
  - Arterial bruits, pulse deficits
- **Pulmonary:**
  - Crackles/rales
- **Neurologic:**
  - Mental status changes, "AAO <4"
  - Focal neurologic deficits

Diagnostic Studies:
- CBC
- Electrolytes
- BUN/creatinine
- Glucose
- U/A (RBC's, casts)
- Cardiac enzymes
- CXR (wide mediastinum, pulmonary edema)
- ECG (ST/T wave changes, Q waves, LVH)

Note: When available, obtain previous ECG/CXR/labs to establish baseline and confirm dynamic changes.

Evidence of acute, ongoing TOD?

YES

NO

Hypertensive Emergency

General Goals:
- Stop progression of TOD.
- Avoid organ *hypoperfusion* during treatment.

Points of Emphasis:
- Parenteral therapy should be initiated immediately. Further diagnostic testing should not delay treatment.
- ICU admission with intra-arterial BP monitoring is preferred.
- In general, one should aim to lower the MAP by no more than 20% within minutes to an hour. Over the next 2–6 hours, one should aim for a goal BP of approximately 160/110 mm Hg if initial reduction was well tolerated.
- The parenteral agents used should be chosen based on the specific hypertensive syndrome being managed as outlined in **Figure 22.1**.
- Begin to plan oral regiment based on medical comorbidities and home medications.
- Start weaning parenteral agents and institute appropriate oral therapy once BP is controlled for 12–24 hours and autoregulation is reestablished.
- After acute treatment has begun, consider initiating workup of secondary causes of hypertension in appropriate patients.

Hypertensive Urgency
- Initiate oral hypertensive therapy based on medical comorbities and home medications.
- Determine level of monitoring required based on clinical substrate and availability of close outpatient follow-up.
- Most patients can be managed as outpatients with goal of lowering MAP by 20% in 1–2 days with further reduction to goal ambulatory levels in weeks to months.
- Outpatient follow-up should be arranged within 48–72 hours to ensure compliance and to emphasize need for long term BP control to lower CV risk.

Proceed to Figure 22.1 for syndrome specific management goals.

HTN, hypertension; BP, blood pressure; HPI, history of present illness; EOD, end-organ damage; CNS, central nervous system; MS, mental status; HA, headache; SOB, shortness of breath; DOE, dyspnea on exertion; PMH, past medical history; Hx, history; Ob/Gyn, obstetrics/gynecology; MAO, monoamine oxidase; OTC, over the counter; HR, heart rate; Sao₂, saturation arterial oxygen; AI, aortic insufficiency; CV, cardiovascular; JVP, jugular venous pressure; "AAO <4", not awake, alert and oriented to either person, place, time, or situation; CBC, complete blood count; BUN, blood, urea, nitrogen; U/A, urinalysis; RBC, red blood cells; CXR, chest x-ray; ECG, electrocardiogram; LVH, left ventricular hypertrophy; ICU, intensive care unit; MAP, mean arterial pressure.

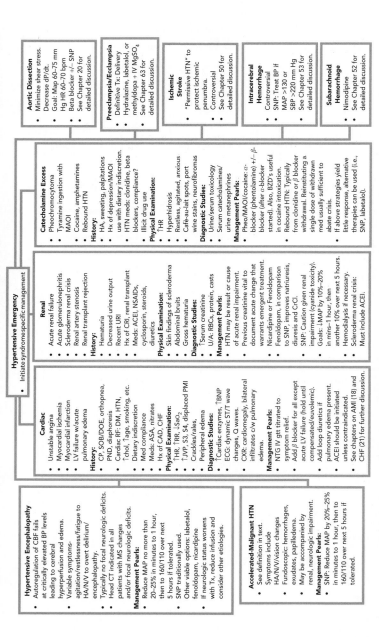

Figure 22.1. Management of Specific Hypertensive Emergencies

CBF, cerebral blood flow; BP, blood pressure; HA, headache; N, nausea; V, vomiting; MS, mental status; MAP, mean arterial pressure; SNP, sodium nitroprusside; Tx, treatment; HTN, hypertension; LV, left ventricle; CP, chest pain; SOB, shortness of breath; DOE, dyspnea on exertion; PND, paroxysmal nocturnal dyspnea; RF, risk factors; DM, diabetes mellitus, chol, cholesterol; ASA, aspirin; CAD, coronary artery disease; CHF, congestive heart failure; HR, heart rate; RR, respiratory rate; Sao$_2$, saturation arterial oxygen; JVP, jugular venous pressure; PMI, point of maximal impulse; BNP, brain natriuretic peptide; CXR, chest x-ray; IV, intravenous; NTG, nitroglycerin; gtt, drip (intravenous); ACEI, angiotensin-converting enzyme inhibitor; AMI, acute myocardial infarction; URI, upper respiratory infection; Hx, history; CRI, chronic renal insufficiency; NSAIDs, nonsteroidal anti-inflammatory drugs; CrCl, creatinine clearance; MAOI, monoamine oxidase inhibitor; pheo, pheochromocytoma; BZDs, benzodiazepines; dP/dt, rate of change in pressure; bpm, beats per minute.

TABLE 22.1 Parenteral Agents Used in Hypertensive Emergencies

Drug	Dose	Onset/Duration	Adverse Effects[a]	Points of Emphasis
Sodium nitroprusside (SNP)	Initial: 0.2–0.50 mcg/kg/min continuous infusion Maint: titrate to goal BP; up to 8–10 mcg/kg/min continuous infusion	Onset: Second Duration: 2–3 min after infusion is stopped	Thiocyanate and cyanide poisoning, nausea, vomiting, ↓BP	■ Potent arterial and venous dilator with rapid onset and offset of effect. ■ Preferred agent for most HTN emergencies. ■ Use with beta-blocker if used in aortic dissection. ■ Administer via continuous infusion in ICU, guided by intra-arterial BP monitoring. ■ Caution in renal or hepatic impairment due to thiocyanate/cyanide accumulation. ■ Signs of toxicity include metabolic acidosis, tremors, seizures, nausea, and vomiting. ■ Thiocyanate levels >10 mg/dL should be avoided. ■ Avoid prolonged use (>24–48 hr) in all patients. Max level infusions should be used for no more than 10 minutes to limit toxicity. ■ Increases intracranial pressure but the simultaneous fall in SVR off-sets this effect. Therefore, it is still recommended in hypertensive encephalopathy.
Labetalol	Bolus: 20 mg × 1, then 20–80 mg q 10 min to maximum dose 300 mg Infusion: 0.5–2 mg/min	Onset: 5–10 min Duration: 3–6 hr	↓HR, HB, HF, Bronchospasm, nausea, vomiting, flushing	■ Combined alpha and beta-adrenergic blocker. ■ Can be given as IV bolus or IV infusion. Excessive BP drops are unusual. ■ Useful in most hypertensive emergencies but avoid in CHF and severe asthma. ■ Commonly used agent (along with hydralazine) in HTN in pregnancy.
Nitroglycerin	Initial: 5 mcg/min Maint: titrate q 3–5 min up to 100 mcg/min	Onset: 2–5 min Duration: 5–15 min	Tolerance, HA, ↓BP, nausea, methemoglobinemia	■ Similar to SNP, but causes mostly venodilation with only modest arteriolar dilation effects at higher doses. ■ Most useful in emergencies complicated by cardiac compromise (i.e., myocardial ischemia/infarct, LV failure/pulmonary edema). ■ Also indicated in management of postoperative HTN following CABG ■ Tolerance will develop with prolonged use.

(continued)

TABLE 22.1 Parenteral Agents Used in Hypertensive Emergencies *(continued)*

Drug	Dose	Onset/Duration	Adverse Effects[a]	Points of Emphasis
Hydralazine	Bolus: 10–20 mg q30min until goal BP	Onset: 10–30 min Duration: 2–4 hr	↓BP, ↑HR, flushing	■ Direct arteriolar vasodilator with no significant venous effects. ■ Caution in patients with CAD or aortic dissection given reflex sympathetic stimulation. Must use with beta-blocker in these patients. ■ Avoid in patients with increased ICP. ■ BP lowering response is less predictable than with above agents and, therefore, use should be limited to HTN in pregnancy if possible.
Enalapril	Initial: 1.25 mg × 1, then 1.25–5 mg q6hr	Onset: 15–30 min Duration: 6–12 hr	↓BP, renal failure, hyperkalemia	■ The only available IV angiotensin-converting enzyme inhibitor. ■ Response to agent is unpredictable and depends on plasma renin activity and volume status of patient. ■ Most useful as an adjunctive agent in patients with CHF or scleroderma renal crisis. ■ Contraindicated in pregnancy and in renal-artery stenosis.
Nicardipine	Initial: 5 mg/hr, increase by 2.5 mg/h q20min up to maximum dose 15 mg/h	Onset: 15–30 min Duration: 1–4 hr	↓BP, ↑HR, HF, HA nausea, flushing	■ Dihydropyridine calcium channel blocker. ■ Can be used effectively in most emergencies, but should be avoided in acute heart failure. ■ Reflex tachycardia may be avoided with addition of beta-blocker.
Fenoldopam	Initial: 0.1 mcg/kg/min Maint: titrate q15min, up to 0.6 mcg/kg/min	Onset: 3–5 min Duration: 30 min	↑HR, HA, nausea, flushing	■ Selective peripheral dopamine-1 receptor agonist causing primarily arterial vasodilation with rapid onset and relatively short offset of effect. ■ Shown to improve renal perfusion; therefore, useful in patients with renal impairment. ■ Contraindicated in patients with glaucoma.
Esmolol	Bolus: 500 mcg/kg, repeat after 5 min Infusion: 50–100 mcg/kg/min, up to 300 mcg/kg/min	Onset: 1–5 min Duration: 15–30 min	↓HR, HB, HF, bronchospasm, nausea, vomiting, flushing	■ Short-acting, cardioselective beta-adrenergic blocker. ■ If concern for significant adverse effects to beta-blockers, short duration of esmolol may be useful.
Phentolamine	Bolus: 5–10 mg, repeat q5–15min Infusion: 0.2–5 mg/min	Onset: 1–2 min Duration: 10–20 min	↑HR, HA, nausea	■ Alpha-adrenergic blocker, used primarily in sydromes associated with excess catecholamines (i.e., pheochromocytoma, tyramine ingestion while on MAOI).

Maint, maintenance; BP, blood pressure; HTN, hypertension; ICU, intensive care unit; SVR, systemic vascular resistance; HR, heart rate; HB, heart block; HF, heart failure; CHF, congestive heart failure; LV, left ventricle; CABG, coronary artery bypass grafting; CAD, coronary artery disease; ICP, intracranial pressure; MAOI, monoamine oxidase inhibitor.

[a]Either common or life-threatening adverse effects of these medications are listed. This does not represent a comprehensive list of all possible adverse effects.

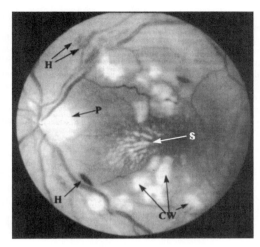

Figure 22.2. Hypertensive neuroretinopathy in malignant hypertension. Fundus photograph in a 30-year-old man with malignant hypertension demonstrates all of the characteristic features of hypertensive neuroretinopathy, including striate hemorrhages (H), cotton-wool spots (CW), papilledema (P), and a star figure at the macula (S). From Nolan CR. The patient with hypertension. In: Schrier RW, ed. *Manual of Nephrology*. Philadelphia: Lippincott Williams & Wilkins; 2000:236, with permission.

Treatment of hypertensive emergencies has a simple goal: stop the progression of TOD. The complexity of management lies in the careful balance that one must maintain between sufficiently and quickly lowering the arterial pressure without causing a precipitous decline that can lead to organ hypoperfusion. This balance is best achieved with parenteral agents that have a rapid onset and short half-life, administered under the guidance of intra-arterial blood pressure monitoring. Sodium nitroprusside is an agent with these desired "on-off" or "light switch" properties; therefore, it is the preferred agent in most hypertensive emergencies (Table 22.1 has details for this and other agents used for hypertensive emergencies). In contrast, sublingual nifedipine, a once commonly used medication for hypertensive crisis, has a variable, unpredictable, and uncontrollable blood pressure-lowering effect that can lead to coronary, renal, and cerebral hypoperfusion. Therefore, its use should be avoided. There are other reasonable alternatives and one must tailor therapy to the particular type of emergency, as outlined in Figure 22.1.

Suggested Reading

Calhoun DA, Oparil S. Treatment of hypertensive crisis. *N Engl J Med.* 1990;323:1177–1183.
  A review of treatment options for the hypertensive crisis.
Choubanian AV, Bakris GL, Black HR, et al. Seventh report of the Joint National Committee on Prevention, Detection, Evaluation and Treatment of High Blood Pressure. Hypertension. 2003;42: 1206–1252.
  JNC VII, a comprehensive expert review of hypertension, including sections dedicated to addressing approach to hypertensive emergencies.
Elliot WJ. Clinical features in the management of selected hypertensive emergencies. *Prog Cardiovasc Dis.* 2006;48:316–325.
  Concise review of definitions, epidemiology, pathophysiology, and syndrome specific treatment options.
Grossman E, Messerli FH, Grodzicki T, et al. Should a moratorium be placed on sublingual nifedipine capsules given for hypertensive emergencies and pseudoemergencies ? *JAMA.* 1996 Oct. 23–30; 276(16):1328–1331.
  A discussion of the potential for adverse outcomes when sublingual nifidepine is used to treat hypertensive emergencies.

Kaplan NM. Hypertensive crises. In: Kaplan NM, ed. *Kaplan's Clinical Hypertension.* 9th ed. Philadelphia: Lippincott Williams & Wilkins; 2006:311–324.

A leader in hypertension provides his approach to management of hypertensive crises. Also embedded elsewhere in text are chapters that address HTN in pregnancy, catecholamine excess states, renal failures, etc. in greater detail.

Rehman SU, Basile JN, Vidt DG. Hypertensive emergencies and urgencies. In: Black HR, Elliot WJ, eds. *Hypertension: A Companion to Braunwald's Heart Disease.* Philadelphia: Saunders-Elsevier; 2007:517–524.

A current review of approach to hypertensive urgencies and emergencies in a comprehensive text dedicated to addressing all aspects of hypertension, written by leaders in the field.

ELECTROLYTE ABNORMALITIES
Kamalanathan K. Sambandam

23

DISORDERS OF SODIUM CONCENTRATION

Hypernatremia and hyponatremia are primarily disorders of *water* balance or *water* distribution across the various fluid compartments in the body. Although alterations in sodium (Na^+) content change Na^+ concentration ($[Na^+]$) transiently, there is a resulting perturbation in total body water osmolarity (osmoles/liter [mOsm/L]), which is detected by hypothalamic osmoreceptors. Compensatory changes in water balance then occur through the action of antidiuretic hormone (ADH, or vasopressin) and the thirst control centers of the hypothalamus, which return $[Na^+]$ to normal. A persistent abnormality in $[Na^+]$ would thus require an alteration in the thirst response, or the action of ADH, both of which commonly occur in critically ill patients. Indeed, the incidence of hyponatremia and hypernatremia in the intensive care unit (ICU) may each be 15% to 30%. The dysnatremias' significance lies not only in their direct clinical effects in the individual patient, but also through their ability to predict mortality. The in-hospital mortality of patients with either hyponatremia or hypernatremia is approximately 30% to 40%, which is significantly greater than normonatremic patients. The increased mortality is generally from the severe underlying disease processes, and not from the dysnatremias, per say.

Hyponatremia

There are four main mechanisms of hyponatremia (Alg. 23.1): (a) dilution from extracellular fluid (ECF) hyperosmolarity, (b) appropriate ADH secretion from either true or effective decreased circulating volume, (c) inappropriate ADH secretion, or (d) hypotonic fluid loading.

Etiologies of Special Importance in the Critically Ill Patient

Hyperglycemia (Hyperosmolar Hyponatremia)
Glucose acts as an osmotically active solute because it is restricted to the ECF. In the marked hyperglycemia of diabetic ketoacidosis and hyperosmolar hyperglycemic state, the ECF

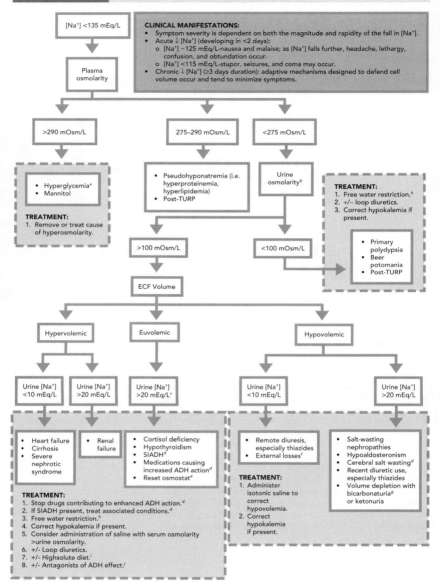

Post-TURP, posttransurethral resection of the prostate; ECF, extracellular fluid; ADH, antidiuretic hormone; SIADH, syndrome of inappropriate antidiuretic hormone. [a]The plasma [Na⁺] falls by 2.4 mEq/L for every 100 mg/dL rise in the plasma [glucose] above normal. [b]Urine specific gravity, although less accurate than a laboratory measurement of urine osmolarity, can be obtained rapidly at the bedside and converted to osmolarity by the following relationship: osmolarity = (specific gravity −1) × 35,000. [c]Urine [Na⁺] may be <20 mEq/L with low Na⁺ intake. [d]See text for details. [e]Urine osmolarity may be <100 mOsm/L after a water load. [f]Includes gastrointestinal losses (vomiting, diarrhea, fistulas), skin losses (burns, sweating), and third spacing (peritonitis, pancreatitis) with concomitant hypotonic fluid replacement. [g]From vomiting-induced contraction alkalosis or proximal renal tubular acidosis. [h]Free water restriction must be to an amount less than the urine output. [i]May include high protein diet or urea administration (30 to 60 g/day). [j]These are used when other measures have failed and may include conivaptan, demeclocycline (300 to 600 mg twice daily), or lithium.

hyperosmolarity (usually >290 mOsm/L) causes water to shift from the intracellular fluid (ICF) compartment to the ECF, and dilutional hyponatremia ensues. The plasma [Na$^+$] falls by 2.4 mEq/L for every 100 mg/dL rise in the plasma [glucose] above normal. In DKA the urinary excretion of anionic ketones contributes slightly to the hyponatremia by obligating renal Na$^+$ loss to maintain urine electroneutrality.

Edematous States (Hypervolemic Hyponatremia)

Heart failure, cirrhosis, and severe nephrotic syndrome result in decreased effective circulating volume (ECV), which non-osmotically stimulates hypothalamic thirst centers and ADH release. Impaired free water excretion occurs as exhibited by a urine osmolarity >100 mOsm/L (Alg. 23.1). If the rise in total body water exceeds the increase in total body Na$^+$, hyponatremia results. The degree of hyponatremia often correlates with the severity of the underlying condition.

Syndrome of Inappropriate ADH (Euvolemic Hyponatremia)

Non-osmotic release of vasopressin (either from the posterior pituitary or an ectopic source) also underlies the pathophysiology of the syndrome of inappropriate ADH (SIADH). However, the presence of euvolemia and a low serum uric acid concentration (<4 mg/dL as opposed to the usually higher values found in states of low ECV) differentiates this from the edematous states previously mentioned. Commonly associated conditions include neuropsychiatric disorders (e.g., meningitis, encephalitis, acute psychosis, cerebrovascular accident, head trauma), pulmonary diseases (e.g., pneumonia, tuberculosis, positive pressure ventilation, acute respiratory failure), malignant tumors (most commonly, small cell lung cancer), and physical/emotional stress and pain. Before making the diagnosis of SIADH, pharmacologic agents that enhance ADH action must be withdrawn.

- Nicotine, carbamazepine, antidepressants, narcotics, antipsychotic agents, and certain anti-neoplastic drugs may stimulate ADH release.
- Chlorpropamide, methylxanthines, and nonsteroidal anti-inflammatory drugs (NSAIDs) potentiate the action of ADH.
- Oxytocin and desmopressin acetate are ADH analogs.

Cerebral Salt Wasting (Hypovolemic Hyponatremia)

Neurosurgery and central nervous system trauma, especially subarachnoid hemorrhage, at times may be associated with excessive renal Na$^+$ excretion. Although poorly understood, the mechanism may involve the release of a brain natriuretic peptide and/or the loss of renal sympathetic tone. The loss of Na$^+$ causes volume depletion, which leads to the nonosmotic release of ADH. This volume depletion is the main feature that distinguishes cerebral salt wasting from SIADH. The hyponatremia, however, does not always correct with volume resuscitation, perhaps as a result of concomitant ADH release from the damaged brain. In some cases, the use of fludrocortisone has ameliorated the decline in [Na$^+$].

Treatment

Hyponatremia treatment is outlined in Algorithms 23.1 and 23.2. The hyponatremia in hyperosmolar or iso-osmolar states is usually of little clinical significance as fluid shifts to the ICF compartment and neuronal cell swelling does not occur. Likewise, mild asymptomatic hyponatremia, as is often seen with disorders such as reset osmostat, does not require specific treatment. When more significant hypo-osmolar hyponatremia occurs, management involves three steps: (a) determine the required rate of [Na$^+$] correction, (b) correct the hypo-osmolarity at the rate desired, and (c) correct the underlying disorder. Although acute hyponatremia (<2 days in duration) may be corrected rapidly, adaptive mechanisms designed to defend cell volume that occur in hyponatremia of longer duration (>2 days) necessitate slower correction to avoid precipitating central pontine myelinolysis (CPM). In its most overt form, CPM is characterized by flaccid paralysis, dysarthria, and dysphagia. In more subtle presentations it can be confirmed by computed tomography scan or magnetic resonance imaging of the brain. The risk of precipitating CPM is increased with correction of the [Na$^+$] by >12 mEq/L in a 24-hour period. The absolute magnitude of the

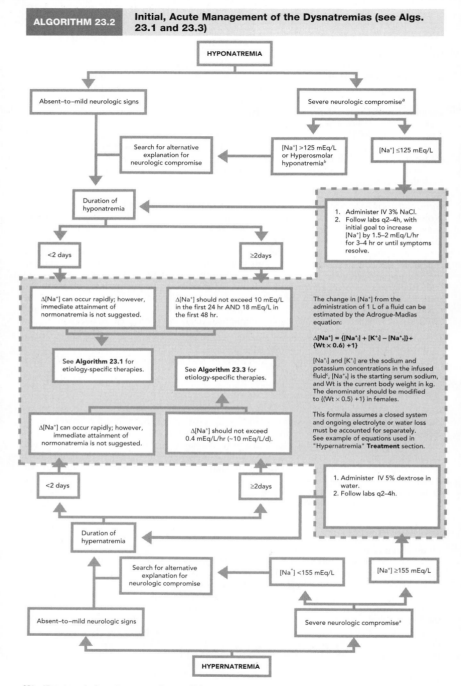

ALGORITHM 23.2   Initial, Acute Management of the Dysnatremias (see Algs. 23.1 and 23.3)

HYPONATREMIA

Absent–to–mild neurologic signs

Severe neurologic compromise[a]

Search for alternative explanation for neurologic compromise

[Na+] >125 mEq/L or Hyperosmolar hyponatremia[b]

[Na+] ≤125 mEq/L

Duration of hyponatremia

1. Administer IV 3% NaCl.
2. Follow labs q2–4h, with initial goal to increase [Na+] by 1.5–2 mEq/L/hr for 3–4 hr or until symptoms resolve.

<2 days

≥2days

Δ[Na+] can occur rapidly; however, immediate attainment of normonatremia is not suggested.

Δ[Na+] should not exceed 10 mEq/L in the first 24 hr AND 18 mEq/L in the first 48 hr.

See **Algorithm 23.1** for etiology-specific therapies.

See **Algorithm 23.3** for etiology-specific therapies.

Δ[Na+] can occur rapidly; however, immediate attainment of normonatremia is not suggested.

Δ[Na+] should not exceed 0.4 mEq/L/hr (~10 mEq/L/d).

The change in [Na+] from the administration of 1 L of a fluid can be estimated by the Adrogue-Madias equation:

$$\Delta[Na^+] = \{[Na^+_i] + [K^+_i] - [Na^+_s]\} + \{Wt \times 0.6) + 1\}$$

$[Na^+_i]$ and $[K^+_i]$ are the sodium and potassium concentrations in the infused fluid[c], $[Na^+_s]$ is the starting serum sodium, and Wt is the current body weight in kg. The denominator should be modified to $\{(Wt \times 0.5) + 1\}$ in females.

This formula assumes a closed system and ongoing electrolyte or water loss must be accounted for separately. See example of equations used in "Hypernatremia" **Treatment** section.

<2 days

≥2days

1. Administer IV 5% dextrose in water.
2. Follow labs q2–4h.

Duration of hypernatremia

Search for alternative explanation for neurologic compromise

[Na+] <155 mEq/L

[Na+] ≥155 mEq/L

Absent–to–mild neurologic signs

Severe neurologic compromise[a]

HYPERNATREMIA

[a]Significant confusion, stupor, or seizure activity.
[b]Plasma osmolarity >290 mOsm/L in the setting of marked hyperglycemia or mannitol infusion.
[c][Na+] in hypertonic saline is 513 mEq/L, in normal saline it is 143 mEq/L, and in 5% dextrose in sterile water it is 0 mEq/L.

correction in 24 hours appears to be more important than the rate, such that an initially rapid rate of correction tapering off after several hours incurs less risk than a slow, steady correction that exceeds 12 mEq/L in 1 day. Risk factors for precipitating CPM include the presence of hypoxemia and pre-existing hypokalemia, malnutrition, or alcoholism. It must be kept in mind that simple water restriction in primary polydipsia or saline resuscitation in hypovolemic patients may lead to overly rapid correction of hyponatremia. This can be prevented by the administration of free water or the use of the vasopressin analog desmopressin acetate to slow the rate of free water excretion.

The change in $[Na^+]$ from the administration of 1 L of a fluid can be estimated by the Adrogue-Madias equation (see Alg. 23.2 and the example of its application in the hypernatremia treatment section). Severe neurologic dysfunction should generally be treated with a 3% NaCl solution. However, any saline solution that is hyperosmolar to the urine can increase the $[Na^+]$ when oral water intake is restricted. A crystalloid with an osmolarity less than urine osmolarity may actually worsen the hyponatremia, even if the fluid's $[Na^+]$ is greater than the serum $[Na^+]$: For example, a patient with a $[Na^+] = 108$ mEq/L and urine osmolarity persistently >500 mOsm/L from SIADH is given normal saline (NS) to attempt to correct the hyponatremia. The 308 mOsm contained in 1 L of NS will be excreted in 0.6 L of additional urine output (308 mOsm ÷ 500 mOsm/L) and 0.4 L of free water (1 − 0.6 L) will be retained. The $[Na^+]$ will thus fall further.

The simultaneous administration of an intravenous (IV) loop diuretic to promote further free water excretion can counteract this seemingly paradoxic effect.

Hypernatremia

There are three main mechanisms of hypernatremia (Alg. 23.3): (a) primary Na^+ gain, and, much more commonly, (b) extrarenal or (c) renal hypo-osmolar fluid loss.

Etiologies of Special Importance in the Critically Ill Patient

Insensible Free Water Loss
In ambulatory adults at room temperature, hypotonic fluid loss occurs from the skin and respiratory tract at a rate of approximately 400 to 500 mL/day each. However, insensible water losses greatly depend on respiratory rate, body temperature, ambient temperature, and humidity. These variables make losses much more difficult to predict in the ICU patient who may be mechanically ventilated and either hypo- or hyperthermic. In general, water losses increase by 100 to 150 mL/day for each degree of body temperature more than 37°C. Still, fluid losses from the skin can vary enormously (100 to 2,000 mL/hour) with sweating or in the setting of severe burns. If these insensible losses are not matched in addition to sensible-free water loss, hypernatremia will ensue.

Primary Na+ Gain
Critically ill patients often require the administration of hypertonic saline solutions. Common examples of this occur with large-volume 0.9% NaCl resuscitation or the administration of several ampules of $NaHCO_3$ (which is hypertonic to plasma) during cardiopulmonary resuscitation. Because of the kidney's capacity to greatly increase renal Na^+ excretion in response to hypervolemia, hypernatremia arising from this mechanism alone is less common than that occurring with hypotonic fluid loss.

Diabetes Insipidus
The appropriate renal response to hypernatremia is excretion of a small volume (<800 mL/day) of concentrated urine (>800 mOsm/L). These responses are diminished in central diabetes insipidus (CDI) and nephrogenic diabetes insipidus (NDI) in which there is, respectively, either impaired ADH secretion or resistance to its effect. The most common cause of CDI is damage to the neurohypophysis as a result of trauma, neurosurgery, granulomatous disease, neoplasms, vascular accidents, or infection. In some cases, CDI is idiopathic and may occasionally be hereditary. NDI may also rarely be inherited. Acquired NDI can be classified into disorders associated with intrinsic renal diseases (e.g., sickle cell nephropathy,

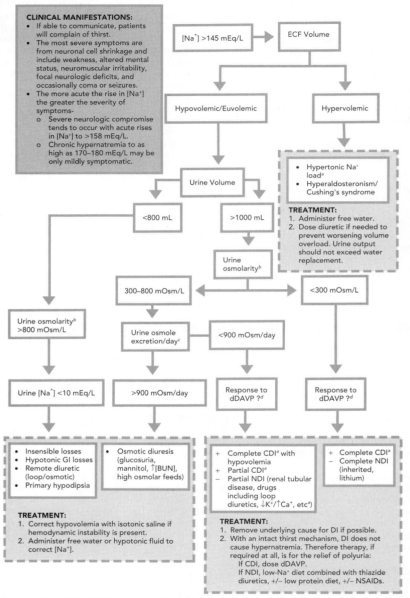

ALGORITHM 23.3 Clinical Manifestations of Hypernatremia and Approach to the Diagnosis and Treatment (see Alg. 23.2)

CLINICAL MANIFESTATIONS:
- If able to communicate, patients will complain of thirst.
- The most severe symptoms are from neuronal cell shrinkage and include weakness, altered mental status, neuromuscular irritability, focal neurologic deficits, and occasionally coma or seizures.
- The more acute the rise in [Na⁺] the greater the severity of symptoms-
  - Severe neurologic compromise tends to occur with acute rises in [Na⁺] to >158 mEq/L.
  - Chronic hypernatremia to as high as 170–180 mEq/L may be only mildly symptomatic.

[Na⁺] >145 mEq/L → ECF Volume

Hypovolemic/Euvolemic → Hypervolemic

Hypervolemic:
- Hypertonic Na⁺ load[a]
- Hyperaldosteronism/Cushing's syndrome

TREATMENT:
1. Administer free water.
2. Dose diuretic if needed to prevent worsening volume overload. Urine output should not exceed water replacement.

Urine Volume → <800 mL / >1000 mL

>1000 mL → Urine osmolarity[b]

Urine osmolarity[b]: 300–800 mOsm/L / <300 mOsm/L

<800 mL → Urine osmolarity[b] >800 mOsm/L → Urine [Na⁺] <10 mEq/L

300–800 mOsm/L → Urine osmole excretion/day[c]: <900 mOsm/day / >900 mOsm/day

<300 mOsm/L → Response to dDAVP?[d]

<900 mOsm/day → Response to dDAVP?[d]

- Insensible losses
- Hypotonic GI losses
- Remote diuretic (loop/osmotic)
- Primary hypodipsia

- Osmotic diuresis (glucosuria, mannitol, ↑[BUN], high osmolar feeds)

+ Complete CDI[a] with hypovolemia
+ Partial CDI[a]
− Partial NDI (renal tubular disease, drugs including loop diuretics, ↓K⁺/↑Ca⁺, etc[a])

+ Complete CDI[a]
− Complete NDI (inherited, lithium)

TREATMENT:
1. Correct hypovolemia with isotonic saline if hemodynamic instability is present.
2. Administer free water or hypotonic fluid to correct [Na⁺].

TREATMENT:
1. Remove underlying cause for DI if possible.
2. With an intact thirst mechanism, DI does not cause hypernatremia. Therefore therapy, if required at all, is for the relief of polyuria:
   If CDI, dose dDAVP.
   If NDI, low-Na⁺ diet combined with thiazide diuretics, +/− low protein diet, +/− NSAIDs.

ECF, extracellular fluid; dDAVP, desmopressin acetate; GI, gastrointestinal; BUN, blood, urea, nitrogen; CDI, central diabetes insipidus; NDI, nephrogenic diabetes insipidus; K⁺, potassium; Ca⁺, calcium; NSAIDs, nonsteroidal anti-inflammatory drugs; (+), conditions with increase in urine osmolarity in response to desmopressin acetate; (−), conditions with little increase in urine osmolarity in response to desmopressin acetate. [a]See text for details. [b]Urine specific gravity, although less accurate than measurement of urine osmolarity, can be obtained rapidly at the bedside and converted to osmolarity by the following relationship: osmolarity = (specific gravity − 1) × 35,000. [c]Daily urinary osmolar excretion can be measured by timed urine collection or estimated by spot urine osmolarity × average urine volume per 24 hours. [d]Determined by administering desmopressin (10 mcg intranasally) after careful water restriction. The urine osmolarity should increase by at least 50% in complete CDI and does not change in NDI.

polycystic kidney disease, obstructive nephropathy, Sjogren), drugs (e.g., lithium, demeclo-cycline, amphotericin, glyburide), electrolyte disorders (hypercalcemia and hypokalemia), and conditions that reduce renal medullary hypertonicity (e.g., osmotic diuresis, excessive water intake, and the use of loop diuretics).

Osmotic Diuresis

Increased renal free water loss is necessitated by high solute loads reaching the lumen of the distal nephron. Osmotic diuresis very commonly results from poorly controlled diabetes mellitus and its associated glucosuria. IV mannitol administration, azotemia out of proportion to the decrease in glomerular filtration rate (as can occur in the catabolic ICU patient with moderate renal insufficiency on high-protein feeds and stress-dose steroids), or large enteral solute loads with high osmolar feeds, can also result in an osmotic diuresis. This cause of hypernatremia can be confused for DI, but can be distinguished from it by quantifying the number of osmoles excreted in the urine per day (Alg. 23.3).

Treatment

Hypernatremia treatment is outlined in Algorithms 23.2 and 23.3. The management of hypernatremia involves three steps: (a) determine the rate of correction, (b) correct the water deficit and hypovolemia at the rate desired, and (c) correct the underlying disorder. As for hyponatremia, the desired rate of correction of hypernatremia depends on the acuity of its development and whether associated neurologic dysfunction is present. Acute hypernatremia (<2 days duration) may be corrected rapidly, but overaggressive correction of hypernatremia of longer duration causes a rapid shift of water into neuronal cells that have adapted to the hyperosmolarity. Seizures or permanent neurologic damage may result. Thus, in hypernatremia of >2 days in duration, the decrease in [Na^+] should be limited to 0.4 to 0.5 mEq/L/hr (~10mEq/L/d), which allows for a margin of error from the observed safe rate of correction of 12 mEq/L/d (note the similarity to the treatment of hyponatremia).

In general, when severe neurologic compromise is present, the hyperosmolarity should initially be reduced with IV 5% dextrose in sterile water (D5W). Once neurologic improvement occurs, the remaining free-water deficit can be replaced with enteral water flushes, continued IV D5W, or IV ¼ NS with or without K^+ additive. The last fluid may be more appropriate in situations of both water and electrolyte losses as occurs with gastrointestinal and diuretic-induced losses. The change in [Na^+] that occurs with fluid administration can, as with hyponatremia, be predicted by the Adrogue-Madias equation (Alg. 23.2). The formula assumes a closed system and requires separate account of ongoing losses.

For example, a 70-kg woman with 2 L/day diarrhea presents with lassitude and [Na^+] = 160 mEq/L, [K^+] = 3.0. Her urine output averages 0.7 L/day. The chosen replacement fluid is ¼ NaCl with 20 mEq KCl/L. The estimated [Na^+] from 1 L of this fluid would be –2.8 mEq/L ([38.5 {sodium concentration in ¼ NaCl} + 20 − 160] ÷ [(70 × 0.5) + 1]). In a closed system, one can predict that 3,600 mL ([10 mEq/L] ÷ [2.8 mEq/L per 1,000 mL of infused fluid]) of this crystalloid per day would reduce the patient's [Na^+] by 10 mEq/day. Because 0.7 L/day of urine output and 2 L/day of ongoing diarrhea must also be accounted for, an estimated 6.3 L (3.6 L + 0.7 L + 2 L) of this fluid should be given at 260 mL/hr during the next 24 hours. As this is only an approximation, the [Na^+] should be followed closely and therapy adjusted accordingly. Note that accounting for ongoing electrolyte-free water loss in the treatment of hyponatremia is harder to do and would reduce the amount of hypertonic fluid to give rather than augment it.

DISORDERS OF POTASSIUM CONCENTRATION

The total body potassium (K^+) content in a normal adult is approximately 3,000 to 4,000 mEq, 98% of which is intracellular. The normal serum K^+ concentration ([K^+]) is 3.5 to 5 mEq/L, whereas that inside cells is approximately 150 mEq/L. Thus, the ECF compartment from which we measure the serum [K^+] contains only 2% of the total body K^+. Perturbations in the serum [K^+] therefore are misleading as to the degree of the total K^+ deficit or excess. With the major effector organ of K^+ excretion being the kidney, K^+ balance is regulated primarily by two physiologic stimuli; aldosterone and the K^+ concentration itself. Aldosterone is secreted in response to high angiotensin II, or hyperkalemia, and increases renal K^+ wasting. The plasma $[K^+]$ can also directly affect urinary K^+ excretion independent of aldosterone.

Hypokalemia

There are three main mechanisms of hypokalemia (Alg. 23.4): (a) shift of K^+ to the ICF, (b) inappropriate renal wasting, and (c) extrarenal K^+ loss.

Etiologies of Special Importance in the Critically Ill Patient

Transcellular Shift
Movement of K^+ into cells may transiently decrease the plasma $[K^+]$ without altering total body K^+ content. The magnitude of the change is relatively small, often <1 mEq/L, but it may amplify hypokalemia from other causes. Triggers of intracellular shift include alkalemia, insulin, and catecholamines (either produced endogenously through the stress response or administered exogenously). Marked anabolism can also result in K^+ translocation into cells. The most common example of this occurs with the refeeding syndrome, when nutritional support is initiated after a prolonged period of starvation.

Gastrointestinal K^+ Loss
In general, gastrointestinal fluids have a significant K^+ content and excessive enteral losses will result in hypokalemia. When the lower gastrointestinal tract is the source of the loss, there is often a concomitant metabolic acidosis from bicarbonate loss. When losses are from the upper tract, metabolic alkalosis is usually present.

Renal K^+ Loss
Urinary K^+ wasting may be caused by factors that augment the distal nephron tubular flow rate or by factors that increase the distal tubular fluid $[K^+]$. Augmented distal flow occurs with diuretic use, osmotic diuresis, DI, and the polyuric phase of acute tubular necrosis. Increased distal nephron $[K^+]$ occurs with thiazide and loop diuretics, hyperaldosteronism of any cause (most commonly decreased ECV), the urinary excretion of anions (which necessitates the coexcretion of cations, including K^+), hypomagnesemia, and amphotericin B. Thus, the hypokalemia often seen with diabetic ketoacidosis results from several mechanisms: the osmotic diuresis caused by glucosuria, the hyperaldosteronism from volume depletion, the urinary excretion of anionic ketones, and the intracellular shift resulting from insulin therapy. Similarly, in the hypokalemia associated with vomiting or nasogastric suction, renal loss of K^+ results from volume depletion and alkalosis-induced bicarbonaturia (as HCO_3^- is negatively charged), in addition to the gastric loss of K^+ and the transcellular shift from alkalemia.

Treatment

Hypokalemia treatment is outlined in Algorithm 23.4. Rapid correction of hypokalemia is required when symptoms or electrocardiographic changes are present. In these cases and when patients are unable to take enteral medications, IV repletion is appropriate. Otherwise it is generally safer to correct hypokalemia via the enteral route, and larger doses can be administered orally given the limitations on the rate of IV infusion of K^+. KCl is usually the preparation of choice regardless of the route of administration as it promotes more rapid correction of hypokalemia and concomitant metabolic alkalosis than the other preparations. Potassium bicarbonate or citrate may be useful in correcting the hypokalemia and acidosis associated with chronic diarrhea or renal tubular acidoses. Hypomagnesemia should be sought in all hypokalemic patients and corrected prior to or concurrently with K^+ repletion (see "Hypomagnesemia: Treatment"). Without Mg^+ repletion, reduced renal K^+ absorption in the loop of Henle and collecting duct would result in the prompt loss of administered K^+. Although there are rules to estimate the total K^+ deficit present, mechanisms of transcellular shift are difficult to predict and the degree of K^+ depletion does not correlate well with the serum $[K^+]$. The serum $[K^+]$ should therefore be monitored frequently during therapy.

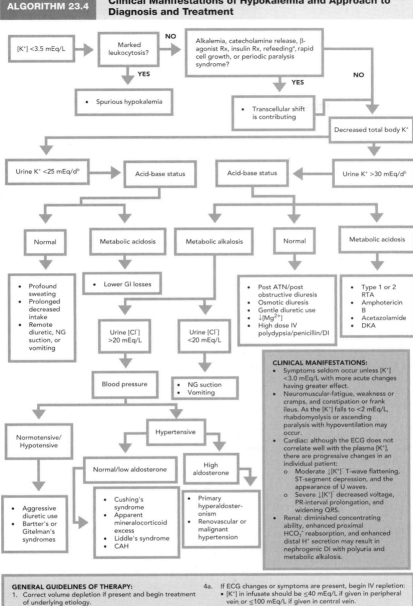

ALGORITHM 23.4 — Clinical Manifestations of Hypokalemia and Approach to Diagnosis and Treatment

[K+] <3.5 mEq/L → Marked leukocytosis?

- YES → Spurious hypokalemia
- NO → Alkalemia, catecholamine release, β-agonist Rx, insulin Rx, refeeding[a], rapid cell growth, or periodic paralysis syndrome?
  - YES → Transcellular shift is contributing
  - NO → Decreased total body K+

Decreased total body K+ →
- Urine K+ <25 mEq/d[b] → Acid-base status
- Urine K+ >30 mEq/d[b] → Acid-base status

Urine K+ <25 mEq/d — Acid-base status:

- Normal
  - Profound sweating
  - Prolonged decreased intake
  - Remote diuretic, NG suction, or vomiting
- Metabolic acidosis
  - Lower GI losses
- Metabolic alkalosis
  - Urine [Cl−] >20 mEq/L → Blood pressure
    - Normotensive/Hypotensive
      - Aggressive diuretic use
      - Bartter's or Gitelman's syndromes
    - Hypertensive
      - Normal/low aldosterone
        - Cushing's syndrome
        - Apparent mineralocorticoid excess
        - Liddle's syndrome
        - CAH
      - High aldosterone
        - Primary hyperaldosteronism
        - Renovascular or malignant hypertension
  - Urine [Cl−] <20 mEq/L
    - NG suction
    - Vomiting

Urine K+ >30 mEq/d — Acid-base status:

- Normal
  - Post ATN/post obstructive diuresis
  - Osmotic diuresis
  - Gentle diuretic use
  - ↓[Mg2+]
  - High dose IV polydypsia/penicillin/DI
- Metabolic acidosis
  - Type 1 or 2 RTA
  - Amphotericin B
  - Acetazolamide
  - DKA

CLINICAL MANIFESTATIONS:
- Symptoms seldom occur unless [K+] <3.0 mEq/L with more acute changes having greater effect.
- Neuromuscular-fatigue, weakness or cramps, and constipation or frank ileus. As the [K+] falls to <2 mEq/L, rhabdomyolysis or ascending paralysis with hypoventilation may occur.
- Cardiac: although the ECG does not correlate well with the plasma [K+], there are progressive changes in an individual patient:
  o Moderate ↓[K+] T-wave flattening, ST-segment depression, and the appearance of U waves.
  o Severe ↓[K+] decreased voltage, PR-interval prolongation, and widening QRS.
- Renal: diminished concentrating ability, enhanced proximal HCO3− reabsorption, and enhanced distal H+ secretion result in nephrogenic DI with polyuria and metabolic alkalosis.

GENERAL GUIDELINES OF THERAPY:
1. Correct volume depletion if present and begin treatment of underlying etiology.
2. Search for and treat hypomagnesemia.[c]
3. Estimate the K+ deficit:
   • A decrement of 1 mEq/L represents an estimated total body deficit of 200–400 mEq.
4a. If ECG changes or symptoms are present, begin IV repletion:
   • [K+] in infusate should be ≤40 mEq/L if given in peripheral vein or ≤100 mEq/L if given in central vein.
   • Infusion rate should be ≤20 mEq/hr unless paralysis or malignant ventricular arrhythmias are present.
4b. If no ECG changes or symptoms, begin PO repletion.
5. Monitor [K+] frequently during therapy.

Rx, medication; NG, nasogastric; GI, gastrointestinal; ATN, acute tubular necrosis; IV, intravenous; DI, diabetes insipidus; RTA, renal tubular acidosis; DKA, diabetic ketoacidosis; ECG, electrocardiogram; CAH, congenital adrenal hyperplasia; PO, by mouth. [a]See text for details. [b]The total daily K+ excretion can be estimated by multiplying a spot urine [K+] by the daily urine output. Alternatively, a spot urine [K+] alone may be used (urine [K+] <20 mEq/L suggests appropriate K+ avidity during extrarenal loss), but is less accurate in situations of either polyuria or oliguria. [c]See Table 23.7 for the treatment of hypomagnesemia.

Hyperkalemia

There are three main mechanisms of hyperkalemia (Alg. 23.5): (a) reduced glomerular filtration, (b) effective hypoaldosteronism, and (c) transcellular shift. Sustained hyperkalemia almost always requires the first of these mechanisms as normal kidneys have a tremendous capacity for K^+ excretion.

Etiologies of Special Importance in the Critically Ill Patient

Transcellular Shift

The movement of K^+ from the ICF to the ECF may transiently increase the plasma $[K^+]$ without altering total body K^+ content, often amplifying the hyperkalemia resulting from other causes. Potential causes of extracellular shift include insulin deficiency, ECF hyperosmolarity, acidemia, intense exercise, and cell lysis (such as occurs in the tumor lysis syndrome, rhabdomyolysis, and intravascular or extravascular hemolysis). Diabetic ketoacidosis may promote hyperkalemia through these first three mechanisms of K^+ shift, despite patients being total body-K^+ depleted. Medications that cause extracellular shift include nonselective beta-blockers, overdosed digitalis, and succinylcholine. The hyperkalemia that occurs with succinylcholine is usually small (~0.5 mEq/L) and brief (resolving within 10 to 15 minutes). But it can be significantly accentuated in patients with massive trauma, burns, or neuromuscular disease.

Insufficient Renal Function

The diseased kidney responds to progressive renal insufficiency with increased K^+ excretion per functioning nephron over time. If low K^+ intake is maintained, this adaptation is usually able to maintain normal $[K^+]$ until the glomerular filtration rate falls to the point of oliguria. Thus, when hyperkalemia develops in a nonoliguric patient, there is usually a second contributing mechanism or the renal injury is severe and has occurred over a short time period. Diminished distal tubular fluid delivery, as occurs in states of decreased ECV, is a common contributing mechanism in the critically ill patient. In such situations, little salt and water is present in the distal nephron lumen to allow for sufficient K^+ secretion to occur in exchange for Na^+ absorption.

Drugs

Anti-kaliuretic medications are another common component of the usual multifactorial hyperkalemia that occurs in the ICU patient. Heparin, ketoconazole, angiotensin-converting enzyme inhibitors, and angiotensin II receptor antagonists decrease aldosterone production, and spironolactone is a competitive aldosterone antagonist. NSAIDs inhibit renin secretion, a process that is several steps upstream of aldosterone release. NSAIDs also decrease glomerular filtration through the inhibition of vasodilatory renal prostaglandins in afferent arterioles, and thus reduce distal solute delivery. Cyclosporine may both lower renin levels and attenuate the effect of aldosterone. K^+-sparing diuretics, trimethoprim, and pentamidine all block Na^+ reabsorption in exchange for K^+ secretion by the distal nephron.

Treatment

Hyperkalemia treatment is outlined in Algorithm 23.5 and Table 23.1. The presence of symptoms or electrocardiogram changes associated with hyperkalemia necessitates the prompt initiation of measures capable of rapidly lowering the serum $[K^+]$ (Table 23.1). It must be remembered that mechanisms of outward K^+ shift from the large intracellular pool may dramatically increase the serum $[K^+]$, and that can be rapidly reversed (such as the marked hyperosmolarity and acidemia of diabetic ketoacidosis) can allow sufficient correction of life-threatening hyperkalemia without additional therapy. Calcium, although it does not reduce the $[K^+]$, serves to stabilize the cardiac myocyte membrane. This is given simultaneously with therapies that shift K^+ to the ICF (insulin and albuterol) while mechanisms of increasing K^+ excretion (sodium polystyrene sulfonate, diuretics, and/or hemodialysis) are initiated as well.

Notably, the use of $NaHCO_3$ to promote intracellular shift is falling out of favor, based on data indicating that large doses of bicarbonate (400 mEq) are required to elicit a

(text continues on page 165)

ALGORITHM 23.5 Clinical Manifestations of Hyperkalemia and Approach to Diagnosis and Treatment

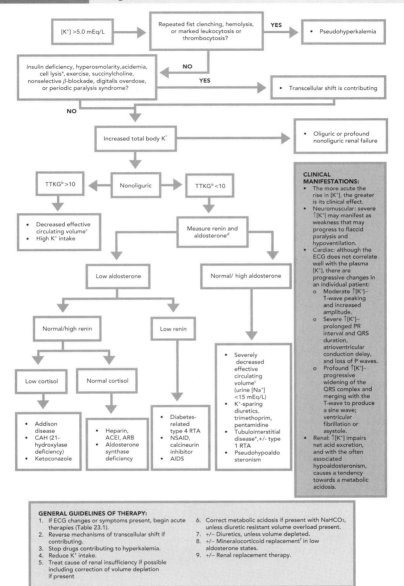

CLINICAL MANIFESTATIONS:
- The more acute the rise in [K+], the greater is its clinical effect.
- Neuromuscular: severe ↑[K+] may manifest as severe weakness that may progress to flaccid paralysis and hypoventilation.
- Cardiac: although the ECG does not correlate well with the plasma [K+], there are progressive changes in an individual patient:
  o Moderate ↑[K+]– T-wave peaking and increased amplitude.
  o Severe ↑[K+]– prolonged PR interval and QRS duration, atrioventricular conduction delay, and loss of P waves.
  o Profound ↑[K+]– progressive widening of the QRS complex and merging with the T-wave to produce a sine wave; ventricular fibrillation or asystole.
- Renal: ↑[K+] impairs net acid excretion, and with the often associated hypoaldosteronism, causes a tendency towards a metabolic acidosis.

GENERAL GUIDELINES OF THERAPY:
1. If ECG changes or symptoms present, begin acute therapies (Table 23.1).
2. Reverse mechanisms of transcellular shift if contributing.
3. Stop drugs contributing to hyperkalemia.
4. Reduce K+ intake.
5. Treat cause of renal insufficiency if possible including correction of volume depletion if present
6. Correct metabolic acidosis if present with NaHCO₃, unless diuretic resistant volume overload present.
7. +/– Diuretics, unless volume depleted.
8. +/– Mineralocorticoid replacement[f] in low aldosterone states.
9. +/– Renal replacement therapy.

TTKG, transtubular K+ gradient; ECG, electrocardiogram; CAH, congenital adrenal hyperplasia; ACEI, angiotensin converting enzyme inhibitor; ARB, angiotensin receptor blocker; RTA, renal tubular acidosis; NSAID, nonsteroidal anti-inflammatory drug; AIDS, acquired immune deficiency syndrome. [a]See text for details. [b]TTKG = ([K+u] ÷ [K+p]) ÷ (Osmu ÷ Osmp), where [K+u] = urine K+ concentration, [K+p] = plasma K+ concentration, Osmu = urine osmolarity, and Osmp = plasma osmolarity. The formula assumes that vasopressin is present and active, assured by confirming Osmu >Osmp. [c]Causes include hypovolemia, heart failure, cirrhosis, and nephrotic syndrome. [d]Renin and aldosterone levels should ideally be measured in a morning specimen while the patient is on a low salt diet and after the administration of a loop diuretic the night before to induce mild volume contraction. [e]Causes include sickle cell anemia, chronic obstruction, renal transplant rejection, lupus. [f]Replacement doses vary from 0.05 to 0.2 mg of fludrocortisone.

TABLE 23.1 Acute Therapies for the Management of Hyperkalemia

Treatment	Dosing	Onset/Duration	Magnitude of [K⁺] Decline	Comments
Ca^{2+}	1 g of 10% calcium gluconate or $CaCl_2$ infused IV over 2–3 min. May repeat if no improvement in ECG by 5 min.	Immediate onset, lasting 30–60 min.	None	$CaCl_2$ should be administered via a central vein to decrease risk of extravasation skin necrosis. Watch for signs of hypercalcemia.
Insulin	10 U of regular insulin IV (with 50 g of dextrose IV if not significantly hyperglycemic).	Onset at 15 min, lasting 6–8 hr.	~1 mEq/L	Watch for hypo- or hyperglycemia (if dextrose given). The latter can offset insulin's K⁺ lowering effect.
Albuterol	10–20 mg given by nebulized inhalation over 15 min OR 0.5 mg in 100 mL of 5% dextrose infused IV over 15 min.	Onset at 10–30 min, lasting 3–6 hr.	1–1.5 mEq/L	Tachycardia and variable effects on blood pressure may result. Hyperglycemia may worsen and offset some K⁺ lowering.
$NaHCO_3$	2–4 mEq/min in drip (three ampules $NaHCO_3$ in sterile water or 5% dextrose) until bicarbonate normalized.	Onset at 4 hr, lasting >6 hr.	0.5–0.75 mEq/L	Not effective unless metabolic acidosis precedes therapy. Watch for volume overload in diuretic resistant states. May lower serum ionized $[Ca^{2+}]$ and make more susceptible to arrhythmias.
Loop +/− thiazide diuretics	Widely variable dose depends on GFR.	Onset at 30–60 min, lasting 4–6 hr (duration prolonged in renal insufficiency).	Variable depending on diuretic response	Avoid in volume-depleted states until euvolemia restored. Saline alone is usually sufficient in cases with normal GFR.
Sodium poly-styrene sulfonate	25–50 g mixed in 100 mL 20% sorbitol PO OR 50 g in 200 mL 30% sorbitol per rectum.	Onset at 1–2 hr, lasting 4–6 hr.	0.5–1 mEq/L	Caution with use in the postoperative patient because of risk of intestinal necrosis. Watch for worsening volume overload or hypernatremia from exchanged [Na⁺].
Hemo-dialysis	Variable, based on starting [K⁺].	Immediate onset, lasting until dialysis completion.	Variable, based on dialysis dose and dialysate [K⁺].	Watch for posttreatment K⁺ rebound beginning immediately after dialysis completion.

IV, intravenous; ECG, electrocardiogram; GFR, glomerular filtration rate; PO, by mouth.

modest and delayed K^+-lowering effect (~0.7 mEq/L decrease occurring only after 4 hours). Dialytic therapies are not always required for severe hyperkalemia if rapid correction of antikaliuretic mechanisms is possible, such as with the prompt reversal of volume depletion. Although a 4-hour hemodialysis treatment might remove approximately 120 mEq of K^+, with normal renal function one can excrete up to 400 mEq/day in hyperkalemia of >2 days in duration.

Another important aspect of therapy is limiting exogenous potassium loads, some of which may not be obvious: Each 8-ounce can of high-protein tube feeds contains approximately 10 mEq of K^+ and a single unit of packed red blood cells with a prolonged storage time may constitute approximately 5 mEq.

DISORDERS OF CALCIUM CONCENTRATION

Approximately 99% of body calcium (Ca^{2+}) is in bone with most of the remaining 1% in the ECF. The ionized Ca^{2+} concentration ($[Ca^{2+}]$), which must lie within a narrow range (4.6 to 5.1 mg/dL) for optimal neuromuscular function, is normally precisely controlled by a negative feedback mechanism involving parathyroid hormone (PTH). PTH increases serum $[Ca^{2+}]$ by stimulating bone resorption, increasing Ca^{2+} reclamation in the kidney, and promoting the renal conversion of 25-hydroxyvitamin D_3 (25[OH]D_3) to its more active form 1,25-dihydroxycholecalciferol (1,25[OH]$_2D_3$; calcitriol), which promotes intestinal Ca^{2+} absorption.

Disorders of Ca^{2+} concentration are common among critically ill patients, particularly hypocalcemia. Low ionized $[Ca^{2+}]$ has been observed in up to 88% of ICU patients. Furthermore, the presence of hypocalcemia serves as a marker of disease severity, showing correlation with both Acute Physiology and Chronic Health Evaluation II (APACHE-II) scores and patient mortality.

Hypocalcemia

There are three main mechanisms in the development of true hypocalcemia (Table 23.2): (a) effective hypoparathyroidism, (b) effective vitamin D deficiency, and (c) chelation of Ca^{2+} from the circulation.

Etiologies of Special Importance in the Critically Ill Patient

Pseudohypocalcemia
Nearly 50% of serum Ca^{2+} exists in its free ionized form, whereas the remainder is complexed to albumin (40%) and anions such as phosphate (10%). Changes in serum albumin and serum anions alter total serum $[Ca^{2+}]$ without affecting the clinically relevant ionized $[Ca^{2+}]$. Hypoalbuminemia is very common in the ICU setting because albumin concentrations fall during the systemic inflammatory response and with large-volume fluid resuscitation. The total serum $[Ca^{2+}]$ is lowered in such situations, but ionized $[Ca^{2+}]$ remains within the normal range. If an ionized $[Ca^{2+}]$ is unavailable, the total $[Ca^{2+}]$ can be corrected for the presence of hypoalbuminemia by the following equation:

$$\text{Corrected } [Ca^{2+}] = [Ca^{2+}] + \{0.8 \times (4.0 - [\text{albumin}])\}.$$

Chelation
An increase in the availability of any anion that combines readily with Ca^{2+} may cause hypocalcemia as ionized Ca^{2+} is chelated by this species. Both extravascular and intravascular chelation may occur. Examples of the former occur during the release of negatively charged fatty acids in severe pancreatitis and with the tremendous deposition of Ca^{2+} and PO_4^{3-} in bone that occurs after rapidly reversing prolonged, severe hyperparathyroidism by parathyroidectomy. The hypocalcemia that results from this "hungry bone syndrome" can persist for months.

Intravascular chelation occurs in several other situations found in the critically ill patient: More anionic side chains on albumin become available to bind Ca^{2+} as H^+

TABLE 23.2	The Differential Diagnosis, Clinical Manifestations, and Treatment of Hypocalcemia ((Corrected $[Ca^{2+}]$ <8.4 mg/dL OR [ionized Ca^{2+}] <4.2 mg/dL) where corrected $[Ca^{2+}]$ = $[Ca^{2+}]$ + {0.8 × (4.0 − [Albumin])}).

Etiology	Characteristic Laboratories
Hypoparathyroidism	
Autoimmune parathyroid destruction (polyglandular immune syndrome I)	Low or inappropriately normal iPTH, ↑$[PO_4{}^{3-}]$
Infiltrative disease (hemochromatosis, Wilson's disease, malignant replacement)	Low or inappropriately normal iPTH, ↑$[PO_4{}^{3-}]$
Iatrogenic (total parathyroidectomy)	Low or inappropriately normal iPTH, ↑$[PO_4{}^{3-}]$
Congenital (familial hypocalcemia, DiGeorge's syndrome)	Low or inappropriately normal iPTH, ↑$[PO_4{}^{3-}]$
Severe hypermagnesemia or severe hypomagnesemia	Low or inappropriately normal iPTH, ↑$[PO_4{}^{3-}]$
Parathyroid Hormone Resistance	
Moderate hypomagnesemia	↑iPTH
Pseudohypoparathyroidism types 1a, 1b, and 2	↑iPTH, ↑$[PO_4{}^{3-}]$
Bisphosphonate, gallium nitrate, or calcitonin therapy	↑iPTH, ↓$[PO_4{}^{3-}]$
Vitamin D Deficiency	
Advanced chronic kidney disease	↑iPTH, ↑$[PO_4{}^{3-}]$, ↓$1,25(OH)_2D_3$
Vitamin D-dependent rickets type 1	↑iPTH, ↓$[PO_4{}^{3-}]$, ↓$1,25(OH)_2D_3$
Low precursor vitamin D intake or malabsorption with limited sun exposure	↑iPTH, ↓$[PO_4{}^{3-}]$, ↓$25(OH)D_3$
Severe hepatic insufficiency	↑iPTH, ↓$[PO_4{}^{3-}]$, ↓$25(OH)D_3$
Severe nephrotic syndrome	↑iPTH, ↓$[PO_4{}^{3-}]$, ↓$25(OH)D_3$
P450 enzyme inducing medication (many anticonvulsants, isoniazid, rifampin)	↑iPTH, ↓$[PO_4{}^{3-}]$, ↓$25(OH)D_3$
Calcium Chelation	
Hyperphosphatemia (rhabdomyolysis, tumor lysis, massive hemolysis, phosphosoda bowel preparation)	↑iPTH, ↑$[PO_4{}^{3-}]$
Hyperoxalemia (ethylene glycol poisoning)	↑iPTH
Pancreatitis	↑iPTH
Post-hyperparathyroid hungry bone syndrome	↓iPTH, ↓$[PO_4{}^{3-}]$
Alkalemia	↑iPTH
Massive transfusion of citrate containing blood products	↑iPTH
Foscarnet therapy	↑iPTH
Other	
Sepsis	variable iPTH
Gadolinium induced pseudohypocalcemia	normal iPTH, normal ionized $[Ca^{2+}]$

CLINICAL MANIFESTATIONS:

Acute, moderate ↓$[Ca^{2+}]$: circumoral or distal paresthesias and tetany, including carpopedal spasms. Latent tetany may be elicited by certain maneuvers:

Trousseau's sign: carpal spasm when a blood pressure cuff is inflated around arm above systolic pressure for 3 minutes.

Chvostek's sign: facial muscle twitching when the facial nerve is tapped anterior to the ear.

Acute, severe ↓$[Ca^{2+}]$: laryngospasm, confusion, seizures, or vascular collapse with bradycardia and decompensated heart failure.

ECG: QT interval prolongation with bradycardia and in some cases complete heart block.

Chronic ↓$[Ca^{2+}]$: may be asymptomatic but also may be associated with cataracts and basal ganglia calcification.

(continued on next page)

TABLE 23.2	The Differential Diagnosis, Clinical Manifestations, and Treatment of Hypocalcemia ((Corrected [Ca^{2+}] <8.4 mg/dL OR [ionized Ca^{2+}] <4.2 mg/dL) where corrected [Ca^{2+}] = [Ca^{2+}] + {0.8 × (4.0 − [Albumin])}). (*Continued*)

GENERAL GUIDELINES OF THERAPY:
1. If ECG changes or symptoms present, begin IV replacement:
   a. Consider early initiation of hemodialysis when caused by hyperphosphatemia or hyperoxalemia.
   b. Bolus 2 g MgSO$_4$ IV over 15 min if known ↓[Mg^{2+}] or empirically if renal function is normal.
   c. Bolus 2g Ca^{2+} gluconate (20 mL or two ampules of 10% Ca^{2+} gluconate; 1 g = 93 mg elemental Ca^{2+}) in 50–100 mL of 5% dextrose or saline IV over 10–15 min.
   d. Begin continuous Ca^{2+} infusion: Dilute 6 g of Ca^{2+} gluconate (or 2 g, 20 mL, or two ampules of 10% CaCl$_2$^{a}; 1 g = 272 mg elemental Ca^{2+}) in 500 mL of 5% dextrose or saline and infuse at 0.5–1.5 mg elemental Ca^{2+}/kg/hr.
   e. Follow ionized [Ca^{2+}] or corrected [Ca^{2+}] Q 6 hours and continue infusion until [Ca^{2+}] normalizes.
   f. Begin to overlap with PO replacement.
2. Dose 1–2 g elemental Ca^{2+} PO TID to QID. Unless concomitantly hyperphosphatemic, dose separate from meals.
3. +/− 0.25–4 mcg/d calcitriol +/− ergocalciferol especially in vitamin D-deficient states.
4. +/− salt restriction and hydrochlorothiazide if hypercalciuria occurs.

ECG, electrocardiogram; iPTH, intact parathyroid hormone.
^{a}Although Ca^{2+} gluconate may be given peripherally, CaCl$_2$ should only be administered through a central vein.

concentrations fall in alkalemia. Massive phosphate loads from any cause (e.g., tumor lysis, rhabdomyolysis) can also lower ionized [Ca^{2+}]. And finally, the administration of large volumes of citrate-containing blood products such as fresh-frozen plasma or packed red blood cells can result in hypocalcemia. This is usually transient but may be more prolonged and severe in situations of hepatic insufficiency when the metabolism of citrate is impaired.

Sepsis

Hypocalcemia occurs commonly in sepsis, particularly when involving a Gram-negative organism. Indeed, in one study, ionized hypocalcemia was found in 30% of cases of Gram-negative septicemia and in none of those cases caused by Gram-positive bacteria. The pathogenesis is incompletely understood, but most patients have elevated PTH and low calcitriol levels. Elevated levels of procalcitonin have been found in many of these patients, suggesting that this hormone precursor may exert a hypocalcemic effect in the critically ill population.

Treatment

Hypocalcemia treatment is outlined in Table 23.2. The management of symptomatic hypocalcemia or that associated with electrocardiogram abnormalities should be prompt and aggressive. Intravenous Ca^{2+} replacement should be initiated in such situations.

Hypomagnesemia, if present, must be treated first in order to effectively correct the hypocalcemia. If the cause of low [Ca^{2+}] is marked hyperphosphatemia or hyperoxalemia, it is important to limit IV replacement to those cases in which cardiac effects or significant symptoms are apparent. Overaggressive repletion in such situations may cause metastatic calcification and later result in rebound hypercalcemia, as has been described following severe rhabdomyolysis. In cases of profound hypocalcemia from hyperphosphatemia or hyperoxalemia, clearance of the chelating species through the early initiation of hemodialysis with higher Ca^{2+} dialysate should be considered. For hypocalcemia occurring in the setting of profound sepsis or other shock states, evidence guiding therapy is lacking. Although increases in cardiac contractility and blood pressure have been observed, there exists some animal data that suggest that reperfusion injury and mortality may be worsened by Ca^{2+} administration.

Asymptomatic hypocalcemia may be managed with oral Ca^{2+} supplements and vitamin D or its active metabolite, calcitriol, to increase intestinal Ca^{2+} absorption. If hypercalciuria develops with chronic therapy at a serum $[Ca^{2+}]$ <8.5 mg/dL (this occurs especially with effective hypoparathyroidism), salt restriction and hydrochlorothiazide can be considered to reduce renal Ca^{2+} excretion.

Hypercalcemia

There are four main mechanisms of hypercalcemia (Table 23.3): (a) effective hyperparathyroidism, (b) effective vitamin D excess, (c) non–PTH-induced bone resorption, and (d) decreased renal Ca^{2+} excretion. Many cases of life-threatening hypercalcemia seen in the critically ill are related to malignancy, with each of the first three of these mechanisms occurring as primary processes in various cancer-induced hypercalcemias. The fourth mechanism is almost always secondarily present as hypercalcemia-induced volume depletion reduces Ca^{2+} excretion.

Etiologies of Special Importance in the Critically Ill Patient

Humoral Hypercalcemia of Malignancy

Cancers may at times produce a hormone that differs slightly from PTH, but retains its biologic activity. This PTH-related peptide has most often been associated with squamous carcinomas of the lung, head and neck, or esophagus, carcinomas of the kidney, bladder, or ovary, and, less commonly, pheochromocytoma. As in cases of primary hyperparathyroidism, hypercalcemia and hypophosphatemia are present, but hypercalcemia is often much more severe and the intact PTH is suppressed. In most cases of humoral hypercalcemia of malignancy, patients usually have advanced, clinically obvious disease.

Tumoral/Granulomatous Calcitriol Production

Active vitamin D can be produced by the lymphocytes of some Hodgkin and non-Hodgkin lymphomas. Mononuclear cell production of calcitriol also occurs in granulomatous diseases such as sarcoidosis and fungal or tuberculous infections. In these conditions, $1,25(OH)_2D_3$ levels are elevated through ectopic production, and increased intestinal Ca^{2+} and phosphate absorption occurs. PTH levels are suppressed by the resultant hypercalcemia, but the elevation in $[Ca^{2+}]$ is usually less severe than in humoral hypercalcemia of malignancy. Again, in most cases the underlying condition is usually easily apparent.

Osteolytic Hypercalcemia of Malignancy

In this form of cancer-associated hypercalcemia, cytokines produced by tumor cells (such as interleukins-1 and -6) act locally to stimulate osteoclast bone resorption. Hypercalcemia and hyperphosphatemia occur only with extensive bone involvement by tumor, and the serum alkaline phosphatase is often significantly elevated. Once more, PTH is suppressed. The most frequently associated malignancies include breast carcinoma, non-small cell lung cancer, myeloma, and lymphoma.

Treatment

Hypercalcemia treatment is outlined in Table 23.4. Rapidly acting therapies for hypercalcemia are warranted if severe symptoms are present or with $[Ca^{2+}]$ >12 mg/dL. First, the anticalciuretic effect of hypovolemia should be corrected with IV isotonic fluid boluses. Continuing maintenance IV saline after achieving euvolemia further promotes Ca^{2+} excretion. Loop diuretics add little to the calciuretic effect of saline administration and may prevent adequate restoration of ECV. However, they are useful if signs of hypervolemia develop. Calcitonin and hemodialysis against a low Ca^{2+} dialysate are the only other means of lowering the serum $[Ca^{2+}]$ within hours.

TABLE 23.3	The Differential Diagnosis and Clinical Manifestations of Hypercalcemia ([Ca^{2+}] >10.3 mg/dL OR [ionized Ca^{2+}] >5.2 mg/dL)

Etiology	Characteristic Laboratories
Hyperparathyroidism	
Primary hyperparathyroidism (85% adenomas, 14% diffuse four-gland hyperplasia, 1% parathyroid carcinoma)	High or inappropriately normal iPTH, ↓[PO$_4^{3-}$], urine Ca^{2+} >200 mg/d or FE Ca^{2+} >1%[a]
Tertiary hyperparathyroidism	High or inappropriately normal iPTH, ↓[PO$_4^{3-}$], urine Ca^{2+} >200 mg/d or FE Ca^{2+} >1%[a]
Lithium use	High or inappropriately normal iPTH, normal [PO$_4^{3-}$], urine Ca^{2+} <200 mg/d or FE Ca^{2+} <1%[a]
Familial hypocalciuric hypercalcemia	High or inappropriately normal iPTH, normal [PO$_4^{3-}$], normal 25(OH)D$_3$[b], urine Ca^{2+} <200 mg/d or FE Ca^{2+} <1%[a]
Humoral hypercalcemia of malignancy[c]	↓iPTH, ↓[PO$_4^{3-}$], ↑parathyroid hormone-related peptide
Vitamin D Excess	
Precursor vitamin D intoxication	↓iPTH, ↑[PO$_4^{3-}$], ↑25(OH)D$_3$
Tumoral calcitriol production[c]	↓iPTH, ↑[PO$_4^{3-}$], ↑1,25(OH)$_2$D$_3$
Extensive granulomatous disease[c]	↓iPTH, ↑[PO$_4^{3-}$], ↑1,25(OH)$_2$D$_3$
Calcitriol overdose	↓iPTH, ↑[PO$_4^{3-}$], ↑1,25(OH)$_2$D$_3$
Acromegaly	↓iPTH, ↑[PO$_4^{3-}$], ↑1,25(OH)$_2$D$_3$
Nonparathyroid-Induced Bone Resorption	
Osteolytic hypercalcemia of malignancy[c]	↓iPTH, ↑[PO$_4^{3-}$], ↑↑alkaline phosphatase
Paget's disease	↓iPTH, ↑[PO$_4^{3-}$], ↑↑alkaline phosphatase
Immobilization	↓iPTH
Vitamin A intoxication	↓iPTH
Hyperthyroidism	↓iPTH
Adrenal insufficiency	↓iPTH, ↑[K$^+$], ↓[HCO$_3^-$]
Decreased Renal Calcium Excretion	
Volume depletion	↓iPTH
Milk alkali syndrome	↓iPTH, ↑[HCO$_3^-$]
Thiazide diuretics	↓iPTH

CLINICAL MANIFESTATIONS:
Signs and symptoms generally present only if the [Ca^{2+}] >12 mg/dL and tend to be more severe if ↑[Ca^{2+}] develops rapidly.
Acute ↑[Ca^{2+}]:
  Renal—polyuria with hypovolemia.
  Gastrointestinal—anorexia, vomiting, constipation, and rarely abdominal pain from pancreatitis.
  Neurologic—weakness, fatigue, confusion, stupor, and coma.
  ECG—shortened QT interval and, with very severe ↑[Ca^{2+}], variable degrees of atrioventricular block
Chronic ↑[Ca^{2+}]:
  Renal—polyuria, nephrolithiasis or nephrocalcinosis with irreversible renal failure.
  Musculoskeletal—fractures with little trauma. Osteitis fibrosa cystica with "brown tumors" and marrow replacement occurs rarely if hyperparathyroidism is profound and prolonged.

ECG, electrocardiogram; FE Ca^{2+}, fractional excretion of calcium; iPTH, intact parathyroid hormone.
[a]FE Ca^{2+} = (urine [Ca^{2+}] × plasma [creatinine]) ÷ (plasma [Ca^{2+}] × urine [creatinine]).
[b]Primary hyperparathyroidism with concomitant vitamin D deficiency must be ruled out.
[c]See text for details.

TABLE 23.4	Treatment of Hypercalcemia		
Treatment	**Dosing**	**Onset/Duration**	**Comments**
Isotonic saline	Bolus isotonic saline until euvolemic (may require up to 3–4 L), then adjust rate to achieve urine output of 100–150 mL/hr.	Onset at 2–4 hr.	Watch for signs of volume overload. Loop diuretics should be held unless incipient volume overload develops.
Calcitonin	4–8 IU/kg IM or SC q6–12h.	Onset at 4–6 hr; tachyphylaxis develops after 2–3 d.	Lowers serum Ca^{2+} 1–2 mg/dL. Side effects include flushing, nausea, and, rarely, allergic reactions.
Bisphosphonates	Zoledronate 4 mg IV over 15 min OR pamidronate 60–90 mg IV over 2–4 hr.	Onset at 2 d with peak effect at 4–6 d; lasts 2–4 wk.	Decrease infusion rate of pamidronate or lower zoledronate dose in renal insufficiency.
Gallium nitrate	100–200 mg/m^2/d continuous infusion for up to 5 d.	Onset after 2 d; lasts 1–2 wk.	Significant risk of nephrotoxicity and it is contraindicated if [creatinine] >2.5 mg/dL.
Glucocorticoids	Prednisone 20–60 mg/d (or equivalent glucocorticoid dose).	Onset in 5–10 d.	Effective only in cases of hematologic malignancies including myeloma, vitamin D excess states, and vitamin A intoxication.
Hemodialysis	Variable based on starting [Ca^{2+}].	Immediate onset, lasting until dialysis completion.	Useful for cases of severe hypercalcemia (>16 mg/dL) and when diuretic resistant volume overload prohibits saline administration.

GENERAL GUIDELINES OF THERAPY:
1. Correct volume depletion which is usually present.
2. If ECG changes or symptoms are present, or if [Ca^{2+}] >12, begin the most rapidly acting therapies (saline, calcitonin, +/− hemodialysis), often in combination.
3. Initiate longer term treatments (bisphosphonates, gallium, glucocorticoids) early as their effects are delayed.

ECG, electrocardiogram.

While initiating the previously mentioned acute therapies, it is often necessary to simultaneously start more long-term measures of Ca^{2+} control. Usually this consists of administering an IV bisphosphonate, which decreases Ca^{2+} resorption from bone by osteoclasts. In situations of effective vitamin D excess and when hypercalcemia occurs as a result of hematologic malignancies such as multiple myeloma, the administration of glucocorticoids is effective for lowering the serum [Ca^{2+}] and can be used alone or with bisphosphonates.

DISORDERS OF PHOSPHORUS CONCENTRATION

Approximately 85% of total body phosphorus (PO_4^{3-}) is in bone, and most of the remainder is within cells. In fact, PO_4^{3-} is the major intracellular anion. Only 1% of total body phosphorus is in the ECF. Thus, serum PO_4^{3-} concentration ([PO_4^{3-}]) may not reflect total body phosphorus stores. In addition to its importance in bone formation, phosphorus is an integral component of adenosine triphosphate and thus critical for normal cellular metabolism. Furthermore, its presence in the red blood cell as 2,3-bisphosphoglycerate makes it important in the regulation of hemoglobin oxygen affinity and therefore tissue oxygen delivery.

Phosphorus balance is determined primarily by four factors: PTH, $[PO_4^{3-}]$, calcitriol, and insulin. PTH lowers serum $[PO_4^{3-}]$ through urinary wasting by decreasing proximal tubular reabsorption of PO_4^{3-}. The $[PO_4^{3-}]$ itself further regulates renal excretion with hyperphosphatemia also decreasing proximal tubular reabsorption. Calcitriol increases serum $[PO_4^{3-}]$ by enhancing intestinal phosphorus absorption. Finally, insulin lowers serum levels by shifting PO_4^{3-} into cells. Hypophosphatemia has been found to occur in 29% of surgical ICU patients. Because renal failure is its major predisposing factor, hyperphosphatemia is also common in the medical ICU.

Hypophosphatemia

There are three main mechanisms of hypophosphatemia (Table 23.5): (a) intracellular shift, (b) reduced intestinal absorption, and (c) renal $[PO_4^{3-}]$ wasting.

Etiologies of Special Importance in the Critically Ill Patient

Intracellular Shift
Respiratory alkalosis is a very common cause of redistributive hypophosphatemia as the intracellular rise in pH stimulates glycolysis and the subsequent phosphorylation of various intermediates in the pathway. The marked anabolism that occurs during the abrupt reversal of negative caloric states with dextrose-containing IV fluids or total parenteral nutrition (i.e., the refeeding syndrome) similarly shifts PO_4^{3-} to the ICF. The surge in insulin that occurs further promotes the intracellular translocation. Refeeding is a major contributor to the hypophosphatemia that occurs among 34% of postsurgical ICU patients after receiving nothing by mouth for as little as 2 days. Finally, severe chronic obstructive pulmonary disease (COPD) patients often are malnourished and total body PO_4^{3-} is depleted. Catecholamines, including the beta-agonists used to treat COPD exacerbations, shift PO_4^{3-} into cells, worsening the hypophosphatemia. Theophylline and corticosteroid therapy both encourage renal PO_4^{3-} wasting, thus exacerbating the phenomenon. It is especially important to be aware of this tendency toward hypophosphatemia in COPD patients as this may contribute to diaphragmatic weakness.

Renal Wasting
Hyperparathyroidism from any cause increases renal PO_4^{3-} excretion. Chronic alcohol consumption also causes renal PO_4^{3-} wasting by an unknown mechanism. This in combination with the usually poor nutritional status of these patients leads to a total body PO_4^{3-} deficit. With possible contributions from intracellular shift from the respiratory alkalosis of liver failure, the increased adrenergic tone of withdrawal, and the refeeding syndrome occurring with dextrose infusions, profound hypophosphatemia can manifest in the hospitalized alcoholic. Increased renal tubular fluid flow from any cause can also lead to urinary PO_4^{3-} wasting. This occurs, for instance, with aggressive volume expansion or with osmotic diuresis, such as occurs with the glucosuria of DKA. Furthermore, insulin therapy in DKA shifts PO_4^{3-} into cells and may worsen the hypophosphatemia.

Treatment

Hypophosphatemia treatment is outlined in Table 23.5. Mild hypophosphatemia (1.9 to 2.5 mg/dL) is common in the hospitalized patient and is often simply caused by transcellular shifts, requiring no treatment except correction of the underlying cause. Severe, symptomatic hypophosphatemia (<1.0 mg/dL), however, may require IV PO_4^{3-} therapy. Although the rapid administration of large doses of IV PO_4^{3-} (0.8 mmol/kg during 30 minutes) to critically ill patients has been shown to be safe and effective, care must be taken with parenteral therapy to avoid hyperphosphatemia, which may cause hypocalcemia and ectopic calcification in tissues. In the presence of renal insufficiency, IV PO_4^{3-} should be given at lower doses (33% of usual doses in severe renal failure) and with even greater care. IV repletion can be transitioned over to oral therapy when the $[PO_4^{3-}]$ is >1.5 mg/dL. Enteral replacement may result in diarrhea and nausea. Because of the need to replenish intracellular stores, 24 to 36 hours of repletion may be required. There has been no demonstrated clear benefit to aggressive repletion of PO_4^{3-} in asymptomatic hypophosphatemia. Studies of PO_4^{3-} therapy in the treatment of DKA for instance, have shown no improved outcomes, and may even suggest increased morbidity, primarily through the precipitation of hypocalcemia.

TABLE 23.5	The Differential Diagnosis, Clinical Manifestations, and Treatment of Hypophosphatemia ([PO₄³⁻] <2.8 mg/dL)

Etiology	Characteristic Laboratories
Transcellular shift	
Insulin Administration[a]	
Refeeding syndrome	FE PO_4^{3-} <5%[b] or urine PO_4^{3-} <100 mg/d
Respiratory alkalosis	FE PO_4^{3-} <5%[b] or urine PO_4^{3-} <100 mg/d
Catecholamine release/β-agonist therapy	
Reduced Absorption	
Phosphate binder (including most antacids) overuse	FE PO_4^{3-} <5%[b] or urine PO_4^{3-} <100 mg/d
Malabsorption/malnutrition	FE PO_4^{3-} <5%[b] or urine PO_4^{3-} <100 mg/d
Vitamin D deficiency[c]	FE PO_4^{3-} >5%[b] or urine PO_4^{3-} >100 mg/d, ↓[Ca²⁺], ↑PTH, ↓25(OH)D₃
Increased Renal Excretion	
Hyperparathyroidism (primary or tertiary)	FE PO_4^{3-} >5%[b] or urine PO_4^{3-} >100 mg/d, ↑[Ca²⁺], ↑PTH, ↑[Ca²⁺]
Osmotic diuresis/ acetazolamide	FE PO_4^{3-} >5%[b] or urine PO_4^{3-} >100 mg/d
Volume expansion	FE PO_4^{3-} >5%[b] or urine PO_4^{3-} >100 mg/d
Chronic alcoholism	FE PO_4^{3-} >5%[b] or urine PO_4^{3-} >100 mg/d
Theophylline use	FE PO_4^{3-} >5%[b] or urine PO_4^{3-} >100 mg/d
Corticosteroid use	FE PO_4^{3-} >5%[b] or urine PO_4^{3-} >100 mg/d
X-linked hypophosphatemic rickets	FE PO_4^{3-} >5%[b] or urine PO_4^{3-} >100 mg/d
Fanconi syndrome	FE PO_4^{3-} >5%[b] or urine PO_4^{3-} >100 mg/d
Oncogenic osteomalacia	FE PO_4^{3-} >5%[b] or urine PO_4^{3-} >100 mg/d
Other	
Sepsis	
Intensive dialysis, especially continuous renal replacement therapy	
Posthyperparathyroid hungry bone syndrome	FE PO_4^{3-} <5%, ↓[Ca²⁺]
Pseudohypophosphatemia (hyperbilirubinemia, some paraproteinemias, mannitol infusions)	

CLINICAL MANIFESTATIONS:
Signs and symptoms typically occur only if total body PO_4^{3-} depletion is present and $[PO_4^{3-}]$ <1 mg/dL.
Muscular: weakness, impaired diaphragmatic function (especially in COPD), ileus, rhabdomyolysis, and heart failure.
Neurologic: paresthesias, dysarthria, confusion, stupor, seizures, and coma.
Hematologic: rarely hemolysis and platelet dysfunction with bleeding.
Chronic ↓[PO_4^{3-}] causes rickets in children and osteomalacia in adults.

(continued on next page)

TABLE 23.5	The Differential Diagnosis, Clinical Manifestations, and Treatment of Hypophosphatemia ([PO₄³⁻] <2.8 mg/dL) (*Continued*)

GENERAL GUIDELINES OF THERAPY:

1. If symptomatic, or intolerant to PO, begin IV replacement (reduce doses in setting of renal insufficiency):
   a. Severe $\downarrow$[PO_4^{3-}] ($\leq$1 mg/dL)- dose 0.6 mmol/kg IBW IV^d over 6 hr. If hypotension ensues, suspect hypocalcemia and discontinue infusion.
   b. Moderate $\downarrow$[PO_4^{3-}] (1–1.8 mg/dL): dose 0.4 mmol/kg IBW IV^d over 6 hr.
   c. Mild $\downarrow$[PO_4^{3-}] (1.9–2.5 mg/dL): dose 0.2 mmol/kg IBW IV^d over 6 hr.
2. If asymptomatic, dose 0.5–1 g elemental phosphorus PO bid-tid. This should correct most deficits by 1 wk. Preparations include:
   a. Neutra-Phos: 250 mg [8 mmol] phosphorus and 7 mEq each of Na^+ and K^+
   b. Neutra-Phos K: 250 mg phosphorus and 14 mEq K^+
   c. K-Phos Neutral: 250 mg phosphorus with 13 meq Na^+ and 1.1 mEq K^+.
3. Treat vitamin D deficiency, if present [see Table 23.2, General Guidelines of Therapy].

iPTH, intact parathyroid hormone; FE PO_4^{3-}, fractional excretion of phosphate; PO, by mouth; IV, intravenous; COPD, chronic obstructive pulmonary disease; IBW, ideal body weight.
^{a}Dextrose infusions may also result in hypophosphatemia in predisposed individuals through the induction of endogenous insulin release.
^{b}FE PO_4^{3-} = (urine [PO_4^{3-}] × plasma [creatinine]) ÷ (plasma [PO_4^{3-}] × urine [creatinine]).
^{c}See Table 23.2 under "Vitamin D Deficiency" for various etiologies, although advanced renal insufficiency is usually associated with hyperphosphatemia.
^{d}Two IV preparations exist: use potassium phosphate if normal renal function and [K^+] <4 mEq/L; use sodium phosphate if renal function is impaired or [K^+] >4 mEq/L.

Hyperphosphatemia

The etiology, laboratory findings, clinical manifestations, and treatment of hyperphosphatemia are outlined in Table 23.6.

DISORDERS OF MAGNESIUM CONCENTRATION

Approximately 60% of body magnesium (Mg^{2+}) is in bone, and most of the remainder is within cells. Only 1% is in the ECF. Mg^{2+} is not exchanged easily between these three pools and there is little buffering of fluctuations in the serum Mg^{2+} concentration ([Mg^{2+}]). Furthermore, the [Mg^{2+}] is a poor predictor of intracellular and total body stores. Unlike the electrolytes discussed to this point, there are no hormones specifically delegated to the regulation of Mg^{2+} balance. The main determinant of Mg^{2+} balance is serum [Mg^{2+}]: hypomagnesemia stimulates renal tubular reabsorption of Mg^{2+}, whereas hypermagnesemia inhibits this process.

Clinically significant hypermagnesemia is rare, in part because of the kidney's capacity to immensely increase Mg^{2+} excretion, unless there is renal insufficiency. However, hypomagnesemia occurs commonly in the ICU. As an important participant in most processes involving Ca^{2+} flux, and a cofactor in reactions consuming adenosine triphosphate, Mg^{2+} is critical for many biologic processes.

Hypomagnesemia

There are three main mechanisms of hypomagnesemia (Table 23.7): (a) urinary Mg^{2+} loss, (b) extrarenal loss, and (c) chelation of Mg^{2+} from the circulation.

TABLE 23.6	The Differential Diagnosis, Clinical Manifestations, and Treatment of Hyperphosphatemia ($[PO_4^{3-}]$ >4.5 mg/dL)

Etiology	Characteristic Laboratories
Transcellular shift	
Rhabdomyolysis	↓$[Ca^{2+}]$, urine PO_4^{3-} >1,500 mg/d[a]
Tumor lysis syndrome	↓$[Ca^{2+}]$, urine PO_4^{3-} >1,500 mg/d[a]
Massive hemolysis	↓$[Ca^{2+}]$, urine PO_4^{3-} >1,500 mg/d[a]
Metabolic acidosis (especially lactic acidosis and ketoacidosis)	
Hypoinsulinemia (such as with diabetic ketoacidosis)	
Increased Intake/Absorption	
Phosphosoda bowel prep	↓$[Ca^{2+}]$, urine PO_4^{3-} >1,500 mg/d[a]
Precursor vitamin D intoxication	↑$[Ca^{2+}]$, urine PO_4^{3-} >1,500 mg/d,[a] ↑$25(OH)D_3$
Tumoral calcitriol production	↑$[Ca^{2+}]$, urine PO_4^{3-} >1,500 mg/d,[a] ↑$1,25(OH)_2D_3$
Extensive granulomatous disease	↑$[Ca^{2+}]$, urine PO_4^{3-} >1,500 mg/d,[a] ↑$1,25(OH)_2D_3$
Calcitriol overdose	↑$[Ca^{2+}]$, urine PO_4^{3-} >1,500 mg/d,[a] ↑$1,25(OH)_2D_3$
Decreased Renal Excretion	
Acute/chronic renal insufficiency	↓$[Ca^{2+}]$, urine PO_4^{3-} <1,500,mg/d
Hypoparathyroidism[b]	↓$[Ca^{2+}]$, urine PO_4^{3-} <1,500,mg/d
Pseudohypoparathyroidism types 1a, 1b, and 2	↓$[Ca^{2+}]$, urine PO_4^{3-} <1,500,mg/d
Acromegaly[c]	mild ↑$[Ca^{2+}]$, urine PO_4^{3-} <1,500,mg/d, ↑$1,25(OH)_2D_3$
Tumoral calcinosis[c]	mild ↑$[Ca^{2+}]$, urine PO_4^{3-} <1,500,mg/d, ↑$1,25(OH)_2D_3$
Other	
Pseudohyperphosphatemia (ex vivo hemolysis, thrombocytosis, rare paraproteinemias)	

CLINICAL MANIFESTATIONS:

Symptoms and signs are those attributable to hypocalcemia (see Table 23.2) and metastatic calcification of soft tissues, including blood vessels, cornea, skin, kidney, and periarticular tissue.
   Calciphylaxis: skin ischemia and necrosis that may occur in chronic kidney disease patients from the calcification of smaller blood vessels and their subsequent thrombosis.

GENERAL GUIDELINES OF THERAPY:

1. Correct underlying cause (If normal renal function and phosphate handling is achieved, ↑$[PO_4^{3-}]$ will usually correct within 12 hrs).
2. Consider forced saline resuscitation +/− acetazolamide (15 mg/kg q4h).
3. For severe ↑$[PO_4^{3-}]$, especially when renal insufficiency is not rapidly reversible, initiate hemodialysis or continuous renal replacement therapy.
4. For chronic ↑$[PO_4^{3-}]$, use phosphate binders (non-Ca^{2+} based if concomitant ↑$[Ca^{2+}]$).

[a]Unless volume depletion or renal insufficiency is present.
[b]See Table 23.2 under "Hypoparathyroidism" for various etiologies.
[c]Also results from increased intestinal phosphate absorption from ↑$1,25(OH)_2D_3$.

TABLE 23.7	The Differential Diagnosis, Clinical Manifestations, and Treatment of Hypomagnesemia ($[Mg^{2+}]$ <1.3 mEq/L or <1.6 mg/dL)

Etiology	Characteristic Laboratories
Reduced Intake/Extrarenal loss	
Starvation	Urine Mg^{2+} <2 mEq/d or FE Mg^{2+} <2%[a]
Malabsorption/diarrhea	Urine Mg^{2+} <2 mEq/d or FE Mg^{2+} <2%[a]
Prolonged gastrointestinal drainage (nasogastric suction, intestinal fistulas, biliary drainage, etc.)	Urine Mg^{2+} <2 mEq/d or FE Mg^{2+} <2%[a]
Burns	Urine Mg^{2+} <2 mEq/d or FE Mg^{2+} <2%[a]
Renal Wasting	
Hypercalcemia	Urine Mg^{2+} >2 mEq/d or FE Mg^{2+} >2%[a]
Osmotic diuresis/polyuric phase of resolving acute tubular necrosis	Urine Mg^{2+} >2 mEq/d or FE Mg^{2+} >2%[a]
Volume expansion	Urine Mg^{2+} >2 mEq/d or FE Mg^{2+} >2%[a]
Chronic tubulointerstitial diseases	Urine Mg^{2+} >2 mEq/d or FE Mg^{2+} >2%[a]
Chronic alcoholism	Urine Mg^{2+} >2 mEq/d or FE Mg^{2+} >2%[a]
Gitelman's (and less commonly Bartter's) syndrome	Urine Mg^{2+} >2 mEq/d or FE Mg^{2+} >2%[a]
Drugs (loop/thiazide diuretics, aminoglycoside, amphotericin B, platinum based chemotherapy, pentamidine, cyclosporine)	Urine Mg^{2+} >2mEq/d or FE Mg^{2+} >2%[a]
Chelation[b]	
Hyperphosphatemia (rhabdomyolysis, tumor lysis, massive hemolysis, phosphosoda bowel preparation)	Urine Mg^{2+} <2 mEq/d or FE Mg^{2+} <2%[a]
Hyperoxalemia (ethylene glycol poisoning)	Urine Mg^{2+} <2 mEq/d or FE Mg^{2+} <2%[a]
Pancreatitis	Urine Mg^{2+} <2 mEq/d or FE Mg^{2+} <2%[a]
Posthyperparathyroid hungry bone syndrome Alkalemia	Urine Mg^{2+} <2 mEq/d or FE Mg^{2+} <2%[a]
Massive transfusion of citrate containing blood products	Urine Mg^{2+} <2 mEq/d or FE Mg^{2+} <2%[a]
Foscarnet therapy	Urine Mg^{2+} <2 mEq/d or FE Mg^{2+} <2%[a]

CLINICAL MANIFESTATIONS:
Symptoms generally do not occur until $[Mg^{2+}]$ <1 mEq/L (<1.2 mg/dL).
Neuromuscular: lethargy, confusion, ataxia, nystagmus, tremor, fasciculations, tetany, and seizures.
Cardiac: atrial and ventricular arrhythmias, especially in patients on digoxin.
ECG: prolonged PR and QT interval with a widened QRS and U waves. Torsades de pointes is the classically associated arrhythmia.
Symptoms and signs associated with $\downarrow[K^+]$ [see Alg. 23.4] and $\downarrow[Ca^{2+}]$ [see Table 23.2] may contribute to the clinical picture.

GENERAL GUIDELINES OF THERAPY:
1. If ECG changes or symptoms present begin IV replacement (reduce doses in renal insufficiency):
   a. 1–2 g $MgSO_4$ (1 g $MgSO_4$ = 96 mg elemental Mg^{2+} = 8 mEq Mg^{2+}) IV over 15 min, followed by an infusion of 6 g MgSO4 in 1 L IV fluid over 24 hr.
   b. Continuous infusion may be required for 3–7 days to replenish total body stores. Follow $[Mg^{2+}]$ q24h (more frequently if renal insufficiency present) and adjust infusion to maintain $[Mg^{2+}]$ <2.5 mEq/L. Check tendon reflexes often for $\uparrow[Mg^{2+}]$.
2. If asymptomatic and no ECG changes:
   a. For mild $\downarrow[Mg^{2+}]$: 240 mg PO elemental[c] Mg^{2+}/d in divided doses.
   b. For severe $\downarrow[Mg^{2+}]$: up to 720 mg PO elemental[c] Mg^{2+}/d in divided doses.
   c. If PO not possible or diarrhea present: 2–6 g IV $MgSO_4$ infused at 1 g/hr or less.
3. For chronic $\downarrow[Mg^{2+}]$ from renal wasting, consider high-dose amiloride.

ECG, electrocardiogram; IV, intravenous; FE Mg^{2+}, fractional excretion of magnesium; PO, by mouth.
[a]FE Mg^{2+} = (urine $[Mg^{2+}]$ × plasma [creatinine]) ÷ (0.7 × plasma $[Mg^{2+}]$ × urine [creatinine]).
[b]Note similarity with causes of hypocalcemia by chelation.
[c]Magnesium oxide = 0.6 mg elemental Mg^{2+}/mg.

Etiologies of Special Importance in the Critically Ill Patient

Gastrointestinal Loss

Intestinal secretions have significant Mg^{2+} content, with more Mg^{2+} present in lower intestinal fluids. Fistulas, prolonged gastrointestinal drainage, or diarrhea can therefore lead to negative Mg^{2+} balance.

Renal Wasting

Chronic alcoholism may lead to renal tubular dysfunction, resulting in inappropriate Mg^{2+} wasting. This is exacerbated by the malnutrition that is often present, but is reversible with 1 month of abstinence. Numerous drugs have similarly been associated with urinary Mg^{2+} wasting. More prolonged dosing of aminoglycosides may cause renal tubular damage with characteristic Mg^{2+} wasting and polyuria. The development of hypomagnesemia may even be delayed until after completion of therapy and the tubular transport defect can persist for months.

Chelation

Because Mg^{2+} is an ion with similar charge and size as Ca^{2+}, all of the same previously listed causes of hypocalcemia from chelation can result in hypomagnesemia, although usually to a lesser degree. This phenomenon has been described, for instance, in cases of severe acute pancreatitis. Hypomagnesemia worsens the hypocalcemia in this setting through its reduction of PTH secretion and PTH effect (Table 23.2).

TABLE 23.8	The Differential Diagnosis, Clinical Manifestations, and Treatment of Hypermagnesemia

Etiology

Excessive administration of Mg^{2+} containing antacids/laxatives, especially in renal insufficiency
Aggressive IV Mg^{2+} administration such as for the treatment of eclampsia/preeclampsia
Theophylline intoxication
Diabetic ketoacidosis
Tumor lysis syndrome
Adrenal insufficiency
Occasionally in primary hyperparathyroidism

CLINICAL MANIFESTATIONS:
Signs and symptoms are seen only if the serum $[Mg^{2+}] >4$ mEq/L (>4.8 mg/dL).
Neuromuscular: hyporeflexia (usually the first sign of Mg^{2+} toxicity), weakness, and lethargy that can progress to somnolence and paralysis; ileus. With diaphragmatic involvement can lead to respiratory failure.
Cardiac: hypotension, bradycardia, and cardiac arrest.
    ECG: $[Mg^{2+}] = 5–10$ mEq/L – bradycardia and prolonged PR, QRS, and QT intervals. $[Mg^{2+}]$ >15 mEq/L – complete heart block or asystole may ensue.

GENERAL GUIDELINES OF THERAPY:
1. Stop additional Mg^{2+} administration.
2. If ECG changes or symptoms are present:
    a. Administer 1–2 g Ca^{2+} gluconate IV over 10 min.
    b. Consider initiation of hemodialysis especially if renal insufficiency is present and not easily reversible.
3. $+/-$ forced saline resuscitation.

IV, intravenous; ECG, electrocardiogram.

Treatment

Hypomagnesemia treatment is outlined in Table 23.7. The route of Mg^{2+} repletion depends on whether clinical manifestations from Mg^{2+} deficiency are present and not on the $[Mg^{2+}]$. Asymptomatic hypomagnesemia without electrogram abnormalities can be treated orally, even if the deficiency is severe, unless malabsorption is present. Oral therapy avoids the abrupt increase in $[Mg^{2+}]$ that occurs with IV repletion and which increases renal excretion of part of the administered dose. The major side effect of enteral therapy is diarrhea. In scenarios with chronic urinary Mg^{2+} wasting, K^+-sparing diuretics like amiloride can be administered to reduce renal losses. Symptomatic hypomagnesemia should be treated parenterally, often with continued oral or IV replacement during 3 to 7 days to replenish intracellular stores. Deep tendon reflexes should be tested frequently during aggressive parenteral dosing as hyporeflexia suggests the development of hypermagnesemia. Reduced doses and more frequent monitoring must be used even in mild renal insufficiency.

Hypermagnesemia

The etiology, clinical manifestations, and treatment of hypermagnesemia are outlined in Table 23.8.

Suggested Reading

Adrogue H, Madias N. Aiding fluid prescription for the dysnatremias. *Intensive Care Med.* 1997;23:309–316.
> *The original paper first presenting the use of the Adrogue-Madias equation for planning initial therapy in the dysnatremias. The concepts underlying the equation and its derivation are presented. Several examples with a comparison to the prior approach are also given.*

Allon M, Shanklin N. Effect of bicarbonate administration on plasma potassium in dialysis patients: interactions with insulin and albuterol. *Am J Kidney Dis.* 1996;28:508–514.
> *The time course of the acute therapies for hyperkalemia are studied and compared. This is one of several papers confirming the relative ineffectiveness of bicarbonate in the acute treatment of hyperkalemia.*

Amanzadeh J, Reilly RF. Hypophosphatemia: an evidence-based approach to its clinical consequences and management. *Nat Clin Pract Nephrol.* 2006;2:136–148.
> *An excellent review of the effects of hypophosphatemia and its treatment based on the available clinical data.*

Fraser CL, Arieff AI. Epidemiology, pathophysiology, and management of hyponatremic encephalopathy. *Am J Med.* 1997;102:67–77.
> *Review describing the pathophysiology of hyponatremia and factors linked with neurologic compromise based on case-control associations. Management guidelines differing from the traditional are offered. Includes a bibliography with most of the papers of significance on this topic.*

Kraft MD, Btaiche IF, Sacks GS. Treatment of electrolyte disorders in adult patients in the intensive care unit. *Am J Health-Syst Pharm.* 2005;62:1663–1682.
> *An extensive topic review on the presentations and management of all of the electrolyte abnormalities touched upon here. Whenever possible clinical studies are cited by an extensive bibliography.*

Palevsky PM, Bhagrath R, Greenberg A. Hypernatremia in hospitalized patients. *Ann Intern Med.* 1996;124:197–203.
> *Describes the incidence of in-hospital hypernatrimia and clinical characteristics, pathophysiologic mechanisms, and outcomes for a cohort of hypernatremic patients.*

Palmer BF. Hyponatremia in patients with central nervous system disease: SIADH versus CSW. *Trends Endocrinol Metab.* 2003;14:182–187.
> *A good review on the difficult topic of cerebral salt wasting.*

Rose B, Post T. *Clinical Physiology of Acid-Base and Electrolyte Disorders.* 5th ed. New York: McGraw-Hill; 2001.
   A textbook which thoroughly describes the renal handling of sodium, potassium, and water, including normal physiology and pathophysiology. Many classic experiments in renal physiology are presented throughout the text to illustrate the described principles.
Zivin JR, Gooley T, Zager RA, et al. Hypocalcemia: a pervasive metabolic abnormality in the critically ill. *Am J Kidney Dis.* 2001;37:689–698.
   A study which defines the high incidence of hypocalcemia in a diverse population of the critically ill. Associations with increased illness severity are highlighted.

Acid-Base Disorders

V

METABOLIC ACID-BASE DISORDERS

Namrata Chawla and Matthew J. Koch

24

Acid-base disorders are commonly encountered in the critical care setting. A stepwise approach to the evaluation of these disorders helps delineate the appropriateness of the homeostatic response, the correct approach to management, and the underlying cause. This section will review the diagnosis and management of metabolic acidosis and alkalosis. Respiratory acidosis and alkalosis are discussed separately (see Chapter 25).

In nonpathologic states, homeostasis is maintained despite the daily production of approximately 15,000 mmol of carbon dioxide (CO_2) and 50 to 100 mEq of hydrogen ions (H^+), resulting from the catabolism of carbohydrates, fats, and proteins. Appropriate acid-base balance is essential because the extracellular H^+ concentration compatible with life is a relatively narrow range (150 to 15 nmol/L and respective pH of 6.8 to 7.8). Disorders of the acid-base system and the appropriate management are best understood by examining the equation for the bicarbonate-carbon dioxide buffer system:

$$H_2O + CO_2 \leftrightarrow H_2CO_3 \leftrightarrow H^+ + HCO_3^-$$

The enzyme carbonic anhydrase catalyzes the reaction of water (H_2O) and carbon dioxide (CO_2) to form carbonic acid (H_2CO_3). Carbonic acid dissociates into bicarbonate (HCO_3^-) and a hydrogen ion (H^+). Bicarbonate is a major extracellular buffer, and acid-base balance is maintained by the renal system through changes in bicarbonate and hydrogen ion production and excretion, and by the respiratory system through compensatory changes in carbon dioxide. Appropriate respiratory compensation for an acute metabolic acidosis is a 1.2 mm Hg decrease in the partial pressure of CO_2 (PCO_2) for each 1 mEq/L decrease in the serum bicarbonate. Compensation begins immediately but may no be complete for 12 to 24 hours. Respiratory compensation for metabolic alkalosis is a 0.7 mm Hg increase in the PCO_2 for each 1 mEq/L increase in the serum bicarbonate (Table 24.1). However, hypoventilation is required for a PCO_2 increase, which is often not possible for critically ill patients with underlying cardiac and pulmonary disorders.

TABLE 24.1	Expected PCO_2 and Respiratory Compensation for Metabolic Acidosis and Alkalosis
Metabolic acidosis	PCO_2 is >10 mm Hg in a single disorder
	$PCO_2 = -1.2$ mm Hg for every 1 mEq/L fall in $[HCO_3^-]$ (below 24 mEq/L)
Metabolic alkalosis	PCO_2 is <60 mm Hg in a single disorder
	$PCO_2 = +0.7$ mm Hg for every 1 mEq/L rise in $[HCO_3^-]$ (above 24 mEq/L)

The following steps are used to evaluate metabolic acid-base disorders (Alg. 24.1).

1. Determine the underlying abnormality—metabolic acidosis and/or metabolic alkalosis.
2. Determine the contributing factors (anion gap acidosis $\pm$ nonanion gap acidosis $\pm$ metabolic alkalosis) and evaluate the delta gap (see later discussion).
3. Evaluate the appropriateness of respiratory compensation.
4. Determine the likely cause of the disorder and whether or not urgent intervention is necessary.

METABOLIC ACIDOSIS

Acidemia is the most common acute metabolic acid-base disturbance presenting in the critical care setting. The four main mechanisms used in an attempt to maintain homeostasis in this setting are:

1. Extracellular buffering primarily via HCO_3^-
2. Intracellular and bone buffering (buffers up to 55% to 60% of the acid load)
3. Renal excretion of H^+ and regeneration of bicarbonate
4. Removal of CO_2 by alveolar ventilation

Metabolic acidosis may present as a single disturbance of either anion gap or nonanion gap etiology. A double disorder would include either of these in combination with a metabolic alkalosis, or the concurrent presence of an anion gap and nonanion gap acidosis. A triple metabolic disorder (combined anion gap and nonanion gap acidosis with a metabolic alkalosis) may be suggested clinically, but is usually not obvious from laboratory data. Inappropriate respiratory compensation in any of these situations may add the additional component of respiratory acidosis or alkalosis.

Anion Gap Acidosis

The anion gap represents the normal serum anions that are not accounted for in the anion gap formula [Serum Sodium (Na^+) − (Serum Chloride (Cl^-) + Serum HCO_3^-)]. The normal anion gap is approximately 8 to 12 mEq/L. The utilization of bicarbonate to buffer significant quantities of an additional, pathologic anion results in an anion gap acidosis. Causes of an anion gap metabolic acidosis include lactic acidosis, toxic ingestions, ketoacidosis, rhabdomyolysis, and renal failure (Tables 24.2 and 24.3).

A decrease in the non-chloride, non-bicarbonate anions (primarily albumin), or the presence of excess non-sodium cations, results in a decrease in the calculated anion gap, as the serum Cl^- concentration $[Cl^-]$ will increase to compensate for the charge difference. Each 1 g/dL decrease in the serum albumin will decrease the calculated anion gap by 2.5 to 3 mEq/L. Thus, a significant anion gap acidosis may be missed in the setting of hypoalbuminemia if this issue is not considered. In addition to hypoalbuminemia, a low (or even negative) calculated anion gap may occur with bromide or lithium intoxication, multiple myeloma, and as a laboratory artifact in severe hypernatremia (levels >170 mEq/l) or hyperlipidemia.

The serum osmolal gap may be of some value when a toxic ingestion (ethanol, methanol, ethylene glycol) is a suspected cause of an anion gap acidosis (Table 24.3). An increased osmolal gap is an otherwise nonspecific finding and may be seen in other forms of anion gap acidosis. The normal osmolal gap is approximately 10 mOsm/kg.

Osmolal gap = Measured serum osmolality − calculated serum osmolality

Calculated serum osmolality = $2 \times [Na^+] + [BUN]/2.8 + [glucose]/18$

ALGORITHM 24.1   **Approach to Metabolic Acidosis and Alkalosis**

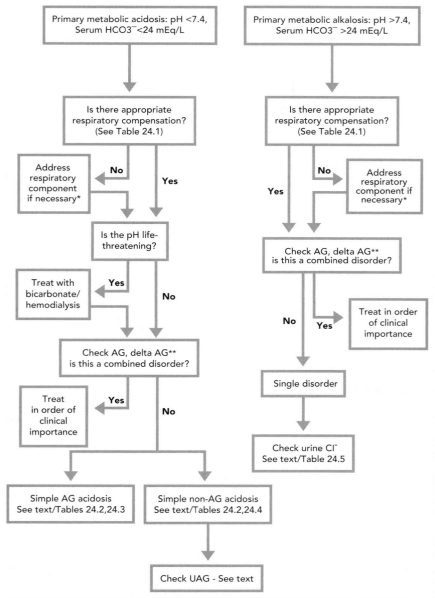

*May require intubation and mechanical ventilation for patients with life-thredtening acid-base disturbances unable to fully hyper- or hypo-ventilate appropriately.
AG, anion gap; UAG, urine anion gap.
**See text for details.

TABLE 24.2	Causes of Anion Gap and Nonanion Gap Metabolic Acidosis	

Mechanism	Increased Anion Gap Acidosis[a]	Normal Anion Gap Acidosis

Increased acid production or administration	Lactic acidosis: lactate, D-lactate
	Ketoacidosis
	Massive rhabdomyolysis
	Intoxications:
	  Methanol/formaldehyde - formate
	  Ethylene glycol - glycolate, oxalate
	  Toluene - hippurate
	  Salicylates
	  Paraldehyde - organic anions
	  L-5 oxoprolinuria
		Ammonium chloride ingestion
		Hyperalimentation fluids/saline infusion

Increased bicarbonate loss or loss of bicarbonate precursors		GI losses (negative UAG)
		  Diarrhea
		  Pancreatic, biliary, intestinal fistulas
		  Ostomy
		  Cholestyramine
		  Sevelamer
		Renal losses
		  Carbonic anhydrase inhibitors
		  Type 2 (proximal) RTA
		Treatment phase of ketoacidosis

Decreased acid excretion (positive UAG)	Chronic renal failure	Acute renal failure Chronic renal failure Type 1 (distal) RTA Hypoaldosteronism (type 4 RTA)

GI, gastrointestinal; UAG, urine anion gap; RTA, renal tubular acidosis.
[a]See Table 24.3 for further discussion.

Nonanion Gap Acidosis

Nonanion gap acidosis occurs in the setting of bicarbonate loss, but without the presence of an additional, pathologic anion. The $[Cl^-]$ is increased to maintain electroneutrality and the calculated anion gap remains normal. In some cases, the presence of limited quantities of an additional, pathologic anion in the setting of normal renal excretion presents as a nonanion gap acidosis. If production or ingestion of the pathologic anion increases significantly or if renal function deteriorates and excretion is limited, an anion gap acidosis will result. The differential of nonanion gap acidosis includes gastrointestinal losses versus a renal etiology (Table 24.2).

The urine anion gap (UAG) is used to discern the source of bicarbonate loss in a nonanion gap acidosis when the cause is not clinically evident.

$$UAG = (Urine\ [Na^+] + Urine\ [K^+]) - (Urine\ [Cl^-])$$

The UAG is normally zero or slightly positive. In the setting of a nonrenal cause of a nonanion gap acidosis, ammonium excretion, as NH_4Cl, appropriately increases and the UAG becomes negative, usually ranging from -20 to -50 mEq/L. In conditions with impaired renal acid excretion, such as chronic kidney disease and distal renal tubular acidosis, the urine anion gap will remain positive or become only slightly negative. The UAG has no utility in the setting of hypovolemia, oliguria, low urine $[Na^+]$, or in anion gap acidosis.

(text continues on page 185)

TABLE 24.3	Causes and Treatment of Anion Gap Metabolic Acidosis

Condition	Cause and Symptoms	Treatment	Comments
Lactic acidosis Pyruvate $\updownarrow$ Lactate	**Increased lactate production** **1.** Increased pyruvate production: enzymatic defects in glycogenolysis or gluconeogenesis **2.** Decreased pyruvate utilization: enzymatic defects in pyruvate dehydrogenase or carboxylase. **3.** Increased conversion of pyruvate to lactate: Increased metabolic rate Grand mal seizure Severe exercise Hypothermic shivering Shock/cardiac arrest/acute pulmonary edema Severe hypoxemia CO poisoning* Cyanide intoxication* **Decreased lactate utilization** Hypoperfusion Alcoholism* Liver disease	Correction of the underlying disorder and reversal of circulatory failure is the primary therapy Role of sodium bicarbonate administration is controversial; may be indicated if severe acidosis-pH <7.1 or loss of buffering capacity (bicarbonate <5 mEq/L). Hemodialysis may be indicated in resistant cases. *Alternative therapies* (clinical efficacy and safety for these have not been demonstrated in randomized controlled human studies). Tham (tromethamine)-inert amino alcohol that buffers acids without generating CO_2. Renally excreted and may produce hyperkalemia, hypoglycemia, and respiratory depression in anuric/oliguric patients. Carbicarb: equimolar mixture of sodium carbonate and sodium bicarbonate. Diminished risk of hypercapnia and intracellular acidosis compared with sodium bicarbonate. Dichloroacetate: activates pyruvate dehydrogenase, and increases oxidation of pyruvate thus decreasing its conversion to lactate.	**Caution with bicarbonate therapy in the following settings:** Volume overload Postrecovery metabolic alkalosis Hypernatremia Increased CO_2 production and possible retention in setting of circulatory failure with worsening of mixed venous PCO_2 Intracellular acidosis Reduction in ionized calcium and worsening of cardiac contractility.
Propylene glycol toxicity*	Converts to pyruvate and lactate. Vehicle for lorazepam and other agents, and continuous infusion may result in lactate accumulation and increased osmolar gap.	Discontinue infusion.	
Ketoacidosis (see Chapter 28)	In the setting of insulin deficiency. Symptoms include vomiting, abdominal pain, severe volume depletion/dehydration.	Insulin and fluids - acidosis will improve with insulin induced metabolism of ketoacids and regeneration of serum HCO_3^-.	

(Continued)

TABLE 24.3	Causes and Treatment of Anion Gap Metabolic Acidosis (*Continued*)

Condition	Cause and Symptoms	Treatment	Comments
Salicylate toxicity*	Toxicity when plasma level >40–50 mg/dL (therapeutic, 20–35 mg/dL). Mixed metabolic acidosis and respiratory alkalosis. Increased ketoacid and lactate production. Diagnosis - plasma salicylate level.	Reduce salicylate levels to avoid neurotoxicity. Alkalinization of plasma to a pH >7.45–7.5 converts salicylate to ionized form which lowers CNS levels. Alkalinization of urine decreases renal tubular reabsorption of ionized salicylate. Consider hemodialysis for plasma concentration >80 mg/dL.	If respiratory alkalosis is the primary disturbance, then further alkalinization is not necessary.
Methanol* ↕ Formaldehyde ↕ Formic acid	Minimal lethal dose is 50–100 mL. Symptoms include weakness, headache, blurred vision and blindness. Diagnosis - plasma methanol assay.	The treatment for both methanol and ethylene glycol is identical. Prompt treatment is necessary and includes: Oral charcoal Sodium bicarbonate Administration of ethanol or fomepizole-competes with or inactivates metabolism, respectively, of parent compound and prevents formation of toxic metabolites. Administration of folic acid, thiamine and pyridoxine. Hemodialysis for removal of toxic metabolites and parent compound.	Simultaneous use of both ethanol and fomepizole is not recommended as fomepizole increases the half-life of ethanol.
Ethylene glycol* ↓ Glycolic and oxalic acid	Component of antifreeze and solvents. Symptoms include neurologic and cardiopulmonary abnormalities, flank pain, and renal failure. Envelope- and needle-shaped oxalate crystals may be visible in the urine. Diagnosis-plasma ethylene glycol assay.		
L-5 oxoproline toxicity	High anion gap acidosis in children secondary to congenital glutathione synthetase deficiency. Acquired oxoprolinuria associated with acetaminophen and other medications. Renal dysfunction and sepsis predispose. Diagnosis-negative toxicity screening and high plasma and urine levels of 5-oxoproline/urine organic acid screen.	Treatment primarily includes cessation of the offending agent. *N*-acetylcysteine may be beneficial; restoration of glutathione stores reduces L-5 oxoproline levels.	
D-Lactic acidosis Glucose ⌐ bacterial │ overgrowth ↳ in the colon D-Lactate	Associated with short gut syndrome and overproduction of D-lactate. Symptoms: episodic anion gap acidosis (usually occurring after high-carbohydrate meals) and neurologic abnormalities including cerebellar ataxia, confusion, slurred speech. Diagnosis: enzymatic assay for D-lactate.	Treatment includes sodium bicarbonate administration and antimicrobial agents.	

*See Chapter 32.

Renal Tubular Acidosis (RTA)

These disorders are characterized by a hyperchloremic metabolic acidosis resulting from diminished net renal H^+ secretion. A diagnosis of RTA cannot be made in the setting of acute renal failure or with moderate-to-severe chronic kidney disease. Although the presence of a pre-existing or developing RTA may complicate the diagnosis and contribute to metabolic acidosis in the critical care setting, it seldom affects acute management. The primary importance of RTA recognition is to prevent attribution of acidosis to an alternate etiology and to allow appropriate management of these primarily chronic conditions (Table 24.4). A detailed discussion of this topic is beyond the intent of this manual.

Treatment

Treatment of the various disorders is outlined in Table 24.3. The primary goal in treating metabolic acidosis is reversal of the underlying process. Administration of bicarbonate is controversial, as some clinical parameters may actually worsen with correction of the acidosis. However, partial correction should be considered in the setting of life-threatening metabolic acidosis (pH <7.1) or when the serum bicarbonate is low enough (i.e., <10 to 12 mEq/L) that loss of effective respiratory compensation would result in life-threatening acidosis. For example; the pH is approximately 7.2, the serum bicarbonate is 8 mEq/L, and the PCO_2 is appropriately compensated at 20 mm Hg. If respiratory compensation becomes inadequate and the PCO_2 increases to 55 mm Hg, the pH will suddenly decrease to approximately 6.9. To decrease the risk of either a further drop in the serum bicarbonate or a sudden inability to achieve appropriate respiratory compensation, a serum bicarbonate target of 10 to 12 mEq/L is recommended.

One caveat is the administration of bicarbonate in the setting of severe circulatory failure. This may result in an apparent improvement in acidosis as measured by the arterial blood gas, but an actual worsening of the overall acidosis if a venous blood gas is obtained (given delayed elimination of the CO_2 produced as a result of the administered bicarbonate). Thus, both arterial and venous values should be monitored when bicarbonate is administered in this setting. Continuous or intermittent hemodialysis may also be used to correct severe, refractory acidosis in the appropriate clinical situation. In the setting of a combined metabolic and respiratory acidosis, correction of the respiratory acidosis component should be addressed prior to administration of bicarbonate or initiation of hemodialysis.

Bicarbonate Deficit

The amount of bicarbonate required to correct a metabolic acidosis can be estimated from the following formula:

Total body weight (kg) $\times$ [0.4 + (2.4/ [HCO_3^-])] = apparent volume of distribution

Apparent volume of distribution $\times$ target change in [HCO_3^-] = mEq of $NaHCO_3$

For example, to increase the serum bicarbonate to 12 mEq/L in a 60-kg patient with a serum bicarbonate level of 5 mEq/L:

60 kg $\times$ [0.4 + 2.4/5] = apparent VD of 53 L

53 $\times$ target change in [HCO_3^-] (12-5 = 7 mEq/L) = 371 mEq

Thus, in a static situation, almost 400 mEq of $NaHCO_3$ would need to be administered in an attempt to increase the [HCO_3^-] to 12 mEq/L. This calculation is obviously an approximation and does not take into account ongoing bicarbonate losses or continued acid production. A standard ampule of sodium bicarbonate contains 50 mEq in 50 mL, given as an intravenous bolus or mixed with 5% dextrose containing sterile water.

METABOLIC ALKALOSIS

Most cases of metabolic alkalosis encountered in the intensive care unit are induced by loss of gastric secretions from gastric suctioning or vomiting, or from diuretic therapy. Other causes include bicarbonate administration, the posthypercapnic state, and citrate associated with centrifugal plasma exchange, massive transfusion, or fresh-frozen plasma administration. The condition is often aggravated by renal insufficiency, which delays bicarbonate

TABLE 24.4 Renal Tubular Acidosis (RTA)

	Distal (Type 1) RTA	Proximal (Type 2) RTA	Hyporeninemic Hypoaldosteronism (Type 4) RTA
Causes	Idiopathic, familial, Sjogren syndrome, hypercalciuria, rheumatoid arthritis, sickle cell anemia, SLE, amphotericin	Idiopathic, multiple myeloma, carbonic anhydrase inhibitors, heavy metals (lead, mercury), amyloidosis, hypocalcemia and vitamin D deficiency	Diabetes, ACE inhibitors, tubulointerstitial nephritis, NSAIDS, heparin, adrenal insufficiency, obstructive uropathy, K^+-sparing diuretics
Defect	Impaired distal tubular H^+ excretion (distal acidification)	Impaired proximal tubular bicarbonate absorption ± associated glycosuria, aminoaciduria, phosphaturia	Aldosterone deficiency or resistance
Plasma HCO_3^-	Variable; usually more severe acidosis with level <10 mEq/L.	Less severe acidosis than distal RTA; usually 12–20 mEq/L	Usually >15 mEq/L
Urine pH during acidemia[a]	>5.3	Variable; >5.3 if serum HCO_3^- is above the reabsorptive threshold. The excessive bicarbonate "spills out" into the urine causing a high urine pH. <5.3 if serum HCO_3^- is below threshold.	Usually <5.3
Plasma K^+	Usually low;–usually corrects with alkali therapy	Low; usually worsened by bicarbonaturia seen with alkali therapy	High
UAG	Positive	Variable; not helpful.	Positive
Associated conditions	Renal stones/nephrocalcinosis	Rickets/osteomalacia/Fanconi syndrome	None
Treatment	Alkali therapy: sodium citrate/potassium citrate/sodium bicarbonate	Alkali therapy: higher doses are needed because of bicarbonaturia. Thiazide diuretics may be tried in resistant cases.	Treat the cause of hypoaldosteronism/ low potassium diet/loop diuretics

SLE, systemic lupus erythematosus; ACE, angiotensin-converting enzyme; NSAIDs, nonsteroidal anti-inflammatory drugs; UAG, urine anion gap.
[a]In metabolic acidosis with intact renal acid excretion, urine pH should be <5–5.3.
Modified from Rose B, Post T. *Clinical Physiology of Acid-base and Electrolyte Disorders.* 2001. 5th ed. New York: McGraw-Hill.

| TABLE 24.5 | Chloride-Responsive and Chloride-Resistant Metabolic Alkalosis |

Chloride Responsive (Urinary Cl$^-$ ≤25 mEq/L)	Chloride Resistant (Urinary Cl$^-$ >25 mEq/L)
Loss of gastric H$^+$ - vomiting or gastric suction Prior loop/thiazide diuretic use Chloride-losing diarrhea: villous adenoma/ some cases of factitious diarrhea due to laxative abuse Cystic fibrosis (high sweat Cl$^-$) Posthypercapnia	Mineralocorticoid excess: primary hyperaldosteronism, Cushing or Liddle syndromes, exogenous steroid use, licorice ingestion Active loop/thiazide diuretic use Bartter or Gitelman syndromes Alkali load: exogenous bicarbonate infusion, citrate-containing blood products, antacids (milk-alkali syndrome) Severe hypokalemia
Treatment includes administration of 0.9% or 0.45% NaCl and repletion of potassium stores.	**Treatment is disease-specific and includes repletion of potassium stores.**

excretion. Metabolic alkalosis may be the primary disorder, but likewise can be associated with an anion gap or nonanion gap acidosis as well as with a respiratory acidosis or alkalosis. Of note, however, is that a slight increase in the anion gap can occur in some cases of metabolic alkalosis, often related to an increased albumin concentration resulting from a contracted volume state. Metabolic alkalosis can be broadly categorized into a chloride-responsive or chloride-resistant process (Table 24.5).

Common Causes of Metabolic Alkalosis

Gastric secretion loss
Loss of gastric secretions occurs from removal of gastric contents by tube drainage or from vomiting. Normally, hydrogen ions released into the stomach reach the duodenum, where they stimulate pancreatic bicarbonate secretion into the gastrointestinal tract, maintaining acid-base balance. When gastric contents are lost, bicarbonate is not secreted, resulting in increased plasma bicarbonate and metabolic alkalosis. Self-induced vomiting is often denied by patients with eating or factitious disorders, and a low urine chloride supports the diagnosis.

Contraction alkalosis
Contraction alkalosis occurs in the setting of excessive loss of chloride-rich, bicarbonate-free fluid. This is most commonly seen with the use of loop or thiazide diuretics, but can also occur with gastric losses or with cystic fibrosis (high sweat [Cl$^-$]). As a result of "contraction" of the extracellular volume, there is a relative increase in the bicarbonate concentration. Despite the relative intravascular volume depletion, there is an obligate urinary loss of sodium with bicarbonate in this setting. Therefore, urine chloride concentration is usually a better predictor of the volume status in this form of metabolic alkalosis than urine sodium.

Posthypercapnic Alkalosis
Chronic respiratory acidosis is associated with an appropriate compensatory increase in the serum bicarbonate concentration. Sudden normalization of a chronically elevated PCO$_2$ via mechanical ventilation can result in an acute, potentially lethal increase in the pH. Therefore, the PCO$_2$ should not be decreased rapidly in the setting of a well-compensated chronic respiratory acidosis.

Refeeding Syndrome
Patients fed a high-carbohydrate diet after a prolonged fast can acutely develop metabolic alkalosis. Intracellular hydrogen ion shift is the proposed mechanism. Refeeding may also be independently associated with hypophosphatemia.

Severe Hypokalemia
Severe hypokalemia via multiple renal mechanisms causes hydrogen ion secretion and bicarbonate reabsorption. The ensuing metabolic alkalosis is refractory to treatment until potassium stores are replaced.

Milk-Alkali Syndrome
Milk-alkali syndrome results from a chronic high calcium intake (usually in the form of calcium-containing antacids) and is usually associated with renal insufficiency.

Treatment

Intravenous sodium chloride fluid administration will reverse chloride-responsive metabolic alkalosis (Table 24.5). Response to treatment can be monitored via urine pH and urine chloride concentration. In cases of severe, refractory alkalosis (usually associated with bicarbonate administration in the setting of renal failure), hydrochloric acid infusion through a central line is rarely needed, but can be used. Other alternatives include the use of intermittent hemodialysis with the bicarbonate bath decreased to the lowest allowable value (limited bicarbonate gradient available with most systems) or a continuous hemofiltration modality using primarily a nonbicarbonate, noncitrate replacement fluid.

Acetazolamide can be considered in cases of worsening metabolic alkalosis associated with volume overload complicated by the need for continued attempts at diuresis (non–chloride-responsive). Acetazolamide inhibits carbonic anhydrase, the enzyme that catalyzes the conversion of carbon dioxide and water into carbonic acid, causing renal excretion of hydrogen ions and retention of bicarbonate. Decreased bicarbonate excretion from carbonic anhydrase inhibition causes a metabolic acidosis to counter the alkalosis. Acetazolamide has minimal diuretic effects as a single agent, but can have additive effects when combined with loop and/or thiazide diuretics if the serum bicarbonate concentration is elevated. Although alkalosis may not improve significantly when acetazolamide is used in combination with other diuretics, it may prevent worsening alkalosis.

MIXED ACID-BASE DISORDERS

The delta anion gap is useful in determining the presence of a combined anion gap and nonanion gap metabolic acidosis or a mixed anion gap acidosis/metabolic alkalosis.

$$\text{Delta Anion Gap } (\Delta/\Delta): \quad \frac{\Delta^* \text{ AG (from normal, which is approximately 10)}}{\Delta^* \text{ HCO}_3 \text{ (from normal, which is approximately 25 mEq/L)}}$$

$*\Delta$ = Change

As a result of non-bicarbonate buffering, the ratio is usually >1 in the setting of an anion gap acidosis (the magnitude of increase in the anion gap is greater than the reduction in serum bicarbonate). A ratio <1 indicates the possibility of a combined anion gap and nonanion gap acidosis, and a markedly increased ratio indicates the possibility of a combined anion gap acidosis with a metabolic alkalosis. The ratio may be 1:1 initially with acute lactic acidosis, given the early absence of significant non-bicarbonate buffering.

Suggested Reading
Arroliga AC, Shehab N, McCarthy K, et al. Relationship of continuous infusion lorazepam to serum propylene glycol concentration in critically ill adults. *Crit Care Med.* 2004;32: 1709–1714.
    Prospective observational study evaluating the dose relationship between lorazepam infusion and propylene glycol accumulation.

Gauthier PM, Szerlip HM. Metabolic acidosis in the intensive care unit. *Crit Care Clin.* 200218:289–308.

An extensive review of diagnostic and therapeutic approach to metabolic acidosis with focus on critical care issues.

Gehlbach BK, Schmidt GA. Bench-to-bedside review: treating acid-base abnormalities in the intensive care unit—the role of buffers. *Crit Care.* 20048:259–265.

This review article extensively discusses the role of bicarbonate therapy as well as alternative therapies in lactic acidosis.

Judge BS. Differentiating the causes of metabolic acidosis in the poisoned patient. *Clin Lab Med.* 2006;26:31–48, vii.

Describes toxicities due to methanol, ethylene glycol and other ingestions, their effects on acid base balance, diagnosis and treatment.

Rose B, Post T. *Clinical Physiology of Acid Base and Electrolyte Disorders.* 5th ed. New York: McGraw Hill.

An extremely comprehensive text book describing pathophysiologic mechanisms, diagnoses and treatment of metabolic acid base disorders.

Tailor P, Raman T, Garganta CL, et al. Recurrent high anion gap metabolic acidosis secondary to 5-oxoproline (pyroglutamic acid). *Am J Kidney Dis.* 2005;46:e4–10.

Case report and discussion of a common but under diagnosed cause of high anion gap acidosis-5 oxoproline toxicity.

25

RESPIRATORY ACID-BASE DISORDERS
Andrew Labelle

Respiratory acid-base disorders are commonly seen in the intensive care unit, and can occur independently or coexist with metabolic acid-base disorders (see Chapter 24). Respiratory acid-base disorders are characterized by altered plasma carbon dioxide levels, measured on arterial blood gas analysis as the partial pressure of carbon dioxide ($PaCO_2$). Respiratory acidosis is characterized by an elevated $PaCO_2$ and decreased pH, and respiratory alkalosis by a decreased $PaCO_2$ and elevated pH. The $PaCO_2$ in healthy adults is 35 to 45 mm Hg and the normal pH is 7.35 to 7.45. For calculation purposes, it is reasonable to use 40 mm Hg as the baseline $PaCO_2$ level and 7.4 as the baseline pH. In general, each *acute* 10 mm Hg change in the $PaCO_2$ causes a 0.08 change in the arterial pH. For example, in a patient with a plasma pH of 7.4, an acute increase in the $PaCO_2$ from 40 to 50 mm Hg would be expected to decrease the plasma pH from 7.4 to 7.32. An acute 10 mm Hg decrease in the $PaCO_2$ from 40 to 30 mm Hg would be expected to increase the pH from 7.4 to 7.48.

In respiratory acid-base disorders, the kidneys compensate for changes in the $PaCO_2$ by increasing the plasma bicarbonate (HCO_3^-) in respiratory acidosis, or decreasing the plasma bicarbonate in respiratory alkalosis. Acute respiratory acid-base disorders result in small changes in the bicarbonate concentration, and cellular buffering predominates. Chronic renal compensation occurs during days to weeks, and results in a larger change in plasma bicarbonate. Table 25.1 shows the expected change in the plasma bicarbonate level in acute and chronic respiratory acidosis and alkalosis. The serum bicarbonate in a healthy adult is approximately 22 to 26 mEq/L. Thus it is reasonable to use a level of 24 mEq/L for calculation purposes. Compensatory change in bicarbonate is associated with a shift in the pH back toward normal. A normal pH is not achieved by compensation alone and *overcompensation does not occur*. Therefore, a mixed respiratory and metabolic disorder is present if the pH is normal and the $PaCO_2$ is altered. For example, a pH of 7.4 with a $PaCO_2$ of 60 mm Hg means that, in addition to the respiratory acidosis, a metabolic alkalosis is present that has moved the pH back to normal (see step 4). Mixed acid-base disorders do not include the renal bicarbonate compensation that occurs for acute and chronic respiratory acid-base disorder.

Evaluation of respiratory acid-base disorders can be relatively straightforward in patients with an isolated acute primary respiratory acidosis or alkalosis, such as occurs in a young patient with an acute asthma exacerbation or in an otherwise healthy patient with anxiety-induced hyperventilation, or more difficult when superimposed metabolic acid-base disorders are present in a critically-ill patient. Further complicating evaluation is the change that occurs in the serum bicarbonate in acute and chronic respiratory acidosis and alkalosis. Algorithm 25.1 and steps 1 through 6 can aid in analyzing a respiratory acid-base disorder. However, these are general rules, and when evaluating a given arterial blood gas in a primary respiratory acid-base disorder, the patient's clinical history and physical examination have to be incorporated to arrive at the correct diagnosis (see step 5 for further explanation).

Respiratory acidosis results from hypercapnia induced by alveolar hypoventilation. The approach to hypercapnia and the differential diagnosis is outlined in Chapter 7, Algorithm 7.1 and includes disorders in any component of the ventilatory mechanism, such as the central or peripheral nervous system, chest wall, respiratory muscles, pleura, upper airway, or lungs.

Respiratory acidosis treatment is directed at the underlying cause, outlined in various other chapters in this manual. In general, treatment is aimed at improving alveolar ventilation and includes bronchodilators for patients with asthma and chronic obstructive

TABLE 25.1	Expected [HCO_3^-] Change in Acute and Chronic Respiratory Acid-Base Disorders (Assume a Baseline [HCO_3^-] of 24 mEq/L)
Acute respiratory acidosis	[HCO_3^-] = +1 mEq/L for every 10 mm Hg increase in Pa_{CO_2} above 40 mm Hg
Chronic respiratory acidosis	[HCO_3^-] = +3[a] mEq/L for every 10 mm Hg rise in Pa_{CO_2} above 40 mm Hg
Acute respiratory alkalosis	[HCO_3^-] = −2 mEq/L for every 10 mm Hg decrease in Pa_{CO_2} below 40 mm Hg
Chronic respiratory alkalosis	[HCO_3^-] = −4[a] mEq/L for every 10 mm Hg decrease in Pa_{CO_2} below 40 mm Hg

[a]Some authors use 3.5 mEq/L for chronic respiratory acidosis and 5 mEq/L for chronic respiratory alkalosis.

pulmonary disease, bilevel positive airway pressure, mechanical ventilation (used with caution in patients with chronic respiratory acidosis with an elevated serum bicarbonate as rapid correction can cause a life-threatening metabolic alkalosis), reversal of drug effects, treatment of pulmonary edema, and addressing neuromuscular diseases. Sodium bicarbonate is not recommended in respiratory acidosis as it may worsen hypercapnia and pulmonary edema, or cause a metabolic alkalosis. Small doses of sodium bicarbonate can be considered in cases of severe acidosis (pH < 7.1) with intractable hypercapnia.

Causes of respiratory alkalosis are listed in Table 25.2; the underlying pathophysiologic mechanism for each is alveolar hyperventilation. Respiratory alkalosis can be associated with a normal or elevated alveolar-arterial oxygen gradient (P[A-a]O_2 gradient, abbreviated A-a gradient, and is discussed in more detail in Chapter 7). In patients with an elevated A-a gradient, the differential diagnosis is the same as for patients with an elevated A-a gradient and hypoxia (see Algorithm 7.2). In patients with a normal A-a gradient, causes include central nervous system disorders such as tumors, encephalitis, anxiety, and fever, hypoxia from altitude or severe anemia, hyperventilation in intubated patients on mechanical ventilatory support, endocrine disorders, and drugs.

TABLE 25.2	Causes of Respiratory Alkalosis	
Normal P(A-a) O$_2$ Gradient		
Mechanical hyperventilation	Drugs	
Central Nervous System	Salicylates	
Psychogenic hyperventilation	Progesterone	
Fever	Catecholamines	
Pain	Hypoxia	
Encephalitis/meningitis	High altitude	
Tumors	Severe anemia	
Pregnancy	Endotoxinemia	
Hyperthyroidism	Cirrhosis	
Elevated P(A-a) O$_2$ Gradient[a]		
V/Q mismatch	Shunt	

P[A-a]O_2, alveolar-arterial oxygen gradient; V/Q, ventilation/perfusion.
[a]The differential diagnosis of respiratory alkalosis with an elevated alveolar-arterial oxygen gradient (P(A-a)O_2) is the same as hypoxia with an elevated P(A-a)O_2 listed in Chapter 7, Algorithm 7.2.

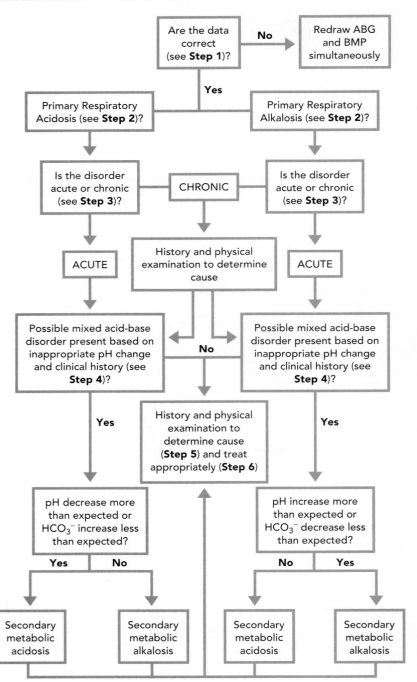

ALGORITHM 25.1 | Approach to Respiratory Acid-Base Disorders (see Steps 1 through 6)

Are the data correct (see **Step 1**)?
— **No** → Redraw ABG and BMP simultaneously

Yes

Primary Respiratory Acidosis (see **Step 2**)?

Primary Respiratory Alkalosis (see **Step 2**)?

Is the disorder acute or chronic (see **Step 3**)?

CHRONIC

Is the disorder acute or chronic (see **Step 3**)?

ACUTE

History and physical examination to determine cause

ACUTE

Possible mixed acid-base disorder present based on inappropriate pH change and clinical history (see **Step 4**)?

No

Possible mixed acid-base disorder present based on inappropriate pH change and clinical history (see **Step 4**)?

Yes

History and physical examination to determine cause (**Step 5**) and treat appropriately (**Step 6**)

Yes

pH decrease more than expected or HCO_3^- increase less than expected?

Yes   **No**

pH increase more than expected or HCO_3^- decrease less than expected?

No   **Yes**

Secondary metabolic acidosis

Secondary metabolic alkalosis

Secondary metabolic acidosis

Secondary metabolic alkalosis

ABG, arterial blood gas; BMP basic metabolic panel

As in respiratory acidosis, respiratory alkalosis treatment is directed at the underlying cause. Causes of hypoxia should be identified and treated. In mechanically ventilated patients, minute ventilation should be decreased by decreasing the respiratory rate and/or tidal volume. In psychogenic hyperventilation, reassurance and anxiolytics can be used. In patients at high altitudes, acetazolamide can be used to induce a metabolic acidosis to compensate for the respiratory alkalosis.

Step 1–Obtain an ABG (see section on arterial cannulation) and ensure the $[HCO_3^-]$ is accurate using the Henderson Equation.*

$$[HCO_3^-] = 24 \times PaCO_2/[H^+]$$

H$^+$ concentration and corresponding pH

pH	[H$^+$] meq/L
7.10	79
7.20	63
7.30	50
7.40	40
7.50	32
7.60	25

*Conversely, obtain ABG and basic metabolic panel simultaneously and compare $[HCO_3^-]$ in the ABG and basic metabolic panel to ensure accuracy. They should agree within 2mmol/L.

Step 2–Determine the underlying abnormality, i.e. a primary respiratory acidosis or alkalosis (metabolic acid-base disorders are discussed separately).

1. A primary respiratory acid-base disorder is present if the $PaCO_2$ is altered and the change in pH is in the opposite direction.
   a. A respiratory acidosis is present if the $PaCO_2$ is >40–45 mmHg and the pH is decreased.
   b. A respiratory alkalosis is present if the $PaCO_2$ is <35–40 mmHg and the pH is increased.

Step 3–Examine the pH, $PaCO_2$, and serum bicarbonate to determine if the respiratory acid-base disorder is acute or chronic.

1. As stated above, each acute change in the $PaCO_2$ of 10 mmHg will change the pH 0.08 (or 0.008 for each 1 mmHg change) in the opposite direction.
2. Each partially metabolically compensated change in the $PaCO_2$ of 10 mmHg will change the pH 0.03-0.08 in the opposite direction.
3. Each fully compensated change in the $PaCO_2$ of 10 mmHg will change the pH approximately 0.03, **but not back to normal.**
4. Table 25.1 shows the expected metabolic compensation for acute and chronic respiratory acid-base disorders, which occurs through changes in serum bicarbonate. Deviations in the serum bicarbonate that are significantly less than or greater than expected suggest a superimposed metabolic acid-base disorder.

Step 4–Determine if a mixed respiratory and metabolic acid-base disorder is present.

1. A superimposed metabolic acid-base disorder is present if the change in pH is **more** than 0.08 in the **opposite** direction of each 10 mmHg change in the $PaCO_2$.
   a. A metabolic acidosis is superimposed on a respiratory acidosis if the decrease in pH is greater than expected based on the $PaCO_2$. For example, pH 7.1 and $PaCO_2$ 60

mm HG. The expected pH for an acute increase in the $PaCO_2$ to 60 mm Hg is 7.24. Thus a superimposed metabolic acidosis is present.

   b. A metabolic alkalosis is superimposed on a respiratory alkalosis if the increase in pH is greater than expected based on the $PaCO_2$. For example, pH 7.55 and $PaCO_2$ 30 mmHg. The expected pH for an acute decrease in the $PaCO_2$ to 30 mm Hg is 7.48. Thus a superimposed metabolic alkalosis is present.

2. A combined acidosis and alkalosis is present if the $PaCO_2$ is increased or decreased and the pH is normal (approx 7.4).

   a. As stated, compensation back to normal does not occur. Therefore a normal pH with an altered $PaCO_2$, regardless of metabolic compensation, supports a superimposed metabolic disorder.

Step 5–Correlate the above steps with the patients clinical history and physical exam to arrive at the correct diagnosis.

For example, consider an ABG with pH 7.20, $PaCO_2$ 80, and plasma bicarbonate 33 meq/L. The primary disorder is a respiratory acidosis, evidenced by the decrease in pH and increase in $PaCO_2$ (**Step 2**). The expected plasma bicarbonate would be 28 meq/L if this were an acute acidosis, or 38 meq/L if it were chronic (**Step 3**). If this were an acute change in the $PaCO_2$, the pH would be 7.08 (0.08 change in pH for each 10 mmHg change in $PaCO_2$). Thus this cannot be a simple acute respiratory acidosis (**Step 4**). However there are multiple valid explanations for these ABG findings. One possibility is that it represents a partially compensated respiratory acidosis. Conversely, this could represent an acute respiratory acidosis with a superimposed metabolic alkalosis (explaining the higher than normal serum bicarbonate). A final possibility is that it represents an acute respiratory acidosis on a compensated chronic respiratory acidosis. Thus, the patient's clinical history and physical exam must be incorporated to determine the correct interpretation. If the patient had severe, compensated COPD complicated by acute cardiogenic pulmonary edema, an acute respiratory acidosis on a chronic compensated respiratory acidosis would seem likely.

Step 6–Once the etiology has been determined, treat appropriately (see end of opening text).

Suggested Reading

Epstein SK, Singh N. Respiratory acidosis. *Respir Care.* 2001;46:366–383.
   Review of the pathophysiology, evaluation, and causes of respiratory acidosis.
Foster GT, Vazin ND, Sassoon CS. Respiratory alkalosis. *Respir Care.* 2001;46:384–391.
   Review of the pathophysiology, evaluation, and causes of respiratory alkalosis.
Kaufman D, Kitching AJ, Kellum JA. Acid-base balance. In: Hall JB, Schmidt GA, Wood LD, eds. *Principles of Critical Care.* 3rd ed online, New York: McGraw Hill 2002; 1202–1208.
   Comprehensive textbook review of acid-base disorders.

Endocrine Disorders

VI

THYROID DISORDERS
William E. Clutter

26

HYPERTHYROIDISM

Major clinical findings in hyperthyroidism are listed in Table 26.1. Cardiac findings may be prominent, including tachycardia, atrial fibrillation, heart failure, and exacerbation of coronary artery disease. Rarely, severe hyperthyroidism may be associated with fever and delirium, sometimes called *thyroid storm*.

Major causes of hyperthyroidism are listed in Table 26.2. Graves disease (which may also cause proptosis) is the most common.

When the diagnosis of hyperthyroidism is suspected in a critically ill patient, plasma thyroid-stimulating hormone (TSH) and free thyroxine (T_4) should be measured. Clinical hyperthyroidism suppresses TSH to <0.1 mcU/mL, so a nonsuppressed plasma TSH excludes the diagnosis of hyperthyroidism. Plasma TSH may also be suppressed by severe nonthyroidal illness (about 10% of patients in intensive care units have plasma TSH <0.1 mcU/mL) and by therapy with dopamine or high-dose glucocorticoids. Thus, a suppressed plasma TSH alone does not establish the diagnosis.

If plasma TSH is suppressed and plasmafree T_4 is elevated, the diagnosis of hyperthyroidism is established. If plasmafree T_4 is not elevated, one of the other causes of suppressed plasma TSH previously listed is more likely. Heparin therapy may artifactually increase plasmafree T_4, so in heparin-treated patients, plasma total T_4 should be measured instead.

Treatment

The etiology of hyperthyroidism determines the best long-term therapy, but differential diagnosis can be deferred in the critically ill patient. Emergency therapy (Table 26.3) is indicated when hyperthyroidism exacerbates heart failure or an acute coronary syndrome, or when thyroid storm is present. It includes rapid inhibition of thyroid hormone synthesis (and conversion of T_4 to tri-iodothyronine [T_3]) by the thionamide propylthiouracil, inhibition of thyroid hormone secretion by iodine, and inhibition of the cardiovascular effects of hyperthyroidism by beta-antagonists. Hydrocortisone is usually recommended because it also inhibits T_4 conversion to T_3.

TABLE 26.1	Major Clinical Findings in Hyperthyroidism

Common	Seen Primarily in Severe Hyperthyroidism
■ Heat intolerance ■ Weight loss ■ Palpitations ■ Sinus tachycardia ■ Atrial fibrillation ■ Brisk tendon reflexes ■ Fine tremor ■ Lid lag ■ Proximal muscle weakness	■ Heart failure ■ Exacerbation of coronary artery disease ■ Fever and delirium ("thyroid storm")

Some authors have advocated treatment of amiodarone-induced hyperthyroidism with glucocorticoids alone, but the regimen described here has a high success rate in this disorder.

Plasma-free T_4 should be measured every 3 to 7 days. When free T_4 approaches the normal range, the doses of propylthiouracil and iodine should be gradually decreased. Iodine can usually be stopped at the time of hospital discharge, and radioactive iodine therapy for Graves disease or toxic multinodular goiter can be scheduled 2 to 3 weeks later.

HYPOTHYROIDISM

Major clinical findings in hypothyroidism are listed in Table 26.4. Severe hypothyroidism may contribute to hypothermia, hypoventilation, bradycardia, hypotension, and hyponatremia in the setting of concomitant critical illnesses.

Major causes of hypothyroidism are listed in Table 26.5. More than 90% of cases are primary hypothyroidism, most often iatrogenic or due to chronic autoimmune thyroiditis. Any pituitary or hypothalamic disorder can cause secondary hypothyroidism, but these disorders are usually clinically apparent because of other manifestations.

When the diagnosis of hypothyroidism is suspected in a critically ill patient, plasma TSH and free T_4 should be measured. Even mild primary hypothyroidism causes elevation of plasma TSH, so a normal plasma TSH excludes this diagnosis. Plasma TSH values >20 mcU/mL establish the diagnosis of primary hypothyroidism. Milder elevations of plasma TSH are usually due to primary hypothyroidism, but may also occur transiently during recovery from severe nonthyroidal illness.

TABLE 26.2	Major Causes of Hyperthyroidism

Associated with increased radioactive iodine uptake
■ Graves disease
■ Toxic multinodular goiter
■ Thyroid adenoma
Associated with decreased radioactive iodine uptake
■ Iodine-induced hyperthyroidism (due to amiodarone or iodine-containing contrast media[a])
■ Painless thyroiditis
■ Subacute thyroiditis
■ Factitious hyperthyroidism (ingestion of thyroid hormone or tissue)

[a]Iodine excess can cause both hyper- and hypothyroidism, depending on the patient's underlying thyroid function and basal iodine consumption.

TABLE 26.3	Emergency Therapy of Hyperthyroidism

Propylthiouracil: 300 mg PO q6h
Iodine (SSKI): 2 drops PO q12h
Beta-antagonist, with the dose adjusted to control tachycardia; initially:
    Propranolol, 40 mg PO q6h, or
    Esmolol, 500 mcg/kg IV followed by 50 mcg/kg/min IV
Hydrocortisone: 50 mg IV q8h

PO, by mouth; q, every; IV, intravenously.

TABLE 26.4	Major Clinical Findings in Hypothyroidism

Common	Seen Primarily in Severe Hypothyroidism
▪ Cold intolerance	▪ Hypothermia
▪ Fatigue	▪ Bradycardia
▪ Somnolence	▪ Hypoventilation
▪ Constipation	▪ Hypotension
▪ Weight gain	▪ Hyponatremia
▪ Slow tendon reflexes	▪ Pericardial or pleural effusion
▪ Nonpitting edema (myxedema)	
▪ Dry skin	

TABLE 26.5	Major Causes of Primary Hypothyroidism

▪ Chronic lymphocytic thyroiditis (Hashimoto's disease)
▪ Iatrogenic (after radioactive iodine therapy or thyroidectomy)
▪ Drugs
    Iodine excess (e.g., amiodarone, iodine-containing contrast media[a])
    Lithium
    Interferon-alpha
    Interleukin-2
▪ Iodine deficiency

[a]Iodine excess can cause both hyper- and hypothyroidism, depending on the patient's underlying thyroid function and basal iodine consumption.

TABLE 26.6	Emergency Therapy of Hypothyroidism
Thyroxine: 50–100 mcg IV q6–8h for 24 hr, then Thyroxine: 75–100 mcg IV q24h until oral intake is possible Hydrocortisone: 50 mg IV q8h	
IV, intravenously; q, every.	

If plasma free T_4 is low and plasma TSH is not elevated, the patient may have secondary hypothyroidism, but in a critically ill patient, this pattern of test results is more likely to be due to functional suppression of TSH and T_4 secretion by the nonthyroidal illness (the "euthyroid sick syndrome"). If the patient has clinical findings that may be due to hypothyroidism, empiric treatment with thyroxine should be started and the diagnosis should be reassessed after recovery. Otherwise, the patient can be observed with periodic measurement of plasma TSH and free T_4 to determine whether the abnormalities resolve with recovery.

Treatment

Emergency therapy of hypothyroidism (Table 26.6) is indicated if the patient has clinical signs that could be contributed to by hypothyroidism, such as bradycardia, hypoventilation, hypothermia, or hypotension. Each of these abnormalities should also be treated in the standard fashion as they are rarely due to hypothyroidism alone. Vital signs and cardiac rhythm should be monitored because treatment can exacerbate underlying heart disease. Hydrocortisone is given because of impaired adrenal function in severe hypothyroidism. No clinical trials have determined the optimum method of emergency treatment of hypothyroidism, but this method (Table 26.6) rapidly alleviates thyroxine deficiency while minimizing the risk of adverse events. There is no evidence to support treatment of the functional suppression of TSH and T_4 by nonthyroidal illness.

Suggested Reading

Cooper DS. Antithyroid drugs. *N Engl J Med.* 2005;352:905–917.
    Comprehensive review of thionamide drugs.
Fliers E, Alkemade A, Wiersinga WM. The hypothalamic-pituitary-thyroid axis in critical illness. *Best Practice Res Clin Endocrinol Metab.* 2001;15:453–464.
    Review of the pathophysiology, diagnosis and management of the changes in thyroid function in nonthyroidal illness
Osman F, Franklyn JA, Sheppard MC, et al. Successful treatment of amiodarone-induced thyrotoxicosis. *Circulation.* 2002;105:1275–77.
    Case series showing a high success rate with thionamide treatment alone.

ADRENAL INSUFFICIENCY IN CRITICAL ILLNESS

27

Timothy J. Bedient and Marin H. Kollef

An increase in circulating and tissue corticosteroid levels during critical illness is an important adaptive response. Normally, severe illness and stress stimulate the hypothalamic-pituitary-adrenal (HPA) axis, causing release of corticotropin releasing hormone (CRH) from the hypothalamus. CRH stimulates the anterior pituitary to release adrenocorticotropic hormone (ACTH or corticotropin), with ACTH causing increased cortisol production by the adrenal cortex's zona fasciculata. With acute illness such as severe infection, trauma, and burns, there is an increase in cortisol production by as much as a factor of six. Normally, circulating cortisol is bound to corticosteroid-binding globulin (CBG), with <10% in the free, bioavailable form. During acute illness, however, CBG levels decrease by as much as 50%, with unbound cortisol levels increasing. Although it is the unbound cortisol that is physiologically active, current laboratory assays only measure total cortisol. In a healthy, unstressed person, the HPA axis undergoes diurnal variation, but this is lost in critical illness. The major physiologic actions of circulating cortisol include increasing blood sugar levels; facilitating the delivery of glucose to cells during stress; facilitating normal cardiovascular reactivity to angiotensin II, epinephrine, and norepinephrine; contributing to the maintenance of cardiac contractility, vascular tone, and blood pressure; and anti-inflammatory and immunosuppressive effects.

Chronic adrenal insufficiency (Addison's disease) is a rare cause of intensive care unit admission and is distinct from the HPA axis dysfunction that occurs during critical illness, which has been termed *critical illness-related corticosteroid insufficiency* (CIRCI). CIRCI is characterized by an inappropriately low increase in cortisol during acute illness, also referred to as *relative adrenal insufficiency*. It is mediated in part by inflammatory cytokine inhibition of (a) CRH and ACTH release, (b) adrenal cortisol synthesis, and (c) glucocorticoid receptor translocation and transcription. In addition to CIRCI, adrenal insufficiency in critical illness may also be separated into two categories: *primary* if it is due to adrenal gland dysfunction, or *secondary* if it caused by central disruption of CRH or ACTH release. Causes or primary adrenal insufficiency in acute illness include direct injury to the adrenal glands from trauma, infarction, infection, malignancy, and hemorrhage; drug-induced suppression of cortisol synthesis; and autoimmune adrenalitis. Secondary causes include discontinuation of exogenous corticosteroids in patients on chronic immunotherapy, central nervous system malignancies, and head trauma. Causes of adrenal insufficiency are listed in Table 27.1.

Signs and symptoms of corticosteroid insufficiency resulting from HPA dysfunction are listed in Table 27.2. In pre-existing hypoadrenalism, these findings may be present before the onset of acute illness. However, in critically ill patients, adrenal insufficiency should be suspected in all patients with hypotension that is unresponsive to intravenous (IV) fluid administration and who require vasopressor support.

Although it is well documented that acute illness increases cortisol through stimulation of the HPA axis, it is less clear what defines an adequate stress response to acute illness. In addition, although CIRCI should be considered in all critically ill patients, most of the studies have focused on patients with severe sepsis and septic shock. Previous studies have suggested that a random serum cortisol >25 to 34 mcg/dL in critically ill patients makes relative adrenal insufficiency unlikely. However, recent studies have suggested that random cortisol measurements may have limited utility in the diagnosis of adrenal insufficiency, except in patients with a baseline cortisol <10 to 15 mcg/dL, and have highlighted the diagnostic value of a cortisol increase of ≤9 mcg/dL 60 minutes after stimulation with 250 mcg of IV cosyntropin (synthetic ACTH) as making adrenal insufficiency likely in critical illness.

TABLE 27.1	Causes of Adrenal Insufficiency

Cause	Example
Infection	Sepsis/septic shock
	HIV
	Cytomegalovirus
	Staphylococcus aureus, toxin-producing strain
	Fungal disorders (histoplasmosis, blastomycosis, cryptococcus)
	Tuberculosis
Medications	Suppressing release of corticotropin releasing hormone from the hypothalamus and pituitary:
	Corticosteroids
	Megestrol acetate
	Inhibition of enzymes involved in cortisol synthesis:
	Etomidate
	Ketoconazole
	Metyrapone
	Increased metabolism of cortisol:
	Rifampin
	Phenytoin
Malignancy	Adrenal metastases
Adrenal hemorrhage	Secondary to shock
	Anticoagulation
	Meningococcemia (Waterhouse-Friderichsen syndrome)
	Disseminated intravascular coagulation
	Antiphospholipid syndrome
Autoimmune	Addison's disease
Hypothalamic and pituitary disorders	Resulting in secondary adrenal insufficiency:
	Infection
	Pituitary tumor or metastases
	Infiltrative disorders (sarcoidosis, histiocytosis)
	Postpartum pituitary necrosis
	Trauma (blunt, radiation, surgical)

HIV, human immunodeficiency virus.

TABLE 27.2	Signs and Symptoms of Adrenal Insufficiency

Sign	Symptoms
Cardiovascular	Hypotension that is usually not responsive to fluid administration requiring use of vasopressors; hyperdynamic hemodynamic profile is common; tachycardia unless severe hypothyroidism is also present
Metabolic/electrolyte	Hypoglycemia, hyponatremia, hyperkalemia, fever
Hematologic	Eosinophelia and anemia
Neuromuscular	Weakness, fatigue, myalgia, arthralgia, headache, memory impairment, depression
Gastrointestinal	Anorexia, diarrhea, nausea, salt craving, weight loss
Cutaneous	Vitiligo, alopecia

In a prospective inception cohort study performed by Annane et al. in 2000 of 189 patients with septic shock, it was noted that an intermediate or poor prognosis occurred in patients with a cortisol increase in response to cosyntropin of ≤9 mcg/dL, with the highest mortality found in those patients who, in addition to a cosyntropin response of ≤9 mcg/dL, had an initial cortisol >34 mcg/dL. Another study by Annane et al. in 2006 of 101 patients with sepsis, 41 patients without sepsis, and 32 healthy controls, the overnight metyrapone stimulation test (Alg. 27.1) was used to investigate the diagnostic value of the cosyntropin test, and found that adrenal insufficiency was likely if the baseline cortisol level was <10 mcg/dL or change in cortisol after cosyntropin was ≤9 mcg/dL, and unlikely when cosyntropin stimulated cortisol levels were ≥44 mcg/dL and the change in cortisol after cosyntropin was ≥16.8 mcg/dL. These diagnostic values were explored further in 2007 by Lipiner-Friedman et al. in the retrospective arm of the CORTICUS study group. This retrospective multicenter cohort study included 477 patients with severe sepsis and septic shock who had undergone an ACTH stimulation test on the first day of sepsis, and found that random cortisol levels ≥15 mcg/dL, regardless of the cutoff, were not independent predictors of shock reversal, hospital mortality, or survival duration. However, patients with a baseline cortisol level <15 mcg/dL or change in cortisol ≤9 mcg/dL after cosyntropin, had a longer duration of shock and a shorter survival time. Corticosteroids were used to treat 44% of patients and were associated with a strong reduction in the risk of dying (OR, 0.21; 98% CI, 0.08 to 0.52). Measuring serum cortisol 30 and 60 minutes after cosyntropin added no significant diagnostic value to checking cortisol at 60 minutes alone.

Randomized studies have been performed to determine if corticosteroid replacement therapy is beneficial in patients with varying diagnostic definitions of adrenal insufficiency. In a placebo-controlled, randomized, double-blind study by Annane et al. in 2002, 300 patients with septic shock were randomized to receive hydrocortisone 50 mg every 6 hours and fludrocortisone 50 mcg once daily for 7 days, or placebo, after undergoing a 250 mcg cosyntropin test. Of the 229 patients with relative adrenal insufficiency (115 placebo and 114 corticosteroid), defined as an increase after cosyntropin of ≤9 mcg/dL, there was significantly reduced mortality (73 patients vs. 60 patients, $p = 0.02$) and withdrawal of vasopressor therapy within 28 days (46 patients vs. 65 patients, $p = 0.001$) in the corticosteroid treated patients, without increasing adverse events. In the 70 patients who had a cosyntropin response ≥9 mcg/dL, corticosteroid replacement therapy had no significant effect on the same outcomes and no trend toward efficacy. These data were supported by two meta-analyses examining glucocorticoids administration in severe sepsis and septic shock showing reduced mortality when glucocorticoids were given at similar dosages. Previous studies showing a survival disadvantage used higher-dose corticosteroids (23,975 mg vs. 1,209 mg) administered for a shorter duration.

However, the preliminary results of the randomized arm of the CORTICUS study, which have not been published at the time of this review, found no benefit to treating patients with septic shock, including the subgroup with a cosyntropin response ≤9 mcg/dL. This study differed from the initial randomized study by Annane in 2002 in that patients in the CORTICUS study were randomized up to 72 hours after the onset of septic shock rather than within 8 hours, patients in the CORTICUS study included those with severe sepsis and septic shock rather than septic shock alone (i.e., could be included in the study without hypotension requiring vasopressors), received 11 days of corticosteroid replacement rather than 7 days, and were not given fludrocortisone. How this study will change clinicians' approach to treating adrenal insufficiency in septic shock has yet to be seen.

Glucocorticoids, however, may not be appropriate for all critically ill patients as highlighted in a case-control study by Britt et al. in 2006 in 100 patients (six with septic shock) in a burn trauma ICU who received steroids, compared with 100 matched control patients, showing that corticosteroid use was associated with increased infection rates, increased ICU and ventilator duration, and a trend toward increased mortality.

Based on these data, there are no definitive diagnostic criteria for relative corticosteroid insufficiency in critically ill patients. Some experts believe the supraphysiologic dose of cosyntropin used in an attempt to increase cortisol production from an already stimulated adrenal gland may be less important than the baseline cortisol alone. However, numerous studies have found benefit from corticosteroid replacement in patients with relative

ALGORITHM 27.1 **Diagnostic and Therapeutic Approach to Adrenal Insufficiency in the Critically Ill Patient**

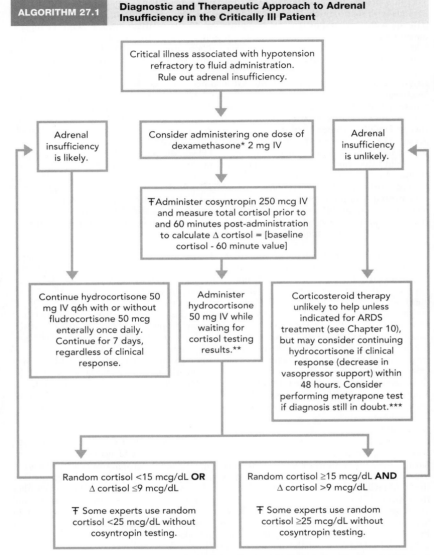

ARDS, acute respiratory distress syndrome; IV, intravenous; Cortisol, change in cortisol level in mcg/dL.
*Dexamethasone does not interfere with the cosyntropin test and 2 mg IV is equivalent to approximately 50 mg of hydrocortisone.
** Administer only if dexamethasone was not given initially.
*** Metyrapone blocks the conversion of 11-deoxycortisol to cortisol by CYP11B1 and causes a rapid fall in cortisol. To test, give metyrapone PO at 30 mg/kg at 12 AM and measure 11-deoxycortisol and cortisol 8 hours later. A normal response is an 8 AM serum 11-deoxycortisol level of 7 to 22 mcg/dL and serum cortisol <5 mcg/dL. Serum 11-deoxycortisol <7 mcg/dL indicates adrenal insufficiency. Patients who undergo metyrapone testing should receive at least 24 hours of corticosteroid replacement. *Metyrapone is not currently available for routine clinic use in the United States.*

adrenal insufficiency defined by cosyntropin stimulated cortisol ≤9 mcg/dL, and there is suggestion, at least in retrospective data, that baseline cortisol levels >10 to 15 mcg/dL may be less important than adrenal reserves as measured with 250 mcg cosyntropin stimulated serum cortisol levels at 1 hour.

Thus, although our understanding of relative adrenal insufficiency in the critically ill continues to evolve, nearly all evidence agrees that adrenal insufficiency is likely when the baseline cortisol is <10 to 15 mcg/dL in critically ill patients, and that cosyntropin stimulation testing may have additional diagnostic value in identifying which patients are likely to respond to corticosteroid replacement, at least in the setting of volume unresponsive hypotension in patients with septic shock. We recommend that critically ill patients with shock unresponsive to IV fluids requiring vasopressor support be evaluated for adrenal insufficiency and treated as illustrated in Algorithm 27.1. Patients may be given dexamethasone 2 mg IV while waiting for cosyntropin testing results, as dexamethasone does not interfere with the cosyntropin test. Otherwise, patients should be started on hydrocortisone immediately following cosyntropin testing while waiting for the results. Once treatment is initiated, the cause of adrenal insufficiency can be explored further. Many patients with adrenal insufficiency related to critical illness can be expected to regain normal function of the HPA axis with recovery from their illness. Some experts, however, still use the random cortisol alone, feeling that adrenal insufficiency is unlikely when the random cortisol is ≥25 mcg/dL and that cosyntropin testing has no additional diagnostic value. Certainly more studies are needed.

Suggested Reading

Annane A, Bellissant E, Bollaert PE, et al. Corticosteroids for severe sepsis and septic shock: a systematic review and meta-analysis. *BMJ.* 2004;329:480–489.
  Meta-analysis of 16 randomized and quasi randomized trials involving 2063 patients with severe sepsis and septic shock showing that long courses (≥ 5 days) with low dose corticosteroids (≤ 300 mg hydrocortisone or equivalent) reduced 28 day and hospital mortality.
Annane D, Maxime V, Ibrahim F, et al. Diagnosis of adrenal insufficiency in severe sepsis and septic shock. *Am J Respir Crit Care Med.* 2006;174:1319–1326.
  An update on the diagnosis of adrenal insufficiency using cosyntropin stimulation.
Annane D, Sebille V, Charpentier C, et al. Effect of treatment with low dose of hydrocortisone and fludrocortisone on mortality in patients with septic shock. *JAMA.* 2002;288:862–871.
  A placebo controlled, randomized, double-blind study showing a 7-day treatment with low doses of hydrocortisone and fludrocortisone in patients with septic shock and relative adrenal insufficiency, significantly reduced the risk of death without an increase in adverse events.
Annane D, Sebille V, Troche G, et al. A 3-level prognostic classification in septic shock based on cortisol levels and cortisol response to corticotropin. *JAMA.* 2000;283:1038–1045.
  A prospective inception cohort study evaluating the prognostic value of cortisol and the cosyntropin stimulation test in patients with septic shock.
Cooper MS, Stewart PM. Corticosteroid insufficiency in acutely ill patients. *N Engl J Med.* 2003;348:727–734.
  A focused review on the pathogenesis and treatment of adrenal insufficiency in the critically ill.
Lipiner-Friedman D, Sprung CL, Laterre PF. Adrenal function in sepsis: The retrospective Corticus cohort study. *Crit Care Med.* 2007;35:1012–1018.
  Retrospective cohort study from 20 European intensive care units examining the relationship between baseline and cosyntropin stimulated cortisol levels and mortality in patients with severe sepsis and septic shock showing that delta cortisol and not basal cortisol levels were associated with clinical outcomes.
Marik P. Mechanisms and clinical consequences of critical illness associated adrenal insufficiency. *Curr Opin Crit Care.* 2007;13:363–369.
  Review of the causes and consequences of adrenal insufficiency in critically-ill patients.
Marik PE, Zaloga GP. Adrenal insufficiency in the critically ill. *Chest.* 2002;122: 1784–1796.
  A general overview of adrenal insufficiency as it occurs in critically ill patients.

28

DIABETIC KETOACIDOSIS AND HYPEROSMOLAR HYPERGLYCEMIC STATE

Timothy J. Bedient, Runhua Hou, and Garry S. Tobin

Diabetic ketoacidosis (DKA) and hyperosmolar hyperglycemic state (HHS) are life-threatening hyperglycemic complications of diabetes mellitus (DM), and common reasons for admission to the intensive care unit. The annual incidence of DKA ranges from 4.6 to 8 episodes per 1,000 patients with DM. The annual incidence of HHS is lower than DKA and accounts for less than 1% of primary diabetic admissions. The mortality rate is <5% in DKA and approximately 15% in HHS, but varies based on severity, age, and underlying illness. Precipitating factors include inadequate insulin treatment or noncompliance, new-onset DM, infections (most commonly pneumonia and urinary tract infections), cardiovascular events, and pregnancy. DKA typically occurs in patients with type 1 DM, but does occur in patients with type 2 DM at a much lower frequency. HHS is typically confined to patients with type 2 DM.

DKA is characterized by hyperglycemia (blood glucose typically ≥250 mg/dL), acidosis (arterial pH ≤7.3), and ketosis (positive urine and plasma ketones), along with dehydration and electrolyte abnormalities in varying degrees. Prominent presenting symptoms include nausea/vomiting, abdominal pain, and polyuria. HHS is characterized by hyperglycemia (blood glucose typically 600 to 1,200 mg/dL), hyperosmolarity (serum osmolarity 320 to 380 mOsm/L), pronounced dehydration (hemodynamic instability, prerenal azotemia, decreased urine output), and neurologic sequelae ranging from mild lethargy to coma. HHS has an insidious onset, typically over weeks, with patients experiencing polyuria, polydipsia, weight loss, and neurologic changes including fatigue, confusion, or coma. Table 28.1 highlights the differences between DKA and HHS.

DKA and HHS are the result of insulin deficiency in patients with DM. In both disorders, insulin deficiency causes increased hepatic glycolysis and gluconeogenesis, and impaired glucose utilization by peripheral tissues, leading to hyperglycemia. In patients with DKA, the absolute lack of insulin causes an increase in counterregulatory hormones (cortisol, growth hormone, catecholamines, and glucagon), which promote lipolysis in adipose tissue and the release of free fatty acids. In the liver, the free fatty acids are converted to ketones. In HHS patients, even in the absence of exogenous insulin, there is typically enough intrinsic insulin production by beta cells to suppress counterregulatory hormone release. Thus, hormone levels are only mildly elevated, and increased hepatic glucose production usually occurs without a significant rise in serum ketones.

The hyperglycemia in both disorders causes an osmotic diuresis. However, in HHS the hyperglycemia is more pronounced, resulting in greater diuresis. The resulting dehydration impairs renal function, decreasing glucose excretion, and worsening hyperglycemia. In contrast, patients with DKA suffer from a metabolic acidosis as a result of the ketones produced by the liver. In both disorders, diuresis causes loss of sodium and potassium, and although initial laboratory values are variable, total body sodium and potassium are depleted.

Treatment of DKA and HHS requires reversal of the hyperglycemia by administering insulin, and replacing the circulating and total body volume and electrolyte deficits as outlined in Algorithm 28.1. Insulin and intravenous (IV) fluids will correct the acidosis in patients with DKA, but can rapidly produce hypokalemia as potassium shifts intracellularly. Successful treatment of both disorders requires frequent monitoring and decision-making based on the patient's clinical condition, and laboratory data as it is becomes available. The factor that precipitated the DKA and HHS should be sought and treated.

TABLE 28.1	Initial Laboratory Values in Diabetic Ketoacidosis and Hyperosmolar Hyperglycemic State			
		DKA		
Value	Mild	Moderate	Severe	HHS
Plasma glucose (mg/dL)	>250	>250	>250	>600
Arterial pH	7.25–7.30	7–7.24	<7	>7.30
Serum bicarbonate (meq/L)	15–18	10–14	<10	>15
Urine and serum ketones	Positive	Positive	Positive	Trace/small
Serum osmolarity (mOsm/L)	<320	<320	<320	330–380
Anion gap	>10	>12	>12	<12
Mental status	Alert	Alert/drowsy	Stupor/coma	Stupor/coma
Sodium (mmol/L)	125–135	125–135	125–135	135–145
Potassium (mmol/L)	Normal to ↑	Normal to ↑	Normal to ↑	Normal
Creatinine (mg/dL)	Slight ↑	Slight ↑	Slight ↑	Moderate ↑

DKA, diabetic ketoacidosis; HHS, hyperosmolar hyperglycemic state.

In patients with DKA and HHS, insulin should be given IV. If IV administration cannot be achieved, an intramuscular or subcutaneous (SC) route is an option. However this is a less reliable method to achieve the insulin levels needed in seriously ill patients. Patients with HHS are often more responsive to insulin than patients with DKA and a lower dose is often used (Alg. 28.1). In both disorders, the blood glucose (BG) should be decreased by 50 to 75 mg/dL/hr. Decreasing the BG more than 75 to 100 mg/dL/hr can cause an osmotic encephalopathy. Glucose lowering in the first 2 hours may be more rapid as a result of initial volume expansion.

When the BG reaches 250 mg/dL, 5% dextrose should be added to the IV fluids to maintain hyperglycemia while keeping insulin in the supraphysiologic range. In DKA, hyperglycemia resolves faster than acidosis and supraphysiologic insulin is needed to suppress lipolysis and hepatic ketone production, and to increase peripheral ketone use. In DKA the blood glucose should be kept between 150 and 200 mg/dL until the anion gap is closed. In HHS, the blood glucose should be kept slightly higher, generally between 250 and 300 mg/dL to allow gradual correction of intracranial fluid shifts. In HHS, values should be kept at 250 to 300 mg/dL until the patient's mental status improves.

When the anion gap is closed (DKA) or the patient's mental status improves (HHS), IV insulin can be converted to SC insulin as listed in Algorithm 28.1. Failure to give SC insulin when the IV insulin is stopped can result in rebound hyperglycemia with worsening mental status in HHS, or acidosis in DKA.

Cerebral edema is a serious complication of both DKA and HHS. This devastating consequence is observed more frequently in children than in adults. Symptoms include headache, altered mental status, or a sudden deterioration in mental status after an initial improvement. The risk factors for cerebral edema are excessive correction with free H_2O and a rapid decline in the BG. Failure of the serum sodium to rise during treatment is a clue to excess hydration with free H_2O. Prompt recognition and treatment with IV mannitol and corticosteroids is essential to prevent neurologic sequelae. Computed tomography imaging can show the presence of cerebral edema. Morbidity and mortality are high once cerebral edema is recognized.

ALGORITHM 28.1	Management of Diabetic Ketoacidosis and Hyperosmolar Hyperglycemic State

INSULIN TREATMENT

1) Bolus 0.1–0.15 U/kg regular insulin intravenously (IV) (subcutaneous [SC]/intramuscular [IM] can be given if no IV access)
2) Start continuous IV insulin infusion via an infusion pump
   Standard infusion is 100 U **regular human insulin** (IV t $^1/_2$ 5–9 minutes) in 100 mL 0.9% NaCl.
   For **DKA** start at 0.1 U/kg/hr
   For **HHS** start at 0.05 U/kg/hr

BLOOD GLUCOSE MONITORING

1) Check initial blood glucose (BG) q1h. **Goal decrease in BG is 50–75 mg/dL/hr.**
2) Once stable (3 consecutive values decreased in target range), change BG monitoring to q2h. Resume q1h BG monitoring for each change in the insulin infusion rate (see below).
3) Add dextrose 5% to IV fluids when BG <250 mg/dL
   For **DKA goal BG 150–200 mg/dL until anion gap closed.**
   For **HHS goal BG is 250–300 mg/dL until mental status improves.**

CHANGING THE INSULIN INFUSION RATE

1) ↓ IV insulin by 50%/hr if BG decreases by >100 mg/dL/hr in any 1 hour period.*
2) ↑ insulin drip by 50%/hr if change in BG is <50 mg/dL/hr.
3) For **DKA and HSS**, when BG decreases to 250 mg/dL, insulin infusion may need to be decreased 50% to maintain glucose at target levels (see Blood Glucose Monitoring above).

Start SC insulin when:
1) Anion gap closed (DKA)
2) Serum bicarbonate increases to >15 meq/L (DKA)
3) Patient able to eat
4) Mental status improves (HHS)

Stop the insulin drip after all of the following are done**
1) Give short acting insulin (aspart or lispro) SC at twice the hourly IV rate (e.g., if IV rate is 5 U/hr, give 10U short acting insulin SC).
2) Give long acting insulin (regular, NPH or glargine) SC at 0.2–0.3 U/kg, or home insulin dose.
3) Ensure patient has a meal and is eating.

*Lowering glucose >100 mg/dL/hr may cause osmotic encephalopathy.
**Failure to give SC insulin may result in rebound hyperglycemia and ketosis due to the short t$^1/_2$ of IV regular insulin (5–9 min).

(continued on the next page)

(continued from previous page)

FLUID MANAGEMENT*

Fluid replacement varies based on age, weight, hemodynamics, and comorbidities. A reasonable approach follows:

1) **Replace intravascular volume**
   Give 1 L 0.9% NaCl over 30–60 min. Give an additional 1–2 L q30–60 min until hemodynamically stable and urine output increased.
2) **Replace total body water deficit**
   Change to 0.45% NaCl and infuse at 150–500 mL/hr.
   When BG <250 mg/dL add dextrose 5% and decrease to 100–200 mL/hr.

*Fluid is replaced over 12–24 hr and patients are generally depleted 3–6 L in DKA and 8–12 L in HHS.
*Monitor urine output, heart rate, blood pressure, and respiratory status. Care must be taken in patients with congestive heart failure and kidney disease.

ELECTROLYTE MANAGEMENT

1) Check basic metabolic panel (BMP), arterial blood gas, magnesium (Mg^{2+}), and phosphorous (PO_4^{3-}).
2) Repeat BMP, Mg, PO_4^{3-} q2–4h depending on degree of electrolyte imbalance.

Potassium (K^+)
K^+ >_5.5 meq/L: leave potassium supplement out of IVF
K^+ 4–5.4 meq/L: add 20 mEq KCl/L to IVF
K^+ 3–3.9 meq/L: add 40 mEq KCl/L to IVF
K^+ <3 meq/L: add 60 mEq KCl/L to IVF
In DKA, if initial K^+ is <3.3 meq/L, **DO NOT** give IV insulin until the serum K^+ is supplemented to >3.3 mmol/L due to the risk of severe hypokalemia.

Sodium (Na^+)
Hypoglycemia causes an artifactually low serum sodium, and the correct value must be calculated. Corrected Na^+ = Measured Na^+ [mmol/L] + (1.6 (Measured BG [mg/dL] − 100)/100)
Na^+ replaced with IV fluids initially as 0.9% NaCl for first 1–3 L and then as 0.45% NaCl (see Fluid Management).

Bicarbonate (HCO_3^-)
Usually in DKA only.
Replacement generally not necessary as insulin will reverse the HCO_3^- deficit with its inhibition of lipolysis.
Consider HCO_3^- in the following situations (see Chapter 24; metabolic acidosis):
   1) Severe acidosis with pH <7 (the HCO_3^- should be stopped once the pH is >7.1)
   2) Severe loss of buffering capacity when serum HCO_3^- <5–10 meq/L
   3) Acidosis induced cardiac or respiratory distress
   4) Severe hyperkalemia

Magnesium and Phosphorus
Severe hypomagnesemia and hypophosphatemia are not common complications of DKA and HHS (see Chapter 23 if they occur) and supplementation is usually not necessary.

PRECIPITATING FACTOR TREATMENT

The cause of the DKA or HHS should be sought and treated. Common precipitants include missed insulin therapy, infections such as pneumonia, sepsis, and urinary and upper respiratory tract infections, trauma, myocardial infarction, pregnancy, or as the initial presentation of DM.

Suggested Reading

Faich GA, Fishbein HA, Ellis SE. The epidemiology of diabetic acidosis: a population based study. *Am J. Epidemiol.* 1983;177:551–558.

A 12 month epidemiologic study conducted from 1979–1980 of all acute care centers in Rhode Island which examined the incidence, mortality rates, precipitating factors, and cost for patients admitted with DKA.

Kitabchi AE, Guillermo EU, Murphy MB, et al. Management of hyperglycemic crises in patients with diabetes. *Diabetes Care.* 2001;24: 131–153.

An extensive review of the definitions, causes, manifestations, pathophysiology, and treatment of DKA and HHS.

Magee MF, Bhatt BA. Management of decompensated diabetes. Diabetic ketoacidosis and hyperglycemic hyperosmolar syndrome. *Crit Care Clin.* 2001;17(1):75–106.

Review of DKA and HHS.

GLUCOSE CONTROL IN THE ICU

Timothy J. Bedient, Runhua Hou, and Garry S. Tobin

29

Hyperglycemia is a common finding in patients in the intensive care unit (ICU), occurring in both diabetic and nondiabetic patients. Factors contributing to hyperglycemia in critically ill patients include increased counterregulatory hormones (cortisol and glucagon), hepatic insulin resistance, decreased physical activity with resultant decrease in insulin-stimulated glucose uptake in heart and skeletal muscle, glucocorticoid therapy, dextrose-containing intravenous fluids, and dense caloric enteral and parenteral nutrition. Numerous observational studies have shown that hyperglycemia is an independent risk factor for morbidity and mortality in patients in the medical, surgical, neurology, and cardiac ICUs, including postoperative cardiac and general surgery patients, patients with acute myocardial infarction and stroke, and general medicine patients.

Until recently, it was less clear if hyperglycemia was a benign, physiologic marker of more severe critical illness, or a treatable cause of worse clinical outcomes. Only a few randomized trials have addressed this question, and they have shown that treating hyperglycemia in critically ill patients reduces morbidity and mortality. However, which patients benefit the most from treatment and the optimal glucose targets still remains unclear. The following discussion addresses the current evidence, recommendations, and areas of uncertainty.

The seminal randomized study treating hyperglycemia in critically ill patients was published by Van den Berghe et al. in 2001 and included 1,548 intubated patients (13% with known diabetes) in a surgical ICU who were randomly assigned to intensive glycemic control with a target glucose between 80 and 110 mg/dL (n = 765), versus a standard care group that was treated with insulin when the blood glucose was >215 mg/dL, with a target glucose between 180 and 200 mg/dL (n = 783). The study found that the intensive care mortality rate was 42% lower (8% vs. 4.6%, p <0.04) in the intensive treatment group, with the benefit reaching statistical significance in patients who remained in the ICU for more than 5 days. The major difference in mortality was attributed to a decrease in the development of multiorgan failure with sepsis.

Van den Berghe et al. addressed nonsurgical patients in 2006 with a follow-up trial limited to patients in a medial ICU, which randomized 1,200 patients (16.9% with known diabetes) to intensive glucose control versus standard care utilizing the same protocol as in their 2001 trial. The study did not replicate the mortality benefit seen in the surgical ICU study. Overall, there was no significant difference in the in-hospital mortality rate (37.3% vs. 40%, p = 0.33). While the study did show decreased in-hospital mortality for the 767 patients who stayed in the ICU ≥3 days (43% vs. 52.5%, p 0.009), there was increased mortality in the patients who stayed in the ICU <3 days (12.9% vs. 9.6%, p=0.41 after correcting for baseline risk factors), although this difference did not reach statistical significance. Despite no overall mortality benefit, there was reduced morbidity in the intensive treatment group, including less newly acquired kidney injury, reduced duration of mechanical ventilation, shorter ICU stay, and shorter hospital stays. There was no significant difference in bacteremia or duration of antibiotics.

In the two trials by Van ben Berghe et al., hypoglycemic episodes were increased in the intensive treatment group (5.2% vs. 0.7% in the surgical ICU, 18.7% vs. 3.1% in the medical ICU). Despite the high incidence of hypoglycemia, serious immediate side effects such as hemodynamic compromise and seizures were not reported. While hypoglycemia is more common in patients with renal and hepatic failure, which may partially explain the increased incidence of hypoglycemia in the medical ICU, hypoglycemia was identified as an

TABLE 29.1	Recommended Target Blood Glucose for Patients in the Intensive Care Unit	
American Diabetes Association		**American College of Endocrinology**
As close to 110 mg/dL as possible; generally <180 mg/dL		<110 mg/dL

independent risk factor for death in the medical ICU. However, the effect was not seen until at least 24 hours after the hypoglycemic episode. The reason for this is unclear.

The Diabetes Insulin-Glucose Infusion in Acute Myocardial Infarction (DIGAMI) study examined intensive versus conventional glucose treatment in diabetic patients hospitalized with acute myocardial infarction. The intensive treatment group received intravenous insulin in the first 24 hours followed by aggressive subcutaneous glucose control for 3 months. The primary outcome was mortality at 1 year, which was found to be 29% lower in the intensive treatment group. It was unclear to what degree inpatient and outpatient glucose control contributed to the mortality benefit, which prompted DIGAMI-2. This study randomized 1,253 patients with diabetes mellitus to intensive inpatient treatment only, intensive inpatient and outpatient treatment, or aggressive outpatient treatment only. Unfortunately, the study did not enroll enough patients and the difference in the mean glucose values was small. Not surprisingly, the study found no significant 1-year mortality difference between the three groups.

Adding to the uncertainty in cardiac patients are two recent observational studies that noted an increased risk of death in patients admitted for acute myocardial infarction who developed hypoglycemia during hospitalization.

The conclusions and current recommendations based on these studies are controversial. Table 29.1 lists the most recent recommendations for glucose control in the ICU by the American Diabetes Association (Position Statement 2006) and the American College of Endocrinology, which includes patients in all ICUs. However, some experts believe these recommendations are too stringent and a reasonable goal for medical and surgical ICU patients is to aim for a glucose value <140 to 150 mg/dL, and possibly <110 mg/dL. In cardiac ICU patients, given the possible increased mortality with hypoglycemia and the lack of evidence for early glucose control, a value <180 mg/dL may be reasonable. Overall, studies support intensive glucose control in patients who are expected to stay in the ICU more than 3 to 5 days. The postulated reason for this is that preventing hyperglycemia prevents complications from hyperglycemia, and complications take time to develop. It seems reasonable to exclude medical ICU patients who are eating and who are expected to be in the ICU <3 days. However, it is not always possible to predict the length of ICU stays, and physician discretion is needed.

In critically ill patients admitted to the ICU, all oral antihyperglycemic agents and subcutaneous insulin should be stopped. Insulin in critically ill patients should be given intravenously. The half-life of intravenous insulin is 5 to 9 minutes, which allows for rapid reversal of hypoglycemia when it occurs. Most ICUs now have standardized glucose algorithms, generally managed by nurses, which have been shown to be valid ways to manage glucose. The most effective glucose algorithms are dynamic and incorporate the rate of glucose change into the insulin dose adjustments. Table 29.2 contains a validated insulin-infusion protocol outlining how to initiate an insulin infusion, monitor blood glucose, and manage hypoglycemia. Algorithm 29.1 shows how to manage the insulin-infusion rate.

In managing glucose, one must make insulin-infusion adjustments based on changes in carbohydrate intake. For example, a change in the dextrose 5% rate from 150 mL/hr (180 g carbohydrates normalized during a 24-hour period) to 75 mL/hr (90 g carbohydrates normalized during a 24-hour period) will require a decrease in the insulin- infusion rate in order to prevent hypoglycemia. In critically ill patients, multiple sources of carbohydrate need to be taken into consideration when calculating the insulin dose such as parenteral nutrition, enteral tube feeds, and glucose containing IV fluid. Nutrition, whether enteral or perenteral , should be given as a continuous infusion rather than intermittent boluses to prevent significant fluctuations in blood glucose. It is often critical to reassess caloric intake every 12 to 24 hours. The patients most at risk for hypoglycemia are those with renal failure and hepatic failure. Close attention to details and a less aggressive titration schedule in patients with liver and renal failure should allow insulin drips to be safely used. Meticulous attention must also be paid to patients with impaired mental status who are unable to perceive and respond to low glucose levels.

The implementation of any protocol, whether taken from the literature or developed locally, especially one as complex as an IV insulin drip protocol, requires a significant amount of education and training. Even under controlled conditions, the protocol can be violated frequently. The violations could be as simple as a missed blood glucose or as serious as a failure to adjust the insulin-infusion rate. Human error has to be taken into consideration when evaluating blood glucose control. Computerized calculation of the drip rate will minimize mistakes and may improve outcome.

Once patients improve and are ready to be discharged from the ICU, intravenous insulin needs to be switched to subcutaneous insulin. Using an insulin sliding scale alone is likely to result in rebound hyperglycemia. Using basal long-acting insulin (NPH or glargine) combined with prandial and sliding scale short-acting insulin (aspart, lispro, glulisine) will lead to better glycemic control. When calculating the dosage, one needs to take into account the prior history of diabetes, type of diabetes, stress level, prior insulin dosage, steroid use and general clinical status. Long-acting insulin needs to overlap with discontinuation of the drip to prevent hyperglycemia. We give short acting insulin at two times the drip rate plus long acting insulin (generally starting with 0.2–0.3 U/kg of body weight/day) and turn the drip off immediately. If short-acting insulin is not given, then the drip should overlap 2 to 3 hours to allow the long-acting insulin to be effective.

In summary, although the current recommendations for glucose targets are controversial, treating hyperglycemia in critically ill patients leads to decreased morbidity and mortality. Available data are limited but suggest medical and postsurgical patients who are in the ICU more than 3 to 5 days are most likely to benefit. Insulin in critically ill patients should be given intravenously to allow rapid reversal of hypoglycemia if it occurs, with early data suggesting that critically ill medical and cardiac patients may be most sensitive to the effects of hypoglycemia. Insulin-infusion protocols implemented by well- trained staff can be effective ways to manage blood glucose. Paying careful attention to changes in patient's clinical condition and nutritional status, as well as vigorous glycemic monitoring by hospital staff, will minimize hypoglycemic events At the time of this publication, several large, randomized clinical studies are under way to further address hyperglycemia in critically ill ICU patients.

TABLE 29.2	Insulin Infusion Protocol

Initiating Insulin Infusion

Standard insulin infusion 100 U **regular human insulin** in 100 mL 0.9% normal saline.

Preferred administration IV (t½ 5–9 minutes) via an infusion pump.

Give initial bolus if blood glucose (BG) >150 mg/dL;

Divide initial BG by 70 and round to nearest 0.5 U (e.g., BG 250: 250/70 = 3.57, rounded to 4, so IV bolus 4 U.)

After bolus, start infusion at same hourly rate as bolus (4 U/hr IV in above example).

If **BG less than 150 mg/dL,** divide by 70 for initial hourly rate with **NO bolus** (e.g., BG 150 would be 150/70 = 2.15, rounded to 2, so start at 2 U/hr IV).

Go to Algorithm 29.1 for instructions on changing the insulin infusion rate.

Blood Glucose Monitoring

Check BG q1h until stable (3 consecutive values in target range).

Once stable can change BG monitoring to q2h.

If stable, q2h for 12–24 hours can change to q3–4h, if

no significant change in nutrition or clinical status

Resume q1h BG monitoring for BG >70 md/dL with any of the following;

Change in insulin-infusion rate.

Initiation or cessation of corticosteroid or vasopressor therapy.

Significant change in clinical status.

Change in nutritional support (initiation, cessation, or rate change).

Initiation or cessation of dialysis of CVVHD.

Hypoglycemia (BG <70 mg/dL)

If **BG <50 mg/dL,** stop infusion and give 25 g dextrose 50% (1 amp D50) IV.

Recheck BG q 10–15 min.

When BG >90 mg/dL, recheck in 1 hour. If still >90 mg/dL after 1 hour, resume insulin infusion at **50% most recent rate.**

If **BG 50–69 mg/dL,** stop infusion.

If symptomatic or unable to assess, give 25 g dextrose 50% (1 amp D50) IV.

Recheck BG q15min.*

If asymptomatic, consider 12.5 g dextrose 50% (1/2 amp D50) or 8 oz. fruit juice PO.

Recheck q15–30min.*

*When, BG >90 mg/dL, recheck in 1 hour. If still >90 mg/dL after 1 hour, resume insulin infusion at **75% most recent rate**.

BG, blood glucose; CVVHD, continuous venovenous hemodialysis; IV, intravenous; PO, by mouth.
Modified from Goldberg PA, Siegel MD, Sherwin RS, et al. Implementation of a safe and effective insulin-infusion protocol in a medical intensive care unit. *Diabetes Care.* 2004;27:461–467, with permission.

ALGORITHM 29.1	Changing the Insulin Infusion Rate

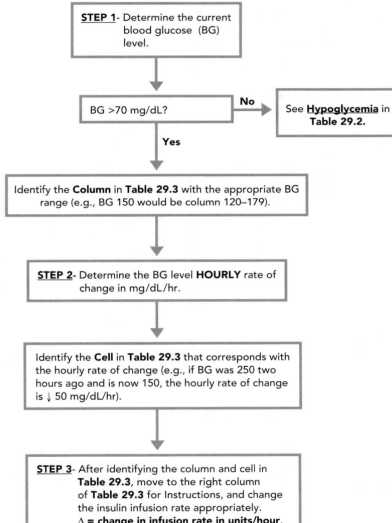

STEP 1- Determine the current blood glucose (BG) level.

BG >70 mg/dL?

No → See **Hypoglycemia** in **Table 29.2.**

Yes

Identify the **Column** in **Table 29.3** with the appropriate BG range (e.g., BG 150 would be column 120–179).

STEP 2- Determine the BG level **HOURLY** rate of change in mg/dL/hr.

Identify the **Cell** in **Table 29.3** that corresponds with the hourly rate of change (e.g., if BG was 250 two hours ago and is now 150, the hourly rate of change is ↓ 50 mg/dL/hr).

STEP 3- After identifying the column and cell in **Table 29.3**, move to the right column of **Table 29.3** for Instructions, and change the insulin infusion rate appropriately. Δ = **change in infusion rate in units/hour**, and is based on the current infusion rate listed in **Table 29.4**. (In the preceeding example with BG 150 mg/dL and down by 50 mg/dL/hr, the Instructions would be to 'decrease Infusion by Δ.' In **Table 29.4** **if** the current infusion rate was 5 U/hr, you would decrease the infusion by 1 U/hr).

TABLE 29.3   Current Blood Glucose Level and Rate of Change[a]

BG 70–89 mg/dL	BG 90–119 mg/dL	BG 120–179 mg/dL	BG >180 mg/dL	Instructions (See Table 29.4 for Δ)
		BG↑ by >40 mg/dL/hr	BG↑	INCREASE INFUSION by 2Δ
	BG↑ by >20 mg/dL/hr	BG↑ by 1–40 mg/dL/hr OR BG UNCHANGED	BG UNCHANGED OR BG↓ by 1–40 mg/dL/hr	INCREASE INFUSION by Δ
BG↑	BG↑ by 1–20 mg/dL/hr, BG UNCHANGED, OR BG↓ by 1–20 mg/dL/hr	BG↓ by 1–40 mg/dL/hr	BG↓ by 41–80 mg/dL/hr	NO INFUSION CHANGE
BG UNCHANGED OR BG↓ by 1–20 mg/dL/hr	BG↓ by 21–40 mg/dL/hr	BG↓ by 41–80 mg/dL/hr	BG↓ by 81–120 mg/dL/hr	DECREASE INFUSION by Δ
BG↓ by >20 mg/dL/hr See below[b]	BG↓ by >40 mg/dL/hr	BG↓ by >80 mg/dL/hr	BG↓ by >120 mg/dL/hr	HOLD INFUSION × 30 min then DECREASE by 2Δ

[a]See Algorithm 29.1 for instructions.
[b]Hold insulin infusion; check BG q15–30 min; when >90 mg/dL, restart infusion at 75% most recent rate.

TABLE 29.4   Changes in Insulin Infusion Rate (Δ) in U/Hr

Current Infusion Rate (U/hr)	Δ = Rate Change (U/hr)	2Δ = 2 × Rate Change (U/hr)
<3	0.5	1
3–6	1	2
6.5–9.5	1.5	3
10–14.5	2	4
15–19.5	3[a]	6[a]
20–24.5[a]	4[a]	8[a]
>25[a]	5[a]	10[a]

[a]Infusions typically range 2–10 U/hr. Doses in excess of 20 U/hr are unusual and a physician should be notified to explore potential contributing factors such as errors in insulin dilution and administration.

Suggested Reading

American Diabetes Association. Standards of medical care in diabetes-2006. Diabetes Care 2006; 28 Supplement 1:4–42.
ADA summary and recommendations for diagnosing and treating diabetes and hyperglycemia.

Garber AJ, Moghissi ES, Bransome ED Jr, et al. American College of Endocrinology position statement on inpatient diabetes and metabolic control. *Endocr Pract.* 2004;10: 77–82.
Summary of the current evidence for glycemic control in hospitalized diabetic and non-diabetic patients, including current ACE recommendations.

Goldberg PA, Siegel MD, Sherwin RS, et al. Implementation of a safe and effective insulin infusion protocol in a medical intensive care unit. *Diabetes Care.* 2004;27:461–467.
Results of a nurse-implemented insulin infusion protocol which incorporated the velocity of glycemic change, showing it to be a safe and effective protocol for managing blood glucose in critically ill patients.

Inzucchi SV. Management of Hyperglycemia in the Hospital Setting. N Eng J Med 2006; 355:1903–1911.
A review of glycemic control in hospitalized and critically ill patients, including evidence for treatment, strategies for glucose control, and current recommendations.

Krinsley JS. Association between hyperglycemia and increased hospital mortality in a heterogeneous population of critically ill patients. *Mayo Clin Proc.* 2003;78:1471–1478.
Retrospective analysis of blood glucose levels in intensive care unit patients showing the lowest hospital mortality (9.6%) among patients with mean glucose values between 80 and 99 mg/dL, with mortality increasing progressively as glucose values increased (42.5% in patients with mean glucose values above 300 mg/dL).

Malmburg K, Ryden L, Efendic S, et al. Randomized trial of insulin-glucose infusion followed by subcutaneous insulin treatment in diabetic patients with acute myocardial infarction (DIGAMI study): effects on mortality at 1 year. *J Am Coll Cardiol.* 1995;26: 57–65.
Randomized trial of patients with acute MI showing a 29% reduction in 1 year mortality in patients assigned to intensive glucose control starting in-hospital and continuing for 3 months when compared with standard glucose control.

Malmberg K, Ryden L, Wedel H, et al. Intensive metabolic control by means o insulin in patients with diabetes mellitus and acute myocardial infarction (DIGAMI 2): effect on mortality and morbidity. *Eur Heart J* 2005;26:650–651.
Randomized trial of patients with acute MI comparing intensive inpatient glucose control to intensive outpatient glucose control compared to standard care which showed no difference in 1 year mortality. However the study was underpowered and the difference in mean glucose values was small.

Pinot DS, Skolnick AH, Kirtane AJ. U-Shaped relationship of blood glucose with adverse outcomes among patients with ST-segment Elevation Myocardial Infarction. *J Am Coll Cardiol.* 2005;46:178–180.
Report on pooled data from the TIMI 10-A/B, LIMIT-AMT, and OPUS studies showing significantly higher 30 day mortality in patients with acute STEMI who had hypoglycemia (BG <81 mg/dL), with only 8.7% of the hypoglycemic patients diagnosed with diabetes.

Van Den Berghe G, Wouters P, Weekers F, et al. Intensive insulin therapy in critically ill patients. *N Engl J Med.* 2001;345:1359–1367.
Randomized trial in a surgical ICU which showed decreased ICU mortality in hyperglycemic patients assigned to intensive glucose treatment (goal 80–110 mg/dL) compared with standard care (goal 180–200 mg/dL).

Van Den Berghe G, Wilmer A, Hermans G, et al. Intensive insulin therapy in the medical ICU. *N Eng J Med.* 2006;354:449–461.
Randomized trial in a medical ICU which showed significantly reduced morbidity but not in-hospital mortality in patients assigned to intensive glucose treatment (goal 80–110 mg/dL) compared with standard care (goal 180–200 mg/dL).

Cancers can cause metabolic, space-occupying, and hematologic complications in which immediate recognition and treatment is required to prevent death or significant morbidity. This chapter reviews the acute management of spinal cord compression, tumor lysis syndrome, superior vena cava syndrome, and leukostasis, which can occur in patients with known malignancy or as presenting complications. Acute management of other severe complications of malignancy such as airway and gastrointestinal obstruction, cardiac tamponade, hypercalcemia, adrenal insufficiency, hematologic abnormalities, increased intracranial pressure, and febrile neutropenia is discussed in other chapters.

SPINAL CORD COMPRESSION

Back pain is the most frequent symptom associated with spinal cord compression and commonly precedes neurologic impairment. The pain may be localized to the back, or radiate unilaterally or bilaterally in the distribution of spinal roots. Coughing or movement can often exacerbate the pain secondary to radiculopathy. Some patients complain of sensory paresthesias such as burning, skin sensitivity, and numbness. Compression of the long sensory tracts in the cervical cord may cause paresthesias to appear in various lower dermatomes. The onset of motor symptoms is variable, and can accompany, precede, or develop after sensory deficits. Common symptoms include weakness or heaviness of the affected limbs, flaccid paralysis, and loss of bladder and bowel control. Cord compression symptoms may present abruptly or progress gradually.

The most important aspect of the patient evaluation is suspicion for the presence of cord compression by the examining health care provider. New-onset back pain in a patient at risk mandates a careful neurologic examination. In cases of gradual cord compression, patients may be unaware of sensory deficits, but they may be detected on neurologic examination. Regions distal to the cord compression may be weak and hyperreflexic with upgoing reflexes in the toes, (extensor plantar, i.e., Babinski) while reflexes at the level of a lesion are decreased. The possibility of urinary retention should be evaluated by obtaining a postvoid bladder residual or by ultrasound examination. Anal sphincter function is usually preserved until late in cord compression, but should be evaluated by digital rectal examination. Acute, severe cord compression can cause spinal shock, with hyporeflexia and flaccid paralysis in all regions below the lesion.

All patients with suspected cord compression should undergo spine imaging. Magnetic resonance imaging (MRI) is the modality of choice when available. Contrast computed tomography (CT) or CT myelography is recommended if MRI is not available or cannot be performed. It is important to image the entire spine, as some patients may have more than one region of compression. Plain films and bone scans have a limited role as they may miss soft tissue components of tumors. If the nature of the compressing mass is uncertain, surgical or image-guided biopsy for tissue diagnosis is essential. When cord compression is the initial presentation of cancer, further evaluation may reveal a lesion such as a lymph node, which may be easier to biopsy.

Treatment

The general approach to the evaluation and management of the patient with spinal cord compression is outlined in Algorithm 30.1. The importance of recognizing spinal cord compression is to preserve or resume patient's neurologic function. This is truly a medical urgency and should receive urgent evaluation and treatment.

Corticosteroids should be administered if spinal cord compression is suspected and may be started in the absence of a tissue diagnosis. Steroids decrease edema associated with spinal cord compression and transiently improve symptoms. One common approach is dexamethasone given as a loading dose of 10 mg intravenously (IV) or orally (PO) followed by 4 mg IV or PO every 6 hours. Patients should receive prophylactic gastric acid suppression (with an H_2 blocker or proton pump inhibitor) to prevent the development of stress ulcers. Dexamethasone should be continued during the initial evaluation and treatment period and then tapered off during the subsequent 2 to 3 weeks, regardless of symptom improvement.

Because early studies of surgical decompression through posterior laminectomy followed by radiation therapy (XRT) seemed equivalent to XRT alone, external-beam XRT became the treatment of choice. Standard radiation doses range from 2,500 to 4,000 cGy delivered in 10 to 20 fractions. Traditional indications for surgical intervention have included the need for a tissue diagnosis, resection of relatively "radioresistant" tumors and tumors primarily treated by surgery (such as sarcomas), and when there is cord compression in a previously irradiated spine. A recent randomized study comparing surgical decompression followed by XRT to XRT alone has caused a major change in the approach to patients with spinal cord compression. The study was stopped after an interim analysis revealed significantly better outcomes for patients treated surgically, with more ambulatory patients remaining ambulatory (84% vs. 57%) and nonambulatory patients regaining the ability to walk (62% vs. 19%). For these reasons, surgery should be considered initially in all patients presenting with cord compression. Our approach at Washington University is to have all patients presenting with spinal cord compression evaluated by spine surgery, radiation oncology, and medical oncology before initiating therapy.

Sudden or very rapid onset symptoms suggests the possibility of vertebral burst fracture causing bony impingement on the cord. This requires urgent surgical intervention to remove bone fragments from the spinal canal. Patients with extensive bony destruction by tumor and vertebral instability may be at risk for further compression fractures and symptom recurrence after completing XRT. These patients should be considered for vertebral stabilization. Surgical patients usually require 7 to 10 days for wound healing before beginning XRT. Systemic therapy using hormonal therapy or chemotherapeutic agents as well as zoledronic acid should be included when appropriate, especially in highly sensitive tumors such as prostate cancer, germ cell tumors, and lymphoma.

TUMOR LYSIS SYNDROME

The tumor lysis syndrome (TLS) refers to the metabolic consequences resulting from the sudden release of potassium, phosphates, and purine metabolites from tumor cells undergoing cell death. TLS is classically associated with malignancies such as acute lymphoblastic

ALGORITHM 30.1

Approach to the Evaluation and Management of Patients with Suspected or Documented Spinal Cord Compression from Cancer

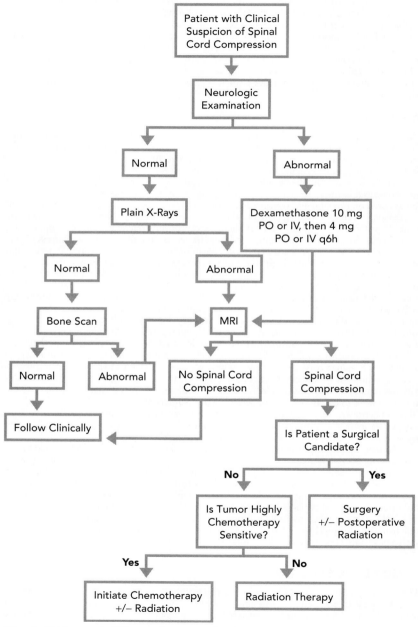

PO, orally; IV, intravenously; MRI, magnetic resonance imaging.

leukemia or Burkitt lymphoma, which are characterized by a high-growth fraction, present with substantial systemic tumor burden, and which respond rapidly to cytotoxic chemotherapy. However, TLS can occur in any situation in which considerable tissue bulk is rapidly destroyed within the body, including cytotoxic chemotherapy, biologic treatments, corticosteroids, radiation, and chemoembolization. Clinical manifestations are variable and cannot be used to monitor the course of TLS, but may include arrhythmias, mental status changes, tetany, stupor, renal failure, and even sudden death from hyperkalemic cardiac arrest. Ideally, the treating physician should anticipate TLS and intervene before the patient develops symptoms or serious metabolic complications.

TLS is diagnosed by blood analysis, which shows acute renal failure, and electrolyte derangements including hyperkalemia, hyperuricemia, hyperphosphatemia, and hypocalcemia. Renal failure occurs from precipitation of phosphate and urate salts in the renal tubules. The resulting renal impairment leads to further accumulation of phosphorus and uric acid, creating an escalating destructive cycle. Patients at risk for TLS often have some degree of renal insufficiency prior to chemotherapy, usually in part from inadequate hydration. Patients at highest risk include those with high-grade or bulky lymphoid malignancies such as Burkitt lymphoma and acute lymphoblastic leukemia. Patients with other "treatment-sensitive" malignancies such as chronic lymphocytic leukemia and small cell lung cancer and high tumor burden should be considered at risk.

Treatment

The general approach to the prevention and management of TLS is summarized in Algorithm 30.2. The best approach to TLS is prevention. Patients at high risk of TLS should be volume-repleted before beginning chemotherapy, and isotonic fluids should be infused at 200 to 300 mL/hr to achieve a brisk diuresis during the first 2 to 3 days of chemotherapy. The goal of hydration is to preserve renal function and to eliminate cellular breakdown products as they are released. Patients should have blood chemistries (especially potassium, phosphorous, calcium, creatinine, uric acid, and lactate dehydrogenase) monitored every 8 to 12 hours during the first 2 to 3 days of treatment. Furosemide may be given to maintain urine output, and may also increase excretion of potassium. The urine pH should be >7 to maintain uric acid and phosphorus in their ionized, soluble form to prevent crystal deposition in the renal tubules. We recommend urine alkalinization with either one ampule of $NaHCO_3$ in 1 Liter 0.45% NaCl or two to three ampules in 1 Liter 5% dextrose containing water. Acetazolamide may be used as an adjunct to alkalinize the urine, but is rarely necessary. Bicarbonate should be cautiously used in severe hyperphosphatemia as this may cause calcium phosphate crystallization in the renal microvasculature and tubules, leading to worsening renal failure.

If the serum uric acid is <8 mg/dL, allopurinol should be given PO at 600 mg/day starting 24 to 48 hours before chemotherapy, as it requires 2 to 3 days to decrease uric acid levels. Allopurinol blocks purine metabolism by preventing the conversion of xanthine to uric acid, leaving xanthines, which are more soluble and easily excreted. The allopurinol dose should be decreased for pre-existing renal insufficiency and as tumor bulk decreases.

Urate oxidase (uricase) is a proteolytic enzyme absent in humans, which converts uric acid into water-soluble allantoin, which is highly soluble and is readily excreted by the kidney. Recombinant urate oxidase (generic name, rasburicase) has recently become available, and should be given to all patients with a serum uric acid level ≥ 8 mg/dL. Dosing is 0.15 to 0.2 mg/kg IV and can be repeated every day up to 7 days for a uric acid level above 8 mg/dL. It induces a rapid decline in serum uric acid levels often with normalization of uric acid levels within 4 hours, and improvement in renal function. More than one dose is occasionally needed. Rasburicase also causes phosphate reabsorption, and calcium phosphate deposition can be a persistent problem, requiring aggressive hydration and diuresis even after uric acid levels are undetectable.

Hyperkalemia may develop rapidly and patients at risk should have serum electrolytes checked at least every 8 to 12 hours, and more frequently if TLS develops. Mild hyperkalemia (<5.5 mmol/L) may be treated with Kayexalate resin and hydration. More serious hyperkalemia (>5.5 to 6 mmol/L or with electrocardiogram changes) may be treated acutely with two ampules of calcium gluconate IV rapidly to stabilize the cardiac membrane potentials,

ALGORITHM 30.2	Prevention and Management of Tumor Lysis Syndrome (TLS) in Patients at High Risk

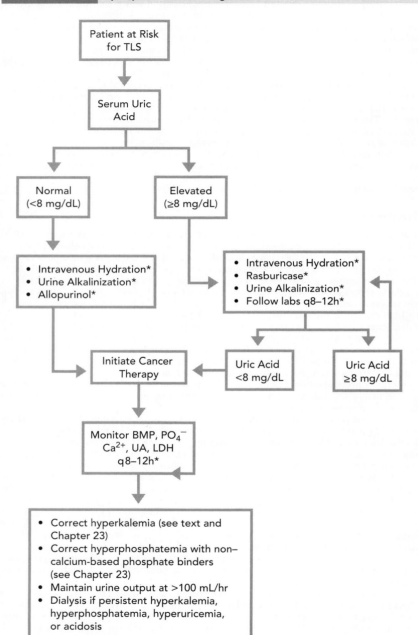

BMP, basic metabolic panel; UA, urinalysis; LDH, lactate dehydrogenase. *See text for details.

followed by 50 mL of 50% glucose solution IV with 10 units regular insulin IV, to transport extracellular potassium intracellularly. This should be followed by Kayexalate to decrease total body potassium as these treatments are only associated with transient improvement in hyperkalemia as potassium shifts intracellularly (see Chapter 23, "Hyperkalemia" for more detailed treatment).

Hyperphosphatemia may be treated with non–calcium-based phosphate binders, and patients should be placed on a renal diet with restricted phosphorous and potassium intake (see Chapter 23, "Hyperphosphatemia" for more detailed treatment).

Indications for hemodialysis include volume overload, serum uric acid >10 mg/dL despite multiple doses of rasburicase, or rapidly rising phosphorus and uncontrolled hyperkalemia. Renal failure caused by TLS is usually reversible, and even patients requiring hemodialysis often regain normal kidney function as the TLS resolves.

SUPERIOR VENA CAVA SYNDROME

Patients with superior vena cava (SVC) syndrome commonly present with dyspnea, cough, swelling of the face, neck, and upper extremities, headache, and chest pain. Symptoms may develop acutely or gradually, and bending forward or lying flat may worsen symptoms. Even in the presence of severe symptoms, patients are rarely critically ill as a result of SVC syndrome alone. Although SVC occlusion is usually not a life-threatening emergency, it can cause significant discomfort and morbidity and should receive immediate attention.

On physical examination, dilated neck veins are usually present, as is edema of the face, arms, neck, and supraclavicular region. Gradual occlusion of the SVC allows the development of collateral veins, which may be easily visible over the upper chest. The chest radiograph often shows a right suprahilar mass or mediastinal widening, but can be normal in some patients.

CT or MRI of the chest can provide information regarding the patency of the SVC and adjacent structures including presence or absence of compressive mass lesions, and is useful in planning subsequent biopsy or therapeutic interventions. A surgical or percutaneous biopsy of an accessible site should be performed in patients who present with SVC syndrome as the initial manifestation of malignancy, patients with a known mass without a prior tissue diagnosis, or for patients in whom the diagnosis of the mass is uncertain (e.g., patients with multiple known malignancies). A tissue diagnosis is essential in the management of SVC syndrome, as specific treatment may be influenced by the tumor type. Only in very rare circumstance should therapy be initiated without a histologic diagnosis.

Treatment

The general approach to the management of SVC syndrome is outlined in Algorithm 30.3. Radiotherapy is the mainstay of treatment for SVC syndrome. Success depends on the tumor type, but 87% of patients respond when treated with regimens delivering 2,000 cGy or more. Patients with "chemoresponsive" tumors, such as germ cell carcinoma, small cell lung cancer, and malignant lymphoma, can be treated with chemotherapy, followed by radiation. Expandable vena caval stents can be helpful in relieving SVC obstruction. Stenting can provide immediate relief to patients who are not expected to have a rapid response to radiation, and to patients who have symptom recurrence after therapy.

A subset of patients develop SVC syndrome from benign causes, and stenting should be considered in these patients. Occlusive SVC thrombosis may occur as a complication of central venous catheters. The central catheter should be left in place to prevent dislodging of the clot and patients should receive therapeutic anticoagulation as with any deep venous thrombosis. Anticoagulation should be continued as long as the patient is thought to have active cancer, and for 6 months after removal of the catheter in patients who are cancer-free. Central vein catheters may also cause stenosis of the SVC, which is treatable with fluoroscopy-guided balloon dilatation with or without stenting.

LEUKOSTASIS

Leukostasis is a syndrome usually associated with high numbers of immature leukocytes (blasts) in the peripheral circulation. Symptoms may include shortness of breath, headache,

ALGORITHM 30.3	Evaluation and Management of Patients with Suspected or Confirmed Superior Vena Cava (SVC) Syndrome

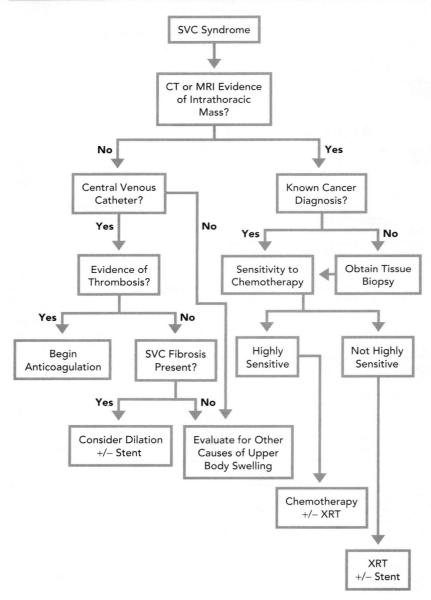

CT, computed tomography; MRI, magnetic resonance imaging; XRT, radiation therapy.

ALGORITHM 30.4	Evaluation and Management of Patients Presenting with Hyperleukocytosis

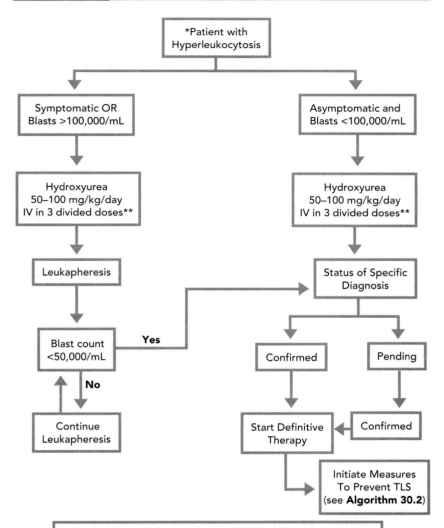

*For all patients;
- If cerebral edema is present, start dexamethasone 10 mg IV, then 4 mg every 6 hours
- If significant hypoxia, monitor in ICU and consider mechanical ventilatory support
- Correct coagulopathy if present

TLS, tumor lysis syndrome; IV, intravenously; ICU, intensive care unit. **Continue as long as the blast count remains above 50,000/mL.

confusion, stupor, or focal neurologic deficits. Leukostasis is a clinical diagnosis as the symptoms are nonspecific, and may be attributed to infection, heart failure, or vascular disease. However, without prompt recognition and treatment, mortality rates may be as high as 40% and can occur within hours of presentation.

Leukostasis is associated with high and rapidly rising blast counts, usually more than 100,000/mL, but may be as low as 50,000/mL. Patients with leukostasis are usually hypoxemic, but spuriously low PaO_2 levels can result from the high metabolic rate of blasts in the arterial blood sample if the specimen is not processed in a timely fashion. A nonspecific diffuse infiltrate is often present on chest radiograph. There may be impairment of other end organs, including the eye, kidney, and liver. Lactic acidosis can be a late event.

Leukostasis is most commonly seen in patients with acute leukemias, especially the myelomonocytic (M4) and monocytic (M5) subtypes, although it has been described in other forms of myeloid leukemias, such as chronic myelogenous leukemia in blast crisis. Despite very high blast counts, which can occur in lymphoid leukemias, leukostasis is not very common in acute lymphoblastic leukemia or chronic lymphocytic leukemia. The classic pathologic finding in leukostasis is occlusive intravascular aggregates of blasts blocking the microcirculation in multiple organs, especially the lungs and brain.

Treatment

The general approach to the patient with hyperleukocytosis is outlined in Algorithm 30.4. Initiation of leukapheresis should not be delayed while a pathologic diagnosis is being determined. Initial management includes IV hydration, allopurinol, and hydroxyurea at a dose of 50 to 100 mg/kg/day in three divided doses as long as the blast count remains above 50,000/mL. Red blood cell transfusion should be resisted, despite frequently coexisting anemia at presentation, as this increases whole-blood viscosity and may exacerbate symptoms of leukostasis. Initial management should be followed rapidly by leukapheresis, with a goal of reducing the blast count to <50,000/mL. Leukapheresis can attenuate or reverse the symptoms of leukostasis, and patients who undergo leukapheresis have a decreased incidence of central nervous system complications. Because blast counts may rebound rapidly after leukapheresis, a definitive treatment plan must be initiated as soon as possible.

Coexisting processes should be sought and reversed. If present, disseminated intravascular coagulation or thrombocytopenia should be corrected to minimize the risk of CNS bleeding. Platelet counts should be monitored closely after leukapheresis, as the procedure often removes a significant number of platelets. Patients suspected of having coexisting infection should have blood drawn for culture and be treated with broad-spectrum antibiotics as local inflammatory processes may increase expression of cellular adhesion molecules and contribute to leukostasis, even in the setting of moderate blast counts.

Suggested Reading

Ahmann, Fredrick R. A reassessment of the clinical implications of the superior vena cava syndrome. *J Clin Oncol.* 1984;2:961–969.
Review of 1986 cases of SVC syndrome where therapy was initiated without a cancer diagnosis, which determined that treatment without a histologic diagnosis was not advised.
Patchell RA, Tibbs PA, Regine WF, et al. Direct decompressive surgical resection in the treatment of spinal cord compression caused by metastatic cancer: a randomized trial. *Lancet.* 2005;366:643–648.
Randomized, multi-institutional, non-blinded trial, which randomly assigned patients with spinal cord compression from metastatic cancer to surgery followed by radiotherapy (n = 50) or radiotherapy alone (n = 51), prematurely stopped after it was found that decompressive surgery with postoperative radiotherapy was superior to treatment with radiotherapy alone (as discussed in text).
Rampello E, Fricia T, Malaguarnera M. The management of tumor lysis syndrome. *Nat Clin Pract Oncol.* 2006;3:438–447.
Review of tumor lysis syndrome management.
Silverman P, Distelhorst CW. Metabolic emergencies in clinical oncology. *Semin Oncol.* 1989;16:504–515.
Review of metabolic complications of malignancy, including tumor lysis syndrome.

Tanigawa N, Sawada S, Mishima K, et al. Clinical outcome of stenting in superior vena cava syndrome associated with malignant tumors. *Acta Radiol.* 1998;39:669–674.

Small study of 33 patients with SVC syndrome with 23 receiving an expandable metallic stent and 10 receiving radiation therapy alone. The study showed no difference in survival, and similar improvements in clinical symptoms.

Wilson E, Lyn E, Lynn A, et al. Radiological stenting provides effective palliation in malignant central venous obstruction. *Clin Oncol (R Coll Radiol).* 2002;14:228–32.

Review of 18 patients presenting with SVC obstruction from tumor or thrombus, all undergoing stenting or thrombolysis, showing a mean duration of palliation of 87 days with no procedure related complications.

Zarkovic M, Kwaan HC. Correction of hyperviscosity by apheresis. *Semin Thromb Hemost.* 2003;29:535–542.

Review of apheresis principles, methods, indications for, and complications.

VIII   *Thermoregulation*

31   TEMPERATURE ALTERATIONS
Derek E. Byers

TEMPERATURE REGULATION

Temperature regulation involves a balance between heat production and dissipation. Basic metabolic processes generate heat, and various adaptive processes ranging from vasodilation and sweating to vasoconstriction and shivering help maintain the normal body temperature at 37°C (98.6°F). Maintenance of euthermia is controlled by the hypothalamus, the brainstem's serotonergic system, and cellular mitochondrial oxidative phosphorylation. Interruption or changes in any of these processes can lead to temperature dysregulation.

FEVER AND HYPERTHERMIA

Fever is a preserved evolutionary response to infection, and involves an increase in the hypothalamic temperature set point with resulting increase in body temperature. Hyperthermia, in contrast, refers to an increase in body temperature associated with normal thermoregulatory center settings, and can be due to increased heat production or decreased heat loss. Studies have shown that immune activity is augmented at elevated temperatures, while bacterial growth is suppressed, and that blocking the body's normal increase in body temperature in response to infection (by forced cooling or antipyretic therapy) may prolong the duration of infectious symptoms. However, high fevers can have undesired consequences including seizures, disseminated intravascular coagulation, renal failure, and death.

A task force that includes societies in critical care medicine and infectious disease define *fever* as a temperature ≥38.3°C (≥101°F) measured from a reliable site (oral, rectal, auditory, or intravenous or bladder thermistor). Temperatures above 38.3°C warrant a thorough physical examination to determine if infection is the cause. At least two sets of blood cultures drawn from two different sterile sites, chest radiograph (especially for intubated patients), and further cultures and testing may be needed, as shown in Algorithm 31.1. The decision to begin antibiotic therapy is based on the patient's clinical stability, likelihood of infection, and immune status. Immunocompromised patients should be

ALGORITHM 31.1   Workup for Fever/Hyperthermia

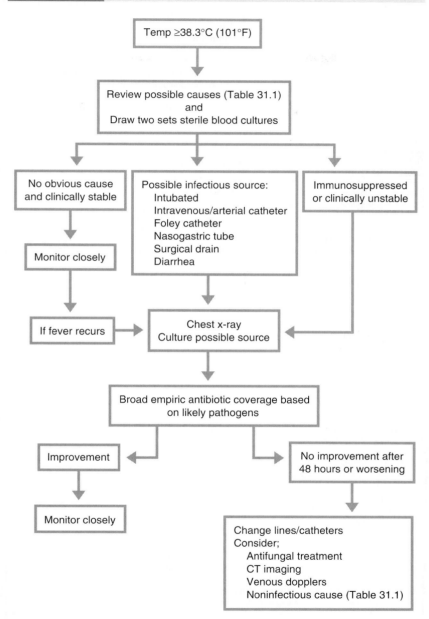

CT, Computed Tomography.

administered empiric broad-spectrum antibiotic coverage (see Chapter 39). Stable patients without an obvious infectious source may be monitored closely for fever recurrence and culture results prior to initiating therapy.

Table 31.1 lists infectious and noninfectious causes of fever and hyperthermia in the intensive care unit (ICU). Most fevers in the ICU are the result of infection, and appropriate antibiotic therapy should lead to improvement within a few days. However, temperatures $\geq 38.3°C$ ($\geq 101°F$) can be associated with several noninfectious sources and workup can lead to futile use of diagnostic testing, antibiotics, and time only to yield negative results. Temperatures $>38.9°C$ ($>102°F$) are uncommon for noninfectious causes, with the exception of drugs (including hyperthermic syndromes), blood transfusions, and hematologic malignancies.

Although numerous drugs can cause hyperthermia, certain drugs cause specific hyperthermic syndromes. Diagnosis of drug-induced hyperthermic syndromes can be made based on medication history and clinical signs.

TABLE 31.1	Causes of Fever and Hyperthermia

Infectious causes
    Ventilator associated pneumonia
    Clostridium difficile colitis
    Intravenous catheter infection
    Urinary tract infection
    Nosocomial pathogen (Gram negative bacteria, *Candida* species)
    Sinusitis
    Abscess formation (intra-abdominal and elsewhere)
    Wound infection (decubitus ulcer)

Noninfectious causes
    Post-transfusion
    ARDS
    Deep vein thrombus
    Chemical thrombophlebitis
    Fat embolism
    Pancreatitis
    Acalculous cholecystitis
    Subarachnoid hemorrhage
    Alcohol/drug withdrawal
    Hyperthyroidism/thyroid storm
    Acute adrenal insufficiency
    Pheochromocytoma
    Transplant rejection
    Rhabdomyolysis/tetanus
    Connective tissue diseases
    Thrombotic thrombocytopenic purpura
    Malignancy ("B symptoms")
    Central/hypothalamic fever
    Drugs (antibiotics, chemotherapeutic agents, cytokines)
    Hyperthermic syndromes:
        Malignant hyperthermia (halothane, isoflurane, succinylcholine)
        Serotonin syndrome (SSRIs, mixed reuptake inhibitors)
        Neuroleptic malignant syndrome (antipsychotic phenothiazines. haloperidol,
            metoclopramide, and prochlorperazine)
        Anticholinergic toxicity (atropine, TCAs, antihistamines)
        Sympathomimetic poisoning (MAOIs, cocaine, amphetamines, methamphetamines)

ARDS, acute respiratory distress syndrome; SSRI, selective serotonin reuptake inhibitors; TCAs, tricyclic antidepressants; MAOIs, monoamine oxidase inhibitors.

Malignant hyperthermia occurs within minutes to hours of exposure to volatile anesthetics (i.e., halothane, isoflurane) or depolarizing muscle relaxants such as succinylcholine. Clinical signs include dramatic temperature elevation, tachycardia, muscle rigidity, and hypercarbia, and can progress to rhabdomyolysis, hemodynamic collapse, and death. Malignant hyperthermia is genetically inherited as a defect in calcium metabolism in skeletal muscle.

Serotonin syndrome typically develops within hours of combined treatment with medications that act on the serotonergic pathway, including selective serotonin-reuptake inhibitors and related antidepressants, tricyclic antidepressants, monoamine oxidase inhibitors, linezolid, dextromethorphan, and meperidine. Clinical diagnosis is based on a triad of cognitive problems (confusion, agitation), autonomic instability, and neuromuscular abnormalities (clonus, hyperreflexia, and tremor). Hyperthermia is found in approximately half of cases and arises from increased muscle activity due to agitation and tremor.

Neuroleptic malignant syndrome usually occurs within several hours to days of starting a new neuroleptic medication (including the antipsychotic phenothiazines). haloperidol, metoclopramide, and prochlorperazine), or acute withdrawal of dopamine agonists such as L-dopa. Clinical signs include hyperthermia, "lead-pipe" muscle rigidity (not clonus in contrast to serotonin syndrome), autonomic instability, and altered mental status (stupor, depression), and it occurs most often in young to middle-aged men. Hyperthermia is the result of muscle rigidity and central hypothalamic dysregulation.

Anticholinergic toxicity is rare and occurs after administration of drugs that block central and peripheral muscarinic receptors, such as antihistamines, atropine, and tricyclic antidepressants. Clinical findings include confusion, tremor, hallucinations, mydriasis, xerostomia, constipation, urinary retention, and coma (see Chapter 32).

Sympathomimetic poisoning can follow ingestion of monoamine oxidase inhibitors and several drugs of abuse including cocaine, amphetamine, and methamphetamine and its derivatives (e.g., ecstasy). Clinical findings include hyperthermia, diaphoresis, tachycardia, ataxia, insomnia, rhabdomyolysis, and seizures. These drugs act largely through serotonergic pathways, but dopaminergic pathways are also involved (see Chapter 32).

Damage to the hypothalamus from trauma, tumor, hemorrhage, or ischemia can raise the hypothalamic temperature set point, causing what is termed a *hypothalamic* or *central fever*. This is a true fever as opposed to a hyperthermic process; clues to suggest a central fever include a plateau fever curve, poor response to antipyretics, lack of sweat, and suspected or confirmed hypothalamic injury. However, hypothalamic lesions are most commonly associated with hypothermia.

Treatment

The decision to treat fever is based on the cause, clinical situation, and severity of temperature elevation. Treatment options are listed in Table 31.2. There is no clear benefit to treating low-grade fevers, and treatment can mask characteristic disease-specific fever patterns (such as tertian and quartan fevers in plasmodium infections, or Pel-Ebstein fevers in patients with lymphoma). Fever significantly increases oxygen consumption, which can have deleterious effects on critically ill patients with severe underlying pulmonary and cardiovascular disease.

Fever can also induce mental status changes and seizures. Treatment of fever is warranted in these situations. Hyperthermic syndromes require removal of the inciting agent and pharmacologic therapy as outlined in Table 31.2. In addition, they do not respond well to antipyretic therapy, and external cooling methods should be started immediately. In severe cases, internal cooling methods may be needed.

HYPOTHERMIA

Hypothermia is defined as core body temperature $<35°C$ ($<95°F$). Table 31.3 lists possible causes. Excessive cold exposure is the most common diagnosis in emergency department settings, but severe sepsis, intoxications, and endocrinopathies are frequent causes seen in the ICU. The majority of cases occur in elderly, debilitated, homeless, or intoxicated patients, and in those with underlying chronic illnesses.

TABLE 31.2	Therapeutic Options for Fever and Hyperthermia

Antipyretics
   Acetaminophen (preferred if no contraindications)
   Nonsteroidal anti-inflammatory drugs
External cooling
   Cooling blankets
   Sponging
   Fans
   Ice baths
Internal cooling
   Gastric or peritoneal lavage
   Intravenous fluid replacement
   Hemodialysis
   Endovascular cooling catheter
Sedation with paralysis if necessary

Drug-induced hyperthermia

Remove inciting agent
Pharmacologic therapy[a]
   Dantrolene: MH and NMS
   Bromocriptine: NMS
   Cyproheptadine: SS
   Physostigmine: AS
   Procainamide should be considered prophylactically for NMS
     due to the high risk of ventricular fibrillation.

[a]See Common Drug Dosages and Side Effects in Appendix
MH malignant hyperthermia, NMS neuroleptic malignant syndrome,
SS serotonin syndrome, AS anticholinergic syndrome

Hypothermia can be divided into three grades based on a reliable core body temperature measurement: mild ($32°C$ to $35°C$ or $90°F$ to $95°F$), moderate ($28°C$ to $32°C$ or $82°F$ to $90°F$), and severe ($<28°C$ or $<82°F$). Mild hypothermia is characterized by shivering, cool extremities, and pallor. Moderate and severe hypothermia are characterized by depressed mental status, ataxia, bradycardia or supraventricular arrhythmias, hyporeflexia, hypoventilation, impalpable pulses, and dilated pupils, and may lead to coma, pulmonary edema, and cardiac arrest. Shivering decreases as hypothermia worsens.

TABLE 31.3	Causes of Hypothermia

Cold exposure
Fulminant sepsis
Drugs (alcohol intoxication, sedatives, general anesthetics,
   antihypertensives)
Hypothyroidism/myxedema coma
Diabetic ketoacidosis
Multisystem trauma
Prolonged cardiac arrest
Kidney failure
Liver failure
Aggressive intravenous fluid replacement
Continuous or intermittent hemodialysis
Hypothalamic lesions (multiple sclerosis)

TABLE 31.4	Therapies for Hypothermia and Expected Change in Core Body Temperature

Warming Method	°C/hr

Passive external
  Blankets
  Warmed ambient environment
  Humidified inspired air
	0.5–4

Active external
  Blankets (prewarmed or heated with forced air or fluid)
  Warm water immersion
  Warm water packs
	1–4

Active internal
  Warmed (42°C) humidified air
  Warmed (42°C) intravenous fluids
  Body cavity lavage with warm saline
    (GI, bladder, peritoneal, pleural)
	Variable

Extracorporeal
  Hemodialysis/hemofiltration
  Continuous arteriovenous rewarming
  Cardiopulmonary bypass
	2–3
	3–4
	7–10

GI, gastrointestinal.
Modified from Aslam AF, Aslam AK, Vasavada BC, et al. Hypothermia: evaluation, electrocardiographic manifestations, and management. *Am J Med.* 2006;119:297–301, with permission.

Laboratory studies may demonstrate acidosis, coagulopathy, and renal and liver abnormalities, but electrolyte changes are unpredictable. End-organ dysfunction is the result of decreased cardiac output and diminished metabolic clearance of toxins and drugs. Electrocardiographic abnormalities include J (Osborn) waves and prolonged PR, QRS, and QT intervals. J waves are positive deflections at the QRS-ST junction in the left ventricular leads and can be found in up to 80% of hypothermic patients, and may be mistaken for new right bundle branch block.

Patients with severe hypothermia are most at risk for developing cardiac arrest, and advanced cardiac life support management is modified for hypothermic cardiac arrest patients. It should be noted that hypothermia-induced bradycardia and peripheral vasoconstriction can make palpation of peripheral pulses difficult. Therefore, hypothermic patients without palpable pulses should be connected to a cardiac monitor quickly to determine the cardiac rhythm. Initial treatment follows the ABCs of advanced cardiac life support, but also aims at aggressive active external and internal rewarming as outlined in Table 31.4. An initial defibrillation attempt is appropriate for ventricular fibrillation and ventricular tachycardia if the core temperature is <30°C, but further attempts should be withheld until the core temperature is increased to >30°C. In addition, cardiovascular drug metabolism is decreased and the effects reduced in hypothermic patients. Thus cardioactive medications are often held at body temperatures <30°C, or if >30°C, the interval between drug administration should be increased to avoid toxic buildup. Induced hypothermia following cardiac arrest is discussed in Chapter 19.

Treatment

Management of hypothermia begins with removal of wet clothing, protection from heat loss, and avoidance of excessive movement to prevent cardiac dysrhythmias. Passive rewarming is usually sufficient for mild hypothermia, but additional active rewarming therapy may be required for moderate and severe cases (Table 31.4). Some experts believe external rewarming can cause temperature "afterdrop" as cold peripheral blood is mobilized to the interior. This can be avoided by the concomitant use of active internal rewarming. Hypotension is also common as patients are rewarmed because of peripheral vasodilation. Thus, patients should be treated with intravenous fluids and the blood pressure should be monitored frequently. Continuous core body temperature monitoring helps to ensure the goal increase of 1°C to 2°C (2°F to 4°F) per hour, and continuous cardiac monitoring and frequent serum electrolyte tests with prompt correction help minimize the risk of arrhythmias. More rapid rewarming is used as noted previously for patients with severe hypothermia and cardiac arrest. Prognosis depends on cause, comorbidities, and complications. Mortality rates up to 100% are reported in the most severe cases. Some experts believe that death cannot be proclaimed with certainty until the patient has been successfully rewarmed.

Frost bitten body parts should be thawed with warm (40-42°C; hot water can cause further damage and should be avoided) water immersion. Avoid manipulating affected areas as this can cause further damage. Blisters often form when tissue is rewarmed and clear blisters should be debrided to avoid continued tissue damage, and hemorrhagic blisters should be left intact to avoid infection. Thawed body parts should be kept on sterile sheets and evaluated by a surgeon to assess tissue viability, though viability can take months to determine. Urgent amputation is rarely needed, though patients should be monitored for development of compartment syndrome.

Suggested Reading

2005 American Heart Association Guidelines for Cardiopulmonary Resuscitation and Emergency Cardiovascular Care, Part 10.4: hypothermia. *Circulation.* 2005;112[Suppl IV]:IV136–IV138.
Current AHA guidelines for modifications of ACLS in hypothermic patients.
Aslam AF, Aslam AK, Vasavada BC, et al. Hypothermia: evaluation, electrocardiographic manifestations, and management. *Am J Med.* 2006;119:297–301.
A review of the causes, diagnostic signs, and management of patients with hypothermia.
Hadad E, Weinbroum AA, Ben-Abraham R. Drug-induced hyperthermia and muscle rigidity: a practical approach. *Eur J Emerg Med.* 2003;10:149–154.
A review of the drug-induced hyperthermic syndromes, help in differential diagnosis, and therapeutic options.
Marik, PE. Fever in the ICU. *Chest.* 2000;117:855–869.
A review of the causes of fever in the ICU and rational approach to management.
O'Grady NP, Barie PS, Bartlett J, et al. Practice parameters for evaluating new fever in critically ill adult patients. *Crit Care Med.* 1998;26:392–408.
Consensus statement from a panel of 13 experts from the Society of Critical Care Medicine and Infectious Disease Society of America that provides a rational and cost-effective approach to diagnosis and management of patients with fevers in the ICU.

Toxicology IX

TOXICOLOGY 32
James A. Driscoll and Steven L. Brody

More than 2.4 million cases of accidental or intentional poisoning were recorded by U.S. poison control centers in 2004, resulting in 1,183 deaths and more than 80,000 intensive care unit admissions. Approximately 83% of cases resulting in death occurred in patients 20 years of age or older. Deaths were most common with intentional overdoses and with ingestions of ethanol, analgesics (especially acetaminophen and aspirin), street drugs of abuse, sedatives/hypnotics/antidepressants, and cardiovascular drugs. Although much of the initial management is provided in the emergency department, critical care physicians must be familiar with the care of the poisoned patient.

KEY STEPS IN THE MANAGEMENT OF THE POISONED PATIENT

Algorithm 32.1 presents the outline for managing a poisoned patient.

1. Before all else, address the "ABCs" (airway, breathing, and circulation):
   - Intubate and mechanically ventilate for airway protection or respiratory failure
   - Give intravenous (IV) crystalloid for hypotension
2. Treat potentially reversible causes of altered mental status or coma with:
   - Rapid glucose assessment or empiric dextrose 25 g IV (one ampule of dextrose 50% in water [D50W])
   - Thiamine 100 mg IV
   - Naloxone 0.4 to 2 mg IV or IM if possible opioid toxicity
3. Give specific antidotes when indicated (see Table 32.4) and call the regional Poison Control Center at 1-800-222-1222 for management advice.
4. Block absorption of toxins when appropriate (see "Gastric Decontamination").
5. Enhance elimination of toxins when appropriate (see "Enhancing Drug Elimination").

EMERGENCY EVALUATION

The initial assessment of the poisoned patient should begin with an assessment of the ABCs: airway, breathing, and circulation. Respiratory depression, loss of airway protective

233

ALGORITHM 32.1   **Key Steps in the Initial Management of the Poisoned Patient**

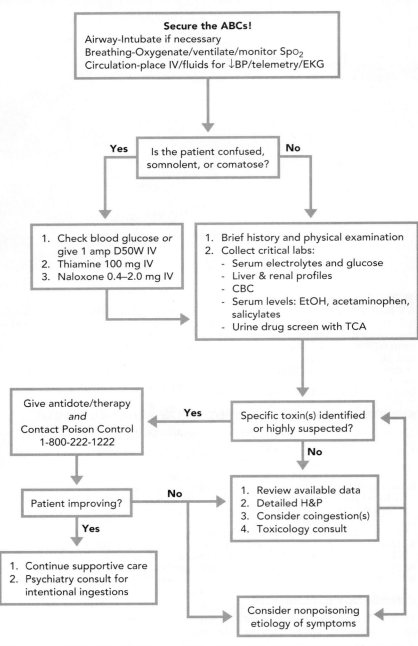

IV, intravenous; D50W, dextrose 50% in water; CBC, complete blood count; EtOH, alcohol; TCA, tricyclic antidepressant; H&P, history and physical examination.

reflexes, and aspirations are common consequences of ingestion. Awake patients may need close monitoring for onset of delayed drug effects, and lethargic or obtunded patients, or those with recurrent seizures may require immediate endotracheal intubation. When in doubt, the airway should be secured by intubation. Care should be taken to clear the airway of secretions or obstruction.

Ventilatory failure in the poisoned patient may be a consequence of respiratory depression (e.g., from sedatives) or muscle paralysis/weakness (e.g., from botulism). Arterial blood gas (ABG) measurement will reveal an elevated $PaCO_2$. Somnolence or obtundation in the setting of a rising $PaCO_2$ is an indication for intubation and assisted ventilation. Bronchospasm may also be seen in cases of inhalational injury and other toxins, and bronchodilators may be useful.

Hypoxemia can result as a consequence of toxin-associated hypoventilation, aspiration, or pulmonary edema. Oxygen should be administered in all lethargic patients during initial workup. Treatment of significant hypoxemia may require mechanical ventilation or high fractions of inspired oxygen (FIO_2). Specific therapies for carbon monoxide poisoning and methemoglobinemia are discussed in separate sections.

Arrhythmias, hypotension, and circulatory failure/shock can occur with poisonings. Venous access should be obtained and IV fluids given for hypotension. Continuous electrocardiogram monitoring should be initiated. Pulseless or hemodynamically unstable patients should receive standard advanced cardiac life support therapies. However, physicians should be aware that toxin-induced cardiac arrest may at times require specific therapies. For example, wide QRS pulseless rhythms due to tricyclic antidepressant (TCA) toxicity should be rapidly treated with sodium bicarbonate, as should hyperkalemic arrests due to salicylate toxicity. Furthermore, some common therapies should be avoided with certain intoxications (e.g., beta-blockers in cocaine intoxication).

All patients (especially the poisoned patient) with altered mental status should be screened for hypoglycemia or treated empirically with IV dextrose (25 g, or one ampule of D50W). Thiamine (100 mg IV) and naloxone (0.4 to 2 mg IV) should also be given to these patients for possible Wernicke encephalopathy and opiate intoxication, respectively. All patients receiving thiamine should also receive IV dextrose.

DIAGNOSTIC STRATEGIES

Important Principles

- All overdoses are polysubstance overdoses until proven otherwise. Ethanol and opiates are common components of polysubstance overdose.
- The following lethal ingestions with specific therapies should always be ruled out:
  Acetaminophen (serum level)
  Tricyclic antidepressants (qualitative urine screen)
  Salicylates (serum level)
- Pre-existing illnesses can confound a "classic" poisoning presentation.
- Toxins screened on "drug screens" vary among institutions. Know your laboratory.
- History, physical examination, and laboratory testing should be directed at identifying or confirming exposure to specific toxins if these are not already known.

Toxidromes

A *toxidrome* is a constellation of signs and symptoms that may be seen after exposure to a specific class of intoxicant (Table 32.1). The physical examination should be performed with particular attention to vital signs, mental status, pupillary size, and psychomotor state that may suggest a specific toxidrome.

Ingestion History

An accurate accounting of the ingestion should be obtained. Specific details including type and quantity of ingestion should be sought, and an outpatient medication profile should be established. Relevant details may come from initial responders (e.g., emergency medical services) or patient contacts. Be aware that the history obtained may be

TABLE 32.1	Clinical Toxidromes	

	Possible Features	Offending Agents
Sympathomimetic	Hypertension, tachycardia, tachypnea, hyperthermia, mydriasis, agitation, hallucinations, diaphoresis	Cocaine Amphetamines Ephedrine Pseudoephedrine Theophylline Caffeine
Anticholinergic "Hot as a hare, dry as a bone, red as a beet, mad as a hatter."	Hypertension, tachycardia, tachypnea, hyperthermia, mydriasis, delirium, hallucinations, dry skin, dry mouth, ileus, urinary retention	Tricyclic antidepressants Antihistamines Atropine Phenothiazines Scopolamine Belladonna alkaloids
Cholinergic "SLUDGE"	Salivation, Lacrimation, Urination, Diarrhea, Gastrointestinal distress, Emesis; also bradycardia, miosis, confusion, coma, bronchoconstriction	Organophosphates Physostigmine Pyridostigmine Edrophonium
Opioid	Hypotension, bradycardia, hypopnea, bradypnea, hypothermia, miosis, CNS depression/coma, decreased bowel sounds, pulmonary edema	Heroin Oxycodone Morphine Meperidine Fentanyl Codeine Methadone
Sedative-hypnotic	Hypotension, bradycardia, hypopnea, bradypnea, CNS depression, coma	Benzodiazepines Barbiturates Alcohols
Extrapyramidal	Rigidity, torticollis, opisthotonos, trismus, oculogyric crisis, dysphoria	Prochlorperazine Haloperidol Chlorpromazine Other antipsychotics

unreliable or incomplete, mandating a rigorous evaluation for possible polysubstance ingestions.

The Optimal Use of Laboratory Tests

Basic tests should include a comprehensive metabolic panel and complete blood cell count. Serum levels of ethanol, acetaminophen, and salicylate, as well as urine screen for common drugs of abuse and TCAs should be sent. Arterial blood should be analyzed by co-oximetry in the presence of respiratory distress, altered mental status, somnolence, coma, or cyanosis. Serum levels of digoxin, lithium, theophylline, phenytoin, and iron may be useful if the patient is known to take or have immediate access to these medicines.

Clues to specific poisonings may be found by attention to the "three gaps": the anion gap, the osmolal gap, and the oxygen saturation gap.

Anion gap elevations may indicate the ingestion of toxins such as ethylene glycol, methanol, or salicylates. The formula for calculating the serum anion gap follows, and causes of an elevated or low anion gap are included in Table 32.2.

$$\text{Anion gap} = [Na^+] - ([Cl^-] + [HCO_3^-])$$

Note: the normal range is 7 to 13 mEq/L, but this may vary among laboratories.

TABLE 32.2	Selected Causes of an Elevated Anion GAP

Toxic ingestions	Other causes
Salicylate	Lactic acidosis
Ethylene glycol	Ketoacidosis
Methanol	Diabetic
Paraldehyde	Starvation
Isoniazid	Alcoholic
Iron	Uremic acidosis
Selected causes of a low anion gap	
Hypoalbuminemia	Lithium
Elevated IgG (e.g., myeloma)	

IgG, immunoglobulin G.

Osmolal gap elevations may be seen with toxic ingestions of alcohols. The serum osmolal gap is the difference between the measured and calculated serum osmolality. Thus, an elevated osmolal gap reflects the presence of an osmotically active substance in the blood that is not accounted for by routine calculation of osmolality. Formulas necessary for calculating the osmolal gap follow, and a list of causes of an elevated osmolal gap are included in Table 32.3.

$$Osm_{calculated} = 2\,[Na^+] + [urea]/2.8 + [glucose]/18 + [ethanol]/4.6$$

where $[Na^+]$ is in mmol/L and [urea], [glucose] and [ethanol] are in mg/dL.

$$Osmolal\ gap = Osm_{measured} - Osm_{calculated}\ (normal <10)$$

Oxygen saturation gap is a term used variably to describe differences between oxyhemoglobin percentage as measured by pulse oximetry (SpO_2) or as estimated from arterial oxygen tension (PaO_2) when compared with the oxyhemoglobin percentage (SaO_2) as measured by co-oximetry. An oxygen saturation gap may indicate poisoning from carbon monoxide, cyanide or hydrogen sulfide, or the presence of an acquired hemoglobinopathy, as occurs with methemoglobinemia. If these toxins are suspected, arterial blood must be analyzed by a co-oximeter, which is capable of measuring the concentrations of oxyhemoglobin, deoxyhemoglobin, methemoglobin, and carboxyhemoglobin in the specimen. By contrast, most pulse oximeters measure absorption of light at only two wavelengths (that correspond to oxyhemoglobin and deoxyhemoglobin). Additionally, some ABG machines will calculate an oxyhemoglobin percentage by plotting the measured PaO_2 on a standard oxygen-hemoglobin dissociation curve. These readings (of SpO_2 or calculated SaO_2) may be misleading indicators of oxygenation in the setting of acquired hemoglobinopathies, emphasizing the need to analyze blood by co-oximetry in these cases.

TABLE 32.3	Selected Causes of an Elevated Osmolal GAP

With normal anion gap	With elevated anion gap
Isopropanol	Methanol
Acetone	Ethylene glycol
Mannitol	Formaldehyde
Diethyl ether	Paraldehyde

TABLE 32.4	Specific Antidotes for Selected Toxins

Toxin	Antidotes
Acetaminophen	*N*-acetylcysteine
Carbon monoxide	100% O_2, hyperbaric O_2 in some cases (see Carbon Monoxide section below)
Cholinesterase inhibitors (e.g., organophosphates)	Atropine 1–5 mg IV, repeat q5–10min for ongoing wheezing or bronchorrhea Pralidoxime 1–2 g IV over 30 minutes, repeat after 1 hour if ongoing weakness or fasciculations
Cyanide	Sodium nitrite 300 mg IV over 2–5 minutes
Digoxin	Digoxin-specific antibody fragments (Fab) Acute: 10–20 vials Chronic: 3–6 vials
Ethylene glycol	Fomepizole 15 mg/kg IV over 30 min (first dose), then 10 mg/kg q12hours × 4 doses, then 15 mg/kg q12hours as needed
Iron	Deferoxamine start at 5 mg/kg/hr, titrate as tolerated to 15 mg/kg/hr, max daily dose 6–8 g/day
Isoniazid	Pyridoxine 1 g for each gram of isoniazid ingested up to 70 mg/kg or 5 g max infused IV at 0.5 g/min until seizures stop, then the remainder infused during 4–6 hours
Methanol	Fomepizole 15 mg/kg IV over 30 min (first dose), then 10 mg/kg q12hours × 4 doses, then 15 mg/kg q12hours as needed
Methemoglobinemia	Methylene Blue 1–2 mg/kg IV over 5 min followed by 30 mL saline flush
Opioids	Naloxone 0.4 – 2 mg IV (IM, SC, or endotracheally)
Sulfonylureas	Octreotide 50 mcg SC q 6 hours

IV, intravenously; IM, intramuscularly; SC, subcutaneously.

TREATMENT STRATEGIES

Antidotes

Specific antidotes are available for relatively few toxins. Although potentially life-saving, many of these antidotes have adverse effects and can be harmful if used inappropriately. Consultation with a poison control center or a medical toxicologist is advised when prescribing an antidote with which one is unfamiliar. A select list of antidotes is included in Table 32.4.

Gastric Decontamination

Among methods for blocking the absorption of drugs in the gastrointestinal (GI) tract, only activated charcoal and whole-bowel irrigation can be recommended for use in certain circumstances. The routine use of gastric lavage, induced emesis (e.g., with syrup of ipecac), and cathartics are not recommended.

Activated charcoal, given orally or through a nasogastric tube, readily adsorbs most toxins, thereby preventing systemic absorption and toxicity. Exceptions that are not well adsorbed by activated charcoal are alcohols, iron, and lithium. The efficacy of activated charcoal is greatest when given within 1 hour of ingestion. A single dose of activated charcoal (1 g/kg) is recommended in adolescents and adults. Multiple-dose activated charcoal may be used as means of drug elimination in the management of certain poisonings and is discussed later. Contraindications to the use of activated charcoal include an unprotected airway and the ingestion of a hydrocarbon. Caution should be taken in the setting of significant GI pathology or recent GI surgery.

TABLE 32.5	Potential Indications for Whole-Bowel Irrigation

Iron poisoning
Lithium poisoning
Sustained-release or enteric coated medication toxicity
Retained illicit drug packets (i.e., from "body packing")

Contraindications

Bowel obstruction	Ileus	Bowel perforation
Unprotected airway	Uncontrolled vomiting	
Hemodynamic instability	Toxic colitis	

Whole-bowel irrigation (WBI) involves the enteral administration of large volumes of an osmotically balanced polyethylene glycol electrolyte solution in order to induce diarrhea with rapid expulsion of unabsorbed toxins from the GI tract. No controlled studies have been published, but WBI may be considered in the management of certain ingestions (Table 32.5). WBI is best performed using a nasogastric tube, and a recommended regimen is 1,500 to 2,000 mL/hr of enterally administered WBI fluid continued at least until a clear rectal effluent is noted. Contraindications include an unprotected airway, bowel perforation or obstruction, ileus, significant GI hemorrhage, toxic colitis, uncontrolled vomiting, and hemodynamic instability.

Gastric lavage involves the serial administration and aspiration of aliquots of water or normal saline (200 to 300 mL) through a large-bore (36 to 40 French) orogastric tube to remove ingested substances that may still be present in the stomach. Effective drug recovery is unlikely if performed more than 1 hour after ingestion, and clinical benefit of gastric lavage has not been demonstrated in the limited number of studies available. Contraindications to gastric lavage include an unprotected airway and ingestion of a corrosive substance or hydrocarbon, a high risk for GI hemorrhage or perforation from known pathology, recent surgery, or coagulopathy. In rare circumstances (e.g., early presentation after ingestion of highly toxic agents), gastric lavage may be considered if no contraindications are identified.

Induced emesis (e.g., using ipecac syrup) is not recommended because of the lack of proven efficacy and interference with enterally administered specific antidotes.

Cathartics are not recommended in the treatment of the acutely poisoned patient.

Enhancing Drug Elimination

Urine alkalinization is a method of enhancing the renal elimination of certain poisons by increasing urine pH to levels ≥ 7.5 through the administration of IV sodium bicarbonate (e.g., 1 to 2 mEq/kg IV during 3 to 4 hours). The strongest indication is moderately severe salicylate toxicity not meeting criteria for hemodialysis. Other possible indications are included in Table 32.6. Potassium supplementation may be required in the setting of

TABLE 32.6	Potential Indications for Urine Alkalinization (with Selected Comments)

Salicylates: Severe cases not meeting criteria for hemodialysis
Methotrexate: Consider hemoperfusion instead
2,4-Dichlorophenoxyacetic acid: Goal urine pH >8 and urine output >600 mL/hr
Chlorpropamide: Dextrose infusion alone usually adequate
Phenobarbital: Multiple dose activated charcoal may be more effective
Diflunisal
Fluoride

Contraindications
Renal failure

TABLE 32.7	Potential Indications for Multiple-Dose Activated Charcoal (Severe Poisoning)

Carbamazepine
Dapsone
Phenobarbital
Quinine
Theophylline

Contraindications
Unprotected airway
Coadministration of cathartic with multiple-dose activated charcoal

hypokalemia to ensure effective urine alkalinization. Urine pH should be monitored frequently (every 1 hour initially) to ensure that the target pH ≥ 7.5 is reached. Serum electrolytes should be monitored every 2 to 4 hours as well. Complications of therapy may include alkalemia and hypokalemia. Renal failure is a contraindication.

Multiple-dose activated charcoal (MDAC) refers to the repeated enteral administration of activated charcoal, which may enhance the elimination of certain toxins (Table 32.7). Dosing regimens vary, but a typical regimen would include a 1 g/kg loading dose, followed by 0.5 g/kg every 2 to 4 hours for at least three doses. Drug elimination occurs by adsorption of toxins that have diffused from the blood into the gut lumen or that have undergone enterohepatic recirculation. Drugs with low volumes of distribution, low protein binding, and long elimination half-lives are the best candidates for MDAC. An unprotected airway is a contraindication to use of MDAC. Cathartics should not be coadministered with MDAC.

Hemodialysis and hemoperfusion are extracorporeal methods of toxin removal that may be required to treat life-threatening toxicity (Table 32.8). General indications for use include clinical deterioration despite intensive alternative therapy, impairment of normal toxin elimination capacity (e.g., as with liver or renal failure), and severe toxicity from drugs that can be removed faster by extracorporeal methods than by endogenous means. Prompt nephrology and medical toxicology consultation should be obtained when hemodialysis or hemoperfusion are being considered.

SPECIFIC POISONINGS

Opioids

Opioid-intoxicated patients present with a syndrome that typically includes sedation, respiratory depression, miosis, and decreased GI motility. Life-threatening manifestations of

TABLE 32.8	Selected Toxins Removable by Hemodialysis or Hemoperfusion with Potential Indications

Hemodialysis	
Salicylates	Significant neurologic symptoms, CV instability, renal failure, level >100 mg/dL
Lithium	Renal failure, coma, seizures, CV instability, myoclonus
Methanol	New visual deficit, severe acidosis, level >50 mg/dL
Ethylene glycol	Severe acidosis, renal failure, level >50 mg/dL
Isopropanol	Hypotension, clinical worsening, level >400 mg/dL; rarely needed
Hemoperfusion	
Barbiturates	Clinical deterioration or renal failure
Carbamazepine	Life-threatening ingestion or clinical deterioration; consider MDAC
Theophylline	Seizures, arrhythmias, persistent hypotension
Valproic acid	Rapid deterioration, hepatic dysfunction, level >1,000 mg/L

CV, cardiovascular; MDAC, multiple-dose activated charcoal.

opioid intoxication are usually due to respiratory depression, which may range from decreases in tidal volume and respiratory rate to complete apnea. ABG analysis will typically reveal an elevated $PaCO_2$ and decreased PaO_2. Hypotension (resulting from histamine release) is more common with certain agents (e.g., meperidine). Noncardiogenic pulmonary edema is not uncommon. Seizures may occur as a result of the accumulation of the neurotoxic metabolites of certain opioids (specifically meperidine, propoxyphene, and tramadol). Acetaminophen or aspirin toxicity may complicate the patient presentation when combination analgesics have been taken.

Management of opioid intoxication is primarily directed at ensuring adequate airway control and ventilation and the early use of naloxone, an opioid antagonist. Naloxone is given initially at doses of 0.4 to 2 mg IV every 2 minutes until effect to a maximum of 10 mg. The duration of naloxone action is 1 to 2 hours, which may be shorter than the activity of the opioid causing intoxication, mandating a several-hour monitoring period after response. Repeated doses of naloxone may be required if the offending opioid is long-acting, and continuous infusions can be considered at a dose of two-thirds the original response dose per hour (consider pharmacist input for dosing assistance). Opioid-dependent patients may suffer opioid withdrawal with naloxone treatment. Pregnant patients may develop uterine contractions and induction of labor with naloxone administration. Oral opiate overdose may be treated with a single dose of activated charcoal, while body packers should be treated with activated charcoal, WBI, and naloxone infusion if symptomatic.

Dextromethorphan is an opioid used as an antitussive in some over-the-counter cough and cold preparations (e.g., Robitussin DM, NyQuil Nighttime Cold Medicine). Dextromethrophan-containing products are often intentionally abused for their psychoactive properties. Intoxicated patients may present with restlessness, mydriasis, ataxia, dizziness, and hallucinations. Stupor, coma, and seizure can occur in more severe cases. Mixed ingestions must be ruled out as over-the-counter cold remedies often contain other ingredients (e.g., acetaminophen, aspirin). Dysphoria associated with dextromethorphan intoxication can be treated with benzodiazepines, and naloxone is partially effective for reversal of respiratory depression. A serotonin syndrome of hyperthermia, hypertension, and muscle rigidity may occur in dextromethrophan-intoxicated patients also taking monoamine oxidase inhibitors. Propoxyphene is an opioid analgesic that can cause significant cardiotoxicity because of myocardial sodium channel blockade, resulting in negative inotropy, QRS prolongation, and arrhythmias. Cardiotoxicity from propoxyphene is best treated with IV sodium bicarbonate in a manner similar to that used for TCA cardiotoxicity (see "Tricyclic Antidepressants").

Acetaminophen

The majority of acetaminophen ingestions cause no significant clinical toxicity, but life-threatening liver injury and even death can occur with overdose. Acute ingestions of 150 mg/kg (or 10 g), or the chronic ingestion of doses in excess of 4 g/day may result in clinical toxicity. The generation of a toxic metabolite, N-acetyl-p-benzoquinoneimine (NAPQI), by the body's cytochrome P-450 mixed-function oxidase system (specifically the CYP2E1 enzyme) in the setting of overwhelmed hepatic glutathione results in hepatic and renal injury. Induction of CYP2E1 (e.g., by ethanol, rifampin, isoniazid, or carbamazepine) or decreased glutathione stores, as occurs with chronic malnutrition from alcoholism, increases the risk for acetaminophen toxicity.

The clinical presentation of acetaminophen overdose depends on the time of presentation and amount of acetaminophen taken. Patients may be entirely asymptomatic, but early symptoms include anorexia, nausea, and vomiting. Liver injury usually occurs within 24 to 36 hours of ingestion as evidenced by elevations in blood levels of aspartate aminotransferase and alanine aminotransferase. Maximal hepatotoxicity is usually seen 72 to 96 hours after ingestion and may result in encephalopathy, coagulopathy, renal failure, hypoglycemia, and shock. Elevations in pancreatic enzymes and acute myocardial injury have also been described.

In all cases of known or possible acetaminophen overdose, the serum level of acetaminophen should be measured 4 hours after ingestion or as soon as possible thereafter and plotted against time using the Rumack-Matthew nomogram (Fig. 32.1).

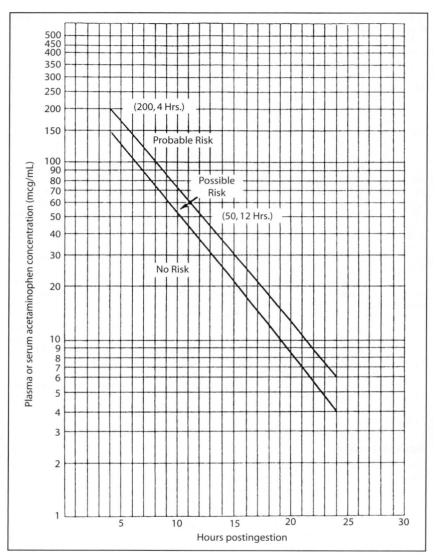

Figure 32.1. Acetaminophen toxicity nomogram .

Plasma concentrations above the lower line ("possible risk") are an indication for treatment with *N*-acetylcysteine (NAC). Administration of NAC should not be delayed while awaiting the serum level in cases of obvious hepatotoxicity or in pregnancy. Repeating the serum acetaminophen level should be considered in cases of ingestion of extended-release products if the initial value is below the treatment line. Although the nomogram assesses risk of toxicity with levels obtained from 4 to 24 hours postingestion, patients who present after 24 hours with detectable acetaminophen levels or elevated liver

TABLE 32.9	Acceptable *N*-Acetylcysteine Protocols for the Treatment of Acetaminophen Toxicity
20-hour IV regimen (continuous infusion)	150 mg/kg IV given over 15 minutes, then 50 mg/kg IV given over 4 hours, then 100 mg/kg IV given over 20 hours
72-hour PO regimen	140 mg/kg PO once, then 70 mg/kg PO q4hours × 17 doses
52-hour IV regimen	140 mg/kg given over 60 minutes, then 70 mg/kg IV q 4 hours × 12 doses
IV, intravenously; PO, orally.	

enzymes should receive NAC therapy while awaiting further data or input from poison control.

NAC enhances both the synthesis of glutathione (which acts as an antioxidant) as well as the conversion of acetaminophen to (nontoxic) acetaminophen sulfate rather than NAPQI. Several different NAC protocols have been used and are of similar efficacy (Table 32.9).

Nausea and vomiting from oral NAC may delay treatment; thus, antiemetic therapy may be required. Vomiting within 1 hour of an administered oral dose requires repeating the dose. IV regimens are associated with higher rates of anaphylactoid responses (e.g., urticaria, bronchospasm, angioedema, and hypotension). These reactions are considered to be related to histamine release and may be treated with decreased infusion rates and antihistamines. On completion of a NAC protocol, the serum acetaminophen and aspartate aminotransferase levels should be measured and therapy continued if within the toxic range. In the setting of liver failure, NAC should be continued after protocol completion.

Severe acetaminophen toxicity resulting in fulminant hepatic failure may result in encephalopathy, shock, hypoglycemia, and coagulopathy. In these cases, early hepatology consultation is advised for assistance in acute management as well as evaluation of candidacy for liver transplantation. A suicide attempt and drug or ethanol abuse alone will not preclude transplantation, but formal psychiatric assessment may be required. Various predictors of the need for liver transplantation after acetaminophen overdose have been used, the best known of which are the King's College Hospital criteria: (a) pH <7.25 in spite of adequate fluid resuscitation or (b) the combination of grade III-IV hepatic encephalopathy, serum creatinine >3.4 mg/dL and prothrombin time >100 seconds are predictive of death without transplantation. Acute renal failure is common in the setting of acetaminophen-induced fulminant hepatic failure and is likely multifactorial in nature. Hemodynamic monitoring may be needed to assess intravascular volume status. Nephrotoxins should be avoided and medications dosed appropriately for renal insufficiency.

Salicylates

Salicylate poisoning can result in significant morbidity or even death. Salicylate toxicity results from both direct corrosive injury to the GI tract and multiple metabolic effects (e.g., respiratory stimulation, uncoupling of mitochondrial oxidative phosphorylation, inhibition of the tricarboxylic acid cycle, enhanced lipolysis with ketone generation). Patients may present with GI symptoms (e.g., abdominal pain, nausea and vomiting, GI bleeding), diaphoresis, respiratory alkalosis with anion gap metabolic acidosis, deranged glucose regulation, tachycardia, ventricular arrhythmias, pulmonary edema/acute lung injury, prolonged prothrombin times, CNS effects (e.g., agitation, confusion, seizures, coma), tinnitus, rhabdomyolysis, and renal failure. The clinical course may be dynamic; for example, with GI symptoms prominent early but metabolic derangements, such as acidosis and renal failure seen later. The finding of coincident CNS changes with tachycardia and diaphoresis suggests severe toxicity and warrants immediate and aggressive action.

The diagnosis of salicylate exposure can be confirmed by obtaining a serum salicylate level. Historically serum levels were plotted on the Done nomogram to predict the degree of

TABLE 32.10	Indications for Hemodialysis in Acute Salicylate Poisoning

Progressive hemodynamic deterioration
Persistent CNS derangement
Severe acid-base or electrolyte disturbances despite appropriate therapy
Renal failure
Acute lung injury
Serum salicylate level >100 mg/dL for acute ingestions

toxicity, but this practice is now discouraged as the nomogram may over- or underestimate toxicity in certain circumstances. Instead, treatment should be based on clinical findings.

Activated charcoal should be administered in cases of suspected or confirmed salicylate poisoning unless a contraindication exists. Serum glucose should be measured or dextrose given empirically if confusion or seizures occur. Benzodiazepines should be administered for recurrent seizures. Fluid deficits may be substantial because of vomiting and insensible losses and should be treated with IV fluid. Additionally, sodium bicarbonate should be given intravenously to a target serum pH of approximately 7.5 (to limit tissue redistribution of salicylate) and urine pH of approximately 8 (to enhance renal elimination of salicylate). Effective alkaluria will require correction of hypokalemia and may even require potassium supplementation in the setting normokalemia. ABG analysis, urine pH, and serum chemistries should be followed serially (every 1 to 4 hours) to guide therapy in the most ill patients. Hemodialysis can effectively remove salicylate, with indications listed in Table 32.10. Delays in initiating hemodialysis when indicated may result in unnecessary morbidity and mortality.

Tricyclic Antidepressants

TCA overdose can result in death. The therapeutic window for these agents is narrow, with doses of >10 mg/kg being potentially life-threatening because of cardiovascular and CNS effects. Toxicity may vary with the class of TCA, but amitriptyline is particularly toxic. Symptoms from TCA toxicity are a result of anticholinergic effects, alpha-adrenergic blockade, inhibition of norepinephrine and serotonin reuptake, and blockade of the fast sodium channels in myocardium, resulting in a quinidine-like effect. Cardiotoxicity may manifest with tachycardia, prolongation of the PR, QRS, or QT intervals, atrioventricular block, arrhythmias, depressed myocardial contractility, or hypotension. Anticholinergic effects may include confusion, sedation, ataxia, coma, impaired sweating, dry mouth, urinary retention, ileus, pupillary dilatation, increased muscle tone, and tremor. Seizures are a common consequence of TCA overdose, and when coupled with impaired sweating, can lead to life-threatening hyperthermia.

TCA overdose should be considered in any patient with confusion or coma, especially if accompanied by tachycardia or QRS interval prolongation on electrocardiogram. A qualitative urine toxicology screen for TCAs should be obtained in cases of suspected poisoning. Specific drug levels are neither valuable nor required to make the diagnosis of acute intoxication.

Initial management of TCA overdose is directed at emergency control of patient airway and breathing, management of hemodynamic instability, and treatment of ongoing seizures. Sodium bicarbonate infusion should be given as an antidote for cardiotoxicity in the setting of ventricular arrhythmias or QRS prolongation >100 msec, or in the presence of hypotension with acidosis (pH <7.20). A typical regimen would be an initial bolus of 1 mEq/kg, followed by an infusion of 150 mEq of sodium bicarbonate in 1 liter of D5W given at 2 to 3 mL/kg/hr IV, adjusted to a target arterial pH of 7.45 to 7.55. The benefits of sodium bicarbonate therapy are multifactorial, related in part to the effect of sodium on myocardial channels. Combination therapy with bicarbonate infusion and hyperventilation should be avoided because of the risk of induction of a life-threatening alkalosis. Type 1a and 1c antiarrhythmics (e.g., procainamide and flecainide) should be avoided in the management of arrhythmias. Benzodiazepines should be used to treat TCA-induced seizures, with phenytoin, barbiturates, and propofol used for refractory cases. Activated charcoal should be given if no contraindication exists. Hemodialysis and hemoperfusion are not thought to be helpful in TCA overdose. Physostigmine is not recommended in the management of TCA overdose because of significant toxicity associated with use.

Beta-Blockers

Beta-adrenergic blockers can result in life-threatening toxicity when taken in doses even two to three times the therapeutic range. Potential cardiovascular manifestations of toxicity include bradycardia and hypotension, atrioventricular block, intraventricular conduction delay, asystole, and cardiogenic shock. CNS toxicity including confusion, seizures, and coma may be seen, particularly with lipid-soluble medications (e.g., propranolol, metoprolol, timolol). Bronchospasm can be life-threatening in patients with underlying chronic obstructive pulmonary disease or asthma. Metabolic derangements such as hypoglycemia and hyperkalemia may also occur. Many beta-blockers have long half-lives, potentially resulting in prolonged effects, and toxicity may even be seen with ocular preparations.

Diagnosis is made based on the clinical presentation and suspected or known history of ingestion. Exposure may be confirmed with qualitative urine screen or by measuring serum levels, although quantitative levels are generally not needed to guide management.

Emergency treatment is directed at the specific clinical manifestation and may include atropine, isoproterenol, or cardiac pacing for bradycardia or heart block, and nebulized bronchodilators for bronchospasm. Refractory bradycardia or hypotension may be treated with glucagon, starting with a 5- to 10-mg IV bolus, followed by continuous infusion at 1 to 10 mg/hr. Nausea, vomiting, hyperglycemia, and hypocalcemia may be seen with glucagon use. Adrenergic agents such as dobutamine, dopamine, and norepinephrine may be ineffective at usual therapeutic doses. External or transvenous pacing should instead be considered early in the management of significant toxicity or large ingestions. Phosphodiesterase inhibitors such as milrinone may be useful in cases of cardiogenic shock. Refractory cases may require hemodynamic support by cardiopulmonary bypass.

Activated charcoal may be useful to block absorption in early presentations. Most beta-blockers have very large volumes of distribution, making them less susceptible to clearance by extracorporeal techniques. Acebutolol, atenolol, and sotalol are exceptions that are amenable to extracorporeal removal in cases of severe toxicity.

Calcium Channel Blockers

Calcium channel blockers can result in significant toxicity, particularly in patients with underlying cardiovascular disease or when coingested with other cardiovascular medicines (e.g., beta-blockers). Clinical manifestations of calcium channel blocker toxicity are primarily cardiovascular. Hypotension is common. Bradycardia and cardiac conduction disturbances may occur, typically with nondihydropyridines. By contrast, dihydropyridines may result in hypotension with reflex tachycardia due to a lack of activity on the sinoatrial and atrioventricular nodes. Noncardiovascular effects include nausea and vomiting, mental status changes, noncardiogenic pulmonary edema, hyperglycemia, and seizures. Sustained-release preparations may result in prolonged or delayed toxicity.

Diagnosis is made based on a typical presentation with a history of ingestion. Comprehensive urine toxicology screening may detect diltiazem and verapamil.

Treatment is directed at the particular manifestation of toxicity. IV fluid should be given initially for hypotension. IV calcium is given for hypotension or cardiac conduction disturbances. A typical dose is 10 mL of 10% $CaCl_2$ given over 2 to 3 minutes, with additional doses every 5 to 10 minutes for ongoing instability, followed by continuous infusion of 10% $CaCl_2$ at 10 mL/hour. IV dopamine or norepinephrine may be needed for refractory hypotension.

Glucagon and phosphodiesterase inhibitors should also be considered in these cases. Insulin-glucose infusions (to a target serum glucose between 100 and 200 mg/dL) may be useful in cases refractory to these measures. Invasive hemodynamic monitoring is encouraged in patients not responding to initial resuscitation measures. Severely poisoned patients may require support using ventricular pacing, ventricular assist devices, and even cardiopulmonary bypass, depending on the scenario.

Activated charcoal may be given to block absorption in early presentations or with sustained release preparations. Most calcium channel blockers have large volumes of distribution and are highly protein-bound, making them poor candidates for removal by hemodialysis. Nicardipine, nifedipine, and nimodipine have lower volumes of distributions and are potentially removable by hemoperfusion in cases of severe toxicity.

Cocaine

Cocaine is a common drug of abuse that may be intranasally insufflated, intravenously injected, or smoked. Acute intoxication can result in life-threatening cardiovascular, pulmonary, and CNS complications. Mechanisms of toxicity include inhibited monoamine reuptake and enhanced catecholamine release (together resulting in increased levels of catecholamines), as well as blockade of Na^+ channel activity. Additionally, cocaine promotes thrombogenesis and vasoconstriction. Many features of cocaine intoxication are shared with amphetamine toxicity, and management is similar. Both substances are commonly coingested with alcohol, which may complicate management.

The clinical presentations of cocaine intoxication can be quite varied. Hyperthermia, hypertension, and tachycardia are commonly seen. Neuropsychiatric presentations may include agitation and confusion ("agitated delirium"), dystonic reactions, acute cerebrovascular accidents, and seizures. Cardiovascular complications include acute myocardial infarction and arrhythmias. Possible pulmonary complications include pulmonary edema (cardiogenic or noncardiogenic), alveolar hemorrhage, inhalational heat or burn injury to the aerodigestive tract mucosa, and barotrauma (e.g., pneumothorax, pneumomediastinum) from coughing against a closed glottis while smoking or intranasally inhaling cocaine. Vasoconstriction can result in intestinal or renal ischemia. Rhabdomyolysis is common among patients presenting to emergency departments. In addition to fetal toxicity, use of cocaine during pregnancy may result in abruptio placentae, spontaneous abortion, and premature labor.

Urine drug of abuse screens may be positive for cocaine for 2 to 3 days after use. False-negative test results can occur, and repeat testing is appropriate in the setting of a negative test finding but with high clinical suspicion. Serum chemistries, renal markers, troponin, and creatine phosphokinase levels as well as urinalysis should routinely be obtained.

Management of cocaine toxicity depends on the presentation. Benzodiazepines (e.g., diazepam 5 to 10 mg every 5 minutes as needed) function as first-line therapy for agitation and most manifestations of toxicity. Treatment of hyperthermia includes adequate sedation and, if necessary, external cooling with misting and fanning. Hypertension is best treated with sedation, and if necessary, calcium channel blockers, sodium nitroprusside, or phentolamine. Pure beta-blockers are contraindicated. Other contraindicated medications are listed in Table 32.11.

Chest pain should be thoroughly evaluated with possible causes to include acute coronary events, aortic dissection, and pneumothorax. If coronary vasospasm or myocardial infarction is suspected, then oxygen, aspirin, nitroglycerin, and benzodiazepines should be given and cardiology consultation considered. Supraventricular arrhythmias can be treated with calcium channel blockers. Ventricular arrhythmias should be treated with benzodiazepines, oxygen, control of ischemia, correction of electrolytes, and if necessary, lidocaine.

TABLE 32.11	**Medications Contraindicated in the Setting of Cocaine Use**

Beta-blockers (absolute contraindication)   Unopposed alpha adrenergic activity may cause HTN or coronary vasospasm
Phenothiazines and butyrophenone antipsychotics (absolute contraindication)   Increase seizure risk, prolong QT interval, promote dystonic reactions
Succinylcholine   May exacerbate rhabdomyolysis induced hyperkalemia
Class Ia antiarrhythmics (e.g., procainamide)   May worsen QRS and QT prolongation and potentiate cocaine effects
HTN, hypertension.

Class Ia antiarrhythmics (e.g., procainamide) should be avoided. Management of body-packing by drug smugglers may include activated charcoal and WBI if asymptomatic, but immediate surgical removal is required in patients with any signs of cocaine intoxication or toxicity that may indicate packet rupture. Attempts to retrieve packets by endoscopy risk drug spillage and are not recommended, particularly in the asymptomatic patient.

Alcohols

Ethanol is widely abused and is a common component of mixed ingestions, particularly in suicide attempts. Toxicity may present with ataxia, dysarthria, CNS depression, respiratory depression, and even death. Diagnosis should be suspected based on presence of characteristic ethanol odor and can be confirmed by measuring the blood ethanol level. Treatment is largely supportive and is directed at ensuring adequate airway control and ventilation. Confused or comatose patients should be screened for hypoglycemia and should routinely be treated with thiamine (100 mg IV) followed by 25 g IV dextrose (one ampule of D50W).

Isopropanol is a component of rubbing alcohol and some other household compounds that may be intentionally abused by alcoholics as an alternative to ethanol. Clinical manifestations include GI irritation, upper GI bleeding, CNS depression, respiratory depression, and ketosis. Diagnosis should be considered in patients with CNS depression, particularly when presenting with fruity breath (due to acetone production), unexplained ketosis, or an elevated serum osmolal gap. The diagnosis can be confirmed by measuring the serum level. As with ethanol intoxication, treatment is largely supportive. Confused or comatose patients should be screened for hypoglycemia and treated with thiamine 100 mg IV followed by 25 g dextrose. Isopropanol may be removed by hemodialysis, but this is rarely necessary. Upper GI bleeding should be managed with adequate volume resuscitation, correction of coagulopathies, and usual therapies for GI mucosal injury (proton pump inhibitors, endoscopic interventions as needed).

Methanol is found in many household solvents and may be abused by alcoholics as a substitute for ethanol. Patients may present initially with inebriation and GI irritation. After a characteristic latent period of 12 or more hours, severe manifestations of toxicity including anion gap acidosis, visual disturbance, blindness, respiratory failure, seizures, and coma may occur. Physical examination should include assessment of the pupillary light reflex. Methanol ingestion should be considered in all cases of elevated anion gap. Diagnosis may be made by measuring the serum methanol level, although later presentations may reveal undetectable methanol levels (but elevated formate levels). Toxicity results when methanol is converted to formaldehyde and then to formate by alcohol dehydrogenase. Fomepizole (or ethanol) should be given as a competitive inhibitor of alcohol dehydrogenase in cases of methanol levels >20 mg/dL, acidemia, or an elevated osmolal gap. Fomepizole is dosed at 15 mg/kg IV over 30 minutes, followed by 10 mg/kg IV every 12 hours for four doses, followed by 15 mg/kg IV every 12 hours as needed until the serum methanol level is <20 mg/dL. If ethanol is used instead, it should be administered to a target serum level of 100 to 150 mg/dL. Folic acid (e.g., 50 mg IV every 6 hours) should be given to promote conversion of formate to CO_2 and water. Hemodialysis should be implemented in cases of visual disturbances, serum methanol levels >50 mg/dL, or severe acidosis.

Ethylene glycol is found in antifreeze and may be ingested during suicide attempts or as a substitute for ethanol by alcoholics. Early toxicity manifests with CNS depression. As with methanol, delayed toxic manifestations (after 4 to 12 hours) are often more severe and may include metabolic acidosis, renal failure, seizures, coma, and death. Toxicity arises from the formation of toxic metabolites (e.g., glycolaldehyde and oxalate) under the action of alcohol dehydrogenase. Ethylene glycol should be considered in all cases of elevated anion gap and elevated osmolal gap. The patient's urine may fluoresce under Wood's lamp or reveal oxalate crystals under microscopy. Diagnosis can be confirmed by measuring the serum level, but treatment should not be delayed if clinical suspicion of ingestion is high. Therapy with fomepizole (or ethanol) should be used in a manner similar to that described for methanol poisoning in patients with serum ethylene glycol levels >20 mg/dL, the presence of acidosis, or an elevated osmolal gap. Hemodialysis should be instituted in the setting of renal failure, serum level >50 mg/dL, or severe acidosis. Seizures should be treated with benzodiazepines and correction of any hypocalcemia, if present.

Carbon Monoxide

Carbon monoxide (CO) is a common environmental contaminant that accounts for significant morbidity and mortality worldwide. Carbon monoxide competes with O_2 for hemoglobin-binding sites (forming carboxyhemoglobin, COHb) and has an affinity for hemoglobin that is >200 times that of O_2. Consequently, COHb dissociates extremely slowly, resulting in inadequate oxygen delivery to peripheral tissues.

Neurologic symptoms of toxicity include headache, altered mental status, vision changes, and coma. Nausea and vomiting are common. Cardiac manifestations include arrhythmias and myocardial ischemia or infarction. Less commonly, rhabdomyolysis, pancreatitis, and hepatic injury may be seen. Pulmonary edema may be seen as a consequence of primary cardiac disturbance or from smoke inhalation. Delayed neurologic manifestations (e.g., impaired concentration, amnesia, and depression) are common.

Carbon monoxide poisoning should be suspected after certain exposures (e.g., smoke or poorly ventilated car exhaust, gas stoves, and space heaters). Diagnosis can be confirmed by analyzing arterial blood by co-oximetry, which will allow measurement of COHb. Symptoms and signs of CO toxicity may correlate poorly with the measured COHb levels. Oxyhemoglobin assessments by pulse oximetry (SpO_2) or by estimates made from the partial pressure of oxygen (as reported by some ABG machines) can be misleading in CO poisoning.

The treatment of CO toxicity is 100% oxygen. The half-life of COHb varies inversely with the inspired partial pressure of O_2. For this reason, hyperbaric oxygen (HBO_2) therapy has been used to treat CO toxicity since the 1960s. The threshold indications to institute HBO_2 therapy are not well defined, but most experts recommend this therapy for patients who have had loss of consciousness or who have neurologic abnormalities. The benefits of HBO_2 therapy are thought to be greatest when administered promptly (e.g., within 6 hours of exposure).

Methemoglobinemia

Methemoglobinemia should be suspected in patients with unexplained cyanosis or low SpO_2. The use of certain medications, including the "caine" topical anesthetics, nitrites, nitroglycerin, sulfonamides, dapsone, phenazopyridine, sulfonamides, and antimalarials may cause methemoglobinemia.

Methemoglobin is an oxidized form of hemoglobin that is incapable of transporting oxygen. Consequently, elevated methemoglobin levels result in impaired tissue oxygen delivery. Patients with methemoglobin levels <15% are typically asymptomatic, although cyanosis may be present. Levels of 20% to 50% may result in headache, fatigue, mental status changes, and shortness of breath. Levels of 50% to 70% can cause metabolic acidosis, stupor, coma, seizures, and arrhythmias. Death may occur with levels >70%. Comorbidities including anemia, cardiovascular disease, pulmonary disease, and hemoglobinopathies may result in more severe presentations at a given methemoglobin level.

Arterial blood from patients with methemoglobinemia will typically be very dark (or "chocolate brown") and may reveal a high PaO_2 on blood gas analysis. This discordance between low SpO_2 and normal or high PaO_2 should raise suspicion of methemoglobinemia. Diagnosis can be made by measuring the blood methemoglobin level (normally <2%) by co-oximetry. In the setting of methemoglobinemia, the SpO_2, although low, may actually overestimate the true arterial oxygen saturation (the measured SaO_2, by co-oximetry).

When methemoglobinemia is identified, any possible causative medications should be stopped. Treatment includes supplemental oxygen to fully saturate normal hemoglobin and methylene blue, which acts as an electron carrier to reduce methemoglobin. A typical dose of methylene blue is 1 to 2 mg/kg IV given over 5 minutes and followed by a saline flush. The dose may be repeated if signs (e.g., cyanosis) or symptoms persist after 20 minutes. Transient decreases in the SpO_2 may be seen after methylene blue administration. Life-threatening methemoglobinemia unresponsive to methylene blue may require treatment with red-blood cell exchange transfusion.

Iron

Iron toxicity results from both direct corrosive effects to the GI mucosa and from impairment of cellular respiration with resultant lactic acidosis. Doses of >60 mg/kg of elemental iron are potentially lethal. Patients may initially present with vomiting, diarrhea, GI bleeding, or hypovolemia. Later manifestations may include shock and multiorgan failure. Diagnosis of iron poisoning can be made based on an ingestion history with an appropriate clinical presentation.

Abdominal radiographs should be obtained in cases of suspected ingestion to evaluate for radiopaque tablets. The serum iron level should be measured on presentation (and can be followed serially up to 12 hours after ingestion), with toxicity likely if ≥450 mcg/dL. WBI is indicated (in the absence of bowel perforation or obstruction) as the first-line method of gastric decontamination as activated charcoal will not adsorb iron. Patients presenting with altered mental status, shock, metabolic acidosis, or serum iron levels ≥500 mcg/dL at 4 to 6 hours after ingestion should be treated with the iron chelator deferoxamine. Deferoxamine is given intravenously at 10 to 15 mg/kg/hr by continuous infusion with a recommended maximum daily dose of 6 to 8 g, and therapy should not be delayed while awaiting iron levels in the setting of clinical toxicity. Rate-related hypotension may be observed with deferoxamine, and adequate IV fluid replacement is needed as prophylaxis against acute renal failure. Pregnancy is not a contraindication to the use of deferoxamine in the setting of life-threatening toxicity. Deferoxamine therapy may be stopped when the serum iron level normalizes (as measured by atomic absorption spectroscopy, as deferoxamine interferes with most routine assays), when systemic toxicity and acidosis resolve, or when the urine is no longer reddish-brown (an indication of the presence of chelated deferoxamine-iron complex). The deferoxamine-iron complex promotes the growth of *Yersinia enterocolitica*, increasing the risk of sepsis from this species. GI or surgical consultation is warranted in cases of tablet concretion/bezoar, massive GI bleeding, or bowel perforation. Intestinal stricture and gastric outlet obstruction may occur as late complications of iron overdose.

Suggested Reading

Barceloux D, McGuigan M, Hartigan-Go K, et al. American Academy of Clinical Toxicology; European Association of Poisons Centres and Clinical Toxicologists. Position paper: cathartics. *J Toxicol Clin Toxicol.* 2004;42:243–253.
This paper indicates that cathartics alone are not useful as a means of GI contamination in poisoning.

Brent J, Wallace KL, Burkhart KK, et al, eds. *Critical Care Toxicology: Diagnosis and Management of the Critically Poisoned Patient.* Philadelphia: Mosby; 2005.
This is an excellent, comprehensive and well-referenced toxicology textbook with a critical care focus.

Chyka PA, Seger D, Krenzelok EP, et al. American Academy of Clinical Toxicology; European Association of Poisons Centres and Clinical Toxicologists. Position paper: single-dose activated charcoal. *Clin Toxicol (Phila).* 2005;43:61–87.
This paper discusses dosages, complications and potential indications for the use of single-dose activated charcoal (i.e., early presentation after potentially toxic ingestions of many poisons).

Flomenbaum NE, Goldfrank LR, Hoffman RS, et al, eds. *Goldfrank's Toxicologic Emergencies.* 8th ed. New York: McGraw Hill, Medical Publishing Division; 2006.
This is the classic reference toxicology textbook, which includes a case study approach to specific poisonings.

Krenzelok EP, McGuigan M, Lheureuz P, et al. American Academy of Clinical Toxicology; European Association of Poisons Centres and Clinical Toxicologists. Position paper: ipecac syrup. *J Toxicol Clin Toxicol.* 2004;42:133–143.
This paper indicates that syrup of ipecac should not be used in the management of poisonings.

Olson KR, ed. *Poisoning and Drug Overdose.* 4th ed. New York: McGraw Hill/Lange Medical Books, Medical Publishing Division; 2004.
This is a thorough, compact and easy to navigate toxicology manual.

Proudfoot AT, Krenzelok EP, Vale JA. Position paper on urine alkalinization. *J Toxicol Clin Toxicol.* 2004;42:1–26.
This paper discusses methods, complications and the few indications for urine alkalinization (e.g., moderately severe salicylate toxicity, 2, 4-dichlorophenoxyacetic acid toxicity).

Tenenbein M, Lheureux P. American Academy of Clinical Toxicology; European Association of Poisons Centres and Clinical Toxicologists. Position paper: whole bowel irrigation. *J Toxicol Clin Toxicol.* 2004;42:843–854.

This paper discusses methods, complications and the limited potential indications for whole bowel irrigation (e.g., sustained release ingestions, iron ingestions, "body-packing").

Vale JA, Kulig K. American Academy of Clinical Toxicology; European Association of Poisons Centres and Clinical Toxicologists. Position paper: gastric lavage. *J Toxicol Clin Toxicol.* 2004;42:933–943.

This paper indicates that gastric lavage should not be employed routinely in the management of poisoning..

Watson WA, Litovitz TL, Rodgers GC Jr, et al. 2004 Annual report of the American Association of Poison Control Centers Toxic Exposure Surveillance System. *Am J Emerg Med.* 2005;23:589–666.

These reports are a primary source of epidemiologic data on poisonings in the US.

Infectious Diseases

X

CENTRAL NERVOUS SYSTEM INFECTIONS
Clare N. Gentry and Keith F. Woeltje

33

Meningitis and encephalitis cause significant morbidity and mortality, often requiring intensive care unit-level care. Approximately 50% of patients with bacterial meningitis require mechanical intubation, usually because of altered mental status. Physiologically, *meningitis* is characterized by inflammation of the meninges surrounding the brain and spinal cord, while *encephalitis* refers to inflammation within the brain parenchyma. Clinically, patients with encephalitis are more likely to have altered level of consciousness or confusion, although the clinical presentations of encephalitis and meningitis overlap considerably. The distinction between meningitis and encephalitis has important implications in the etiology, treatment, and prognosis of the illness. Table 33.1 identifies the most common etiologies of meningitis and encephalitis.

The initial evaluation of patients with any type of suspected central nervous system (CNS) infection usually takes place outside the intensive care unit, but a thorough understanding of the workup is essential. An approach to the initial evaluation of CNS infections is presented in Algorithm 33.1. The sensitivity of the classic triad of fever, stiff neck, and altered mental status in predicting bacterial meningitis is <50%, but the absence of all three symptoms makes CNS infection unlikely. Retrospective studies have shown that almost all patients with bacterial meningitis have at least two of four critical symptoms, including fever, neck stiffness, headache, and altered mental status. Until the diagnosis of CNS infection is confirmed or rejected, antimicrobials should be administered empirically.

There is little evidence to suggest that imaging prior to lumbar puncture impacts management or outcomes in patients with CNS infection. Clinical and historical features suggestive of possible abnormalities on computed tomography include: history of CNS disease, history of recent seizure, altered level of consciousness, new focal neurologic deficits on examination, or neurologic findings in the setting of immunosuppression. Many physicians will perform imaging in the presence of these findings. The presence of an abnormality on imaging is not predictive of brain herniation, a life-threatening complication of lumbar puncture, and the decision to obtain imaging should never delay the initiation of empirical antimicrobial treatment.

TABLE 33.1	Common Etiologies of Meningitis and Encephalitis

Type	Etiology
Bacterial meningitis	*Streptococcus pneumoniae*
	Neisseria meningitidis
	Haemophilus influenzae
	Listeria monocytogenes[a]
Viral meningitis	Enteroviruses[b]
	Herpes simplex virus (HSV)
	Lymphocytic choriomeningitis virus
Encephalitis	Enteroviruses[b]
	HSV
	Arboviruses[b]
	West Nile virus
	St. Louis Encephalitis virus
	Eastern equine virus
	Western equine virus

[a]More common in patients >50 years of age and immunocompromised individuals.
[b]Seasonal predominance in summer and fall.

Because the clinical history and physical examination can be unreliable in diagnosing CNS infection, analysis of cerebrospinal fluid (CSF) is crucial. CSF findings are essential in distinguishing bacterial from viral causes of infection. When performed by an experienced technician, Gram stain of the CSF is positive in approximately 50% to 75% of cases of bacterial meningitis. Sensitivity of the test varies by organism; it is positive in 90% of untreated cases of *Streptococcus pneumoniae* versus 30% to 35% of cases of *Listeria* meningitis. Although receipt of antibiotics prior to lumbar puncture will decrease the sensitivity of the cultures, antibiotic treatment should not be delayed to increase culture yield.

In addition to routine Gram stain and culture, CSF should be examined for glucose and protein quantitation, and cell count should be examined from the last tube of fluid obtained. Although rarely seen, cryptococcal meningitis may present as acute meningitis even in immunocompetent individuals. A cryptococcal antigen assay should be ordered on all patients. Fungal, viral, and acid-fast bacilli cultures are very low yield in the setting of acute meningitis or encephalitis and should not be routinely ordered. The laboratory can hold a quantity of CSF for additional testing if indicated from the initial CSF findings. Typical CSF findings for viral and bacterial meningitis as well as encephalitis are presented in Table 33.2.

Encephalitis caused by herpes simplex virus is most often seen in young children and individuals more than 50 years of age. Patients may present with altered level of consciousness, focal cranial nerve findings, or focal seizures and may have abnormal temporal lobe findings on imaging. Because herpes simplex virus encephalitis is associated with high morbidity and mortality when treatment is delayed, patients age 50 years and more with symptoms of encephalitis should be given acyclovir empirically until results of CSF polymerase chain reaction for herpes virus are obtained. Table 33.3 outlines specific recommendations for empirical and specific treatment regimens of CNS infection.

The use of adjuvant steroids in the treatment of bacterial meningitis is controversial. Improvements in morbidity and mortality have been shown in a subgroup of patients with bacterial meningitis caused by *S. pneumoniae*. In general, patients with suspected or proven *S. pneumoniae* meningitis should receive steroids prior to, or concurrent with, the initial dose of antibiotics. There is no proven benefit to steroid treatment started after antibiotic therapy has been administered.

Nosocomially acquired meningitis accounts for only 0.4% of all hospital infections and almost always occurs in the setting of neurosurgical intervention. In contrast to

ALGORITHM 33.1   **Initial Evaluation for Possible Central Nervous System (CNS) Infection**

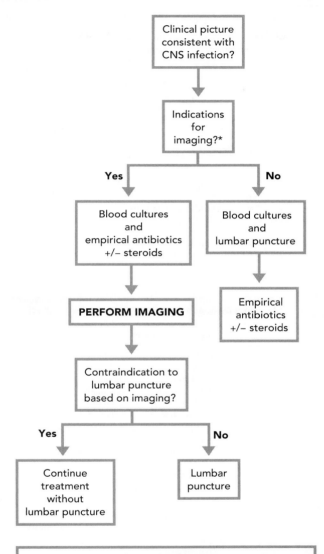

*History of CNS disease, history of recent seizure, altered level of consciousness, new focal neurologic deficits, or neurologic deficits in the setting of immunosuppression

TABLE 33.2	Cerebrospinal Fluid (CSF) Findings in Meningitis and Encephalitis		
CSF Finding	**Bacterial Meningitis**	**Viral Meningitis**	**Encephalitis**
WBC/mm^3	≥1,000	100–10,000	<250
Differential	PMN predominance (≥80%)	Lymphocyte predominance[a] (≥50%)	Lymphocyte predominance[a]
Protein	>250	50–250	<150
CSF to serum glucose ratio	≤0.4	Normal to decreased	>0.5
Opening pressure (mm Hg)	>200	Usually normal	Normal to slightly increased

WBC, white blood cell; PMN, polymorphonuclear cells.
[a]May have neutrophilic predominance initially.

community-acquired bacterial meningitis, nosocomially acquired meningitis is typically caused by Gram-negative organisms, coagulase-negative staphylococcal species, or *Staphylococcus aureus*. Patients should receive empirical treatment with vancomycin for Gram-positive coverage plus ceftazidime or cefepime to cover the possibility of *Pseudomonas* infection.

Recommendations regarding length of treatment are often based on historical practices rather than specific evidence from clinical trials. Given the variable absorption of

TABLE 33.3	Treatment Recommendations for CNS Infection (Adapted from Infectious Diseases Society of America Guidelines)
Etiology	**Suggested Therapy**
Empirical	Vancomycin 10–15 mg/kg IV q8 hours[a] PLUS Ceftriaxone 2 g IV q12 hours Addition of steroids if indicated[b] If ≥50 years, addition of ampicillin 2 g IV q4 hours[a] If suspicion for HSV, addition of acyclovir 10 mg/kg q8 hours[a]
Streptococcus pneumoniae	If PCN MIC ≤1 mcg/mL, ceftriaxone 2 g IV q12 hours If PCN MIC ≥2 mcg/mL OR ceftriaxone MIC ≥1 mcg/mL, vancomycin 10–15 mg/kg IV q8 hours[a] AND Ceftriaxone 2 g IV q12 hours
Neisseria meningitidis	If PCN MIC <0.1 mcg/mL, ampicillin 2 g IV q4 hours[a] If PCN MIC ≥0.1 mcg/mL, ceftriaxone 2 g IV q12 hours
Listeria monocytogenes	Ampicillin 2 g IV q 4 hours[a] If PCN allergy, use trimethoprim/sulfamethoxazole 5 mg/kg q8 hours[c]
Viral meningitis	Supportive measures
Herpes encephalitis	Acyclovir 10 mg/kg IV q8 hours[a]
Other viral encephalitis	Supportive measures

IV, intravenous; HSV, herpes simplex virus; PCN, penicillin; MIC, mean inhibitory concentration
[a]Dose adjustment required for impaired renal function.
[b]Dexamethasone 0.15 mg/kg every 6 hours × 4 days.
[c]Dosing based on trimethoprim component.

TABLE 33.4	Suggested Length of Therapy for CNS Infection by Etiology (Adapted from Infectious Diseases Society of America Guidelines)

Etiology	Length of Treatment (days)
Listeria monocytogenes	≥21
Gram-negative bacilli	21
Group B *Streptococcus*	14–21
HSV Encephalitis	14[a]
Streptococcus pneumoniae	14
Haemophilus influenzae	7
Neisseria meningitidis	7

HSV, herpes simplex virus.
[a]Extend therapy to 21 days if there is immunosuppression.

certain oral antimicrobials, treatment should be given intravenously for the duration of therapy. Suggested lengths of treatment for various CNS infections are shown in Table 33.4.

There is often confusion about the need for isolation in patients diagnosed with meningitis. Two common causes of bacterial meningitis, *Haemophilus influenzae* and *Neisseria meningitidis*, are spread via large particle droplets >5 mcm in size. Infection with either of these organisms warrants droplet precautions for the first 24 hours of treatment. Individuals entering the room should wear standard masks when working within 3 feet of the patient, and patient movement should be limited if possible. If transport is required, the patient should wear a mask to minimize potential spread of infection. Because the etiology of bacterial meningitis is typically unknown at the time of presentation, all patients with suspected meningitis should initially be placed on droplet precautions in addition to standard precautions.

Suggested Reading

deGans J, van de Beek D. Dexamethasone in adults with bacterial meningitis. *N Engl J Med.* 2002; 347: 1549–1556.
A recent randomized, placebo-controlled trial of adjuvant steroid therapy in bacterial meningitis concluding that early steroid therapy decreases mortality and morbidity in patients with bacterial meningitis.

Flores-Cordero JM, Amaya-Villar R, Rincón-Ferrari MD, et al. Acute community-acquired bacterial meningitis in adults admitted to the intensive care unit: clinical manifestations, management and prognostic factors. *Intensive Care Med.* 2003;29:1967–1973.
A focused look at patients with bacterial meningitis requiring admission to the intensive care unit suggesting that clinical course of disease over the first 24 hours of hospitalization is a major predictor of morbidity and mortality.

Hasbun R, Abrahams J, Jekel J, et al. Computed tomography of the head before lumbar puncture in adults with suspected meningitis. *N Engl J Med.* 2001;345:1727–1733.
Large prospective study of CT scan prior to lumber puncture in patients with clinical suspicion of meningitis that shows certain clinical features are predictive of normal head CT in patients with suspected meningitis.

Korinek AM, Baugnon T, Golmard JL, et al. Risk factors for adult nosocomial meningitis after craniotomy: role of antibiotic prophylaxis. *Neurosurgery.* 2006;59:126–33.
Brief review of nosocomial meningitis with evaluation of peri-operative antibiotic prophylaxis. Findings demonstrate antibiotic prophylaxis at the time of neurosurgery improves surgical site infection rates but does not have significant impact on rates of post-operative meningitis.

Palabiyikoglu I, Tekeli E, Cokca F, et al. Nosocomial meningitis in a university hospital between 1993 and 2002. *J Hosp Infect Control.* 2006;62:94–97.

Retrospective evaluation of 51 cases of nosocomial meningitis which showed the major risk factor for hospital-acquired meningitis was neurosurgical procedure. The most common causative organisms were gram-negative bacilli and Straphylococcus species.

Rotbart HA. Viral meningitis. *Semin Neurol.* 2000;20:277–292.

Complete review of all aspects of viral meningitis including epidemiology, pathogenesis, clinical presentations, diagnosis, and treatment options.

Sejvar JJ. The evolving epidemiology of viral encephalitis. *Curr Opin Neurol.* 2006;19: 350–357.

A current look at emerging causes of viral encephalitis which shows ongoing transmission of West Nile Virus in the United States and explores transfusions and transplants as potential sources of transmission for viral encephalitis.

Tunkel AR, Hartman BJ, Kaplan SL, et al. Practice guidelines for the management of bacterial meningitis. *Clin Infect Dis.* 2004;39:1267–1283.

A thorough review of evidence-based treatments for bacterial meningitis with evaluation and treatment guidelines endorsed by the Infectious Diseases Society of America.

van de Beek D, deGans J, Tunkel AR, et al. Community-acquired bacterial meningitis in adults. *N Engl J Med.* 2006;354:44–53.

An up-to-date review of recent studies and advances in bacterial meningitis including management of complications.

COMMUNITY-ACQUIRED PNEUMONIA

Bernard C. Camins

34

Community-acquired pneumonia (CAP) affects about 2 to 3 million patients each year. Although mortality is relatively low (<1%) for nonhospitalized patients, mortality among hospitalized patients can be as high as 30%, with the majority of deaths occurring in patients admitted to the intensive care unit. One of the most important decisions to make is to determine if the patient truly has CAP as opposed to health care-associated pneumonia (HCAP). CAP patients are those patients from whom the first positive bacterial culture is obtained within 48 hours of hospital admission and lack risk factors for HCAP. Please see Chapter 35 for the HCAP criteria.

There is no consensus between the American Thoracic Society and the Infectious Diseases Society of America guidelines if sputum Gram stains and cultures should be obtained from each CAP patient. The American Thoracic Society guidelines recommend sputum Gram stain and culture only on patients who are suspected to have an antibiotic-resistant pathogen, and the Infectious Diseases Society of America recommends obtaining an expectorated sputum sample for Gram stain and culture from all CAP patients. However, both groups are in agreement when recommending the prompt administration of antibiotic treatment. Antibiotic therapy should not be delayed in favor of collecting the sputum sample. The results of the Gram stain should also be interpreted carefully when choosing the initial empiric antibiotic regimen. Sputum culture results are particularly helpful when an organism that is not part of the normal flora is recovered.

Blood cultures should also be obtained, preferably prior to the administration of antibiotics. Obtaining blood cultures within 24 hours of admission has been shown to reduce mortality simply because resistant pathogens are identified earlier with the availability of culture results. Serologies are usually not helpful in the diagnosis of CAP except for *Chlamydophila pneumoniae*, which is an uncommon cause of severe pneumonia requiring admission to the intensive care unit. The diagnosis also may not be made until weeks later when a fourfold increase in the immunoglobulin (Ig) G titers is observed unless acute microimmunofluorescence serologic testing shows an IgM titer ≥1:16. A *Legionella* urine antigen test is recommended for all immunocompromised patients with CAP or any patient with severe CAP. This diagnostic test only detects *Legionella pneumophila* serogroup 1, so a negative result does not rule out *Legionella* pneumonia. A pneumococcal urinary antigen assay may help in the diagnosis of pneumococcal pneumonia. However, this test is not as reliable as the *Legionella* urine antigen assay because it only has a sensitivity of 50% to 80%.

Finally, during influenza season, rapid antigen or polymerase chain reaction assay testing for presence of influenza A or B virus are recommended for both treatment and epidemiologic purposes. Before any empiric antibiotic regimen is selected, a determination needs to be made if the patient truly has CAP or HCAP. Table 34.1. presents information for the treatment of severe CAP. Recently, experts have recommended shorter courses of therapy for CAP. Even in patients with pneumococcal bacteremia from CAP, a 10-day course of therapy may be adequate. A recent randomized controlled trial showed that levofloxacin, 750 mg by mouth daily for 5 days, was equivalent to a 10-day course of the 500-mg dose. However, this study included all hospitalized patients, not only patients with severe CAP. Patients with severe CAP may require at least 10 days of antibiotic therapy. Patients with *Legionella* pneumonia should always be treated with a 14-day course of therapy unless azithromycin is used.

The patient should be clinically stable within 72 hours of initiation of therapy. If there is clinical deterioration after 24 hours of therapy, several possibilities should be considered. First,

TABLE 34.1	Antibiotic Recommendations for the Intensive Care Unit Patient with Community-Acquired Pneumonia

No Risk Factors for *Pseudomonas* Infection	Recommended Antibiotics

Streptococcus pneumoniae including DRSP
Haemophilus influenza
Legionella streptococcus.
Staphylococcus aureus
Streptococcus pyogenes
Less common pathogens
   Klebsiella pneumoniae and other Gram
     negatives
   Mycoplasma pneumoniae
   Respiratory viruses
   Miscellaneous
     Chlamydophila pneumoniae
     Mycobacterium tuberculosis
     Endemic fungi
	β-Lactam[a]
	+
	advanced macrolide[b] OR
	respiratory fluoroquinolone[c]
	OR
	
	respiratory fluoroquinolone,[c] with or
	   without clindamycin if patient has
	   β-lactam allergy

**Risk Factors for *Pseudomonas*
Infection Present[d]**
All the above agents and *Pseudomonas
aeruginosa*
	Recommended Antibiotics
	Antipseudomonal β-lactam[e] with Gram
	   positive coverage + ciprofloxacin
	OR
	Antipseudomonal β-lactam with Gram
	   positive coverage[e] + an aminoglycoside
	   + a respiratory fluroquinolone[c] OR an
	   advanced macrolide[b]
	OR
	Aztreonam + levofloxacin OR
	Aztreonam + moxifloxacin with or without
	   an aminoglycoside if patient has
	   β-lactam allergy

DRSP, drug-resistant *Streptococcus pneumoniae.*
[a]Cefotaxime, ceftriaxone, ampicillin-sulbactam, or ertapenem.
[b]Azithromycin or clarithromycin, but only azithromycin is available intravenously.
[c]Levofloxacin or moxifloxacin.
[d]Severe structural lung disease (e.g., bronchiectasis), recent antibiotic therapy, recent stay in the hospital, malnutrition, chronic corticosteroid therapy (e.g., prednisone >10 mg/day).
[e]Cefepime, piperacillin, piperacillin-tazobactam, imipenem, or meropenem.

a resistant pathogen may be the etiologic agent and the initial empiric therapy may be inadequate. Some patients may have *drug-resistant Streptococcus pneumoniae* or *Pseudomonas aeruginosa* despite the lack of risk factors. Alternatively, unusual bacterial pathogens may be the cause of CAP. There should be a low threshold in screening for human immunodeficiency virus infection and *Pneumocystis jirovecii* pneumonia. Nocardiosis, tuberculosis, or endemic fungi should also be considered in patients who test positive for human immunodeficiency virus. The patient's history should be reviewed again for certain exposures: cattle, sheep, or goat for *Coxiella burnetii*, birds for *Chlamydophila psittaci*, and rabbits for tularemia. Respiratory tract viruses are common causes of pneumonia. Viral pneumonia may be severe in the elderly, immunocompromised, or patients with chronic obstructive lung disease and other comorbid illnesses.

Although the results were varied, previous studies have shown that 4% to 39% of patients hospitalized for CAP had evidence of a viral infection. Severe pneumonia from influenza warrants treatment with an antiviral agent in most situations. Complications of CAP should also be suspected in patients who fail to respond to initial therapy. About 10%

of patients with pneumococcal pneumonia have metastatic disease such as meningitis, arthritis, endocarditis, and peritonitis. A parapneumonic effusion or empyema may require drainage with a chest tube. A repeat chest x-ray or a computed tomography scan may be warranted in patients who fail to respond to therapy. Finally, noninfectious causes such as pulmonary embolus, lung malignancy, hypersensitivity pneumonitis, Wegener's granulomatosis, or eosinophilic pneumonia can be misdiagnosed as CAP.

Suggested Reading

Arbo MD, Snydman DR. Influence of blood culture results on antibiotic choice in the treatment of bacteremia. *Arch Intern Med.* 1994;154:2641–2645.

A randomized controlled trial showing that blood cultures immediately prior to initiation of therapy for CAP leads to improved survival.

Bartlett JG, Breiman RF, Mandell LA, et al. Community-acquired pneumonia in adults: guidelines for management. The Infectious Diseases Society of America. *Clin Infect Dis.* 1998;26: 811–838.

An evidence-based guidelines from the IDSA for the management of CAP in immunocompetent adults.

Dunbar LM, Wunderink RG, Habib MP, et al. High-dose, short-course levofloxacin for community-acquired pneumonia: a new treatment paradigm. *Clin Infect Dis.* 2003;37:752–760.

A randomized controlled trial showing that a short course of levofloxacin at higher doses was as efficacious as the longer course treatment for CAP.

Mandell LA, File TM Jr. Short-course treatment of community-acquired pneumonia. *Clin Infect Dis.* 2003;37:761–763.

A review article advocating shorter courses to avoid the emergence of antibiotic resistance.

Mandell LA, Bartlett JG, Dowell SF, et al. Update of practice guidelines for the management of community-acquired pneumonia in immunocompetent adults. *Clin Infect Dis.* 2003;37:1405–1433.

An update of the evidence-based guidelines from the IDSA for the management of CAP in immunocompetent adults.

Mandell LA, Wunderink RG, Anzueto A, et al. Infectious Diseases Society of America/American Thoracic Society consensus guidelines on the management of community-acquired pneumonia in adults. *Clin Infect Dis.* 2007;44:S27–72.

The latest evidence based recommendations from the ATS for the treatment of immunocompetent adults

35

NOSOCOMIAL PNEUMONIA
Marin H. Kollef

Hospital-acquired pneumonia (HAP) is defined as a nosocomial pneumonia (NP) that occurs 48 hours or more after hospital admission, which was not incubating at the time of hospital admission (Table 35.1). Ventilator-associated pneumonia (VAP) refers to NP that develops more than 48 to 72 hours after endotracheal intubation. It is important to thoroughly evaluate patients with suspected NP in order to exclude other conditions that can mimic the presentation of NP (Table 35.2). HAP is the second most common nosocomial infection in the United States after urinary tract infection, but is the leading cause of mortality attributed to nosocomial infections. The incidence of NP is between 5 and 10 cases per 1,000 hospital admissions and, although the incidence of VAP is difficult to determine because of differences in the case definition, it is estimated that 9% to 27% of patients undergoing mechanical ventilation for >48 hours are affected. "Attributable mortality" from NP is estimated to be between 33% and 50%, with the higher mortality occurring in patients with bacteremia or infections with *Pseudomonas aeruginosa* or *Acinetobacter* species (Table 35.3).

The American Thoracic Society and the Infectious Diseases Society of America published guidelines for the management of adults with HAP, VAP, and health care-associated pneumonia in early 2005. These guidelines provide recommendations for the antibiotic management of NP as summarized in Table 35.4 and Algorithm 35.1. It is important for clinicians treating patients with suspected NP to prescribe initial antimicrobial regimens that are likely to be active against the offending pathogen in order to optimize outcome. Once the pathogens and antimicrobial susceptibilities are known, narrowing or de-escalation of the antimicrobial regimen can occur.

TABLE 35.1	Definitions of Pneumonia[a] (with Focus on Bacterial Pathogens)

Pneumonia Category	Definition
Community-acquired pneumonia	Patients with a first positive bacterial culture obtained within 48 hours of hospital admission lacking risk factors for health care-associated pneumonia
Health care-associated pneumonia	Patients with a first positive bacterial culture within 48 hours of admission and any of the following: admission source indicates a transfer from another health care facility (e.g., hospital, nursing home); receiving hemodialysis, wound, or infusion therapy as an outpatient; prior hospitalization for at least 3 days within 90 days; immunocompromised state due to underlying disease or therapy (human immunodeficiency virus, chemotherapy)
Hospital-acquired pneumonia	Patients with a first positive bacterial culture >48 hours after hospital admission
Ventilator-associated pneumonia	Mechanically ventilated patients with a first positive bacterial culture >48 hours after hospital admission or tracheal intubation, whichever occurred first

[a]Criteria for pneumonia include new or progressive lung infiltrate and at least two of the following clinical criteria: hyperthermia or hypothermia, elevated white blood cell count, purulent tracheal secretions or sputum, and worsening oxygenation.

TABLE 35.2	Noninfectious Causes of Fever and Pulmonary Infiltrates Mimicking Nosocomial Pneumonia

Chemical aspiration without infection
Atelectasis
Pulmonary embolism
Acute respiratory distress syndrome
Pulmonary hemorrhage
Lung contusion
Infiltrative tumor
Radiation pneumonitis
Drug reaction
Bronchiolitis obliterans organizing pneumonia

TABLE 35.3	Most Common Pathogens Associated with Various Pneumonia Categories

Infection Site	Pathogens

I. Pneumonia (immunocompetent)
   1. Community-acquired pneumonia
      (nonimmunocompromised host)
	Streptococcus pneumoniae
	Haemophilus influenzae
	Moraxella catarrhalis
	Mycoplasma pneumoniae
	Legionella pneumophila
	Chlamydia pneumoniae
	Methicillin-resistant *Staphylococcus aureus* (MRSA)
	Influenza virus

2. Health care-associated pneumonia	Methicillin-resistant *S. aureus* *Pseudomonas aeruginosa* *Klebsiella pneumoniae* *Acinetobacter* species *Stenotrophomonas* species *L. pneumophila*
3. Pneumonia (immunocompromised host) a. Neutropenia	Any pathogen listed above *Aspergillus* species *Candida* species
b. Human immunodeficiency virus	Any pathogen listed above *Pneumocystis carinii* *Mycobacterium tuberculosis* *Histoplasma capsulatum* Other fungi Cytomegalovirus
c. Solid-organ transplant or bone marrow transplant	Any pathogen listed above (Can vary depending on timing of infection to transplant)
d. Cystic fibrosis	*H. influenzae* (early) *S. aureus* *Pseudomonas aeruginosa* *Burkholderia cepacia*
4. Lung abscess	*Bacteroides* species *Peptostreptococci* *Fusobacterium* species *Nocardia* (in immunocompromised patients) Amebic (when suggestive by exposure)
5. Empyema	*S. aureus* *S. pneumoniae* Group A Streptococci } Usually acute *H. influenzae* Anaerobic bacteria *Enterobacteriaceae* } Usually subacute or chronic *M. tuberculosis*

| TABLE 35.4 | Antibiotic Recommendations for Nosocomial Pneumonia |

Nonmultidrug-resistant (MDR) Potential Pathogens	Recommended Antibiotics

Streptococcus pneumoniae
Haemophilus influenza
Methicillin-sensitive *Staphylococcus aureus*
Antibiotic-sensitive enteric Gram negative bacilli
  Escherichia coli
  Klebsiella pneumoniae
  Enterobacter species
  Proteus species
  Serratia marcescens
	Ceftriaxone
	OR
	Levofloxacin, moxifloxacin or
	  ciprofloxacin
	OR
	Ampicillin/sulbactam
	OR
	Ertapenem

Potential MDR Pathogens	**Recommended Antibiotics**

Pseudomonas aeruginosa
K. pneumoniae (extended-spectrum β-lactamase +)
Acinetobacter species
Legionella pneumophila
Methicillin-resistant *S. aureus*
	Cefepime, ceftazidime
	OR
	Imipenem or meropenem
	OR
	Pipercillin-tazobactam
	PLUS
	Ciprofloxacin or levofloxacin
	OR
	Amikacin, gentamicin,
	  or tobramycin
	PLUS
	Azithromycin, clarithromycin
	  (if *Legionella* suspected)
	PLUS
	Linezolid or vancomycin

ALGORITHM 35.1   A Step-by-Step Approach to the Management of Nosocomial Pneumonia

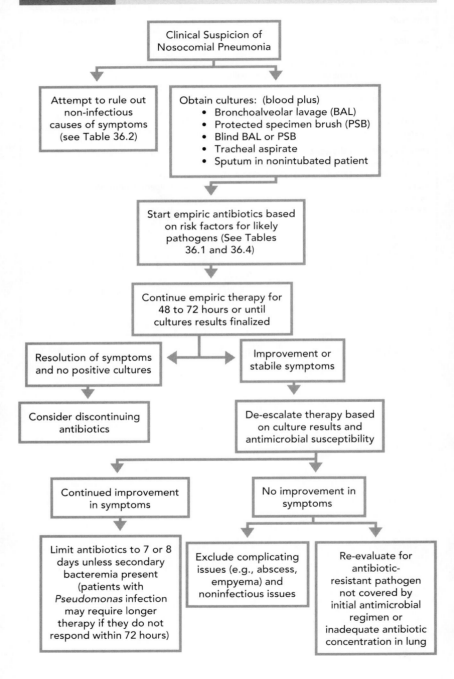

Suggested Reading

American Thoracic Society; Infectious Diseases Society of America. Guidelines for the management of adults with hospital-acquired, ventilator-associated, and healthcare-associated pneumonia. *Am J Respir Crit Care Med.* 2005;171:388–416.
  Management guidelines for nosocomial pneumonia.
Chastre J, Fagon JY. Ventilator-associated pneumonia. *Am J Respir Crit Care Med.* 2002;165:867–903.
  State of the art review of nosocomial pneumonia.

36

CELLULITIS/FASCIITIS/MYOSITIS
Kevin W. McConnell, John P. Kirby, and Craig M. Coopersmith

Skin and soft tissue infections can occur anywhere in the body. They may be characterized either on the basis of anatomic criteria or whether a necrotizing infection is present.

ANATOMIC CLASSIFICATION

Although infections have traditionally been stratified by the depth of tissue involvement, this classification has limited prognostic value. Nonetheless, terminology based on anatomic depth continues to be widely used and therefore retains relevance in clinical practice (Fig. 36.1). Superficial infections involving only the epidermis and dermis—such as pyoderma, impetigo, erysipelas, folliculitis, furuncles, and carbuncles—have limited clinical consequence in the intensive care unit. In contrast, deep soft tissues infections including cellulitis, fasciitis, and myositis may be associated with significant morbidity and mortality, depending on the clinical situation.

Cellulitis is an acute bacterial infection involving the upper subcutaneous tissue, including the superficial fascia. The disease primarily affects the lower extremities, although other areas that may be involved include the periorbital regions, areas near body piercings, incisions, puncture wounds ("skin-popping"/illicit drugs), bites, and areas with any preexisting skin condition such as venous stasis, ischemia, or decubitus ulcers. Intensive care unit patients also have increased susceptibility because of their impaired immune status and altered skin flora. The most common causative organisms are *Streptococcus pyogenes* and *Staphylococcus aureus*. Less common causes of cellulitis may be suspected based on the patient's history or comorbidities (Table 36.1).

Fasciitis involves the subcutaneous tissue and deep fascia. The clinical presentation may be masked, as the overlying skin may be involved only later in the disease process. Trauma is the most common cause; however, approximately 20% of cases of necrotizing fasciitis occur in healthy patients with no known injury, source, or predisposition.

Myositis involves infection down to muscle and is generally differentiated into myonecrosis or pyomyositis. Myonecrosis is associated with gas gangrene and clostridial infections, and pyomyositis is usually the result of a puncture wound with abscess formation. The distinction is vital, as myonecrosis necessitates immediate operative debridement and pyomyositis may be amenable to antibiotics and percutaneous drainage.

NECROTIZING INFECTIONS

Although anatomic location may be used to name the process, the distinction between necrotizing and nonnecrotizing skin and soft tissue infections is more important clinically. Regardless of depth of infection, nonnecrotizing infections usually respond to antibiotics. However, necrotizing infections require immediate surgical debridement, and early diagnosis and intervention represents the most important factor in patient outcome from necrotizing soft tissue infections.

Determining whether or not a necrotizing infection is present can be challenging because physical examination can often be unreliable (Table 36.2). Patients with these

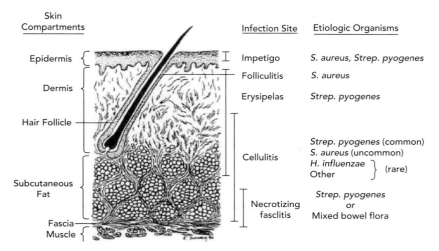

Figure 36.1. Anatomic classification of soft tissue infections.

infections frequently have normal overlying skin, and overt signs of necrotic tissue, such as crepitus, occur in only 30% of patients. It has recently been demonstrated in a small cohort of patients that serum sodium <135 mmol/L or a white blood cell count >15,400 cells/mm^3 carries a sensitivity of 95% and specificity of 94% for predicting the presence of necrotizing infection. Using these criteria, 18/19 patients with necrotizing infection and no obvious clinical signs of necrosis were identified.

Radiographic imaging may also assist in the diagnosis of necrotizing soft tissue infections. Plain radiography shows soft tissue gas in only 15% to 30% of necrotizing infections; thus, magnetic resonance imaging (MRI) is the preferred study. The absence of gadolinium enhancement on MRI indicates nonperfused tissue. Soft tissue gas is also diagnostic of a

TABLE 36.1	Less Common Sources of Soft Tissue Infections

History	Source
Immunosuppressed or neutropenic	Gram negative rods (*Pseudomonas, Escherichia coli*)
Fresh water swim with laceration or abrasion	*Aeromonas hydrophilia*
Salt water swim or sea food contamination of wound	*Vibrio* species (especially *Vibrio vulnificus*)
Cat/dog bite	*Pasteurella multocida,* polymicrobial anaerobes
Human bite	*Bacteroides fragilis, Eikenella* spp., polymicrobial anaerobes
HIV	*Haemophilus influenzae*, fungus, infected Kaposi's sarcoma
Diabetes, pregnancy, cirrhosis	Group B *Streptococcus*

HIV, human immunodeficiency virus.

TABLE 36.2	Characteristics of Necrotizing Infections

Signs/Symptoms Associated with Increased Likelihood That a Necrotizing Infection Is Present

Pain out of proportion to examination
Bullae
Systemic toxicity
Serum sodium <135 mmol/L
WBC >15,400 cell/mm^3
Tenderness beyond the area of erythema
Crepitus
Cutaneous anesthesia
Cellulitis refractory to antibiotic therapy

WBC, white blood count.

necrotizing infection. Sensitivity of MRI varies from 89% to 100%, but specificity ranges from 46% to 86%. Biopsy, frozen section, and culture may also be needed, in light of the limited specificity. An alternative means of establishing the severity of the infection is to make a bedside incision under local anesthesia large enough to permit an examination of the subcutaneous tissue or fascia in any area of concern. A digital examination of the tissue planes may detect the characteristic separation of necrosis and the patient may proceed to the operating room. A management algorithm for distinguishing necrotizing from nonnecrotizing infections is presented in Algorithm 36.1.

Targeted antibiotic therapy against *Streptococcus* and *Staphylococcus* has traditionally been the initial therapy for nonnecrotizing soft tissue infections in which atypical organisms are not suspected. However, antimicrobial management of nonnecrotizing infections is evolving as more infections are caused by resistant organisms such as methicillin-resistant *S. aureus*, including highly aggressive variants that are positive for Panton-Valentine Leukocidin. A recent prospective study of 11 university hospitals demonstrated that 59% of patients presenting with acute soft tissue infections had methicillin-resistant *S. aureus*; therefore, it is appropriate to initiate antimicrobial therapy that has activity against this organism.

Necrotizing infections require immediate surgical debridement and adjuvant antibiotic therapy but still represent a potential lethal disorder, with a 20% to 30% mortality. Hyperbaric oxygen should be considered as an adjunct to surgical debridement and antibiotics, should the therapy not subject the patient to additional risks. Its benefits include a reduction in alpha-toxin production, improved tissue demarcation, and diminished tissue loss. Timely diagnosis, effective surgical debridement, appropriate initial antibiotic coverage, and consideration for adjunctive hyperbaric oxygen are the keys for optimizing patient outcome in necrotizing skin and soft tissue infections.

ALGORITHM 36.1   **Algorithm for Managing Soft Tissue Infections**

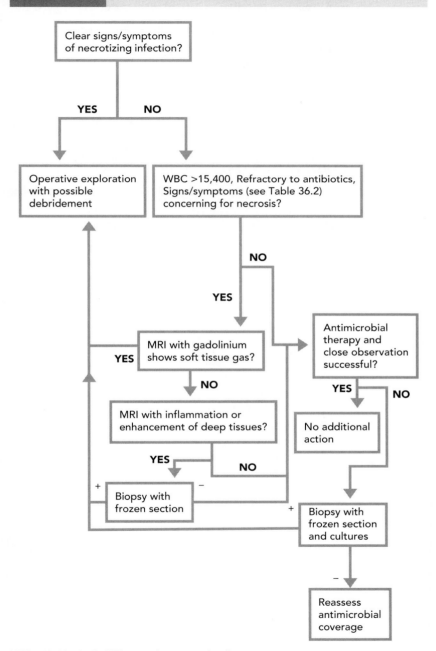

WBC, white blood cells; MRI, magnetic resonance imaging.

Suggested Reading

Brothers TE, Tagge DU, Stutely JE, et al. Magnetic resonance imaging differentiates between necrotizing and non-necrotizing fasciitis of the lower extremity. *J Am Coll Surg.* 1998;187:416–421.
> *A small prospective study showing the utility MRI in diagnosing necrotizing soft tissue infection.*

Feldmeier J. Hyperbaric oxygen: indications and results. The hyperbaric oxygen therapy committee report. Undersea and hyperbaric medicine society, 2003.
> *Evidenced-based review on hyperbaric oxygen usage include indications for usage in soft tissue infection.*

Lopez FA, Lartchenko S. Skin and soft tissue infections. *Infect Dis Clin North Am.* 2006;20;759–772.
> *A review article which emphasizes microbiology and emergence of MRSA in soft tissue infection.*

Malangoni MA, McHenry R. Approach to the patient with soft tissue infection. Wilmore DW, Fink MP, Jurkovich GJ, et al, eds. *ACS Surgery: Principles and Practice 2007.* 2007. <Http://www.webmd.com/>. *This is a comprehensive review with emphasis on indentification of necrotizing infections.*

Moran GJ, Krishnadasan A, Gorwitz RJ, et al. Methicillin-resistant *S. aureus* infections among patients in the emergency department. *N Engl J Med.* 2006;355:666–674.
> *Multicenter trial showing the emergence of MRSA in soft tissue infections.*

Wall DB, Klein SR, Black S, et al. A simple model to help distinguish necrotizing fasciitis from nonnecrotizing soft tissue infection. *J Am Coll Surg.* 2000;191:227–231.
> *This article describes the use of serum sodium and white blood cell count to identify patients with necrotizing infections.*

BACTEREMIA AND CATHETER-RELATED BLOODSTREAM INFECTIONS

Jeffrey C. Jones and David K. Warren

37

Bacteremia is a common complication in the critically ill. Bloodstream infection can develop from an uncontrolled site of localized infection, spontaneously without an obvious source, or originate from the increasing number of percutaneous implanted devices used in critical care. Central venous catheters (CVCs) provide a unique opportunity for pathogens to enter the bloodstream. CVCs become infected through multiple mechanisms. Organisms may invade via the skin insertion site. More commonly, the intra- and extraluminal portions of the catheter or the catheter hub(s) become colonized by bacteria that then enter the bloodstream. Potentially, hematogenous seeding from bacteremia originating at another source can occur. Rarely, contaminated intravenous solutions can create outbreaks of bacteremia with uncommon pathogens. Successful treatment of catheter-associated bloodstream infection is more difficult than simple bacteremia, as organisms on intravascular catheters usually exist within a slimelike biofilm, reducing their susceptibility to antimicrobial therapy and host defenses.

Local infection of the catheter insertion site presents as inflammation and purulent drainage from the entry site. However, local signs of infection are typically absent in catheter-associated bacteremia. Embolic phenomena distal to the catheter (e.g., septic pulmonary emboli) are also highly suggestive of a catheter-associated infection, although not commonly seen. More often the clinician is faced with a critically ill patient who is febrile without an obvious source and has a CVC in place.

Determining if a CVC is the source of a new fever presents a diagnostic and management challenge. A conservative strategy of removing all catheters and replacing them at new sites at the first sign of fever would benefit some patients, but also leads to the removal of many uninfected CVCs, exposing patients to the risks of line replacement unnecessarily. A reasonable approach would be to draw two sets of blood cultures (at least one from a peripheral venipuncture), and then immediately remove the catheter if there are obvious signs of local infection or the patient is in septic shock. If a thorough evaluation does not reveal a source of infection and the patient is stable, it is reasonable to leave the catheter in place, follow the blood cultures, and start empirical antibiotics at the clinician's discretion. If the cultures become positive, the catheter can be removed and a new catheter placed at a different site.

Because the sensitivity and specificity of blood cultures alone are imperfect, multiple strategies have been studied in an attempt to improve the diagnosis of catheter-associated bloodstream infection. Currently, only two methods are practical for widespread application. The first takes advantage of the continuous monitoring system for blood cultures used in most modern microbiology laboratories. Blot et.al. found that, in cases of catheter-associated bloodstream infection, a blood culture drawn from a catheter became positive for growth faster than a paired sample from a peripheral venipuncture. If a catheter-drawn blood culture becomes positive for growth at least 2 hours earlier than a peripherally drawn culture obtained at the same time, this strongly suggests the catheter as the source of the bacteremia. The other common method is culturing segments of catheters after their removal. A variety of techniques have been studied, but the semiquantitative roll plate technique described by Maki et al. in 1977 remains the most common. Documenting significant colonization of a catheter with the same organism isolated from blood cultures provides strong evidence that the catheter is the source of infection. An approach to suspected catheter-associated bloodstream infection in the intensive care unit is presented in Algorithm 37.1.

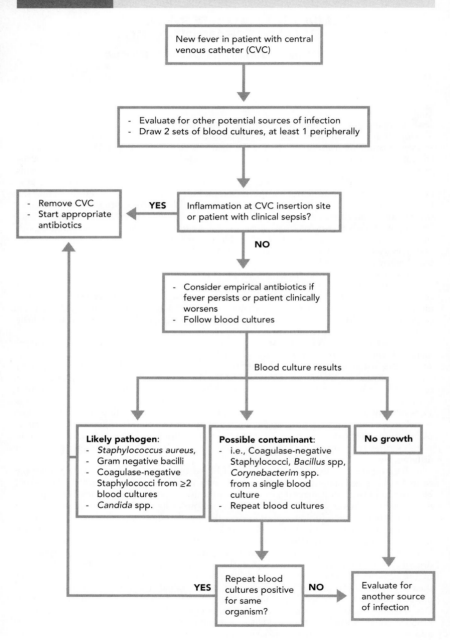

ALGORITHM 37.1   **Evaluation of Suspected Catheter-Associated Bacteremia**

New fever in patient with central venous catheter (CVC)

- Evaluate for other potential sources of infection
- Draw 2 sets of blood cultures, at least 1 peripherally

Inflammation at CVC insertion site or patient with clinical sepsis?

YES →
- Remove CVC
- Start appropriate antibiotics

NO

- Consider empirical antibiotics if fever persists or patient clinically worsens
- Follow blood cultures

Blood culture results

Likely pathogen:
- *Staphylococcus aureus*,
- Gram negative bacilli
- Coagulase-negative Staphylococci from ≥2 blood cultures
- *Candida* spp.

Possible contaminant:
- i.e., Coagulase-negative Staphylococci, *Bacillus* spp, *Corynebacterim* spp. from a single blood culture
- Repeat blood cultures

No growth

Repeat blood cultures positive for same organism?

YES → (Remove CVC / Start appropriate antibiotics)

NO → Evaluate for another source of infection

TABLE 37.1	Management of Bloodstream Infections by Common Pathogens

Staphylococcus aureus
Use β-lactams (oxacillin or nafcillin) for susceptible strains
Use vancomycin for MRSA only
Linezolid and daptomycin are acceptable alternatives for MRSA if unable to tolerate vancomycin
Transesophageal echocardiogram (TEE) recommended, if possible, evaluating for endocarditis
Remove catheters, especially in complicated infections
If endocarditis ruled out by TEE and catheter removed, treat for 14 days
Treat complicated infections (endocarditis, septic thrombophlebitis, prolonged bacteremia) for 4–6 weeks

Coagulase-negative Staphylococci
If catheter removed, treat with vancomycin for 7 days after removal
If catheter must be retained, treat for 14 days with vancomycin, consider antibiotic lock, and repeat blood cultures if signs/symptoms recur

Enterococci
Ampicillin for susceptible isolates
Vancomycin for ampicillin-resistant, vancomycin-sensitive isolates
Linezolid or daptomycin for vancomycin-resistant, ampicillin-resistant isolates
Consider addition of synergy-dosed gentamicin (1 mg/kg IV q8h)
Remove catheters
Treat for 14 days for uncomplicated infection

Gram negative bacilli
Empiric therapy should include agents active against *Pseudomonas aeruginosa*
Tailor antibiotics to sensitivity results
Remove catheter, especially with *Pseudomonas, Acinetobacter, Stenotrophomonas* spp.
If catheter removed treat for 10–14 days, if catheter must be retained consider antibiotic lock therapy

Candida species
Fluconazole (400–800 mg q24h), Amphotericin B deoxycholate (0.6–1 mg/kg q24h) or an echinocandin are all acceptable choices for empirical therapy
Fluconazole should not be used initially if patient has recently received an azole antifungal (e.g., for prophylaxis in high-risk patients)
Antifungal susceptibility can be inferred from the species identification
Repeat blood cultures until negative
Remove catheters
Ophthalmologic examination to exclude endophthalmitis
Treat for 14 days after first negative culture in uncomplicated infections

MRSA, methicillin-resistant *Staphylococcus aureus;* IV, intravenous.

Management strategies for specific pathogens can be found in Table 37.1. Special care should be taken in the case of *Candida* species (discussed in Chapter 38) and *Staphylococcus aureus,* given their ability to establish metastatic foci of infection. *S. aureus* bacteremia should prompt a thorough examination for metastatic sites of infection. High rates of endocarditis have been reported in catheter-associated *S. aureus* bacteremia, and transesophageal echocardiography should be considered in all cases, if not contraindicated.

The decision to remove a tunneled catheter or implanted port in the face of bacteremia is more difficult, given the expense and risk involved. In general, these devices should be removed when there is evidence of soft tissue infection around the tunnel or pocket, complications such as septic thromboembolic disease, endocarditis, or other metastatic foci of infection (when the pathogen is *S. aureus* or *Candida* spp.), and in the case of prolonged bacteremia not responding to appropriate antibiotic therapy. If salvage of the catheter is deemed necessary, there is evidence that use of high-concentration antibiotic lock therapy may improve success rates. Consultation with an infectious diseases specialist is recommended for complicated cases.

Suggested Reading

Beutz M, Sherman G, Mayfield J, et al. Clinical utility of blood cultures drawn from central vein catheters and peripheral venipuncture in critically ill medical patients. *Chest.* 2003;123:854–861.
Blood cultures drawn from central venous catheters or from peripheral venipuncture had similar positive and negative predictive values for detected bloodstream infection.
Blot F, Schmidt E, Nitenberg G, et al. Earlier positivity of central-venous- versus peripheral-blood cultures is highly predictive of catheter-related sepsis. *J Clin Microbiol.* 1998;36:105–109.
Paired sets of blood cultures from a catheter and peripheral venipuncture can be used to diagnose catheter-related bacteremia.
Fowler VG Jr., Li J, Corey GR, et al. Role of echocardiography in evaluation of patients with Staphylococcus aureus bacteremia: experience in 103 patients. *J Am Coll Cardiol.* 1997;30:1072–1078.
Transeophageal echocardiography found a surprisingly high rate of endocarditis in patients with S. aureus bacteremia who had negative transthoracic echocardiograms.
Maki DG, Weise CE, Sarafin HW. A semiquantitative culture method for identifying intravenous-catheter-related infection. *N Engl J Med.* 1977;296:1305–1309.
The original paper describing the commonly used roll plate culture technique.
Mermel LA, Farr BM, Sherertz RJ, et al. Guidelines for the management of intravascular catheter-related infections. *Clin Infect Dis.* 2001;32:1249–1272.
The most recent evidence based guidlines for managing catheter-associated bacteremia.
Stewart PS, William Costerton J. Antibiotic resistance of bacteria in biofilms. *Lancet.* 2001;358:135–138.
A review of possible mechanisms of bacterial resistance within biofilms
Weinstein MP, Towns ML, Quartey SM, et al. The clinical significance of positive blood cultures in the 1990s: a prospective comprehensive evaluation of the microbiology, epidemiology, and outcome of bacteremia and fungemia in adults. *Clin Infect Dis.* 1997;24:584–602.
A prospective study of bacteremia from 3 large medical centers; appropriate antibiotic therapy was associated with lower mortality.

INVASIVE FUNGAL INFECTION

Joseph M. Fritz and Keith F. Woeltje

38

Invasive fungal infections are a significant cause of morbidity and mortality worldwide. The incidence of these infections is steadily increasing. In addition, strains resistant to many commonly used antifungal agents are becoming more prevalent.

Candida species are by far the most common fungal pathogens encountered in the intensive care unit. *Candida* is now the fourth most common cause of nosocomial bloodstream infection. The term *invasive candidiasis* comprises several conditions including candidemia, endocarditis, meningitis, and other forms of deep organ involvement (e.g., endophthalmitis, hepatosplenic candidiasis). The attributable mortality for an episode of invasive candidiasis has been reported to be as high as 40% to 50%.

Perhaps the strongest risk factor for invasive candidiasis is length of intensive care unit stay, with most studies revealing peak incidence at approximately day 10. Colonization with *Candida* (e.g., rectal, sputum, urine, or superficial wound colonization) is also considered a risk factor for the development of invasive disease. The importance of multifocal colonization remains an area of debate. Multiple single-center studies have suggested that multifocal colonization carries higher predictive value for development of invasive disease; however, one of the largest multicenter prospective trials done to date did not show a significant relationship between the number of colonized sites and the development of invasive disease. Other risk factors are listed in Table 38.1.

Candida albicans remains the most common species isolated from patients, accounting for 44% to 71% of disease. However, an epidemiologic shift toward non-*albicans* species is occurring, with the most common non-*albicans* isolates being *Candida glabrata*, *Candida parapsilosis*, *Candida tropicalis*, and *Candida krusei*. This shift has particularly important implications for therapy because of intrinsic fluconazole-resistance carried by *C. glabrata* and *C. krusei*.

The presence of *Candida* in a blood culture should never be perceived simply as a contaminant and should always prompt further investigation for possible sources. Although *Candida* grows readily in current blood culture bottles, blood cultures are positive in only 50% to 70% of patients with invasive candidiasis. However, a positive culture from a nonsterile site often provides little evidence to distinguish between infection and colonization. Biopsy of a specific lesion (from a normally sterile site) demonstrating characteristic histopathology can be considered definitive, but this is often not feasible in critically ill patients. Because of these limitations, a reliable, non–culture-based method has been vigorously sought. Unfortunately, none of the currently available tests have adequate sensitivity and specificity for reliable diagnosis. For this reason, empiric therapy for invasive candidiasis is often appropriate for the critically ill patient, with risk factors, who is not improving with appropriate antibacterial agents. Furthermore, recent evidence suggests a decrease in mortality when antifungal therapy is started early in high-risk hosts showing clinical signs of disease rather than holding therapy until definitive diagnosis (i.e., *Candida* growth in blood culture). Although no major conclusions can be drawn from this limited analysis, we believe that early empiric therapy in high-risk patients pending culture results is justifiable.

Evidence-based guidelines regarding general management and treatment of candidiasis were published by the Infectious Diseases Society of America in 2004; these are currently under revision. According to these guidelines, first-line agents include fluconazole, caspofungin, and amphotericin B. Fluconazole is an appropriate choice for nonneutropenic,

TABLE 38.1	Risk Factors for Invasive Candidiasis

Prolonged ICU stay
Candida colonization
Central venous catheterization
Broad-spectrum antimicrobials
Renal failure
Hemodialysis
Diabetes
Parenteral nutrition
Malignancy
Chemotherapy/immunosuppressive medications
Surgery (particularly abdominal)
Transplantation
APACHE II score $\geq$20
Acute pancreatitis

ICU, intensive care unit; APACHE, Acute Physiology and Chronic Health Evaluation.

hemodynamically stable patients unless there is high suspicion for a fluconazole-resistant species (e.g., previous colonization with *C. glabrata, C. krusei,* or prior prophylaxis/treatment with fluconazole). If fluconazole is used for empiric therapy, a relatively high dose (e.g., 800 mg intravenously daily, adjusted for renal function) should be used until species identification is made. In patients who are neutropenic, hemodynamically unstable, or who are being treated in units with high rates of infection with fluconazole-resistant species (regardless of immune function or hemodynamic status), it is reasonable to treat with an echinocandin or amphotericin B formulation until species identification of the *Candida* isolate is made (Alg. 38.1). It should be noted that since the publication of these guidelines, other agents have been approved for treatment of various forms of invasive candidiasis, including voriconazole (a broad-spectrum azole) and anidulafungin (an echinocandin). In the case of candidemia, the standard duration of therapy is 14 days from the last positive blood culture. Recommended treatment may be considerably longer, depending on the site of involvement. Additional components of management include immediate removal of intravascular catheters and ophthalmologic examination to exclude endophthalmitis.

Because fungal pathogens represent a growing proportion of nosocomial infections, prophylaxis with antifungal agents in high-risk patients has been implemented at several centers. The few trials performed to date have shown a nonsignificant risk reduction with the use of either fluconazole or ketoconazole as prophylaxis; however, these studies were limited by relatively small numbers. Although these results are encouraging, they have not led to definitive recommendations for antifungal prophylaxis. Antifungal prophylaxis may be a reasonable approach in select high-risk patients.

Although a much less common cause of invasive disease, *Aspergillus* species remain an important consideration in a certain subset of patients, particularly those who are immunosuppressed (Table 38.2). Sinopulmonary involvement is the most common manifestation of invasive disease; however, dissemination can occur virtually anywhere, including the skin, central nervous system, eyes, and abdominal viscera. Computed tomography may suggest the diagnosis with findings such as the "halo sign," a haziness surrounding a nodular pulmonary infiltrate. However, this feature can be seen with other angioinvasive infections, so it is far from diagnostic. The organism will grow on culture; however, its presence in samples from nonsterile sites may indicate colonization rather than true infection. The sensitivity of the serum galactomannan assay varies widely in the literature between 29% and 100% and the specificity is typically greater than 85%. False-positive results may also occur in patients receiving piperacillin-tazobactam. The assay potentially can be used as a diagnostic adjunct but should not be used as sole criterion for diagnosis. Demonstration of the organism on biopsy is considered the gold standard for diagnosis.

ALGORITHM 38.1 **Empiric Treatment of Candidemia**

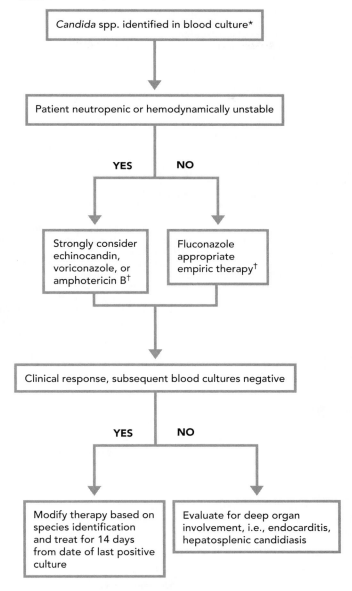

Candida spp. identified in blood culture*

↓

Patient neutropenic or hemodynamically unstable

YES | **NO**

Strongly consider echinocandin, voriconazole, or amphotericin B†

Fluconazole appropriate empiric therapy†

↓

Clinical response, subsequent blood cultures negative

YES | **NO**

Modify therapy based on species identification and treat for 14 days from date of last positive culture

Evaluate for deep organ involvement, i.e., endocarditis, hepatosplenic candidiasis

*Removal of central lines and ophthalmologic exam recommended with diagnosis of candidemia when clinically stable.
†Also consider echinocandin, voriconazole, or amphotericin B for patients colonized with C*andida glabrata* or C*andida krusei*, those residing in units with high rates of infection with these organisms, and recipients of previous fluconazole prophylaxis or therapy.

TABLE 38.2	Risk Factors for Invasive Aspergillosis

Prolonged neutropenia (>10 days)
Hematopoietic stem cell transplantation
Solid organ transplantation
Corticosteroid/other immunosuppressive therapy
Advanced HIV
Chronic granulomatous disease

HIV, human immunodeficiency virus.

In a recent study comparing amphotericin B and voriconazole as initial therapy for invasive aspergillosis, voriconazole was associated with improved survival (71% vs. 58%, respectively). Based on this trial, we recommend the use of voriconazole as first-line therapy. The echinocandins have in vitro activity against *Aspergillus* but are not approved for as primary therapy. Combination therapy has received much attention in recent years and is often used in these patients. In the largest study to date, the combination of voriconazole and caspofungin was compared with voriconazole alone in patients (hematopoietic stem cell transplantation recipients or those with hematologic malignancy treated with cytotoxic chemotherapy) with invasive aspergillosis who failed therapy with amphotericin B formulations. Although the numbers in each arm were small, the combination of caspofungin and voriconazole was associated with a statistically significant improved 3-month survival when compared with voriconazole alone. This trial has not led to definitive consensus, but we believe that combination therapy is appropriate in this population.

Zygomycosis, also commonly referred to as *mucormycosis,* is a general term describing infections with a group of molds belonging to the class Zygomycetes. There are multiple organisms within this general classification, and those most commonly isolated include *Rhizopus, Rhizomucor, Absidia,* and *Mucor.* These organisms are known for their predilection of immunocompromised hosts and typically present with relatively rapid-onset angioinvasive disease. Predisposing factors include diabetes, acidosis, solid-organ and bone marrow transplantation recipients, iron overload, deferoxamine treatment, and other forms of immunosuppression.

TABLE 38.3	Activity of Antifungal Agents

Fungus	Fluconazole	Voriconazole	Echinocandin[a]	Amphotericin B
Candida albicans	+	+	+	+
Candida parapsilosis	+	+	+/−	+
Candida tropicalis	+	+	+	+
Candida glabrata	DD/−	+/−	+	+
Candida krusei	−	+	+	+
Aspergillus spp.[b]	−	+	+	+
Cryptococcus spp.[c]	+	+	−	+
Zygomycetes	−	−	−	+
Fusarium spp.	−	+	−	+/−

+, susceptibility; −, resistance; DD, dose-dependent susceptibility.
[a]Only caspofungin and anidulafungin approved for candidemia.
[b]*Aspergillus terreus* often resistant to amphotericin B.
[c]In vitro data suggest susceptibility to voriconazole, although no clinical trials have been performed to demonstrate efficacy.

The most common presentation is that seen in the diabetic, acidotic patient manifesting as rhinocerebral disease. Pulmonary involvement is the more typical presentation in the posttransplant immunosuppressed host. Although the incidence of zygomycosis remains relatively low, it has shown a definite increase in recent years because of the increasing pop-

TABLE 38.4	Indications/Dosing of Commonly Used Antifungal Agents	

Agent	Dose	Dosing adjustment necessary
	Invasive candidiasis	
Fluconazole	400–800 mg/day, IV or PO	Renal insufficiency
Voriconazole	IV: 6 mg/kg every 12 hr for 2 doses followed by 3–4 mg/kg every 12 hr PO: <40 kg–100 mg every 12 hr ≥40 kg–200 mg every 12 hr	Hepatic dysfunction IV vehicle may accumulate in renal insufficiency
Caspofungin	70 mg loading dose followed by 50 mg/day, IV	Hepatic dysfunction
Anidulafungin	200 mg loading dose followed by 100 mg/day, IV	None
Amphotericin B deoxycholate[a]	0.6–1 mg/day, IV	None, careful monitoring renal and liver function
Amphotericin B lipid formulations[a] ▪ Colloidal dispersion (Amphotec) ▪ Lipid complex (Abelcet) ▪ Liposomal (AmBisome)	3–5 mg/kg/day, IV	None, careful monitoring renal and liver function
	Invasive aspergillosis	
Itraconazole	IV: 200 mg every 12 hr for 4 doses followed by 200 mg/day PO: 200–400 mg/day	Multiple drug interactions IV not recommended for CrCl <30 mL/min
Voriconazole	As listed above	As listed above
Amphotericin B deoxycholate[a]	1–1.5 mg/kg/day	As listed above
Amphotericin B lipid formulations[a]	5 mg/kg/day, IV	As listed above Higher doses sometimes used
Caspofungin	As listed above	As listed above Not approved as first-line therapy
	Zygomycosis	
Amphotericin B deoxycholate[a]	1–1.5 mg/kg/day	As listed above
Amphotericin B lipid formulations[a]	≥5 mg/kg/day, IV[b]	As listed above Higher doses sometimes used

IV, intravenous; PO, by mouth; CrCl, creatine clearance.
[a]Bolus infusion of normal saline with dose recommended to decrease incidence of nephrotoxicity. Premedication with acetaminophen and diphenhydramine may decrease infusion-related reactions. In severe cases, hydrocortisone 50–100 mg IV may also be administered.
[b]Recommended start dose. Higher doses of 7.5–10 mg/kg/day are sometimes used, although there are no prospective trials of efficacy in zygomycosis.

ulation with immunosuppression. Furthermore, there has been an association between zygomycosis and those high-risk patients receiving long-term voriconazole as posttransplant prophylaxis, although a direct causal link has not been established. The organism can be difficult to grow on standard laboratory media; thus, diagnosis is often made based on biopsy demonstrating characteristic histopathology.

The typical broad-spectrum antifungal classes, echinocandins and azoles (including voriconazole), are not effective against Zygomycetes. High-dose amphotericin B is considered standard first-line therapy (e.g., amphotericin B deoxycholate 1 to 1.5 mg/kg/day or amphotericin B lipid formulations at doses of at least 5 mg/kg/day [Table 38.4]). Higher doses are often used (e.g., 7.5 to 10 mg/kg/day) although the efficacy of this approach has not been validated. Because of the angioinvasive nature and propensity to rapidly progress, urgent surgical intervention is always required for rhinocerebral disease and often for pulmonary disease. Posaconazole, recently approved for fungal prophylaxis in the severely immunosuppressed patient, has shown activity against Zygomycetes as salvage therapy in case reports; however, it is not currently approved by the Food and Drug Administration as standard treatment.

Suggested Reading

Blumberg HM, Jarvis WR, Soucie JM, et al. Risk factors for candidal bloodstream infections in surgical intensive care unit patients: the NEMIS Prospective Multicenter Study. *Clin Infect Dis.* 2001;33:177–186.
Multi-center prospective cohort study assessing risk factors for developments of candidemia.
Chayakulkeeree M, Ghannoum MA, Perfect JR. Zygomycosis: the re-emerging fungal infection. *Eur J Clin Microbiol Infect Dis.* 2006;25:215–229.
Review of zygomycosis including epidemiology, risk factors, diagnosis, and treatment.
Herbrecht R, Denning DW, Patterson TF, et al. Voriconazole versus amphotericin B for primary therapy of invasive aspergillosis. *N Engl J Med.* 2002;347:408–415.
Randomized, unblinded trial showing improved outcomes with voriconazole compared to amphotericin B as primary therapy for invasive aspergillosis
Marr KA, Boeckh M, Carter RA, et al. Combination antifungal therapy for invasive aspergillosis. *Clin Infect Dis.* 2004;39:797–802.
Retrospective analysis showing improved 3-month survival with combination of voriconazole and caspofungin when used as salvage therapy.
Mennink-Kersten MA, Donnelly JP, Verweij PE. Detection of circulating galactomannan for the diagnosis and management of invasive Aspergillosis. *Lancet Infect Dis* 2004;4 (6):349–357.
Review of utility of aspergillus galactomannan assay.
Morrell M, Fraser VJ, Kollef MH. Delaying the empiric treatment of *Candida* bloodstream infection until positive blood culture results are obtained: a potential risk factor for hospital mortality. *Antimicrob Agents Chemother.* 2005;49:3640–3645.
Retrospective cohort analysis showing higher mortality with delay in antifungal therapy.
Ostrosky-Zeichner L, Pappas PG. Invasive candidiasis in the intensive care unit. *Crit Care Med.* 2006;34:857–863.
Review of current epidemiologic trends and management strategies for invasive candidiasis in the ICU.
Pappas PG. Invasive candidiasis. *Infect Dis Clin North Am.* 2006;20:485–506.
Review of invasive candidiasis, including pathogenesis, epidemiology, clinical presentation, diagnosis, and treatment of invasive candidiasis.
Pappas PG, Rex JH, Sobel JD, et al. Guidelines for treatment of candidiasis. *Clin Infect Dis.* 2004;38:161–189.
Evidence-based review and treatment recommendations
Playford EG, Webster AC, Sorrell TC, et al. Antifungal agents for preventing fungal infections in non-neutropenic critically ill and surgical patients: systematic review and meta-analysis of randomized clinical trials. *J Antimicrob Chemother.* 2006;57:628–638.
Meta-analysis of twelve studies evaluating efficacy of antifungal prophylaxis in high-risk patients.
Segal BH, Walsh TJ. Current approaches to diagnosis and treatment of invasive aspergillosis. *Am J Respir Crit Care Med.* 2006;173:707–717.
Review of invasive aspergillosis including risk factors, diagnosis, and treatment strategies.

The care of the immunocompromised individual requires an understanding of the patient's form of immunosuppression and its relation to infection by opportunistic pathogens (Table 39.1). A broad differential diagnosis is often needed, and intensive care admission often necessitates empiric therapy until results of diagnostic testing are available. Management of infectious complications in this population is often best accomplished in conjunction with infectious disease consultation.

THE NEUTROPENIC PATIENT

Neutropenic sepsis is a major complication in individuals receiving chemotherapeutic agents, chronic immunosuppressive agents, or those with hematologic malignancies. Gram negative organisms, such as *Pseudomonas aeruginosa* and *Klebsiella* species, have been the leading cause of bacteremia in neutropenic patients. However, Gram positive organisms such as methicillin-resistant *Staphylococcus aureus*, resistant *Streptococcus viridans*, and *Enterococcus* species are being increasingly identified as causes of bacterial sepsis in immunocompromised populations, particularly in individuals with indwelling catheters or mucositis. Empiric broad-spectrum antibiotic coverage, including antipseudomonal coverage, should be initiated immediately after cultures have been obtained.

Although bacterial pathogens are the most common cause of sepsis, septic shock also occurs with fungal infections. There are multiple risk factors for fungemia, including prolonged neutropenia, presence of an indwelling catheter, and previous antibiotic exposure. *Candida albicans* is the most common fungal pathogen causing septic shock. When considering empiric therapy for candidemia, one must consider the institutional prevalence of fluconazole-resistant *Candida* species, especially in individuals who have previously received antifungal prophylaxis (Chapter 38). See Algorithm 39.1 for management of febrile neutropenia.

SOLID-ORGAN AND HEMATOPOIETIC STEM CELL TRANSPLANTATION

The risk of specific infectious complications in patients who have undergone transplantation often follows a temporal pattern (Table 39.2). Nosocomial infections, often relating to surgical and central venous catheter sites, predominate in the first month following transplantation. After the first month, immunosuppressive agents significantly increase the risk of opportunistic infections, with the transplanted organ often being the site of infection (Table 39.3). This risk is relative to the degree of immunosuppression required, typically lasting 3 to 6 months posttransplantation.

Graft-versus-host disease in allogeneic transplant recipients or graft rejection in solid-organ transplant recipients often necessitates further immunosuppression and prolongs this period of increased susceptibility. The routine use of prophylactic antibiotics and antivirals

TABLE 39.1	Common Opportunistic Pathogens Associated with Various Immunocompromised States

Host and source of infection	Pathogens
I. HIV-1 infection (CD4 = CD4$^+$ lymphocytes/mm^3)	
1. Pneumonia	▪ Bacterial pneumonia
	▪ *Pneumocystis jiroveci* (CD4 <200/mm^3)
	▪ Disseminated mycobacterial infection or histoplasmosis (CD4 <50/mm^3)
2. CNS infections	▪ *Cryptococcus* (CD4 <50/mm^3)
	▪ Toxoplasmosis (CD4 <100/mm^3)
	▪ EBV-associated lymphoma (CD4 <100/mm^3)
	▪ JC virus/PML (CD4 <50/mm^3)
	▪ CMV (CD4 <50/mm^3)
II. Solid-organ or bone marrow transplant	
1. Pneumonia	▪ Bacterial
	▪ CMV
	▪ *Aspergillus* sp
	▪ *Pneumocystis jiroveci*
2. CNS infections	▪ *Aspergillus* sp
	▪ *Nocardia* sp
	▪ *Listeria*
	▪ *Toxoplasma gondii*
	▪ HHV-6
	▪ VZV
	▪ Adenovirus
III. Asplenia	▪ *Encapsulated bacteria*
IV. Immunosuppressive medications	
1. Corticosteroids (>10 mg/day) / Methotrexate	▪ *Candida* sp
	▪ *Pneumocystis jiroveci*
	▪ *Nocardia* sp
	▪ *Mucor and Rhizopus* sp
	▪ *Aspergillus* sp
2. Anti-TNF agents	▪ *Mycobacterium tuberculosis*

EBV, Epstein-Barr virus; PML, progressive multifocal leukoencephalopathy; CMV, cytomegalovirus; HHV, human herpes virus; VZV, varicella-zoster virus; TNF, tumor necrosis factor.

can shift the onset of opportunistic infections to the time when prophylaxis is discontinued (especially with cytomegalovirus disease).

HUMAN IMMUNODEFICIENCY VIRUS

Patients with human immunodeficiency virus (HIV) represent another commonly encountered class of immunocompromised individuals. The CD4$^+$ lymphocyte count remains an accurate predictor of susceptibility to opportunistic infection in patients with HIV-1 infec-

ALGORITHM 39.1   **Management of Febrile Neutropenia**

Fever $\geq 38.3°C$ or persistently $\geq 38.0°C$ for at least 1 hr **AND** ANC $\leq 500/mm^3$ or ANC $\geq 500/mm^3$ with expected decline to $\leq 500/mm^3$

- Blood cultures $\times$ 2, urinalysis and urine culutre, chest radiograph
- Empiric Gram negative antibiotics*
- Vancomycin 1 g q12hr $\times$ 72 hr if indicated **

If suspected *intra-abdominal source*, consider adding Metronidazole 500 mg IV q8hr

New temp after afebrile ≥ 48 hr **OR** persistently febrile ≥ 72 hr and cultures negative

If *clinically unstable* consider adding double Gram negative coverage with aminoglycoside $\times$ 72 hr

Discontinue aminoglycoside if cultures negative after 72 hr

Clinically stable
- Culture negative: continue same regimen
- Culture positive: per culture and sensitivities

Clinically unstable
- Change Gram negative coverage
- Consider addition of Vancomycin **

(**) Indications for Vancomycin
- Severe mucositis
- Clinical evidence of catheter-related infection
- Known colonization with resistant streptococci or staphylococci
- Sudden temperature spike of $>40°C$
- Hypotension

Discontinue Vancomycin after 72 hr if cultures negative for coagulase negative staphylococci, methicillin-resistant *Staphylococcus aureus*, or cephalosporin-resistant streptococci

Persistently febrile ≥ 5 days and cultures negative
Consider addition of Vancomycin or antifungal agent (see Chapter)

(*) Gram-negative coverage

Cefepime 1 g IV q8hr **OR** Meropenem 500 mg IV q6hr **OR** Piperacillin-tazobactam 3.375 g IV q6hr

Penicillin allergy
Ciprofloxacin 400 mg IV q12 hr **OR** Aztreonam 2 g IV q8hr

ANC, absolute neutrophil count; IV, intravenous. (Adapted from Barnes-Jewish Hospital Stem Cell Unit Febrile Neutropenia Pathway.)

TABLE 39.2	Temporal Sequence of Infections after Transplantation		
Pathogen class	**1st Month**	**1–6 Months**	**6 Months and more**
Viral	HSV	CMV	CMV (if prophylaxis stopped)
		Adenovirus	Varicella-zoster virus
Fungal	*Candida*	*Aspergillus* species	*Cryptococcus neoformans*
		Pneumocystis jiroveci	
Bacterial	Nosocomial	*Nocardia* species	Encapsulated bacteria
	bacteria	*Listeria monocytogenes*	Mycobacteria

HSV, herpes simplex virus; CMV, cytomegalovirus.

tion. The advent of highly active antiretroviral therapy (HAART) has led to a significant decrease in intensive care unit admission and mortality resulting from infectious causes. If it is necessary to discontinue HAART medications (e.g., drugs cannot be given orally, dangerous potential drug interactions, or if the critical illness is suspected to be caused by these drugs themselves), then all antiretrovirals should generally be stopped simultaneously to reduce the risk of developing antiretroviral resistance.

Overall, bacterial pneumonia remains the most common pulmonary infection in patients with HIV. *Pneumocystis* pneumonia becomes more prevalent in patients with a CD4$^+$ lymphocyte count below 200 cells/mm^3. Patients not adherent to trimethoprim/sulfamethoxazole *Pneumocystis* pneumonia prophylaxis, or those receiving alternative regimens (e.g., dapsone, atovaquone, or inhaled pentamidine) may present with breakthrough infections. Disseminated fungal (particularly *Histoplasma capsulatum*) and mycobacterial pathogens should also be considered, especially in patients with a CD4$^+$ lymphocyte count <50 cells/mm^3.

Some HAART medications are associated with life-threatening toxicities. Nucleoside reverse transcriptase inhibitors, particularly stavudine (d4T), didanosine (ddI), and zidovudine (AZT) have been associated with severe lactic acidosis. Abacavir is associated with a 3% to 5% incidence of hypersensitivity manifested by malaise, gastrointestinal symptoms, and hypotension with or without rash, which is often life-threatening on rechallenge. Nevirapine has been implicated as a cause of fulminant hepatic failure and Stevens-Johnson syndrome.

Radiographic patterns of pulmonary infections and opportunistic infections of the central nervous system are discussed in Table 39.4 and 39.5 respectively. Table 39.6 addresses the diagnosis and treatment of opportunistic infections.

TABLE 39.3	Infections of Particular Importance in Transplant Recipients
Transplant site	**Infection**
Lung	Gram negative bacteria (especially *Pseudomonas aeruginosa*), CMV, *Aspergillus* species pulmonary infections
Cardiac	*Toxoplasma gondii* myocarditis
Liver	Hepatic abscesses with secondary candidal infections
HSCT	CMV, *Aspergillus*; oral, cutaneous, and enteric bacteria in setting of GVHD

CMV, cytomegalovirus; HSCT, hematopoietic stem cell transplantation; GVHD, graft-versus-host disease.

TABLE 39.4	Radiographic Patterns of Pulmonary Infections

Radiographic pattern	Pathogen
Focal infiltrate	**Bacteria,** *Aspergillus* sp, *Pneumocystis jiroveci*
Nodular infiltrates	**Bacteria** (*Staphylococcus aureus, Nocardia* sp, *Legionella spp*), **fungus** (*Aspergillus* sp, *Mucor* sp, *Coccidioides immitis*), typical and atypical **mycobacteria**
Diffuse interstitial	**Virus** (CMV, HSV, VZV, RSV, influenza, adenovirus), *Pneumocystis jiroveci* *Toxoplasma gondii*, bacteria (*Legionella* sp), fungus (*Aspergillus* sp, *Histoplasma capsulatum*)

CMV , cytomegalovirus; HSV, herpes simplex virus; VZV, varicella-zoster virus; RSV, respiratory syncytial virus.

TABLE 39.5	Opportunistic Pathogens of the Central Nervous System[a]

Bacterial	*Listeria monocytogenes*	*Nocardia sp*
Viral	**CMV**	*VZV*
	HSV	Enteroviruses
	HHV-6	**JC Virus (PML)** (CD4 $<50/mm^3$)
	Adenovirus	**EBV-lymphoma** (CD4 $<50/mm^3$)
Fungal	*Aspergillus*	**Cryptococcus** (CD4 $<50/mm^3$)
	Candida sp	
Other	Mycobacteria	Toxoplasmosis (CD4 $<50/mm^3$)

CMV, cytomegalovirus; VZV, varicella-zoster virus; HSV, herpes simplex virus; HHV, human herpes virus; PML, progressive multifocal leukoencephalopathy; EVB, Epstein-Barr virus.
[a]Items in **bold** predominate in human immunodeficiency virus-infected patients; *italicized* items predominate in transplant patients.

| TABLE 39.6 | Methods of Diagnosis and Treatment of Opportunistic Pathogens |

Pathogen	Diagnosis	Treatment
Bacteria		
Legionella sp	Sputum/BAL culture, urine antigen	Azithromycin, clarithromycin, respiratory fluoroquinolone
Nocardia sp	Sputum/biopsy modified AFB stain and culture	TMP/SMX
Mycobacterium tuberculosis	Induced sputum/BAL AFB stain and culture	Four-drug therapy
Non-Tb mycobacteria	Blood/biopsy AFB stain and culture	Variable
Fungi		
Pneumocystis jiroveci	Induced sputum/BAL DFA	TMP/SMX, add corticosteroids if Pao_2 <70 mm Hg
Candida sp	Blood culture, biopsy	See Chapter 38
Cryptococcus neoformans	Serum/CSF antigen, fungal isolator blood culture	Amphotericin B/flucytosine (acute)
Histoplasma capsulatum	Fungal isolator blood culture, urine antigen, histologic visualization	Amphotericin B/itraconazole
Aspergillus sp	BAL/TBB/sputum/biopsy fungal stain and culture, galactomannan antigen, histologic visualization	See Chapter 38
Viruses		
CMV	Blood CMV PCR or PP65 antigen, BAL/biopsy, shell vial culture; histological visualization	Ganciclovir or foscarnet
EBV	CSF PCR	Lymphoma chemotherapy
RSV	Nasopharyngeal swab/BAL DFA and culture	Palivizumab
HSV	CSF/Blood PCR	Acyclovir
HHV-6	CSF DNA PCR	Ganciclovir or foscarnet
Adenovirus	Nasopharyngeal swab/BAL DFA and culture	Cidofovir
Influenza	Nasopharyngeal swab/BAL DFA and culture	Oseltamivir/zanamivir
VZV	BAL/CSF PCR, histologic visualization	Acyclovir
Parasites		
Toxoplasma	CSF/Blood PCR	Pyrimethamine/sulfadiazine

BAL, bronchoalveolar lavage; AFB, acid-fast bacilli; TMP-SMX, trimethoprim-sulfamethoxazole; Tb, tuberculosis; DFA, direct fluorescent antibody testing; CSF, cerebrospinal fluid; TBB, transbronchial biopsy; CMV, cytomegalovirus; PCR, polymerase chain reaction; EBV, Epstein-Barr virus; RSV, respiratory syncytial virus; HSV, herpes simplex virus; HHV, human herpes virus.

Suggested Reading

Fishman JA, Rubin RH. Infection in organ-transplant recipients. *N Engl J Med.* 1998;338: 1741–1751.

A summary article discussing the risk and timetable of infection after transplantation as well as principles of therapy for infections of particular importance.

Gea-Banacloche JC, Opal SM, Jorgensen J et al. Sepsis associated with immunosuppressive medications: an evidence-based review. *Crit Care Med.* 2004;32[Suppl]:S578 –S590.

A review of immunosuppressive medications, their mechanism of action, and the diagnosis and management of specific infection.

Nichols WG. Management of infectious complications in the hematopoietic stem cell transplant recipient. *J Intens Care Med.* 2003;18:295–312.

A review article which includes discussion of etiologies and syndromic approach to infection with an emphasis on pulmonary presentations.

Picazo J. Management of febrile neutropenic patient: a consensus conference. *Clin Infect Dis.* 2004:39[Suppl 1]:S1–S6.

A review article that includes a discussion of the etiology and management of patients with neutropenic fever.

Rosen MJ, Narashimhan M. Critical care of immunocompromised patients: human immunodeficiency virus. *Crit Care Med.* 2006;34[9 Suppl]:S245–250.

A review of etiologies of ICU admission in HIV-positive individuals with an emphasis on pulmonary and medication-related complications.

40 PREVENTION OF INFECTION IN THE INTENSIVE CARE UNIT
Amy M. Hueffmeier

Infections acquired in the intensive care unit (ICU) are a significant contributor to morbidity and mortality in hospitalized patients. ICU-acquired infections increase patient length of stay and can lead to excess costs well beyond $50,000 per occurrence. Multiple measures to prevent the transmission of organisms within the ICU are necessary. Transmission-based precautions—including contact, droplet, and airborne—should be instituted when necessary, and health care worker compliance should be monitored. Contact precautions (gowns and gloves) should be instituted for those with antibiotic-resistant organisms such as methicillin-resistant *Staphylococcus aureus*, vancomycin-resistant *Enterococcus*, multiple-drug resistant Gram negative bacterium, and *Clostridium difficile*. Droplet precautions (donning a surgical mask) are necessary for large droplet infectious agents such as influenza and the meningococcus. Airborne precautions (N95 respirator and negative-pressure ventilation) are used for airborne infectious agents such as *Mycobacterium tuberculosis* and varicella. To prevent exposure to health care workers and other patients, transmission-based precautions must be instituted on first clinical suspicion. Infection Control should be consulted in cases in which a patient or health care worker exposure may have taken place.

Hospital-acquired infections that are device-associated, such as ventilator-associated pneumonia (VAP) and catheter-related bloodstream infections (BSI), pose the greatest risk to hospitalized patients. VAP is reported by the Centers for Disease Control (CDC) as the second most common hospital-acquired infection after Foley catheter-associated urinary tract infections. Central venous catheter-related BSIs are also a concern and can lead to other infectious complications such as endocarditis, septic thrombophlebitis, and osteomyelitis. Both the CDC and the Institute for Healthcare Quality Improvement (IHI) have published evidence-based guidelines for the prevention of device-associated infections and are summarized in Tables 40.1 and 40.2.

Foremost in prevention of device-associated infections is adequate hand hygiene prior to placing and/or handling an invasive device. Alcohol-based hand rubs placed at the bedside have been shown to increase compliance as well as maintain the skin integrity of health care workers' hands and should be encouraged. Alcohol hand rubs can be used whenever hands are not visibly soiled. Antimicrobial soaps should also be available in the ICU setting for use when hands are soiled or following a body substance exposure.

Invasive devices allow organisms a portal of entry during a time when the patient is particularly susceptible to infection. Therefore, general prevention measures should include a daily review of the necessity of all invasive devices and removing them as soon as possible. Clinician-driven ventilator-weaning protocols have been shown to be effective in decreasing VAP rates and are reviewed in Chapter 16.

Additional prevention measures are aimed at the placement and maintenance of the device. Recommendations to prevent VAP are aimed at preventing microaspiration and contamination of the ventilator circuit. Maintaining the head of the patient's bed at a minimum of 30 degrees assists with prevention of aspiration of gastric contents. Providing peptic ulcer disease prophylaxis with H_2-antagonists or proton pump inhibitors is also recommended to decrease VAP. CDC recommendations and IHI recommendations differ in that sucralfate is not preferred for prophylaxis by the IHI. In addition, the ventilator circuit should remain closed as much as possible and in-line suctioning devices should be collected after use.

TABLE 40.1	Summary of Recommendations for the Prevention of Ventilator-Associated Pneumonia

Education and training

Educate health care workers regarding the epidemiology of, and infection control procedures for, preventing health care-associated bacterial pneumonia in such manner as to ensure worker competency according to the worker's level of responsibility in the health care setting.

Hand hygiene and aseptic technique

Decontaminate hands with soap and water or with a waterless antiseptic agent after contact with mucous membranes, respiratory secretions, or objects contaminated with respiratory secretions, before and after contact with a patient who has an endotracheal or tracheostomy tube in place, before and after contact with any respiratory device that is used on patients, between contacts with different patients, after handling respiratory secretions or objects contaminated with secretions from one patient and before contact with another patient, object, or environmental surface; and between contacts with a contaminated body site and the respiratory tract of, or respiratory device on, the same patient.

When soiling with respiratory secretions from a patient is anticipated, wear a gown and change it after soiling occurs and before providing care to another patient. Use only sterile or pasteurized fluid to remove secretions from the suction catheter if the catheter is to be used for re-entry into the patient's lower respiratory tract. If the closed-system suction is used, change the in-line suction catheter when it malfunctions or becomes visibly soiled.

Prevention of aspiration

Remove devices such as endotracheal, tracheostomy, and/or enteral (i.e., oro- or nasogastric, or jejunal) tubes from patients and discontinue enteral-tube feeding as soon as the clinical indications for these are resolved.

As much as possible, avoid subjecting patients who have received mechanically assisted ventilation to repeat endotracheal intubations.

Use sucralfate, H_2-blockers, and/or proton-pump inhibitors for stress-bleeding prophylaxis in a patient receiving mechanical ventilation.

Unless contraindicated by the patient's condition, perform orotracheal rather than nasotracheal intubation.

If there is no medical contraindication, elevate at an angle of 30 to 45 degrees the head of the bed of a patient at high risk for aspiration pneumonia, e.g., a person receiving mechanically assisted ventilation and/or who has an enteral tube in place.

Routinely assess the patient's intestinal motility (e.g., by auscultating for bowel sounds and measuring residual gastric volume or abdominal girth) and adjust the rate and volume of enteral feeding to avoid regurgitation.

Routinely verify appropriate placement of the feeding tube.

Remove devices such as endotracheal, tracheostomy, and/or enteral (i.e., oro- or nasogastric, or jejunal) tubes from patients and discontinue enteral-tube feeding as soon as the clinical indications for these are resolved.

Ventilator circuits

Do not change routinely, on the basis of duration of use, the ventilator circuit (i.e., ventilator tubing, exhalation valve, and the attached humidifier) that is in use on an individual patient. Rather, change the circuit when it is visibly soiled or mechanically malfunctioning.

Periodically drain and discard any condensate that collects in the tubing of a mechanical ventilator, taking precautions not to allow condensate to drain toward the patient.

Use an endotracheal tube with a dorsal lumen above the endotracheal cuff to allow drainage (by continuous suctioning) of tracheal secretions that accumulate in the patient's subglottic area.

Before deflating the cuff of an endotracheal tube in preparation for tube removal, or before moving the tube, ensure that secretions are cleared from above the tube cuff.

Abbreviated and adopted from Tablan OC, Anderson LJ, Besser R, et al. Guidelines for preventing health-care-associated pneumonia, 2003. *MMWR.* 2004;53:RR03.

TABLE 40.2	Summary of Recommendations for the Prevention of Bloodstream Infection

Education and training

Educate health care workers regarding the indications for intravascular catheter use, proper procedures for the insertion and maintenance of intravascular catheters, and appropriate infection control measures to prevent intravascular catheter related infections.

Assess knowledge of and adherence to guidelines periodically for all persons who insert and manage intravascular catheters.

Designate trained personnel for the insertion and maintenance of intravascular catheters and designate personnel who have been trained and exhibit competency in the insertion of catheters to supervise trainees.

Hand hygiene and aseptic technique

Observe proper hand-hygiene procedures either by washing hands with conventional antiseptic-containing soap and water or with alcohol-based gels or foams. Observe hand hygiene before and after inserting, replacing, accessing, repairing, or dressing an intravascular catheter. Use of gloves does not obviate the need for hand hygiene.

Use aseptic technique including the use of a cap, mask, sterile gown, sterile gloves, and a large sterile sheet, for the insertion of CVCs (including peripherally inserted CVCs) or guidewire exchange.

Wear clean or sterile gloves when changing the dressing on intravascular catheters.

Disinfect clean skin with an appropriate antiseptic before catheter insertion and during dressing changes. Although a 2% chlorhexidine-based preparation is preferred, tincture of iodine, or 70% alcohol can be used.

Allow the antiseptic to remain on the insertion site and to air dry before catheter insertion. Allow povidone iodine to remain on the skin for at least 2 minutes, or longer if it is not yet dry before insertion

Do not apply organic solvents to the skin before insertion of catheters or during dressing changes.

Use either sterile gauze or sterile, transparent, semipermeable dressing to cover the catheter site. Replace catheter-site dressing if the dressing becomes damp, loosened, or visibly soiled.

Do not use topical antibiotic ointment or creams on insertion sites (except when using dialysis catheters) because of their potential to promote fungal infections and antimicrobial resistance.

Site and catheter selection

Select the catheter, insertion technique, and insertion site with the lowest risk for complications (infectious and noninfectious) for the anticipated type and duration of IV therapy. Use a subclavian site (rather than a jugular or a femoral site) in adult patients to minimize infection risk for nontunneled CVC placement when not contraindicated.

Use a CVC with the minimum number of ports or lumens essential for the management of the patient

Do not routinely replace central venous or arterial catheters solely for the purposes of reducing the incidence of infection.

Catheter discontinuation and replacement

Promptly remove any intravascular catheter that is no longer essential.

Replace any short-term CVC if purulence is observed at the insertion site.

Do not use guidewire exchanges to replace catheters in patients suspected of having catheter-related infection or routinely to prevent infection.

Pressure monitoring

Use disposable, rather than reusable, transducer assemblies when possible.

Replace disposable or reusable transducers at 96-hour intervals. Replace other components of the system (including the tubing, continuous-flush device, and flush solution) at the time the transducer is replaced.

When the pressure monitoring system is accessed through a diaphragm rather than a stopcock, wipe the diaphragm with an appropriate antiseptic before accessing the system

CVC, central venous catheter; IV, intravenous.
Abbreviated and adopted from O'Grady NP, Alexander M, Dellinger EP, et al. Guidelines for the prevention of intravascular catheter-related infections. *MMWR*. 2002;51:RR10.

Recommendations to prevent BSI include placing the central venous catheter (CVC) while observing aseptic technique and using maximal sterile barriers including sterile gown, sterile gloves, mask, and a full drape. Chlorhexidine is the preferred agent for skin antisepsis prior to CVC placement, as well as preparation during dressing changes. When selecting a site for insertion, the subclavian vein has the least instance of infection and should be favored when placing a CVC for purposes other than dialysis. A summary of CDC and IHI recommendations for CVC placement and maintenance can be viewed in Table 40.2. Clinical management of catheter-related BSIs is described in Chapter 37.

Finally, surveillance for ICU-acquired infections using standardized definitions should take place on a routine basis in order to monitor patient outcomes of care. Infection rates should be provided to ICU medical and nursing staff for review, and immediate action taken in times of increased rates. Additionally, prevention measures should be monitored regularly for consistency of application. For optimal reduction in the transmission of infections, all evidence-based prevention methods for each infection must be applied together. Such a concept is the basis for the IHI prevention of infection "bundles."

Suggested Reading

Ely EW, Meade MO, Haponik EF, et al. Mechanical ventilator weaning protocols driven by nonphysician health-care professionals: evidence-based clinical practice guidelines. *Chest.* 2001;120[6 Suppl]:454S–463S.
Recommendations based on four randomized controlled trials and 11 nonrandomized control trials for the protocol driven weaning of patients from mechanical ventilation.

O'Grady NP, Alexander M, Dellinger EP, et al. Guidelines for the prevention of intravascular catheter-related infections. *MMWR.* 2002;51:RR10.
CDC guidelines discussing the microbiology, pathogenesis, and prevention of intravascular catheter related infections.

Tablan OC, Anderson LJ, Besser R, et al. Guidelines for preventing health-care-associated pneumonia, 2003. *MMWR.* 2004;53:RR03.
CDC update discussing the prevention of HCAP, including prevention of transmission of bacterial, viral, and fungal pathogens.

The Hospital Infection Control Practices Advisory Committee. Guideline for isolation precautions in hospitals. Part II. Recommendations for isolation precautions in hospitals. *Am J Infect Control.* 1996;24:24–52.
The Centers for Disease Control and Prevention and the Hospital Infection Control Practices Advisory Committee's revised recommendations for isolation policies/procedures regarding hospital infection control.

Renal Disorders

ACUTE KIDNEY INJURY
Seth Goldberg and Anitha Vijayan

DEFINITION

Acute kidney injury (AKI) is primarily a disease of hospitalized patients. Although a precise definition is lacking, a general consensus defines acute kidney injury as a doubling in serum creatinine (or drop in glomerular filtration rate >50%) from baseline or a urine output of <0.5 mL/kg/hr for 12 hours, corresponding to the second stage in the RIFLE classification (Risk, Injury, Failure, Loss, End stage) of AKI (Table 41.1). AKI affects approximately 5% to 15% of patients in the intensive care setting, and is associated with mortality in excess of 50%. Prognosis depends on multiple factors, including comorbid conditions, sepsis, oliguria, and the need for renal replacement therapy. Oliguria is defined as urine output of <0.3 mL/kg/hr and is associated with a much poorer prognosis, with mortality rates in excess of 75%. Prognosis is also worse in the group that requires renal replacement therapy. Therefore, a timely diagnosis is critical, as identification and prompt treatment of the cause of renal injury may hasten recovery and avoid the need for dialysis.

DIAGNOSTIC APPROACH

In using an algorithmic approach in the evaluation of AKI, a key step early in the process is to delineate whether the insult is prerenal, intrinsic, or postrenal (Alg. 41.1). In many cases, the patient's history and careful review of the hospital course can provide the necessary information in making such a determination. It is important to look for the presence or absence of hypotension, blood loss, recent intravenous contrast administration, crush injury, new medications (particularly antibiotics), or recent invasive vascular procedures. In patients with mental status changes, obtaining history from a relative or friend is crucial as it can provide clues regarding overdose (e.g., acetaminophen or other medications) or accidental or deliberate ingestion (e.g., ethylene glycol, methanol). On examination, a careful assessment of the patient's volume status often yields valuable clues as to the nature and degree of renal dysfunction. The finding of lower abdominal distention makes bladder outlet obstruction highly likely as the cause of AKI. Systemic signs such as arthritis, rash, and mental status

TABLE 41.1	RIFLE[a] Classification	
Category	GFR and Serum creatinine criteria	Urine output
Risk	GFR down by >25% Creatinine up 1.5 times baseline	<0.5 mL/kg/hr for 6 hr
Injury	GFR down by >50% Creatinine up 2 times baseline	<0.5 mL/kg/hr for 12 hr
Failure	GFR down by >75% Creatinine up 3 times baseline	<0.3 mL/kg/hr for 24 hr or anuria for 12 hr
Loss	Persistent complete loss of kidney function for >4 wk	
End stage	End-stage kidney disease (>3 mo)	

GFR, glomerular filtration rate.
[a]RIFLE = risk, injury, failure, loss, and end stage.

changes also give valuable clues as these can be associated with systemic illnesses such as connective tissue disorders or vasculitides. Objective laboratory and radiologic data that are essential include renal function panel, urinalysis, fresh spun urine sediment, calculated fractional excretion of sodium (FENa), and, when obstruction is suspected, a renal ultrasound. Physician examination of the urinary sediment is essential as this has been shown to be superior to the laboratory examination. Based on the initial suspicion, additional diagnostic tests such as serologic studies or renal ultrasound with Doppler can be ordered. Renal biopsy is necessary to make a diagnosis when glomerulonephritis is suspected and is also used to make a definitive diagnosis of interstitial nephritis. The diagnosis of acute tubular necrosis (ATN) should be based on clinical findings and supporting laboratory data.

PRERENAL DISORDERS

In a prerenal process, there is no single diagnostic laboratory finding. The diagnosis is suspected from the history and physical examination. The kidney function is diminished secondarily through a decrease in the effective circulating volume. This includes not only systemic hypotension, but also congestive heart failure or advanced liver disease. Hypoperfusion may also result from the abdominal compartment syndrome, characterized by an intra-abdominal pressure exceeding 20 mm Hg. This may be secondary to intestinal ischemia or obstruction, massive intra-abdominal hemorrhage, or ascites under pressure.

Diagnosis

In prerenal AKI, the urine sediment is typically bland, lacking cells, crystals, and casts. The calculated fractional excretion of sodium (FENa) is <1%, reflecting the appropriate tubular response to hypoperfusion, retaining sodium and water in order to produce a concentrated urine (osmolality >500 mOsm/kg) of low sodium content. This test is most useful for oliguric patients not exposed to loop diuretics. For patients taking diuretics, the fractional excretion of urea (FEUrea) has been demonstrated to be vastly superior, with a specificity and sensitivity >95%. A FEUrea of <35% would suggest renal hypoperfusion. Other useful parameters in differentiating prerenal problems from tubular dysfunction include the blood urea nitrogen to creatinine ratio (>20:1) and the urine sodium (<20 mEq/L).

Management

Urgent reversal of the cause of renal hypoperfusion is critical because prolonged renal ischemia leads to renal tubular injury (Alg. 41.2). In cases of hypovolemia, or hypotension associated with anaphylaxis, sepsis, or other underfill conditions, volume resuscitation with normal saline, blood products, or other colloids should be administered without delay. Generally, a central venous pressure target of 8 to 12 mm Hg is used. In conditions associated

ALGORITHM 41.1   **Features to Distinguish Among the Three Categories of Acute Kidney Injury**

ACUTE KIDNEY INJURY

Bland urine sediment
- *FENa <1%*
- *FEUrea <35%*

- *Postvoid residual volume >100 mL*
- *Presence of hydronephrosis on renal ultrasound*

PRERENAL

- *FENa >1%*
- *FEUrea >50%*
- *Presence of cells or casts on urine microscopy*

POSTRENAL

Assess volume status

INTRINSIC

- Granular casts
- Recent ↓ BP
- Recent toxin/drug exposure

- WBC casts
- Urine eosinophils
- Peripheral eosinophilia
- New medication
- Skin rash

Dry mucosal membranes, decreased JVP, low CVP, absence of edema, low PCWP, negative fluid balance: VOLUME DEPLETION

Edema with hypotension, elevated JVP, respiratory compromise: DECREASED CARDIAC OUTPUT

Cold extremities, low SVR, high cardiac output, low PCWP: SEPSIS

- RBC casts
- Dysmorphic RBCs
- Pulmonary hemorrhage
- Systemic illness

TUBULAR: Acute tubular necrosis

INTERSTITIAL: Acute interstitial nephritis

GLOMERULAR: Vasculitic, microvascular, and immune complex disorders

FENa, fractional excretion of sodium; FEUrea, fractional excretion of urea; BP, blood pressure; WBC, white blood cell; JVP, jugular venous pressure; CVP, central venous pressure; PCWP, pulmonary capillary wedge pressure; SVR, systemic vascular resistance; RBC, red blood cell.

ALGORITHM 41.2   **Management of Prerenal Causes of Acute Kidney Injury**

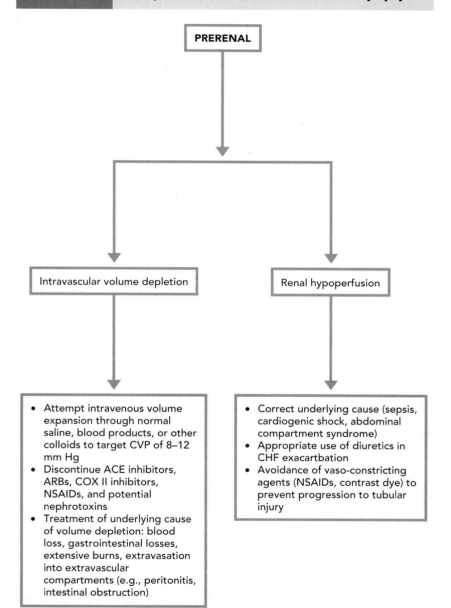

CVP, central venous pressure; ACE, angiotensin-converting enzyme; ARBs, angiotensin II receptor blockers; COX, cyclo-oxygenase; NSAIDs, nonsteroidal anti-inflammatory drugs; CHF, congestive heart failure.

TABLE 41.2	Hepatorenal Syndrome
Subtypes	Type 1: Rapidly progressive form, with doubling of serum creatinine to a level >2.5 mg/dL in <2 wk Type 2: Milder form with gradual, but steady, decline in kidney function, typically with GFR <40 mL/min and serum creatinine >1.5 mg/dL
Physical and laboratory findings	Oliguria (urine output <500 mL/day) Urine sodium <10 mEq/L Serum sodium <130 mEq/L
Medical management	Type 1: Splanchnic (octreotide) and peripheral (midodrine) vasoconstrictors combined with a volume expander (albumin) have shown short-term efficacy. Therapy should continue until renal function has reached plateau for 3–4 days, and may require total course of 2–3 wk. Suggested doses are listed below. Octreotide 25–50 mcg/hr intravenously Midodrine 5–7.5 orally, three times daily Albumin 1 g/kg/day (up to 100 g) intravenously Type 2: Avoid further renal or hepatic injury. During a therapeutic paracentesis, intravenous albumin (8 g/L of ascites removed) should be given. Other conservative measures include sodium restriction (60–90 mEq/day) and diuresis with spironolactone and furosemide (usually given in a 100:40 ratio of spironolactone to furosemide).

GFR, glomerular filtration rate.

with overfill situations, such as congestive heart failure or cardiogenic shock, treatment is directed at maximizing cardiac function, particularly with arterial afterload reduction. In severe liver disease, hepatorenal syndrome (HRS) can develop and lead to acute oliguric kidney injury. HRS is an atypical form of prerenal AKI as volume resuscitation does not result in reversal of the condition. Return of liver function, either spontaneously (e.g., acute hepatitis B, acetaminophen overdose) or through liver transplantation, results in renal recovery. HRS can be triggered by sepsis, spontaneous bacterial peritonitis, large-volume paracentesis, massive gastrointestinal hemorrhage, or an acute hepatic injury superimposed on cirrhosis.

The management of HRS is outlined in Table 41.2. Given the grim prognosis with or without renal replacement therapy, dialysis is generally reserved for patients with reversible conditions or waiting for liver transplantation. The molecular adsorbent recirculating system is a recent innovation found to improve short-term survival and perhaps serve as a bridge to transplantation. With this modified dialysis technique, an albumin-containing dialysate allows for the daily removal of water-soluble and albumin-bound toxins, along with inflammatory cytokines such as tumor necrosis factor-alpha and interleukin-6. The albumin in the dialysate can then be recirculated, avoiding the need for massive amounts of this expensive compound.

POSTRENAL DISORDERS

A postrenal process occurs when the glomerular filtration rate is decreased secondarily by an impediment to urine outflow. The increased pressure in the urinary tract is conveyed proximally from the obstruction, resulting in an increased intratubular hydrostatic pressure and therefore a decreased glomerular filtration rate. The diagnosis is typically made by finding hydronephrosis on renal ultrasound, and should be performed early if obstruction is suspected. In the intensive care setting, unless there is high index of suspicion based on the clinical picture (e.g., recent abdominal surgery, history of malignancy, anticholinergic medications), the yield from renal ultrasound is low. When obstruction is present, its location in the urinary tract frequently determines the method by which the obstruction is relieved (bladder catheterization, ureteral stenting, nephrostomy tubes). A simple method to rule out distal obstruction is to measure the postvoid residual urine volume. Postvoid residual urine volume of 100 mL is consistent with bladder outlet obstruction. In the intensive care unit, obstruction of the Foley catheter with clots should also be considered, and this is ruled out either by flushing the catheter or replacing it with a new one. Absence of hydronephrosis on renal ultrasound does not completely exclude obstruction. In the setting of severe volume depletion, extensive stone burden, or retroperitoneal fibrosis, dilatation of the calyces may not occur and ultrasound may be falsely negative. Patients with a single kidney, such as kidney transplant recipients or kidney donors, or those with prior nephrectomy for other conditions are especially vulnerable to AKI from obstruction, and ultrasound should be obtained as soon as possible. Ultrasound is also useful in documenting the presence of two kidneys, detecting other structural anomalies (polycystic kidneys), and measuring kidney size to aid in assessing the chronicity of the renal disease.

INTRINSIC RENAL DISORDERS

Intrinsic renal disease is present when the injury is at the level of the kidney parenchyma. Further classification depends on the area of involvement: glomeruli, microvasculature, tubules, or interstitium. Such differentiation can frequently be achieved by careful analysis of the urine sediment. Granular casts represent intact and degraded tubular cells and are most often seen in ATN. Red blood cell casts and dysmorphic red blood cells suggest a glomerular origin, and white blood cell casts are found when inflammation is present in the interstitium as in acute interstitial nephritis and pyelonephritis. It is important to note that red and white blood cell casts are fragile and that their absence alone does not necessarily eliminate their associated disorders from the differential diagnosis.

Acute Tubular Necrosis

Diagnosis
The most common cause of AKI in the ICU is ATN. This can result from prolonged prerenal states (e.g., volume depletion, hypotension, medications) or toxins (e.g., intravenous contrast, aminoglycosides, antiviral and antifungal medications, myoglobin).

Usually, the insults are sequential or simultaneous and no single precipitating factor can be identified (Table 41.3 contains a list of common causes of ATN). In the early stages of ischemic injury, tubular function is preserved and presentation is with the typical prerenal parameters of low FENa and bland sediment. However, with severe or prolonged injury, the renal tubules lose their ability to retain sodium and concentrate urine. The FENa is usually above 1% and the FEUrea is >50% with a serum blood urea nitrogen to creatinine <20:1. Examination of the urine sediment can reveal muddy brown granular casts. Because the glomeruli and interstitium are typically spared, other urinary findings such as heavy proteinuria and hematuria are absent.

Although the FENa is a useful indicator to differentiate between prerenal states and ATN, as noted, there are some exceptions to the rule. Certain conditions that result in ATN can demonstrate a low FENa. Contrast-induced nephropathy (CIN) typically manifests as nonoliguric AKI, occurring 3 to 5 days after a radiocontrast study. Early in the course of the renal injury, the FENa is low (<1%) despite the absence of systemic volume depletion. This is a result of the profound renal vasoconstriction caused by release of endothelin induced by intravenous contrast. Rhabdomyolysis and severe hemolysis release pigments (myoglobin and hemoglobin, respectively) that are toxic to the tubules, but may also present early in the course with a low FENa secondary to renal vasoconstriction.

Prevention
Preventive measures are the mainstay of management in AKI secondary to ATN. The majority of the preventive techniques have been studied in the area of CIN. Various intravenous hydration regimens have been shown to reduce the risk of renal injury in patients undergoing radiocontrast procedures, with regimens consisting of normal saline or sodium bicarbonate based intravenous fluids being most effective. "Renal-dose" dopamine infusions have *not* shown to be beneficial in prevention nor aid in recovery from renal injury. In fact, some studies have suggested increased risk for AKI, and thus there is no role for this

| TABLE 41.3 | Common Causes of Acute Tubular Necrosis |

Cause	Description
Ischemia	Can result from prolonged prerenal state (hypovolemia, sepsis, cardiogenic shock)
	Treat by addressing underlying cause and maximizing renal perfusion
Intravascular iodinated contrast	Initially causes profound vasoconstriction giving prerenal parameters (FENa <1%)
	Risk of renal failure is greater with pre-existing renal dysfunction, diabetes, large volume of contrast, volume depletion, high-osmolarity contrast
	Hydration with intravenous sodium chloride or sodium bicarbonate shown to be beneficial
	N-acetylcysteine orally or intravenously may help in prevention
Rhabdomyolysis	May result from crush injury, prolonged immobilization, status epilepticus, hyperthermia, statin medication, cocaine use, hypophosphatemia, snake venom
	Urine dipstick may show heme pigment in absence of RBCs on urine sediment
	FENa <1% in early stage secondary to potent vasoconstriction
	Creatine kinase peaks within 48 hr
	Treat with vigorous hydration (may require up to 10 liters of normal saline during 24 hr)
Hemoglobinuria	May result from hemolytic processes
	Urine dipstick may show heme pigment in absence of RBCs on urine sediment
	FENa <1% in early stage secondary to potent vasoconstriction
	Lactate dehydrogenase elevated, haptoglobin decreased, and unconjugated bilirubin elevated
	Treatment similar to rhabdomyolysis and focus on underlying cause
Aminoglycosides	Typically presents 5–7 days after initiating drug
	Length of treatment correlates with increased incidence of nephrotoxicity
	FENa >1% in most cases
	Usually nonoliguric
	Significant magnesium, potassium, and calcium lost in urine
	Recovery may take several weeks, even if drug is promptly discontinued
Amphotericin B	Effect is cumulative
	Causes intense renal vasoconstriction as well as direct toxicity to tubules by disrupting cell membrane
	Liposomal preparations have lower incidence of nephrotoxicity
Intravenous acyclovir	Insoluble precipitation in renal tubules resulting in obstruction
	Needle-shaped crystals may be seen on sediment
	Discontinuation of medicine usually reverses renal injury
Cisplatin	Dose-related and cumulative effect
	Profound renal magnesium wasting; also with hypokalemia
	Vigorous fluid hydration should be given prior to medication to increase urine flow
Ethylene glycol/methanol	Toxicity can result from ingestion of wood alcohol (methanol) or anti-freeze radiator fluid (ethylene glycol)
	Elevated osmol gap
	Anion gap metabolic acidosis presents later in course
	Oxalate crystals (envelope-shaped) are present in the urine sediment with ethylene glycol but not with methanol intoxication
	Fomepizole antidote is loaded as 15 mg/kg over 30 minutes, then 15 mg/kg every 12 hr
	Hemodialysis may be required to treat refractory metabolic acidosis

(continued)

TABLE 41.3	Common Causes of Acute Tubular Necrosis (*Continued*)

Cause	Description
Tumor lysis syndrome	Results after large numbers of neoplastic cells are rapidly killed after cancer treatment or tumor autolysis
	Intracellular contents are released into the circulation, including potassium, phosphate, and uric acid
	Most often seen 48–72 hr after cancer treatment
	Renal injury is through uric acid precipitation in the acidic environment of the tubules
	Hyperphosphatemia can lead to calcium-phosphate crystal formation and nephrocalcinosis
	Patients are typically oliguric; may require temporary dialysis, although usually reversible if addressed early
	Treatment is with aggressive hydration, allopurinol, rasburicase, and urinary alkalinization with isotonic sodium bicarbonate at 100 mL/hr

FENa, fractional excretion of sodium; RBCs, red blood cells.

agent in the prevention or treatment of AKI. N-acetylcysteine has been studied in small randomized trials, and its combination with intravenous hydration may result in a lower incidence of CIN. Although this advantage has not been clearly defined, N-acetylcysteine can be considered for use in high-risk patients undergoing contrast administration, given its low cost, safety, and potential benefit.

Management and Prognosis
There is no specific treatment for ATN once it has occurred. Therapy is generally supportive and includes the use of renal replacement if necessary. Management should also focus on avoiding additional nephrotoxic insults and adjusting drug doses appropriately for the level of renal function. Attempts to reverse the initial insult should be made, as well as avoiding further injury by restricting the use of iodinated contrast studies and nephrotoxic medications, if at all possible. Depending on the cause and severity, as well as the baseline renal function, renal recovery takes days, weeks, or even months, if at all. Generally, renal recovery can be expected in >90% of patients who previously had normal baseline function.

Glomerular and Microvascular Processes

Glomerular causes of intrinsic renal injury are much less common in an acute intensive care setting (Table 41.4). However, the pulmonary-renal syndromes of Wegener's granulomatosis and Goodpasture's disease should be considered in anyone presenting with simultaneous respiratory and renal dysfunction as they are universally fatal if not recognized and treated in a timely manner. The presence of red blood cell casts specifically suggests a glomerular origin. In the appropriate clinical setting, such findings should trigger a search for vasculitic and nephritic disorders. Serologic tests are helpful in these cases, although kidney biopsy may ultimately be necessary for a definitive diagnosis.

The anti-glomerular basement membrane antibody is a highly sensitive (95%) and specific test (99%) for Goodpasture's disease. In Wegener's granulomatosis, the serine proteinase 3 antibody (c-ANCA, cytoplasmic antineutrophil cytoplasmic antibody) is elevated in >75% of cases; approximately 20% have an elevated myeloperoxidase antibody (p-ANCA) and <5% are ANCA-negative. Treatment of these syndromes is with immediate intravenous corticosteroids (methylprednisolone at 7 mg/kg/day for 3 days followed by oral prednisone at 1 mg/kg/day up to 60 mg) and with cytotoxic immunosuppressants (cyclophosphamide at 2 to 3 mg/kg/day). Therapeutic plasma exchange is also employed in the treatment of Goodpasture's disease. In ANCA-positive vasculitis with advanced renal failure, one study demonstrated that the single predictive factor associated with long-term independence from dialysis was the use

TABLE 41.4	Selected Glomerular and Microvascular Disorders in the Intensive Care Unit	

Cause	Characteristics	Treatment
Immune complex	Hypocomplementemia seen with postinfectious GN, MPGN, SLE, endocarditis, and cryoglobulinemia	Treat the underlying cause in the secondary glomeru-lonephropathies
Pauci-immune	Pulmonary hemorrhage syndromes may have positive serum c-ANCA (Wegener's), or p-ANCA or anti-GBM antibody (Goodpasture's)	Supportive therapy for pulmonary compromise, mechanical ventilation if necessary Corticosteroids and cytotoxic agents
	Dysmorphic RBCs in urine suggest glomerular origin	Plasma exchange for Goodpasture or vasculitis with pulmonary hemorrhage or advanced renal failure
Microvascular	HUS and TTP with low platelets, hemolytic anemia, and schis-tocytes on peripheral smear Atheroembolic disease 3–5 days after invasive vascular procedure, with livedo reticularis and transient peripheral eosinophilia	TTP requires emergent plasma exchange Supportive care for HUS Refractory TTP may benefit from immunosuppression with prednisone and/or rituximab Atheroembolic disease: avoid anticoagulation and further vascular procedures

GN, glomerulonephritis; MPGN, membranoproliferative glomerulonephritis; SLE, systemic lupus erythe-matosus; c-ANCA, cytoplasmic antineutrophilic cytoplasmic antibody; p-ANCA, perinuclear antineu-trophilic cytoplasmic antibody; GBM, glomerular basement membrane; RBCs, red blood cells; HUS, hemolytic-uremic syndrome; TTP, thrombotic thrombocytopenic purpura.

of therapeutic plasma exchange. Therapeutic plasma exchange is also recommended for the management of pulmonary hemorrhage associated with ANCA-positive vasculitis. The differential diagnoses of pulmonary-renal syndromes include community-acquired pneumonia with sepsis and ATN, systemic lupus erythematosus with lung involvement and lupus nephritis, sarcoidosis, infections such as leptospirosis, legionella, ehrlichiosis (pneumonia with acute interstitial nephritis or ATN), and pancreatitis with pneumonia and ATN.

Hemolytic-uremic syndrome (HUS) and thrombotic thrombocytopenic purpura (TTP) are two distinct thrombotic microangiopathies that can result in renal injury. Although distinct clinical entities, they share several common precipitating factors such as human immunodeficiency virus infection, malignancy, calcineurin inhibitors, pregnancy, and chemotherapeutic agents. Ticlopidine and, less commonly, clopidogrel are more closely associated with TTP. In the diarrheal form of HUS, a Shiga-like toxin enters the circulation through compromised colonic epithelium and results in inflammation, endothelial injury, and thrombosis in the renal microvasculature. Therapy is supportive for HUS, with no proven efficacy of antibiotics, anticoagulation, immunoglobulin, or plasmapheresis. In the case of TTP, daily plasma volume exchange is a life-saving therapy and thus must not be delayed. In resistant cases, immunosuppression with high-dose prednisone and rituximab can be used. Splenectomy has been attempted in refractory cases, but is of unproven benefit.

Another microvascular process affecting the kidneys is atheroembolic disease. As hospitalized patients frequently undergo invasive vascular procedures, a high index of suspicion for atheroembolic disease should be maintained in the appropriate clinical setting. These patients demonstrate renal dysfunction days to weeks after aortic manipulation and follow a slowly progressive course. Transient peripheral eosinophilia may be present in >65% of cases. Skin findings are highly variable and may include livedo reticularis of the extremities

TABLE 41.5	Selected Causes of Acute Interstitial Nephritis in the Intensive Care Unit	

Agent	Diagnosis	Course
Methicillin	Hypersensitivity symptoms predominate with fever in 85% Urinary symptoms also very common, as >80% of patients with hematuria, pyuria, eosinophilia, eosinophiluria, or non-nephrotic proteinuria	Most patients recover renal function within 2 months, although nearly one-fifth require temporary dialysis CKD remains in only 10%
Rifampin	Gastrointestinal symptoms (nausea, vomiting, abdominal pain) Oligoanuria in nearly all patients Eosinophilia uncommon although other hematologic abnormalities such as hemolysis (25%) and thrombocytopenia (50%) may occur Elevation of liver enzymes seen in one-quarter of patients Anti-rifampin antibodies in almost all patients Renal biopsy rarely shows immune complex deposition at tubular basement membrane	Occurs 24 hr following dose with prior exposure (up to 1 year prior) Temporary dialysis required in almost all cases CKD remains in only 3%
Other antibiotics (sulfonamides, fluoroquinolones, beta-lactams)	Fever less common than with methicillin (45%), but with rash and flank pain in almost 50%; oliguria in 40% Urinary findings less common than with methicillin	Mean exposure to antibiotic is 10 days CKD remains in approximately 40%
NSAIDs	Hypersensitivity symptoms uncommon More than one-third with nephrotic range proteinuria Renal biopsy may show minimal change disease	Exposure is frequently months before presentation CKD remains in half of patients
Allopurinol	Hypersensitivity symptoms very common and robust with accumulation of metabolite oxypurinol Eosinophilia and hepatitis are common Renal biopsy may show immune complex deposition at tubular basement membrane	Mortality may be as high as 25%

(continued)

TABLE 41.5	Selected Causes of Acute Interstitial Nephritis in the Intensive Care Unit (*Continued*)	

Agent	Diagnosis	Course
Leptospiral nephropathy	Fever and jaundice are very common Other findings may include hepatomegaly, gingival and gastrointestinal bleeding, macroscopic hematuria, conjunctival suffusion, altered mental status; oligoanuria in nearly all patients Rhabdomyolysis, cholestatic hepatitis, hemolytic anemia, and thrombocytopenia are common findings Confirm with positive blood/ urine culture or serology Renal biopsy shows inflammation predominantly at proximal tubules, and may also show interstitial hemorrhage	Nephropathy occurs in 40% of leptospirosis Mortality is approximately 25% CKD remains in only 10%
Sarcoidosis	Extrarenal symptoms predominate, most commonly affecting lungs, eyes, and skin Eosinophilia seen in one-quarter of patients Hypercalcemia common despite advanced renal failure Hilar adenopathy on chest radiograph ACE levels not reliable with renal involvement Renal biopsy can show non-caseating granulomas and giant cells	Often remitting and relapsing course CKD remains in 90%

CKD, chronic kidney disease; NSAIDs, nonsteroidal anti-inflammatory drugs; ACE, angiotensin-converting enzyme.

or digital necrosis with gangrene (blue toe syndrome). Distal pulses are typically present as the occlusion is at the level of smaller arteries and arterioles. The general rule from the renal standpoint is a slow decline in renal function during months, with a third of the patients requiring dialysis. In multivisceral atheroembolic disease, manifested by intestinal ischemia, pancreatitis, and other systemic manifestations, 1-year mortality can be as high as 70%. Specific treatment options are limited but discontinuation of anticoagulation is essential because anticoagulation is a known trigger. Avoidance of further vascular procedures along with judicious control of blood pressure, use of angiotensin-converting enzyme inhibitors, and nutritional support have also been associated with better prognosis. A case series has noted a possible benefit from statin therapy in improving the long-term renal outcome.

Interstitial Processes

Acute interstitial nephritis (AIN) is an inflammatory process caused by medications or by infections. The classic triad of rash, eosinophilia, and fever is not commonly seen. Urinary findings suggestive of AIN include white blood cells, white blood cell casts, and eosinophils.

Eosinophiluria, however, has a sensitivity of only 67% and a specificity of 82%. Renal biopsy may be necessary to establish a definitive diagnosis. Beta-lactam antibiotics are common culprits, although nearly every antibiotic and many nonantibiotic medications have been implicated. Table 41.5 lists some of the more common causes of AIN in the ICU.

Removal of the offending agent or treatment of the underlying infectious disease is the mainstay of therapy. Recovery of renal function may occur during days to weeks, and sometimes during several months. Corticosteroid therapy can be used in severe cases, although there are no randomized trials to support this approach. Cyclophosphamide, mycophenolate mofetil, or other immunosuppressants can be considered in corticosteroid nonresponders after 2 to 3 weeks of therapy.

SUMMARY

An algorithmic approach to acute kidney injury can help uncover the etiology and devise a treatment plan. Early in the investigation, it is important to determine if the insult is prerenal, intrinsic, or postrenal in nature, using the history, physical examination, and laboratory and imaging studies. Physician examination of the urine sediment is of high value in identifying the underlying the renal disorder and may help in further classifying some disorders. Once a specific diagnosis is made, one can initiate specific treatment and, in many cases, achieve successful reversal of kidney injury

Suggested Reading

Arroyo V, Gines P, Gerbes AL, et al. Definition and diagnostic criteria of refractory ascites and hepatorenal syndrome in cirrhosis. *Hepatology*. 1996;23:164–176.
  Review of diagnostic criteria for hepatorenal syndrome.
Bellomo R, Ronco C, Kellum JA, et al. Acute renal failure. Definition, outcome measures, animal models, fluid therapy, and information technology needs: the second international consensus conference of the Acute Dialysis Quality Initiative (ADQI) Group. *Crit Care*. 2004;8:204–212.
  Consensus committee report for defining and managing renal injury.
Keyserling HF, Fielding JR, Mittelstaedt CA. Renal sonography in the intensive care unit: when is it necessary? *J Ultrasound Med*. 2002;21:517–520.
  Retrospective study of the efficacy of renal sonography in making a diagnosis.
Marenzi G, Assanelli E, Marana I, et al. N-acetylcysteine and contrast-induced nephropathy in primary angioplasty. *N Engl J Med*. 2006;354:2773–2782.
  Randomized controlled trial comparing high and low doses of N-acetylcysteine in preventing contrast-induced nephropathy.
Markowitz GS, Perazella MA. Drug-induced renal failure: a focus on tubulointerstitial disease. *Clin Chim Acta*. 2005;351:31–47.
  Review of pattern of drug-induced renal injury.
Merten GJ, Burgess WP, Gray LV, et al. Prevention of contrast-induced nephropathy with sodium bicarbonate: a randomized controlled trial. *JAMA*. 2004;291:2328–2334.
  Randomized study evaluating efficacy of sodium bicarbonate in preventing renal injury.
Mueller C, Buerkle G, Buettner HJ, et al. Prevention of contrast media-associated nephropathy: randomized comparison of 2 hydration regimens in 1620 patients undergoing coronary angioplasty. *Arch Intern Med*. 2002;162:329–336.
  Randomized study comparing different intravenous fluids in preventing renal injury.
Ruggenenti P, Noris M, Remuzzi G: Thrombotic microangiopathy, hemolytic uremic syndrome, and thrombotic thrombocytopenic purpura. *Kidney Int*. 2001;60:831–846.
  Review of TTP and HUS.
Tsai JJ, Yeun JY, Kumar VA, et al. Comparison and interpretation of urinalysis performed by a nephrologists versus a hospital-based clinical laboratory. *Am J Kidney Dis*. 2005;46:820–829.
  Blinded study comparing ability of different examiners in evaluating urinalyses.
Tublin ME, Murphy ME, Tessler FN. Current concepts in contrast media-induced nephropathy. *Am J Roentgenol*. 1998;171:933–939.
  Review of contrast-induced renal injury.

42

RENAL REPLACEMENT THERAPY
Seth Goldberg and Anitha Vijayan

The principal strategy regarding acute kidney injury, particularly in the intensive care setting, is prevention. Once it occurs, the presentation and course are variable and treatment is generally supportive. The optimal time to initiate renal replacement therapy remains unknown.

INDICATIONS

Conventional factors that trigger renal replacement therapy include metabolic acidosis, hyperkalemia, volume overload, and severe uremic symptoms refractory to medical management.

Acidosis

Refractory metabolic acidosis is an acute indication for dialytic therapy in the severely ill patient. Progressive acidemia can develop as the kidneys lose their ability to reclaim bicarbonate and excrete organic acids. More commonly in the intensive care setting, tissue hypoperfusion with multiorgan system failure results in a severe lactic acidosis. Aggressive alkali therapy is controversial in this setting and also frequently encounters problems with volume overload. Initiation of renal replacement therapy would obviate the concern over volume overload and could restore the blood pH to its physiologic range.

Hyperkalemia

Electrolyte disturbances, especially hyperkalemia, can be rapidly fatal and need to be addressed promptly. Temporizing measures include intravenous calcium to stabilize the myocardial cell membrane as well as insulin (with dextrose 50% in water), sodium bicarbonate, and inhaled beta-agonists to promote an intracellular shift in potassium. Elimination of potassium from the body can be achieved with enteric binding resins, but this effect is unpredictable and inefficient.

In the volume-depleted patient, aggressive fluid resuscitation can enhance sodium delivery to the distal nephron and encourage kaliuresis at the sodium-potassium exchanger (see Chapter 23 for further discussion). When these efforts are unsuccessful, urgent dialytic therapy becomes necessary. A dialysate potassium concentration as low as 0 mEq/L can be used in order to achieve an acute reduction in plasma potassium. Continuous renal replacement therapies with high flow rates of dialysate and replacement fluid solutions (35 mL/kg/hr) using 0 mEq/L potassium solutions can also achieve a significant reduction in potassium rapidly.

Volume Overload

Volume overload is another frequently encountered problem in an intensive care unit. Although studies investigating the use of diuretics in this setting have shown conflicting results as to benefit as well as to harm, it is not unreasonable to offer a trial of high-dose loop diuretics prior to initiating renal replacement. However, randomized trials studying the use of diuretics in acute kidney injury have not demonstrated any survival advantage, improvement in renal recovery, or avoidance of dialytic therapy. Respiratory compromise with pulmonary edema or significant soft tissue edema that impairs the barrier defense of the skin is the most common subjective criteria for initiating renal replacement in the oliguric patient. If diuretics are being attempted, then a high dose of loop diuretic (160 to 200 mg of furosemide) should be given intravenously in order for the drug to be delivered to the tubules. If there is no improvement in urine output in 24 hours, then diuretics should be discontinued.

Uremia

With progressive renal dysfunction, there is an impaired ability to excrete nitrogenous wastes and glycosylated end-products. It is generally accepted that blood urea nitrogen (BUN) levels can serve as a surrogate marker for toxin accumulation. Unfortunately, many signs and symptoms commonly found in the uremic syndrome do not always correlate with BUN levels and therefore there is no established objective cutoff beyond which dialytic therapy is recommended. Rather, acute indications for initiating urgent renal replacement therapy center on the presence of specific clinical findings, namely uremic encephalopathy and uremic pericarditis. The latter possesses a high risk of converting into hemorrhagic pericarditis with cardiac tamponade. There are some retrospective case series that suggest that initiation of hemodialysis with a BUN level <60 mg/dL offers survival benefit over those initiated later. However, this has to be studied and confirmed in randomized trials before this policy can be recommended universally.

MODALITIES

Once the decision has been made to initiate renal replacement therapy, one needs to select a modality. The available modalities are intermittent hemodialysis (IHD), continuous renal replacement therapy (CRRT), or peritoneal dialysis. The choice depends on the availability of therapies at the institution, physician preference, the patient's hemodynamic status, and the presence of comorbid conditions. Patients with sepsis or hepatic failure may have potential benefits with continuous therapies. Intermittent modalities generally cause greater fluctuations in blood pressure and produce greater fluid shifts in a short amount of time. Continuous modalities allow for the same solute clearance and fluid removal, but spread out during a 24-hour period, and thus are favored in hemodynamically unstable patients. With slower flow rates, CRRT requires continuous anticoagulation, generally accomplished with heparin. In patients intolerant to heparin, citrate anticoagulation is used with calcium replacement given via a central venous line. It is important to closely monitor ionized calcium levels when citrate is used.

In the United States, CRRT is performed in approximately 30% of patients with acute kidney injury and has almost completely replaced peritoneal dialysis in these patients. However, although CRRT has some potential benefits over IHD, as seen in randomized trials, CRRT has not shown improved survival over IHD in critically ill patients. Likewise, randomized trials have not shown a difference in time to renal recovery or length of intensive care unit or hospital stay between groups treated with IHD versus CRRT. Table 42.1 lists the advantages and disadvantages of the different modalities.

The ideal dose of dialytic therapy in critically ill patients has not yet been conclusively determined. Evidence from end-stage, dialysis-dependent patients suggests that a thrice-weekly regimen should be performed with a urea reduction of approximately 70% per session. However, in the acutely ill intensive care population, these calculations are not always equivalent. The actual clearances are approximately 25% lower what would be expected in a stable chronic dialysis patient, and thus it has been proposed that additional benefit may be derived from higher treatment doses, more frequent treatments, or greater fluid hemofiltration. A few small studies have shown a survival advantage in critically ill patients who underwent either high-flow CRRT (35 mL/kg/hr) or more frequent dialysis. The question of whether intensive dialytic therapy improves survival is currently being studied in a large multicenter clinical trial.

DRUG DOSING IN CRRT

Various factors affect the dosing of medications in the setting of CRRT. Unlike IHD, the clearance of medications is continuous, controlled, and predictable. Patient, drug, and dialysis characteristics determine appropriate dosing schedules to be used.

Total clearance of any compound depends on its elimination by nonrenal, residual renal, and CRRT functions. Generally, the nonrenal clearance is taken to be constant,

TABLE 42.1	Renal Replacement Modalities

Modality	Advantages	Disadvantages
Intermittent hemodialysis (IHD)	High-efficiency transport of solutes when rapid clearance of toxins or electrolytes is required Allows time for off-unit testing	Hemodynamic intolerance secondary to fluid shifts "Saw-tooth" pattern of metabolic control between sessions
Continuous renal replacement therapy	Gentler hemodynamic shifts than IHD Steady solute control	Continuous need for specialized nursing Requires continuous anticoagulation (heparin vs. citrate)
Peritoneal dialysis	Gentler hemodynamic shifts than IHD	Requires invasion of peritoneal cavity, which may not be possible in postoperative patients Less predictable fluid removal rates

although in critically ill patients with multiorgan system failure, this component may be less than predicted. Therapeutic doses have been calculated for a variety of drugs used in the intensive care unit. The recommended doses of some of the more commonly prescribed antibiotics are listed in Table 42.2.

COMPLICATIONS OF RENAL REPLACEMENT THERAPY

As with any procedure, there are certain complications and adverse events that can be associated with renal replacement therapies. Vigilance for such complications and their immediate rectification are essential to prevent life-threatening situations, especially in the vulnerable

TABLE 42.2	Dosing of Common Antimicrobial Agents During Continuous Renal Replacement Therapy (CRRT)[a]

Medication	Dosing In CRRT
Vancomycin	500 mg q day or bid
Cefepime	2,000 mg q day or bid
Ceftazidime	500–1,000 mg bid
Cefotaxime	2,000 mg bid
Ceftriaxone	2,000 mg q day
Imipenem	250–500 mg tid or qid
Ciprofloxacin	200 mg q day or bid
Metronidazole	500 mg tid
Piperacillin	4,000 mg tid
Amikacin	250 mg q day or bid
Tobramycin	100 mg q day
Fluconazole	100–200 mg q day
Acyclovir	3.5 mg/kg q day

bid, two times a day; tid, three times a day.
[a]Ultrafiltration rates of 20–30 mL/min.

population of the intensive care unit. Some are related to the procedure itself, and others are a result of fluid removal or electrolyte and acid-base disturbances. In addition, the necessity for a central venous catheter places the patient at risk for infections complications.

Hypotension

Intradialytic hypotension can occur in all clinical settings with all modalities, although it is more commonly seen with IHD. Volume-depleted and septic patients are at heightened risk, and careful attention to the physical examination and invasive hemodynamic monitoring when indicated can help ensure adequate volume resuscitation prior to initiating the dialysis session. A target central venous pressure of 8 to 12 mm Hg can be used in these settings and may dictate a reduction or stoppage of fluid ultrafiltration. Other factors can also result in intradialytic hypotension. The rapid clearance of uremic solutes can lower the serum osmolality and lead to a fluid shift toward the intracellular space, depleting the intravascular volume. A normal saline bolus of 250 mL or administration of 25% albumin in 100 mL can be used as initial management steps in the treatment of intradialytic hypotension, and ultrafiltration may need to be turned off. The dialysate temperature can be decreased to promote vasoconstriction. Patients who are persistently hypotensive may need to switch to a continuous modality.

Arrhythmias

Cardiac arrhythmias can occur in the setting of rapid electrolyte shifts in acute hemodialysis. In chronic dialysis, a bath with a potassium concentration of 2 to 3 mEq/L is frequently used. However, when hyperkalemia necessitates a dialysate with a potassium concentration of 0 to 1 mEq/L, it is important to monitor hourly potassium levels. A low-potassium dialysate should not be used longer than 1 hour unless the serum potassium remains critically elevated. Patients on digitalis are especially sensitive to hypokalemia. Supraventricular arrhythmias can also be triggered during the placement of the dialysis catheter, by a malpositioned dialysis catheter, and sometimes during dialysis. If the arrhythmia is resulting in hemodynamic compromise, then therapy is discontinued immediately and cardioversion should be attempted.

CENTRAL VENOUS CATHETER PROBLEMS

The dialysis catheter itself can also pose problems. When needed acutely, a nontunneled catheter can be inserted into a central vein at the bedside. When infection and bacteremia occur, prompt catheter removal is generally recommended unless vascular access is especially difficult. Thrombus or fibrin sheaths can form around or inside the catheters causing inadequate blood flows for dialysis. Even though heparin is usually instilled into the hub of the catheter after each dialysis, this does not necessary prevent the clot formation. An attempt at clot lysis can be made by instilling 2 mg of alteplase into each catheter lumen. The catheter is then capped for 2–3 hours and the medication is aspirated before dialysis is attempted. Alteplase should not be administered systemically for this purpose. If the catheter malfunctions, then it may be changed over guidewire or replaced completely.

In patients with chronic kidney disease, subclavian veins are not used for dialysis catheters as there is a high risk of subclavian venous stenosis, which can prevent the future placement of an arteriovenous fistula for dialysis in that extremity. There are no data to suggest that tunneled catheters are more beneficial regarding infection rates or adequacy of dialysis in intensive care patients with acute kidney injury. Tunneled catheters are typically used in patients with multiple malfunctioning temporary catheters, poor chance for early renal recovery, or for those being transferred out of the intensive care unit to a different facility. For clotted tunneled catheters, interventional radiology consultation is required to perform endoluminal brushing to dislodge thrombi and fibrin sheaths.

Dialyzer Reactions

Dialyzer reactions are rare during hemodialysis. Type A reactions are estimated to occur in 4 of every 100,000 sessions and present in the first few minutes once the blood in the circuit returns to the patient. Symptoms are varied and may include urticaria, flushing, chest pain, back pain, dyspnea, vomiting, and chills. Severe cases can progress to hypotension, cardiac arrest, and death. The cause for this reaction is believed to be related to inadequate rinsing of the dialyzer (to clear ethylene oxide used for sterilization) prior to its first use or from contamination with bacterial toxins. Type A reactions are treated by immediately discontinuing the dialysis session and discarding the blood in the circuit. Further therapy with epinephrine or bronchodilators depends on the severity of the reaction.

Type B reactions are more common, and are distinguished from Type A reactions in that they are usually less severe and present later, usually after the first 15 minutes. They occur in 3% to 4% of sessions and also present with chest pain, back pain, dyspnea, or gastrointestinal symptoms. If the symptoms are not severe, then dialysis is continued and the symptoms slowly resolve. Treatment is supportive, with appropriate use of intravenous saline, analgesics, and antiemetics.

Problems Associated with CRRT

One of the advantages of CRRT over IHD is that the slower blood flow rates place a gentler hemodynamic burden on unstable patients. However, hypotension can still occur in this group, especially when high ultrafiltration rates are attempted. Some adverse events are specific to continuous modalities, mostly related to electrolyte abnormalities. Uninterrupted high-flow CRRT can cause dramatic hypophosphatemia. Hypokalemia and hypomagnesemia can also result from CRRT and serum electrolytes need to be monitored at least twice daily to avoid such complications.

Given its lower flow rates, CRRT requires some form of anticoagulation to prevent clotting in the extracorporeal circuit. Heparin is the preferred anticoagulant. In cases of heparin-induced thrombocytopenia, the direct thrombin inhibitor argatroban can be used. When systemic anticoagulation is contraindicated, citrate can be used regionally in the dialysis circuit. Citrate chelates calcium in the serum and inhibits activation of the coagulation cascade. The citrate is quickly metabolized to bicarbonate in the liver and thus does not result in systemic anticoagulation. Calcium is replaced through a separate central venous line and this process requires close monitoring of serum ionized calcium levels. With the breakdown of citrate to bicarbonate, the development of a metabolic alkalosis is another concern with this form of anticoagulation. Metabolic alkalosis can be treated by changing the replacement fluid to sodium chloride from a bicarbonate-based product.

Hypothermia is a well-known complication of CRRT. Significant amounts of heat are lost from the slow-flowing extracorporeal circuit and can cause drops in body temperature of 2°C to 5°C. This can be addressed by warming the replacement fluid being infused or by rewarming the blood returning to the patient through specialized devices that can be attached to the machine. However, this poses a problem regarding the detection of fever. Unpublished reports have shown no advantage to checking routine cultures; therefore, reliance on the other clinical signs of infection is needed.

SUMMARY

Renal replacement therapy is initiated when more conservative medical management has failed to control the fluid, electrolyte, and metabolic complications of acute kidney injury. Several modalities are available to the clinician, and selection between intermittent and continuous forms depends on the availability at the institution, the patient's hemodynamic stability, and comorbid illnesses. Despite the overall safety of these procedures, complications and adverse events can occur, requiring meticulous attention and, in some cases, frequent laboratory monitoring to anticipate and prevent their occurrence.

Suggested Reading

Brause M, Nuemann A, Schumacher T, et al. Effect of filtration volume of continuous venovenous hemofiltration in the treatment of patients with acute renal failure in intensive care units. *Crit Care Med.* 2003;31:841–846.
Prospective pilot study comparing patients dialyzed with different target Kt/V.

Cho KC, Himmelfarb J, Paganini E, et al. Survival by dialysis modality in critically ill patients with acute kidney injury. *J Am Soc Nephrol.* 2006;17:3132–3138.
Multicenter observational study comparing continuous and intermittent dialysis.

Kellum J, Angus DC, Johnson JP, et al. Continuous versus intermittent renal replacement therapy: a meta-analysis. *Intens Care Med.* 2002;28:29–37.
Meta-analysis comparing continuous and intermittent dialysis.
Kroh UF, Holl TJ, Steinhauber W. Management of drug dosing in continuous renal replacement therapy. *Semin Dial.* 1996;9:161–165.
Review of factors determining drug dosing in CRRT.
O'Reilly P, Tolwani A. Renal replacement therapy III: IHD, CRRT, SLED. *Crit Care Clin.* 2005;21:367–378.
Review of replacement options.
Palevsky PM. Renal replacement therapy I: indications and timing. *Crit Care Clin.* 2005;21: 347–356.
Review of dialytic indications.
Ricci Z, Ronco C. Renal replacement therapy II: dialysis dose. *Crit Care Clin.* 2005;21: 357–366.
Review of dialysis dosing.
Ronco C, Bellomo R, Homel P, et al. Effects of different doses in continuous veno-venous haemofiltration on outcomes of acute renal failure: a prospective randomised trial. *Lancet.* 2000;356:26–30.
Randomized study comparing patients assigned to different ultrafiltration doses.
Schiffl H, Lang SM, Fischer R. Daily hemodialysis and the outcome of acute renal failure. *N Engl J Med.* 2002;346:305–310.
Randomized study comparing daily and intermittent conventional dialysis.
Vinsonneau C, Camus C, Combes A, et al. Continuous venovenous haemodiafiltration versus intermittent haemodialysis for acute renal failure in patients with multiple-organ dysfunction syndrome: a multicentre randomised trial. *Lancet.* 2006;368:379–385.
Multicenter randomized study comparing continuous and intermittent dialysis.

XII   Hepatic Diseases

43   ACUTE FULMINANT HEPATIC FAILURE
Sumeet Asrani and Jeffrey S. Crippin

Fulminant hepatic failure (FHF) is a rare entity characterized by coagulopathy, encephalopathy, and acute hepatic failure in the absence of pre-existing cirrhosis (Table 43.1). Exceptions to the absence of pre-existing liver disease include autoimmune hepatitis and Wilson's disease, if the disease has only been recognized within the last 26 weeks. Approximately 2,000 cases of FHF are reported per year, with high morbidity and mortality noted in patients who do not receive hepatic transplantation.

PROGNOSTIC INDICATORS

The timing of the manifestations of FHF can predict prognosis. Jaundice preceding encephalopathy by at least 1 week portends a poorer prognosis. FHF for >2 weeks is associated with a higher likelihood of portal hypertension and mortality. Degree of encephalopathy is another strong predictor of outcome (Table 43.2). Patients with grade II encephalopathy have a 65% to 70% chance of survival, whereas patients with grade III or IV have a 30% to 50% and 20% chance of survival, respectively. The King's College Criteria (Table 43.3) are important prognostic indicators. In patients with nonacetaminophen- associated FHF, the presence of a single factor is associated with a mortality rate of 80% and the rate is 95% with any three factors. In patients with acetaminophen hepatotoxicity and FHF, a single risk factor is associated with a mortality of 55%, and the presence of severe acidosis confers a 95% mortality.

CAUSES AND DIAGNOSIS

Because of the high morbidity and mortality associated with FHF, it is imperative to ascertain the etiology of the liver failure as it can further dictate etiology-specific treatment. A prospective multicenter review of 308 patients enrolled between 1998 and 2001 by the Acute Liver Failure Study Group found the following distribution of causes:

TABLE 43.1	Diagnosis and Causes of Acute Liver Failure

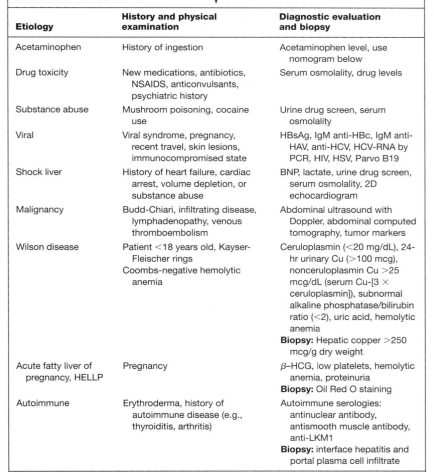

- Acute hepatic disease <26 weeks without evidence of pre-existing cirrhosis
- Encephalopathy
- Coagulopathy (INR >1.5)

Etiology	History and physical examination	Diagnostic evaluation and biopsy
Acetaminophen	History of ingestion	Acetaminophen level, use nomogram below
Drug toxicity	New medications, antibiotics, NSAIDS, anticonvulsants, psychiatric history	Serum osmolality, drug levels
Substance abuse	Mushroom poisoning, cocaine use	Urine drug screen, serum osmolality
Viral	Viral syndrome, pregnancy, recent travel, skin lesions, immunocompromised state	HBsAg, IgM anti-HBc, IgM anti-HAV, anti-HCV, HCV-RNA by PCR, HIV, HSV, Parvo B19
Shock liver	History of heart failure, cardiac arrest, volume depletion, or substance abuse	BNP, lactate, urine drug screen, serum osmolality, 2D echocardiogram
Malignancy	Budd-Chiari, infiltrating disease, lymphadenopathy, venous thromboembolism	Abdominal ultrasound with Doppler, abdominal computed tomography, tumor markers
Wilson disease	Patient <18 years old, Kayser-Fleischer rings Coombs-negative hemolytic anemia	Ceruloplasmin (<20 mg/dL), 24-hr urinary Cu (>100 mcg), nonceruloplasmin Cu >25 mcg/dL (serum Cu-[3 × ceruloplasmin]), subnormal alkaline phosphatase/bilirubin ratio (<2), uric acid, hemolytic anemia **Biopsy:** Hepatic copper >250 mcg/g dry weight
Acute fatty liver of pregnancy, HELLP	Pregnancy	β–HCG, low platelets, hemolytic anemia, proteinuria **Biopsy:** Oil Red O staining
Autoimmune	Erythroderma, history of autoimmune disease (e.g., thyroiditis, arthritis)	Autoimmune serologies: antinuclear antibody, antismooth muscle antibody, anti-LKM1 **Biopsy:** interface hepatitis and portal plasma cell infiltrate

INR, international normalized ratio; NSAIDs, nonsteroidal anti-inflammatory drugs; HBsAg, hepatitis B surface antigen; IgM, immunoglobin M; HBc, hepatitis B core antigen; HAV, hepatitis A virus; HCV, hepatitis C virus; PCR, polymerase chain reaction; HIV, human immunodeficiency virus; HSV, herpes simplex virus; BNP, brain natriuetic peptide; 2D, two-dimensional; β–HCG, beta-human chorionic gonadotropin; LKM1, liver kidney microsomal type 1.

TABLE 43.2	West Haven Criteria for Semiquantative Grading of Mental State

Grade	Criteria
I	■ Trivial lack of awareness ■ Euphoria or anxiety ■ Shortened attention span ■ Impaired performance of addition
II	■ Lethargy or apathy ■ Minimal disorientation for time or place ■ Subtle personality change ■ Inappropriate behavior ■ Impaired performance of subtraction
III	■ Somnolence to semistupor, but responsive to verbal stimuli ■ Confusion ■ Gross disorientation
IV	■ Coma (unresponsive to verbal or noxious stimuli)

From Atterbury C, Maddrey VV, Conn H Neomycin-sorbitol and lactulose in the treatment of acute portal-systemic encephalopathy *Am J Dig Dis*. 1978;23:398–406, with permission.

acetaminophen overdose (39%), indeterminate (17%), idiosyncratic drug reactions (13%), and viral hepatitis with hepatitis A virus or hepatitis B virus (12%). Table 43.1 delineates possible cause of FHF as well as the diagnostic evaluation to determine the cause. The timing of the presentation is also important. An illness of <1 week suggests ischemic hepatopathy or acetaminophen overdose. An illness >4 weeks suggests an unknown or viral etiology. On presentation, initial laboratory analysis should include electrolytes, liver biochemistries, serum creatinine, prothrombin time and international normalized ratio, complete blood cell count, arterial blood gas, acetaminophen level, acute viral hepatitis panel, and toxicology screen. Table 43.1 provides additional guidance for diagnostic evaluation.

TABLE 43.3	King's College Hospital Criteria for Liver Transplantation in Fulminant Hepatic Failure

Acetaminophen-induced disease	Arterial pH <7.30 *OR* Prothrombin time >100 seconds *AND* Creatinine >3.4 mg/dL *AND* Grade III or IV encephalopathy
Nonacetaminophen-induced disease	Prothrombin time >100 seconds (regardless of encephalopathy grade) *OR* Any three of the following (regardless of encephalopathy grade): ■ Age <10 years or >40 years ■ Etiology: non-A, non-B viral hepatitis, halothane hepatitis, or idiosyncratic drug reaction ■ Duration of jaundice before onset of encephalopathy >7 days ■ Prothrombin time >50 seconds ■ Serum bilirubin >18 mg/dL

MANAGEMENT OF SYSTEMIC COMPLICATIONS

Central Nervous System

Cerebral edema and increased intracranial pressure are serious complications of FHF, seen in up to 80% of patients who die in the setting of FHF. The risk of cerebral edema increases with progression of encephalopathy, with a >75% risk in patients with grade IV encephalopathy. An ammonia level of >200 mcmol/L has been associated with cerebral herniation. Advanced cerebral edema can lead to uncal herniation and death.

Management of neurologic complications is outlined in Algorithm 43.1. Patients with grade I or II encephalopathy should be transferred to a liver transplant center. Patients with grade III-IV encephalopathy should be intubated for airway protection. Frequent neurologic examinations are imperative, and clinical clues such as systemic hypertension, bradycardia, posturing, and decreased pupillary reflexes can suggest impending herniation.

Intracranial pressure (ICP) monitoring should be strongly considered for patients with rapidly progressive encephalopathy and those listed for liver transplantation. ICP monitoring is currently used by approximately 50% of liver transplant programs. There are three types of catheters used for monitoring ICP: epidural, subdural, and parenchymal. A review of 262 patients showed a complication rate of 4% with epidural transducers and approximately 20% with subdural and parenchymal monitors. The most common complications include bleeding in the setting of coagulopathy, infection, and volume overload resulting from correction of coagulopathy. Recombinant factor VII has been used in a small trial to aid with placement of ICP transducers with favorable results. ICP should be maintained at a level <20 mm Hg, with a cerebral perfusion pressure (mean arterial pressure minus ICP) >40 to 60 mm Hg.

Once increased ICP or cerebral edema is present, aggressive measures should be undertaken to prevent herniation. Minimal sedation, avoidance of sensory stimulation, and raising the head of the bed can be helpful. Therapies focus on decreasing cerebral edema by osmosis (mannitol or hypertonic saline) or decreasing cerebral blood flow (hyperventilation or hypothermia).

Mannitol is administered as a bolus dose (0.5 to 1 g/kg of a 20% solution). The dose can be repeated twice; however, administration is limited by maintaining a serum osmolality <320 mOsm/kg. If patients have concomitant renal failure, hemofiltration should be considered. Hyperventilation has only a short-term benefit, but can be used with a goal of reducing $PaCO_2$ to 25 mm Hg. A study of 30 patients with ICP monitoring randomized to 3% hypertonic saline with a goal serum sodium concentration of 145 to 155 mmol/L showed a significant decrease in ICP and incidence of increased ICP without an increase in survival. Hypothermia (32°C to 34°C) has been associated with a beneficial effect in uncontrolled trials. Patients with FHF may have seizure activity, but prophylactic phenytoin has not proven to be effective in improving survival based on two conflicting trials. Dexamethasone is not effective at prolonging survival. Barbiturate coma can be attempted for refractory increased intracranial pressure.

Coagulopathy

Management of coagulopathy is outlined in Algorithm 43.1. Synthesis of coagulation factors I, II, V, VII, IX, and X is depressed in patients with FHF. Sources of bleeding include procedure sites, stress ulcers, lungs, and the oropharynx. Proton pump inhibitors should be used for stress ulcer prophylaxis. Platelets should only be transfused for counts <10,000/mcL or in the face of active bleeding. Fresh-frozen plasma should not be transfused unless there is active bleeding or a planned procedure. Packed red blood cells can be transfused for symptomatic anemia or to replace blood loss secondary to hemorrhage.

Factor VII is the initiator of coagulation when tissue factor has been exposed at the site of injury. The role of recombinant factor VII has been evaluated during the placement of ICP monitors. In an unblinded study comparing patients with FHF given recombinant factor VII with a cohort of historic controls, patients with the recombinant factor VII all had successful placement (7/7 vs. 3/8). The patients receiving recombinant factor VII also had a significant decrease in mortality and anasarca from fluid overload.

ALGORITHM 43.1 Management of the Complications of Fulminant Hepatic Failure

Management of Complications

Hypotension

- Resuscitation: Albumin or saline
- MAP <55–60 mm Hg
- Dopamine or norepinephrine
- Maintenance: Dextrose based IV fluids

Coagulopathy

Bleeding?

- Control bleeding:
  - Vitamin K 5–10 mg SC × 3 d
  - Transfuse FFP and platelets, as indicated

- Prophylaxis:
  - PPI
  - Platelets if <10,000/mm^3

Planned procedure?

- Give platelets to >50,000/mm^3
- Consider FVII if renal insufficiency or volume overload

Infection

- Obtain surveillance cultures
- Low threshold for prophylactic broad spectrum antibiotics
- No role for bowel decontamination

If there is ascites perform paracentesis

PMNs >250/mm^3

Treat with:
- Cefotaxime 2 g q8h AND
- Albumin 1.5 g/kg day 1 and 1 g/kg day 3

Renal

- Fluid challenge
- Avoid nephrotoxins

Worsening failure?

CRRT better than IHD

Metabolic

- Initiate early enteral or parenteral nutrition
- Replete electrolytes
- Replete glucose

CNS

See Algorithm 43.2

SC, subcutaneously; FFP, fresh-frozen plasma; Cx, MAP, mean arterial pressure; inh, inhibitors; plts, platelets; PMN, polymorphonuclear leukocyte; CVVHD, continuous venovenous hemodialysis; HD, hemodialysis; D5%, 5% dextrose; CRRT, continuous renal replacement therapy; IHD, intermittent hemodialysis

ALGORITHM 43.2   **CNS Complications of Fulminant Hepatic Failure**

Increased intracranial pressure as indicated by:

- ICP >20–25 mm Hg, CPP <50–60 mm Hg
- Clinical findings: Cushing's reflex, irregular respirations, dilated pupils, decerebrate posturing, ammonia >200 mcmol/L

General Considerations

- CT head to rule out hemorrhage
- Decrease sedation, HOB 30 degrees, avoid valsalva, avoid stimulation, sedation
- Grade III–IV encephalopathy: Intubate
- Agent of choice unknown

- Consider epidural transducer for ICP monitoring; consider FVII for placement
- Goal ICP <20–25 mm Hg, CPP >50–60 mm Hg

Intervention	Administration	Comments
Mannitol	Bolus 0.5–1 g/kg. Can repeat twice.	No role in prophylaxis Keep serum osmolality <320 mOsm/kg; monitor for hyperosmolality Side effects: hypernatremia, volume overload
Hyperventilation	Titrate to p_{CO_2} to 25–30 mm Hg	No role in prophylaxis Temporary measure to prevent acute decompensation
Hypertonic saline	Titrate to serum sodium of 145–155 mmol/L	Prophylactic level 145–155 mmol/L can prevent rise in intracranial pressure without survival benefit
Barbiturates	Thiopental 185–500 mg/15 minutes OR Pentobarbital bolus 3–5 mg/kg followed by continuous infusion of 0.2–1 mg/kg/hr	Can decrease ICP in failed cases Side effects: Severe hypotension
Corticosteroids	Dexamethasone 10 mg IV q6hr	Only indicated for CNS infection or brain tumor Does not increase survival in acute liver failure
Hypothermia	Goal 32°–34°C	Uncontrolled trials suggest benefit Side effects: arrhythmias, infection and coagulopathy

CT, computed tomography; HOB, head of bed; ICP, intracranial pressure; FVII, factor VII; CPP, cerebral perfusion pressure; IV, intravenous.

Hypotension

Hypotension is multifactorial in patients with FHF, resulting from volume depletion, third spacing, infection, gastrointestinal bleeding, or as a result of overall low systemic vascular resistance and a hyperkinetic cardiovascular state. Fluid resuscitation should be balanced with avoidance of volume overload and the theoretical risk of increasing ICP. Maintenance fluid should be glucose-based because of the hypoglycemia associated with liver failure. Although not compared directly in trials, dopamine or norepinephrine can be used for vaso-pressor support. In a small study, dopamine led to a significant increase in cardiac output, systemic oxygen delivery, and hepatic and splanchnic blood flow when used to increase mean arterial pressure by 10 mm Hg. Although systemic oxygen consumption was increased, splanchnic oxygen consumption was decreased. A small trial evaluating the role of norepinephrine in FHF noted an increase in mean arterial pressure, although it was not associated with an increase in cardiac index and actually resulted in a decrease in systemic oxygen consumption, likely from a further decrease in splanchnic oxygen consumption compared with dopamine. Resuscitation with colloid is theoretically better than crystalloid, given that albumin induces a more effective expansion of the central blood volume, but has not shown mortality benefit.

Infection

Infections are found in 80% of patients with FHF, with 25% of patients developing docu-mented bacteremia. Infection at admission is associated with worsening hepatic encephalopathy. Systemic fungal infections are found in one third of infected patients. Although not associated with a survival advantage, prophylactic antibiotics should be strongly considered and a low threshold should be maintained for initiation of empiric broad-spectrum coverage because of the potential interference with transplantation serious infection may pose, as well as the increased risk of hepatic encephalopathy.

Renal Failure

Renal failure is multifactorial in patients with FHF because of the direct toxic effect of ingested substances, volume depletion, hypotension, acute tubular necrosis, and/or the hepatorenal syndrome. In contrast to acute tubular necrosis, renal failure due to the hepa-torenal syndrome is characterized by a low urinary sodium (<10 mEq/L), progressive hyponatremia, and a lack of improvement with volume expansion. In a randomized trial in critically ill patients with hepatic and renal failure, continuous renal replacement therapy was associated with better cardiovascular dynamics than daily intermittent hemodialysis.

Metabolic Complications

Metabolic complications include hypoglycemia resulting from diminished glucose synthesis and lactic acidosis due to anaerobic glucose metabolism. Patients benefit from glucose mon-itoring and treatment of hypoglycemia with dextrose-based solutions. Electrolytes such as phosphorus, potassium, and magnesium usually have abnormal levels and should be repleted as needed. Hyponatremia is also common. A recent Cochrane database review did not find convincing evidence of a beneficial role of branched amino acids in the treatment of patients with hepatic encephalopathy.

MANAGEMENT OF ETIOLOGY-SPECIFIC FHF (See Algorithm 43.3)

Acetaminophen Toxicity

Acetaminophen toxicity is the leading cause of FHF. Indications for empiric treatment include a high suspicion for acetaminophen overdose, known ingestion of >10 g/day, or an elevated acetaminophen level based on the accepted nomogram (Figure 32.1). A single dose of 150 mg/kg or more carries a risk of liver damage, but even smaller doses can be damaging. If ingestion is known to have occurred within 4 hours of presentation, activated charcoal (1 g/kg) was found to be significantly more effective in lowering the plasma acetaminophen level than gastric lavage, ipecac, or supportive treatment. A Cochrane database review reported

ALGORITHM 43.3   Etiology-Specific Management of Fulminant Hepatic Failure

Etiology-Specific Management

Other

- Acute ischemic injury → Maintain perfusion
- Drug-induced hypersensitivity → Consider corticosteroids
- Acute hepatitis B → Consider lamivudine 100 mg po qd
- Autoimmune hepatitis → Prednisone 40–60 mg po qd
- Wilson's disease → Urgent transplant evaluation → Consider chelation with D-Penicillamine 250–500 mg/d OR trientine 750–1,500 mg/d in 3 divided doses
- Herpes virus → Acyclovir
- Mushroom poisoning → Urgent transplant evaluation / Gastric lavage and activated charcoal 1g/kg →
  - Penicillin 300,000–1,000,000 IU/kg IV qd
  - Silibinin/silymarin 30–40 mg/kg qd IV or PO

Acetaminophen

- Within 1–4 hr → Activated Charcoal 1g/kg
- Within 48 hr → Toxic levels on nomorgam or high suspicion
  - Unable to take PO → NAC: IV load150 mg/kg in DSW then 50 mg/kg over 4 hr and then 100 mg/kg over 16 hr
  - Tolerate PO → NAC: Loading dose 140 mg/kg then 70 mg/kg PO q4h ×17 doses

PO, by mouth; DSW, dextrose 5% water; NAC, N-acetylcysteine; IV, intravenous.

that N-acetylcysteine (NAC) may reduce mortality (odds ratio, 0.26) in patients with FHF. NAC is administered if there is a high suspicion of ingestion or if the serum concentration is above the nomogram risk line (Figure 32.1). Administration of activated charcoal prior to treatment with NAC does not reduce its efficacy. The traditional NAC dose is 140 mg/kg by mouth or nasogastric tube diluted to 5% solution, followed by 70 mg/kg by mouth every 4 hours for 17 doses. Intravenous administration is a loading dose of 150 mg/kg in 5% dextrose during 15 minutes with 50 mg/kg during 4 hours and then 100 mg/kg during 16 hours. NAC should be administered as early as possible, although its effect is seen even 48 hours after ingestion. In a review of transplantation for acetaminophen overdose, there was no difference in survival rate between use of oral and various intravenous protocols of NAC administration.

Viral Hepatitis

Hepatitis B accounts for >50% of viral causes of FHF. Treatment with lamivudine (100 mg/day) has been used anecdotally in patients with acute hepatitis B and may result in seroconversion of the hepatitis B e antigen, but there is no current recommendation for acute treatment and duration of therapy has not been ascertained. Hepatitis E is a more common cause in immigrants from countries in which it is endemic. Treatment for acute hepatitis A is supportive.

Transplantation

Liver transplantation is a proven treatment for FHF, although limited by the availability of donors. Posttransplant survival rates are as high as 80% to 90%. The decision to pursue transplantation versus continuing medical therapy (such as NAC) is difficult. Factors to consider include the realistic possibility of spontaneous recovery, the feasibility of transplantation, and assessment of contraindications to transplantation. Prognostic models such as the King's College Criteria (Table 43.3) and the Acute Physiology and Chronic Health Evaluation (APACHE) II score help in determining the need for liver transplantation. For patients with acetaminophen-associated FHF, a recent meta-analysis reported that the King's College Criteria had a sensitivity of 0.59 and specificity of 0.92 in determining the need for transplantation. An APACHE II score of >15 was associated with a specificity of 0.81 and sensitivity of 0.92 in determining the need for transplantation. The APACHE II score had a higher positive likelihood ratio of 16.4 and negative likelihood ratio of 0.19 (one study) versus the King's criteria with a positive and negative likelihood ratio of 12.33 and 0.29, respectively, based on six pooled studies.

FUTURE THERAPIES

Artificial liver support systems and bioartificial livers have been studied as a possible treatment for FHF. A recent Cochrane database review, however, concluded that support systems did not reduce mortality or serve as effective bridges to transplantation when compared with standard medical therapy. In a subgroup analysis, mortality was reduced by 33% in patients with acute on chronic liver failure, but not in acute liver failure.

Suggested Reading

Brok J, Buckley N, Gluud C. Interventions for paracetamol (acetaminophen) overdose. *Cochrane Database Syst Rev.* 2006;CD003328.
   This meta-analysis provides a comprehensive review of proven and unproven therapies for the leading cause of fulminant hepatic failure.
Hoofnagle JH, Carithers RL, Shapiro C, et al. Fulminant hepatic failure: summary of a workshop. *Hepatology.* 1995;21:240–252.
   This paper summarizes issues in the management of fulminant hepatic failure.
Kulkarni S, Cronin DC. Fulminant hepatic failure. In: Hall JB, Schidt GA, Wood LD, eds. *Principles of Critical Care.* 3rd ed. New York: McGraw-Hill Professional; 2005; 1279–1288.
   This chapter provides an excellent overview of the pathophysiology and management issues in fulminant hepatic failure.

Polson J, Lee WM. AASLD position paper: the management of acute liver failure. *Hepatology.* 2005;41:1179–1197.

This paper provides guidelines by the American Association for the Study of Liver Diseases on the management of fulminant hepatic failure.

Raghavan M, Marik PE. Therapy of intracranial hypertension in patients with fulminant hepatic failure. *Neurocrit Care.* 2006;4:179–189.

This paper provides an excellent overview of treatment for intracranial hypertension and reviews the current understanding of the mechanisms leading to this life threatening complication.

Yee HF Jr, Lidofsky SD. Acute liver failure. In: Feldman M, Scharschmidt BF, Sleisenger MH ed. *Sleisenger & Fordtran's Gastrointestinal and Liver Disease.* 7th ed. Philadelphia: Saunders; 2002;1567–1576.

This chapter provides as excellent overview of the pathophysiology and management issues in fulminant hepatic failure.

44 HYPERBILIRUBINEMIA
Sumeet Asrani and Jeffrey S. Crippin

PHYSIOLOGY

Heme is a breakdown constituent of senescent erythrocytes. It is converted to biliverdin by heme oxygenase and further reduced by biliverdin reductase to bilirubin in the reticuloendothelial system. Unconjugated bilirubin is tightly bound to albumin and transferred to the liver. It is transported into the hepatocytes by carrier-mediated mechanisms, transferred to the endoplasmic reticulum bound by cytosolic proteins, and converted to a water-soluble form by the addition of uridine diphosphate glucuronic acid. An adenosine triphosphate-dependent export pump transfers it to the biliary canaliculi, where it is added to bile. Bile drains into the gallbladder and small intestine. It is excreted into stool or metabolized by ileal and colonic bacteria to urobilinogen. Urobilinogen is absorbed in the small intestine and enters the portal circulation. A small portion is excreted into the stool and urine. Hyperbilirubinemia results from disruption of bilirubin metabolism or obstruction of biliary drainage (Alg. 44.1).

INDIRECT HYPERBILIRUBINEMIA

An indirect bilirubin fraction >80% of the total bilirubin is consistent with unconjugated hyperbilirubinemia, resulting from prehepatocyte abnormalities. This may be caused by increased bilirubin production or decreased hepatocyte uptake. Hemolysis is a frequent cause of unconjugated hyperbilirubinemia. Hemolysis may be precipitated by medications, autoimmune disease, malignancy, or infection. It is characterized by an elevated reticulocyte count, schistocytes or spherocytes on the peripheral blood smear, a positive Coombs test, an increased lactate dehydrogenase level, and a decreased haptoglobin. A decrease in hepatocyte uptake is the result of inhibition of uptake mechanisms or enzymatic defects in conjugation. Competitive inhibition of bilirubin uptake may be caused by medications, such as rifampin. A common enzymatic defect causing decreased activity of bilirubin-uridine diphosphate-glucuronyl transferase results in asymptomatic unconjugated hyperbilirubinemia, better known as *Gilbert's syndrome*.

DIRECT HYPERBILIRUBINEMIA

Conjugated or direct hyperbilirubinemia is usually secondary to hepatocellular dysfunction, biliary obstruction, or biliary dysfunction. Hepatocellular dysfunction, whether acute or chronic, can cause reflux of conjugated bilirubin into the circulation. Acute hepatocellular dysfunction is suggested by an elevated bilirubin in association with elevated aminotransferases. Common causes of chronic hepatocellular dysfunction include chronic viral hepatitis and alcoholic liver disease.

Biliary dysfunction results from (a) obstruction of the extrahepatic biliary ducts, (b) nonobstructive inflammation, or (c) infection of the intrahepatic biliary ducts. Imaging is required for diagnosis and guided therapy. Imaging modalities include ultrasound, computed tomography, endoscopic retrograde cholangiopancreatography, percutaneous transhepatic cholangiography, and magnetic resonance cholangiopancreatography (Alg. 44.1). A direct bilirubin fraction >50% of the total bilirubin suggests a hepatobiliary etiology and, if accompanied by an elevated alkaline phosphatase and gamma-glutamyl transpeptidase, favors biliary obstruction.

ALGORITHM 44.1 Evaluation and Management of Hyperbilirubinemia

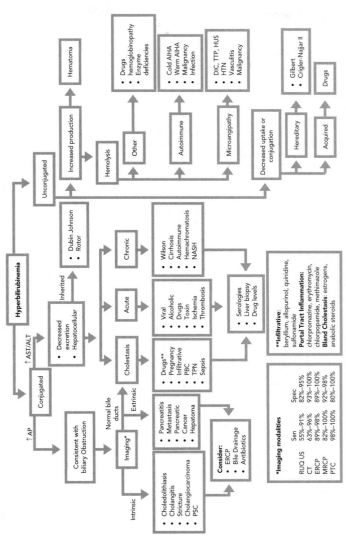

AST, aspartate aminotransferase; ALT, alanine aminotransferase; PSC, primary sclerosing cholangitis; PBC, primary biliary cirrhosis; TPN, total parenteral nutrition; NASH, nonalcoholic steatohepatitis; ERCP, endoscopic retrograde cholangiopancreatography; AIHA, autoimmune hemolytic anemia; DIC, disseminated intravascular coagulation; TTP, thrombotic thrombocytopenic purpura; HUS, hemolytic-uremic syndrome; HTN, hypertension; RUQ US, right upper quadrant ultrasound; CT, computed tomography; MRCP, magnetic resonance cholangiopancreatography; PTC, percutaneous transhepatic cholangiography.

321

Common causes of intrinsic obstruction include choledocholithiasis, biliary strictures, and cholangiocarcinoma. Extrinsic compression can be secondary to pancreatic masses (tumor, fibrosis, pseudocyst, or abscess) or lymphadenopathy. An abdominal ultrasound or computed tomography, both with high specificity, can confirm an obstructive process. Ultrasound is a more sensitive technique for detecting stones within the gallbladder, whereas both techniques are less apt at identifying choledocholithiasis. An ultrasound is less helpful in obese patients and when overlying bowel gas is present. If these studies fail to reveal a cause of biliary obstruction, magnetic resonance cholangiopancreatography gives better visualization of the intrahepatic ducts. Once an obstructive process is confirmed, cholangiography can provide direct access to the biliary tree. Endoscopic retrograde cholangiopancreatography gains access to the proximal biliary tree, and percutaneous trans-hepatic cholangiography, starting at the peripheral bile ducts, allows visualization of the biliary tree. Either study allows decompression of obstructive processes via sphincterectomy and stone retrieval, stricture dilation, or stent placement.

Nonobstructive intrahepatic biliary disease also presents with elevated alkaline phosphatase, an elevated gamma-glutamyl transpeptidase, and direct hyperbilirubinemia without imaging evidence of obstruction. Causes include infiltrative liver disease, inflammation or infection of the bile ductules, autoimmune biliary disease, drug hepatotoxicity, and sepsis. Tuberculosis, fungal infections, hepatic malignancies, and systemic diseases such as amyloidosis and sarcoidosis can lead to biliary ductal inflammation and dysfunction secondary to infiltration. Total parenteral nutrition and drugs such as estrogens and anabolic steroids can produce nonspecific intrahepatic cholestasis. Inflammation of the bile ductules is seen in primary biliary cirrhosis. Inflammation of the portal tracts leading to cholestasis is caused by multiple drugs, including methimazole. If no obstruction is found and a cholestatic pattern still persists, cholangiography may be useful to delineate biliary anatomy. Computed tomography imaging can reveal infiltrative disease. A liver biopsy is often required to further define the amount and type of liver injury.

Suggested Reading

Greenberger NJ, Paumgartner G. Diseases of the gallbladder and bile ducts. In: Kasper DL, Braunwald E, Fauci AS, et al, eds. *Harrison's Principles of Internal Medicine.*16th ed. New York: McGraw-Hill; 2005;1880–1890.
   This chapter discuss common causes of biliary dysfunction and provides an approach to diagnosing biliary disease.
Lidofsky S. Jaundice. In: Feldman M, Scharschmidt BF, Sleisenger MH, ed. *Sleisenger & Fordtran's Gastrointestinal and Liver Disease.* 7th ed. Philadelphia: Saunders; 2002; 249–264.
   This chapter provides a systematic approach to evaluating a patient with jaundice and compares the various imaging modalities to evaluate biliary disease.
Pratt DS, Kaplan MM. *Jaundice.* In: Kasper DL, Braunwald E, Fauci AS, et al, eds. *Harrison's Principles of Internal Medicine.* 16th ed. New York: McGraw-Hill; 2005; 238–242.
   This chapter also provides a systematic approach to evaluating a patient with jaundice.
Summerfield JA. Diseases of the gallbladder and biliary tree. In: Warren DA, Cox TM, Firth JD, et al, eds. *Oxford Textbook of Medicine.* 4th ed. Oxford: Oxford University Press; 2003;697–713.
   This source provides an excellent overview of investigations in biliary disease.
Wolkoff A. The hyperbilirubinemias. In: Kasper DL, Braunwald E, Fauci AS, et al, eds. Harrison's Principles of Internal Medicine. 16th ed. New York: McGraw-Hill; 2005; 1817–1821.
   This chapter provides a great review of the pathophysiology and disorders of the biliary system.

END-STAGE LIVER DISEASE

Kevin M. Korenblat

45

The shared outcome of most untreated, chronic liver diseases is the development of cirrhosis. The resulting clinically evident liver disease is commonly referred to as *decompensated cirrhosis* and is characterized by both portal hypertension and hepatic synthetic dysfunction. These complications typically coexist in patients with cirrhosis and are the major cause of liver disease-related morbidity and mortality. The common complications of portal hypertension are ascites, portal hypertensive-related bleeding, hepatic encephalopathy, and thrombocytopenia. Intensive care unit admissions for these complications are a common occurrence, and successful management depends on prompt diagnosis and treatment.

Ascites describes the accumulation of a serous fluid in the peritoneal cavity. It is the most frequent manifestation of decompensated cirrhosis and it is associated with a 2-year mortality rate of 50%. Cirrhotic ascites is identified by its low albumin content and a >1.1 g/dL difference between serum and ascites albumin concentrations (serum ascites-albumin gradient). Sampling of the ascites is required in all patients with new-onset ascites or in those with a change in their clinical condition, such as confusion, renal dysfunction, or gastrointestinal bleeding. Paracentesis is a safe procedure that can be done even in patients with coagulopathy and thrombocytopenia (Fig. 45.1). The ascites should be analyzed for albumin, cell count and differential, and the fluid inoculated directly into blood culture media. Although ascites is best managed with oral furosemide and spironolactone, diuretics may need to be withheld in intensive care unit patients who frequently have renal dysfunction or hypovolemia. Intravenous diuretics should be avoided in cirrhotic patients as these agents can precipitate renal failure. Hepatic hydrothorax occurs in as many as 13% of patients with ascites, is typically right-sided, and occurs as a result of defects in the diaphragm that permit passage of ascites into the pleural space. This complication can be managed by thoracentesis, diuretics, and, when refractory to medical therapy, transjugular intrahepatic shunt (TIPS) placement. Tube thoracostomy should be avoided because volume losses can be substantial and precipitate renal dysfunction.

The most important complication of ascites is the development of spontaneous bacterial peritonitis (SBP). There is no typical presentation of SBP, and signs such as abdominal pain, fever, or leukocytosis are frequently absent. The diagnosis is established by the finding of >250/mL polymorphonuclear cells in the ascites or the growth of organisms in a culture of ascites fluid. SBP should be differentiated from secondary bacterial peritonitis as a consequence of bowel perforation or nonperforating abdominal abscess (Alg. 45.1). SBP should be treated with prompt parenteral antibiotics. Second- and third-generation cephalosporins (cefotaxime, 1 g intravenously [IV] every 8 hours, or ceftriaxone, 1 g IV every 24 hours) have proven effective in the management of SBP. Renal dysfunction occurs in as many as one third of patients with SBP despite adequate antibiotic treatment. Discontinuation of diuretics and the administration of IV albumin (25%) given at a dose of 1.5 g/kg body weight on day 1 and 1 g/kg day 3 was shown in randomized, controlled studies to reduce the rates of renal dysfunction. This intervention should be strongly considered in all patients with SBP, and particularly those with jaundice and pre-existing renal insufficiency.

The hepatorenal syndrome (HRS) is a clinical diagnosis based on the development of progressive renal failure in cirrhosis. The syndrome can be subdivided into a rapidly progressive (type 1 HRS) and a slower (type 2 HRS) form. Diagnostic criteria have been devised by consensus to assist in the diagnosis (Table 45.1). Treatment of HRS requires intravascular volume expansion. Albumin (25%) is a particularly potent volume expander,

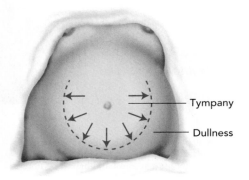

Tympany

Dullness

Figure 45.1. Areas of dullness in both right and left lower abdominal quadrants are ideal sites for diagnostic paracentesis.

and support for its role is provided by the success of albumin in conjunction with vasoactive agents in improving HRS compared with vasoactive agents and saline.

Encephalopathy is a common complication of cirrhosis. Early symptoms are often subtle and can include changes in mood and insomnia that can progress to agitation and coma. Its development should prompt a search from precipitants that commonly include infection, gastrointestinal hemorrhage, or medication exposures. The mediators of hepatic encephalopathy are unknown, and serum ammonia is, at best, a casual marker of hepatic encephalopathy. Treatment options include cathartics (lactulose, 30 mL by mouth [PO] every 2 to 8 hours, or lactulose retention enemas) or enterically active antibiotics (neomycin, 500 mg PO every 6 hours, or rifaximin, 400 mg PO 3 times daily).

Variceal hemorrhage has an annual incidence rate of 20% in cirrhotic patients, and each episode carries a 20% to 40% mortality rate. There is no typical presentation of variceal bleeding, and this should be suspected in those with known chronic liver disease and gastrointestinal hemorrhage. The initial steps in the management of acute variceal bleeding involve resuscitation of hemorrhage shock and protection of the airway (Table 45.2). Volume resuscitation in the form of packed red blood cells should be

TABLE 45.1	Diagnostic Criteria for the Hepatorenal Syndrome

Major criteria
  Advanced, chronic hepatic failure and portal hypertension
  Serum creatinine >1.5 mg/dL or 24-hr urine creatinine clearance <40 mL/min
  Absence of shock, exposure to nephrotoxic agents, hypovolemia, or ongoing sepsis
  No sustained improvement in renal function following diuretic withdrawal and volume
    expansion with 1.5 liters of isotonic saline
  Proteinuria <500 mg/dL
  No evidence of obstructive uropathy or parenchymal renal disease

Minor criteria
  Urine volume <500 mL/day
  Urine sodium <10 mEq/L
  Urine osmolality >plasma osmolality
  Urine RBCs <50 per HPF
  Serum sodium <130 mEq/L

RBCs, red blood cells; HPF, high-power field.

ALGORITHM 45.1   Algorithm for the Assessment of Cirrhotic Ascites

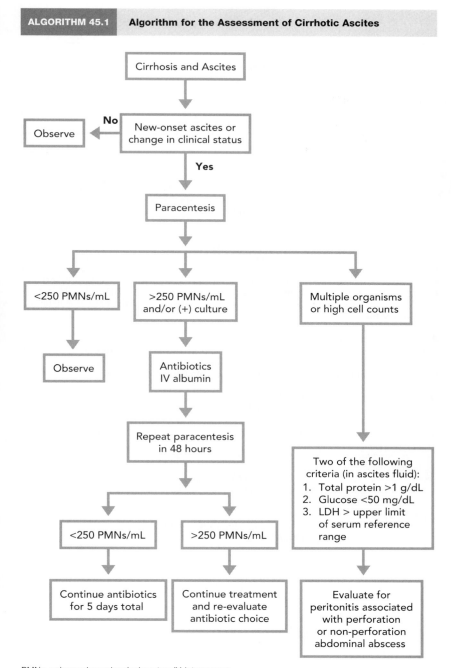

PMNs, polymorphonuclear leukocytes; IV, intravenous.

TABLE 45.2	Guidelines for the Management of Variceal Hemorrhage

Resuscitate hypovolemic shock
Assessment of airway and intubation if airway protection necessary
Octreotide, 50 mcg IV bolus followed by 50 mcg/hr IV infusion
Blood and urine culture; diagnostic paracentesis
Prophylactic parenteral antibiotics
Upper endoscopy
TIPS or Blakemore tube for variceal bleeding refractory to endoscopic management

IV, intravenous; TIPS, transjugular intrahepatic shunt.

first priority over other blood products. Octreotide (50 mcg IV bolus followed by 50 mcg/hr IV infusion) should be started. Diagnostic paracentesis should be performed and prophylactic parenteral antibiotics should be administered because variceal hemorrhage can occur in the setting of bacteremia and can result in bacterial translocation. Upper endoscopy should be performed promptly as both band ligation and sclerotherapy can result in effective hemostasis for esophageal varices. TIPS is an option for esophageal variceal bleeding that is refractory to endoscopy or for bleeding gastric varices. Balloon tamponade devices (Blakemore tube) can also be inserted temporarily in cases in which either TIPS or endoscopy is delayed or unsuccessful. Nonselective beta-blockers are effective at reducing the risk of initial and recurrent variceal bleeding; however, they should be introduced only after acute bleeding is controlled and the patient is hemodynamically stable.

Suggested Reading

Arroyo V, Gines P, Gerbes AL, et al. Definition and diagnostic criteria of refractory ascites and hepatorenal syndrome in cirrhosis. *Hepatology.* 1996;23:164–176.

Gines P, Guevara M, Arroyo V, et al. Hepatorenal syndrome. *Lancet.* 2003;362: 1819–1827.

Moore KP, Wong F, Gines P, et al. The management of ascites in cirrhosis: report on the consensus conference of the International Ascites Club. *Hepatology.* 2003;38:258–266.
Guidelines for the management of cirrhotic ascites by an international expert panel.

Runyon, B A. Management of adult patients with ascites due to cirrhosis. *Hepatology.* 2004;39:841–856.
Practice guidelines of the American Association for the Study of Liver Disease for the management of ascites.

Sort P, Navasa M, Arroyo V, et al. Effect of intravenous albumin on renal impairment and mortality in patients with cirrhosis and spontaneous bacterial peritonitis. *N Engl J Med.* 1999;341:405–409.
A randomized, controlled trial demonstrating that the administration of intravenous albumin can reduce the risk of renal insufficiency associated with the development of spontaneous bacterial peritonitis.

UPPER GASTROINTESTINAL BLEEDING
Chandra Prakash   **46**

Acute upper gastrointestinal bleeding (UGIB) is a common medical emergency that frequently results in emergency department evaluations and intensive care unit admissions. The annual incidence of acute UGIB is estimated to range between 100 and 200 cases per 100,000 population, carrying a mortality rate of 6% to 12%. In recent years the incidence has declined in younger populations, possibly because of lower *Helicobacter pylori* incidence and widespread use of (PPIs). Concurrently, incidence has risen in older populations from increased use of nonsteroidal anti-inflammatory drugs (NSAIDs). Common causes of acute UGIB are listed in Table 46.1.

One of the first assessments in any patient with acute gastrointestinal bleeding is determining the severity of the bleeding episode (Alg. 46.1). Bleeding is considered massive with loss of one fifth to one fourth of the circulating volume if a previously normotensive or hypertensive patient develops resting hypotension. In the absence of resting hypotension, evidence of postural or orthostatic hypotension (drop of systolic blood pressure of 15 mm Hg or increase in heart rate of 20 beats per minute) indicates loss of 10% to 20% of the circulating volume. Bleeding is considered minor if neither of these conditions are met, indicating loss of <10% of circulating volume. In all instances, two large-bore intravenous (IV) lines or a central line are urgently placed, and normal saline or lactated Ringer's solution administered intravenously. Rapid repletion of circulating volume is crucial when blood loss approaches massive, and transfusion of packed red blood cells needs to be arranged. Therefore, blood is drawn for blood count, metabolic profile, coagulation parameters, blood typing, and cross-matching. When type-specific blood is not immediately available, O negative blood may need to be transfused, using rapid infusing devices if necessary. Oxygen is administered by nasal cannula to improve oxygen-carrying capacity of blood, and vital signs and urine output are constantly monitored.

Factors propagating bleeding can be rapidly assessed during this initial evaluation. Patients receiving heparin infusion, thrombolytic therapy, or newer antithrombotic agents (Alg. 46.1) need to be assessed to determine if it is safe to temporarily discontinue these medications. Oral anticoagulants are held, and the anticoagulation reversed with vitamin K and/or fresh-frozen plasma, if possible.

TABLE 46.1	Etiology of Upper Gastrointestinal Bleeding

Peptic ulcer disease (accounts for ~50%)
   Gastric ulcers
   Duodenal ulcers
   Gastric erosions and gastritis
Esophageal and/or gastric varices (accounts for 10%–20%)
Stress ulcers
Mallory Weiss tear
Esophagitis and esophageal ulcers
Vascular abnormalities (angiodysplasia, Dieulafoy lesion, telangiectasia)
Portal hypertensive gastropathy
Neoplasms, benign and malignant
Hemobilia (bleeding into bile ducts)
Hemosuccus (bleeding into pancreatic ducts)
Aortoenteric fistula

Once the patient is stabilized hemodynamically, further evaluation can resume (Alg. 46.1). A history of hematemesis or coffee-ground emesis establishes the diagnosis of UGIB. Melena (passage of dark, tarry, sticky, foul-smelling stool) typically indicates a proximal gut source for blood loss, but melena can develop from bleeding sites as far distal as the proximal or even middle colon. Nevertheless, the presence of melena points to upper endoscopy as the starting point of investigation of the bleeding episode. An upper gastrointestinal source of bleeding may be identified in as many as 10% to 11% of patients presenting with hematochezia and altered hemodynamic parameters. Therefore, in the presence of significant hemodynamic compromise, upper gastrointestinal tract evaluation is indicated even if the bleeding presentation resembles lower gastrointestinal bleeding.

Aspiration of bloody gastric contents through a nasogastric tube establishes the diagnosis of UGIB, and can help triage the need for emergent endoscopy. The aspiration of brighter shades of red blood may indicate ongoing bleeding, wherein urgent endoscopy with endoscopic therapy may lower morbidity. On the other hand, dark blood or coffee grounds that clear quickly on nasogastric tube lavage may indicate that active bleeding has ceased, and elective endoscopy within 24 hours may be adequate (Table 46.2). Early indicators for the need for intensive care unit admission include massive bleeding, hemodynamic compromise, variceal bleeding, bleeding onset while hospitalized for an unrelated illness, and the presence of factors that predict a poor outcome (Table 46.3).

Acute UGIB consists of two broad categories: acute variceal UGIB and acute nonvariceal UGIB (Alg. 46.2). These categories require differing investigative and therapeutic approaches, and may be associated with varied short- and long-term morbidity and mortality. For instance, variceal UGIB is associated with a higher rate of rebleeding (30% to 40% vs. 15% to 20% for nonvariceal bleeding), and a significantly higher mortality (20% to 30% vs. 6% to 9%, respectively). Acute nonvariceal UGIB that develops in patients hospitalized for an unrelated illness is associated with worse morbidity and mortality (estimated at 35%) compared with patients admitted through emergency departments for acute bleeding.

Initial management of acute variceal UGIB includes IV infusion of octreotide, and IV PPI administration is considered routine in nonvariceal UGIB. Early clinical evaluation of acute UGIB should therefore include an assessment to determine which category the patient falls into, with the understanding that such an assessment may not always be accurate or even possible.

The initial mode of therapy for acute UGIB is pharmacologic (Alg. 46.2). Octreotide, a somatostatin analog, lowers splanchnic and portal venous pressure in the short term, with slowing or cessation of variceal UGIB. Early administration of octreotide is encouraged

ALGORITHM 46.1   **Initial Management of Acute Gastrointestinal (GI) Bleeding**

RESUSCITATION
- Establish 2 large-bore IVs or central line
- Obtain blood for blood typing, CBC, CMP, INR, PTT
- Infuse isotonic saline, Ringer's lactate, or 5% hetastarch
- Blood transfusion: O negative if extremely urgent
- Oxygen by nasal canula

$\downarrow$

FACTORS PROPAGATING BLEEDING
- Discontinue anticoagulants (warfarin, heparin), thrombolytic agents
- Discontinue antiplatelet agents if possible (aspirin, clopidogrel)
- Discontinue antithrombotic agents* if possible
- Correct prolonged PT/INR with FFP infusions and/or vitamin K injection
- Correct prolonged PTT with protamine infusion if necessary

$\downarrow$

LEVEL OF BLEEDING[†]
- Hematemesis, coffee ground emesis indicate upper GI bleeding
- Melena usually indicates upper GI bleeding, but can originate more distally
- Maroon stool, red blood in the stool typically indicate lower GI bleeding
- Any bleeding in the presence of hemodynamic compromise can be upper GI in origin

$\downarrow$

ETIOLOGY OF BLEEDING[†]
- Presence of cirrhosis may indicate variceal bleeding
- Hypotension or shock preceding bleeding may indicate ischemic colitis
- Recent polypectomy may indicate postpolypectomy bleeding
- Prior aortic graft surgery may indicate aortoenteric fistula
- Prior radiation therapy may indicate radiation enteritis or proctopathy
- Prior emesis may indicate Mallory-Weiss tear

CBC, complete blood count; CMP, complete metabolic panel; INR, international normalized ratio; PTT, partial thromboplastin time; PT, prothrombin time; FFP, fresh-frozen plasma. *Antithrombotic agents can also propagate bleeding, and include glycoprotein IIb/IIIa receptor antagonists (abciximab [ReoPro], eptifibatide [Integrilin], tirofiban [Aggrastat]) and direct thrombin inhibitors (argatroban, bivalirudin).
[†]These will dictate the nature of further investigation.

TABLE 46.2	Triage of Patients with Acute Upper Gastrointestinal Bleeding

Admission to intensive care unit
  Hypotension at presentation
  Moderate-to-severe bleeding onset while admitted for an unrelated illness
  Ongoing hemodynamic instability despite resuscitation
  Absence of adequate hematocrit increase despite blood transfusion
  Low initial blood count (hematocrit <25% with cardiopulmonary disease or stroke, <20% otherwise)
  Bright or dark red NG tube aspirate, especially if it does not clear with lavage
  Prolonged coagulation parameters (prothrombin time >1.2 times the control value)
  Myocardial infarction, stroke, or other systemic complications of rapid blood loss
  Any unstable comorbid disease, including altered mental status
  Variceal bleeding
  Evidence of active oozing, spurting, or visible vessel on endoscopy

Admission to regular hospital floor
  Stable hemodynamic parameters after initial resuscitation
  Mild hematocrit drop <5% from baseline and/or baseline hematocrit >30%)
  Stable coagulation parameters
  Coffee grounds on NG tube aspirate that clears with lavage
  No systemic complications from blood loss
  No bleeding source found on upper endoscopy
  Nonvariceal bleeding source without active bleeding; bleeding lesion with a clean base or pigmented base

Emergent or urgent upper endoscopy
  Suspected or known variceal bleeding
  Hemodynamic instability despite resuscitation
  Bright red or dark red NG aspirate, especially if it does not clear with lavage
  Absence of appropriate hematocrit increase despite blood transfusion

NG, nasogastric.

(25 to 50 mcg bolus, followed by 50 to 100 mcg/hr infusion) when acute variceal UGIB is suspected. Intravenous antibiotics with coverage of enteric pathogens are administered for 7 to 10 days in patients with variceal bleeding to prevent infectious complications, particularly spontaneous bacterial peritonitis. In all other instances, PPIs are administered to suppress gastric acid (Table 46.4) as clot formation and stabilization is facilitated in an alkaline milieu. Intravenous administration is recommended in patients with ongoing bleeding, or

TABLE 46.3	Factors of Predicting Poor Outcome After Acute Upper Gastrointestinal Bleeding

Age >65 years
Comorbid medical illnesses (liver disease, COPD, renal failure, coronary artery disease, malignancy)
Variceal bleeding
Systolic blood pressure <100 mm Hg at presentation
Large peptic ulcers >3 cm
Active bleeding (spurting blood vessel) at endoscopy
Multiple units of blood transfusion
Onset of acute bleeding when hospitalized for unrelated illness
Need for emergency surgery for bleeding control

COPD, chronic obstructive pulmonary disease.

ALGORITHM 46.2 — Management of Acute Upper Gastrointestinal (GI) Bleeding

- Hematemesis: emesis of blood or coffee grounds
- Blood or coffee grounds in NG tube aspirate
- Melena
- Maroon or red blood in stool with hemodynamic compromise

VARICEAL BLEEDING
Clinical indicators
- History of varices/variceal bleeding
- History of liver disease/cirrhosis
- Spider angiomata
- Caput medusa
- Ascites
- Splenomegaly
- Hepatic encephalopathy
- Pancytopenia, low albumin

NONVARICEAL BLEEDING
Clinical indicators
- Absence of liver disease
- History of peptic ulcers
- History of *Helicobacter pylori*
- History of retching/vomiting
- NSAID/aspirin use
- Chronic renal disease
- Valvular heart disease
- History of hereditary hemorrhagic telangiectasia

Initial resuscitation
- Consider elective intubation for airway protection
- Tamponade (Sengstaken-Blakemore tube) if endoscopic therapy is delayed or not immediately available

Blood pressure tends to run low in cirrhotic patients, caution against over hydration and fluid overload

Pharmacologic therapy
Octreotide bolus and infusion
Vasopressin infusion is an alternative, but side effects may be limiting; rarely used
IV antibiotics to prevent SBP

Endoscopic therapy
- Variceal band ligation
- Variceal sclerotherapy
- Glue injection for gastric varices
Can be repeated if bleeding recurs

Angiography
- Placement of TIPS if endoscopic therapy fails
- Early TIPS for gastric varices from portal hypertension

Surgery
- Splenectomy for gastric varices from splenic vein thrombosis
- Surgical shunts for portal hypertension

Initial resuscitation

Pharmacologic therapy
Intravenous PPI bolus or infusion OR
High-dose oral PPI bid if oral intake tolerated

Endoscopic therapy
Therapy based on presence of stigmata of recent bleeding

Angiography
If endoscopy fails or if bleeding is too fast for adequate endoscopic localization and therapy

Surgery
- As an alternative to angiography if endoscopy fails
- Neoplasms, both benign and malignant
- Isolated vascular abnormalities, e.g., Dieulafoy lesion
- Aortoenteric fistula; emergent surgery

NG, nasogastric; IV, intravenous; SBP, spontaneous bacterial peritonitis; TIPS, transjugular intrahepatic portosystemic shunt; NSAIDs, nonsteroidal anti-inflammatory drugs; PPI, proton pump inhibitor.

TABLE 46.4	Doses of Antisecretory Medication	

Medication	Oral therapy (mg)	Parenteral therapy (mg)
Cimetidine[a]	300 qid 400 bid 800 qhs	300 q6hr
Ranitidine[a]	150 bid 300 qhs	50 q8hr
Famotidine[a]	20 bid 40 qhs	20 q12hr
Nizatidine[a]	150 bid 300 qhs	
Omeprazole	20 qd	
Esomeprazole	40 qd	20–40 q24hr
Lansoprazole	15–30 qd	30 q12–24hr
Pantoprazole	20 qd	40 q12–24hr or 80 IV, then 8 mg/hr infusion

qid, four times daily; bid, two times daily; qhs, at bedtime; qd, daily.
[a]Dosage adjustment required in renal insufficiency.

patients who cannot tolerate oral administration. IV bolus administration (omeprazole, 40 mg every 12 hours IV or equivalent) is favored, but IV infusion (omeprazole, 6 to 8 mg/hr by continuous infusion or equivalent) has been advocated by some for rapid ongoing bleeding. Double-dose PPI (omeprazole, 40 mg or equivalent) administered twice daily has been demonstrated to reduce the likelihood of rebleeding or the need for surgery in acute peptic ulcer bleeding, even when endoscopic therapy was not administered. Stable patients without active ongoing bleeding can tolerate oral PPI administration, and double-dose two times daily may be beneficial at least until endoscopy is performed; some centers administer this higher dose for 5 days.

A crucial adjunct to pharmacologic therapy is endoscopy (Alg. 46. 2), both for definitive diagnosis of the bleeding lesion and for administration of endoscopic therapy to lower the risks for rebleeding, other morbidity including surgery, and mortality. Timing of endoscopy depends on the degree of bleeding, whether bleeding is ongoing, and the patient's overall condition (Table 46.2). Urgent endoscopy is generally indicated in any patient with significant or ongoing bleeding. Hemodynamic parameters should be in the process of being normalized when endoscopy is performed. Conscious sedation can be administered when hemodynamic stability is achieved and the patient is no longer hypotensive. Rapid bleeding or the presence of blood or clots within the upper gastrointestinal tract may preclude complete examination. Administration of a prokinetic agent such as metoclopramide (5 to 10 mg IV) or erythromycin (250 mg IV) may induce gastric-emptying and allow a cleaner endoscopic field. Lavage using large-bore, double-lumen orogastric tubes can be performed to clear the stomach of blood and clots. Positioning the patient so that the intraluminal blood pool is away from the area of interest during endoscopy can be useful. In some instances, especially if large volumes of luminal blood or massive intraluminal clots are encountered, endoscopy may need to be repeated at a later time, or angiography used for bleeding localization. Therapy administered during endoscopy can include variceal band ligation, sclerotherapy, or glue injection for variceal UGIB, and epinephrine injection, thermal cautery, bi- or monopolar cautery, hemoclip deployment, and sclerosant injection for nonvariceal UGIB. Rebleeding rates are typically high in variceal bleeding, to the order of 30% to 40%. Rebleeding rates approximate 15% to 20% in nonvariceal bleeding, stratified by the presence or absence of stigmata of recent hemorrhage in the case of peptic ulcer bleeding (Table 46.5).

TABLE 46.5	Outcome After Endoscopic Therapy of Peptic Ulcers		
Endoscopic finding	**Risk for rebleeding (%)** (after treatment)	**Mortality (%)** (after treatment)	
Clean ulcer base	<5	2	
Flat pigmented spot	10 (<1)	3 (<1)	
Adherent clot	22 (5)	7 (<3)	
Visible vessel	43 (15)	11 (<5)	
Active bleeding	55 (20)	11 (<5)	

Modified from Laine L, Petersen WL. Bleeding peptic ulcer. *N Engl J Med.* 1994;331:717–727.

Short- and long-term outcomes of therapy depend on the cause of the lesion. Rebleeding rates are typically high with variceal bleeding. Nonselective beta-blocker therapy is initiated if the patient tolerates the approach. Repeat variceal band ligation or sclerotherapy can be considered when bleeding recurs. When access to definitive therapy is not immediately available, placement of a Sengstaken-Blakemore or similar tube can tamponade the varices and temporarily stabilize the patient (Table 46.6). Rebleeding refractory to endoscopic therapy is managed by the placement of a transjugular intrahepatic portosystemic shunt. Gastric varices related to portal hypertension are managed with a transjugular intrahepatic portosystemic shunt earlier in the course, and those resulting from splenic vein thrombosis may require splenectomy for successful management. Rebleeding from peptic ulcers can be treated endoscopically, reserving angiographic measures (such as embolization) or surgery for repeated endoscopic failures. Eradication of *H. pylori* accelerates healing of peptic ulcers (Alg. 46.3, Table 46.7). When NSAIDs or aspirin are the etiologic factors, discontinuation, substitution of a less toxic NSAID or a cyclo-oxygenase-2 inhibitor, continuous acid suppression with a PPI, or addition of a mucosal protective agent such as misoprostol may reduce the risk for recurrence of bleeding. Bleeding from neoplastic lesions responds poorly to endoscopic or angiographic hemostasis, and surgery is frequently required. Isolated vascular lesions such as Dieulafoy lesion can be successfully treated endoscopically, angiographically, or surgically with low likelihood for recurrence. On the other hand, angiodysplasia or telangiectasia can redevelop after endoscopic ablation, or may be present elsewhere in the luminal gut, and blood loss frequently recurs.

ALGORITHM 46.3   **Management of Peptic Ulcers**

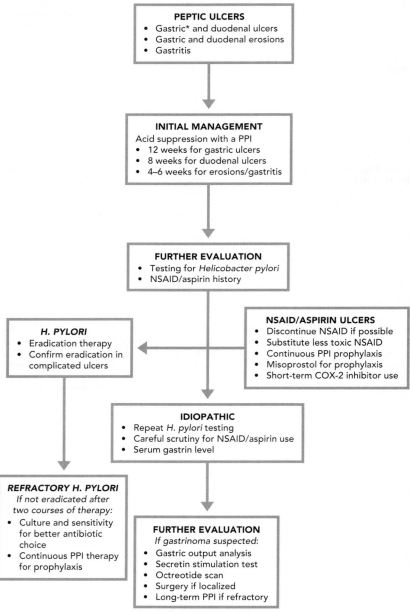

PPI, proton pump inhibitor; NSAID, nonsteroidal anti-inflammatory drug; COX-2, cyclo-oxygenase-2.
*Evaluation with endoscopy or barium contrast study is repeated at 3 months in all patients with gastric ulcers to confirm healing. If the ulcer is not completely healed, multiple biopsies are taken to exclude other nonpeptic causes, including malignancy.

TABLE 46.6	Balloon Tamponade for Variceal Bleeding

Indications
    Temporary control of variceal bleeding (gastric, esophageal or both)
    Access to endoscopic or radiologic therapy not immediately available, to stabilize patient for transport
    Efficacy is thought to be better when combined with pharmacologic therapy (Algorithm 46.2)

Equipment
    Sengstaken-Blakemore tube (three lumen), Minnesota tube (four lumen), Linton-Nachlas tube (gastric balloon alone) or similar tube
    Nasogastric tube when three-lumen tube or gastric balloon alone are used
    Soft restraints
    Traction mechanism (typically a football helmet, weights, or orthopaedic traction system)
    Manometer
    Tube clamps, surgical scissors
    Topical anesthetic, tube connectors, syringes

Technique
    Patient needs to be intubated and sedated, with soft restraints in place
    Test balloons, check intraluminal pressures at full inflation using manometer
    Gastric lavage till clear through nasogastric tube, which is then removed
    Introduce lubricated tube through mouth
    When gastric juice or blood is aspirated through gastric lumen, check tube position radiographically
    With manometer attached to measuring port, fill gastric lumen with air in 100-mL increments to recommended volume for particular tube (typically 450–500 mL)
        If rapid pressure increase noted on manometer, tube may have been inflated in esophagus; deflate immediately, advance tube, reinflate
    Clamp air inlet for gastric balloon, pull back, secure to traction device
    If esophageal balloon inflation is desired, inflate esophageal balloon to 30–45 mm Hg pressure as measured by manometer on measuring port
    Further traction can be applied if bright red blood continues to be aspirated through gastric port
    With three-lumen tubes, place nasogastric tube so tip is 3–4 cm above esophageal balloon, connect to intermittent suction
    Deflate balloons for 5 minutes every 5–6 hours to reduce risk of pressure necrosis
    Keep balloons inflated for up to 24 hours as needed
    Efficacy is around 80% when correctly placed

Complications
    Complications occur in 15%–30%; mortality rate is around 6%
    Major complications include asphyxia, airway occlusion, esophageal rupture, esophageal and gastric pressure necrosis
    Aspiration pneumonia, epistaxis, pharyngeal erosions are other complications

TABLE 46.7	Regimens for *Helicobacter pylori* Eradication

Medications	Dose	Comments[a]
Clarithromycin	500 mg bid	First line
Amoxicillin	1 g bid	
PPI[b]	bid	
Pepto-Bismol	524 mg qid	First line in penicillin-allergic patients
Metronidazole	250 mg qid	Salvage regimen if three-drug regimen fails
Tetracycline	500 mg qid	
PPI[b] or H2RA[c]	bid	
Clarithromycin	500 mg bid	Alternate regimen, if four-drug therapy is
Metronidazole	500 mg bid	not tolerated
PPI[b]	bid	
Levofloxacin	250 mg bid	Alternate salvage regimen
Amoxicillin	1 g bid	
PPI[b]	bid	
Rifabutin	300 mg qd	Alternate salvage regimen
Amoxicillin	1 g bid	
PPI[b]	bid	

bid, twice daily; PPI, proton pump inhibitor; qid, four times daily; H2RA, H_2-receptor antagonists.
[a]Duration of therapy: 10–14 days. When using salvage regimens after initial treatment failure, choose drugs that have not been used before.
[b]Standard doses for PPI: omeprazole, 20 mg; lansoprazole, 30 mg; pantoprazole, 40 mg, rabeprazole 20 mg, all twice daily. Esomeprazole is used as a single 40 mg dose once daily.
[c]Standard doses for H2RA: ranitidine, 150 mg; famotidine, 20 mg; nizatidine, 150 mg; cimetidine, 400 mg; all twice daily.

Suggested Reading

Barkun A, Bardou M, Marshall JK. Consensus recommendations for managing patients with nonvariceal upper gastrointestinal bleeding. *Ann Intern Med*. 2003;139:843–857.

Ferguson CB, Mitchell RM. Nonvariceal upper gastrointestinal bleeding: standard and new treatment. *Gastroenterol Clin North Am*. 2005;34:607–621.

Laine L, Peterson WL. Bleeding peptic ulcer. *N Engl J Med*. 1994;331:717–727.

Leontiadis GI, McIntyre L, Sharma VK, et al. Proton pump inhibitor treatment for acute peptic ulcer bleeding. *Cochrane Database Syst Rev*. 2004;3:CD002094.

Zaman A, Chalasani N. Bleeding caused by portal hypertension. *Gastroenterol Clin North Am*. 2005;34:623–642.

Acute lower gastrointestinal bleeding (LGIB) is traditionally defined as bleeding originating distal to the ligament of Trietz. Acute LGIB is about one-fifth as frequent as acute upper gastrointestinal bleeding (UGIB), with an annual incidence of hospitalization estimated at 20 to 30 per 100,000 population. Similar to trends with acute UGIB, the incidence is higher among older populations. In contrast to UGIB, acute LGIB is associated with less hemodynamic compromise, fewer transfusion requirements, and lower mortality (5%). Typically, acute LGIB is self-limiting, but bleeding can be intermittent and recurrent. Similar to acute UGIB, patients who develop acute LGIB while hospitalized for an unrelated illness have a worse outcome, with estimated mortality of 23%. In recent years, advances in endoscopic and radiologic techniques in actively bleeding patients (such as hemoclip use, superselective embolization of the bleeding vessel) have reduced the need for emergent surgery, leading to lowered rebleeding rates and morbidity in acute LGIB.

Presentation can range from scant bright red blood around formed stool or on toilet tissue to massive uncontrolled bloody bowel movements with hemodynamic compromise and shock. The color of bloody stool has been demonstrated to be a good predictor of the location of the bleeding source in patients without hemodynamic collapse. Patients pointing to a bright red or a dark red color on a color card had the highest positive predictive value for acute LGIB in one study, higher than physician reports of the same color data. Colonic bleeding is clinically indistinguishable from small bowel bleeding, but because colonic sources (Table 47.1) are identified more frequently compared with small bowel sources, and because the colon is much more accessible than the small bowel for investigative procedures, the workup initially focuses on the colon. Bloody diarrhea is sometimes interpreted as acute LGIB by patients, and a few questions usually resolve the issue. If the presentation is bloody diarrhea rather than acute LGIB, stool culture, including culture for *Escherichia coli* O157:H7, and stool *Clostridium difficile* toxin are ordered. Parasitic infestations such as amebiasis may need to be considered and ameba serology ordered, when relevant. In immunosuppressed patients, cytomegalovirus colitis can present with bloody diarrhea. Bleeding presentations of inflammatory bowel disease (Crohn's disease, ulcerative colitis) are more often bloody diarrhea than acute LGIB. The upper gastrointestinal tract can also be the source for bright or dark red blood in the stool if bleeding is massive. The small bowel is investigated if an alternate source is not apparent or identified elsewhere in the luminal gut. Therefore, the spectrum of acute LGIB is broad.

Initial resuscitation and early management of acute gastrointestinal bleeding does not vary by location (see Alg. 46.1, Chapter 46). In addition to the placement of two large-bore intravenous lines, infusions of normal saline, lactated Ringer's solution, or blood products may be appropriate depending on severity of bleeding and acuity of presentation. Anticoagulants, antiplatelet agents, and medications that affect the coagulation cascade are discontinued if possible. When clotting parameters are significantly abnormal, infusions of fresh-frozen plasma, injections of vitamin K, and protamine are administered as indicated.

Certain clinical and laboratory features at presentation may identify patients at risk for higher short-term morbidity, including continued and recurrent bleeding, hemodynamic compromise, syncope, aspirin or anticoagulant use, more than two comorbid medical conditions, and continued bleeding 4 hours after initial presentation. Others have

TABLE 47.1	Causes of Acute Lower Gastrointestinal Bleeding

Colonic sources
Diverticulosis
Angiodysplasia
Neoplasia: includes large polyps and cancers
Post polypectomy bleeding
Colitis: includes inflammatory and infectious causes
Ischemia
Anorectal causes: hemorrhoids, anal fissure
Radiation proctopathy and colopathy
Aortoenteric fistula (rare)
Dieulafoy lesion (rare)

Small bowel sources
Angiodysplasia
Neoplasia: includes cancers, stromal tumors, lymphoma
Enteritis: includes inflammatory and infectious causes
Radiation enteritis and enteropathy
Meckel diverticulum
Aortoenteric fistula (rare)

TABLE 47.2	Triage of Patients with Acute Lower Gastrointestinal Bleeding

Admission to intensive care unit
Hypotension (systolic blood pressure <115 mm Hg) at presentation
Moderate-to-severe bleeding onset while admitted for an unrelated illness
Ongoing hemodynamic instability despite resuscitation
Absence of adequate hematocrit increase despite blood transfusion
Low initial blood count (hematocrit <25% with cardiopulmonary disease or stroke, <20% otherwise)
Prolonged coagulation parameters (prothrombin time 1.2 times the control value or more)
Myocardial infarction, stroke, or other systemic complications of rapid blood loss
Any unstable comorbid disease, including altered mental status
Ongoing significant bleeding 4 hours after presentation
Evidence of active oozing, spurting, or visible vessel on endoscopy
Requirement of angiography for localization or control of bleeding

Admission to regular hospital floor
Stable hemodynamic parameters after initial resuscitation
Mild hematocrit drop <5% from baseline and/or baseline hematocrit >30%)
Stable coagulation parameters
No systemic complications from blood loss
Absence of ongoing bleeding 4 hours after presentation
Emergent *upper* endoscopy in patients with bloody stool
Bright red or dark red blood in stool with hemodynamic compromise
Bloody NG aspirate
Suspicion of aortoenteric fistula (distal duodenum needs to be evaluated)

NG, nasogastric.

identified prolongation of prothrombin time >1.2 times the control value, and altered mental status as additional predictors of poor outcome. These characteristics are useful in making triage decisions, especially in identifying patients who could benefit from admission to an intensive care unit and patients who need urgent investigative procedures (Table 47.2).

As many as 10% of hemodynamically unstable patients presenting with bright shades of blood in their stool may have a bleeding source within reach of an upper endoscope. It is important that these patients be evaluated with the initial intent to exclude an upper source, as upper endoscopy is infinitely easier to perform compared with a colonoscopy in the setting of an acute bleed. A nasogastric tube can be placed and aspiration performed, looking for a bloody aspirate. However, a clear aspirate does not exclude bleeding just distal to the pylorus, and if suspicion is high, an upper endoscopic examination is indicated. Patients with acute bleeding in the setting of past aortic graft repair need an emergent upper endoscopy for evaluation of the distal duodenum, the commonest location for an aortoenteric fistula.

Further evaluation of the patient depends on several factors: the severity and acuity of bleeding, hemodynamic state of the patient, coagulation parameters, and investigative facilities available at the institution. In patients with minimal bleeding with historical features suggesting a distal source (red blood coating outside of formed stool, pain with defecation, tenesmus, passage of fresh clots), inspection of the perianal area, anal canal, rectum, and sometimes the distal colon may be a useful initial step. This can be achieved with anoscopy and/or flexible sigmoidoscopy. However, sigmoidoscopy rarely replaces full colonoscopy after a bowel preparation, as a concurrent more proximal bleeding source cannot be excluded with this approach alone.

Colonoscopy may provide a high rate of identification of the bleeding source if performed within the first 24 hours (45% to 95%), but the feasibility and quality of bowel preparation will impact whether colonoscopy can be successfully performed (Alg. 47.1). Bowel preparation may not be possible unless the patient is hemodynamically stable and able to use the bathroom. Therapeutic maneuvers may not be safe unless coagulation parameters have been brought close to normal. If a bleeding lesion is identified during colonoscopy, therapeutic measures including epinephrine injection, thermal therapy, and mechanical therapy with hemoclips can be successfully attempted. Sometimes, a definitive lesion cannot be identified, but bleeding can be localized to a segment of bowel. At other times, a potential bleeding lesion (such as diverticulosis or angiodysplasia) is visualized, but without active bleeding or stigmata of recent hemorrhage. This provides only circumstantial evidence for localization of the bleeding source, unless a prior radiologic study localized bleeding to the same area of the colon as the potential bleeding lesion on colonoscopy. Early colonoscopy has been demonstrated to shorten the duration of hospitalization and reduce treatment costs.

When early colonoscopy cannot be performed because of rapid bleeding, hemodynamic instability, significantly impaired coagulation parameters, comorbid illnesses, or inability to tolerate a bowel preparation, a tagged red blood cell (RBC) scan helps triage actively bleeding patients to more invasive procedures such as mesenteric angiography and angiotherapy. In the research setting, bleeding rates as low as 0.1 to 0.5 mL/min are picked up by tagged RBC scans, but in the clinical setting, only 45% of tagged RBC scans demonstrate extravasation. Rapidly positive scans have the highest accuracy and predict the best likelihood of identification of the bleeding site at subsequent angiography. A positive tagged RBC scan may identify a population of acute LGIB patients with higher in-hospital morbidity and rebleeding. Delayed positive scans have a much lower sensitivity in accurately localizing the bleeding source, as intestinal peristalsis may impact the reading. A high rate of false localization (22% to 42%) makes a tagged RBC scan unreliable in localizing bleeding for subsequent surgery. The test continues to be used as a screening test prior to more invasive testing such as angiography, although some suggest that the test unnecessarily delays more definitive studies and reduces chances of early bleeding localization. If a rapidly bleeding site is identified on angiography, vasopressin can be infused after selective catheterization of the bleeding vessel. This may induce vasoconstriction and cessation of bleeding. Alternatively, selective embolization of the bleeding vessel can be attempted. Complications of angiography can be dye-related (renal failure), procedure-related (hematoma formation,

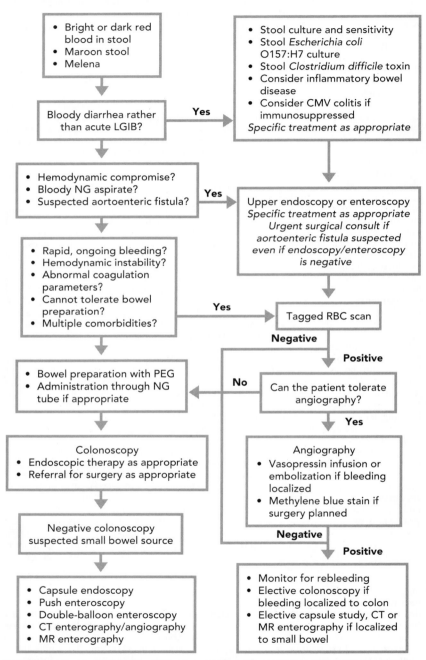

ALGORITHM 47.1   Investigation of Acute Lower Gastrointestinal Bleeding

- Bright or dark red blood in stool
- Maroon stool
- Melena

- Stool culture and sensitivity
- Stool *Escherichia coli* O157:H7 culture
- Stool *Clostridium difficile* toxin
- Consider inflammatory bowel disease
- Consider CMV colitis if immunosuppressed
Specific treatment as appropriate

Bloody diarrhea rather than acute LGIB? — **Yes** →

- Hemodynamic compromise?
- Bloody NG aspirate?
- Suspected aortoenteric fistula?

Yes →

Upper endoscopy or enteroscopy
Specific treatment as appropriate
Urgent surgical consult if aortoenteric fistula suspected even if endoscopy/enteroscopy is negative

- Rapid, ongoing bleeding?
- Hemodynamic instability?
- Abnormal coagulation parameters?
- Cannot tolerate bowel preparation?
- Multiple comorbidities?

Yes →

Tagged RBC scan

Negative — **Positive**

- Bowel preparation with PEG
- Administration through NG tube if appropriate

No ← Can the patient tolerate angiography?

Yes

Colonoscopy
- Endoscopic therapy as appropriate
- Referral for surgery as appropriate

Angiography
- Vasopressin infusion or embolization if bleeding localized
- Methylene blue stain if surgery planned

Negative colonoscopy suspected small bowel source

Negative — **Positive**

- Capsule endoscopy
- Push enteroscopy
- Double-balloon enteroscopy
- CT enterography/angiography
- MR enterography

- Monitor for rebleeding
- Elective colonoscopy if bleeding localized to colon
- Elective capsule study, CT or MR enterography if localized to small bowel

LGIB, lower gastrointestinal bleeding; CMV, cytomegalovirus; NG, nasogastric; RBC, red blood cell; PEG, polyethylene glycol; CT. computed tomography; MR, magnetic resonance.

retroperitoneal bleeding, intestinal ischemia), or as a result of vasopressin infusion (arrhythmias, myocardial infarction).

When blood is seen throughout the colon as well as within the terminal ileum, or if a potential colonic source is not evident despite a careful and adequate examination, the bleeding source could reside in the small bowel. Conventional contrast radiologic studies such as the small bowel follow-through series or enteroclysis have a very low yield for identification of a bleeding source in this setting. Capsule endoscopy has now become the test of choice in situations in which a small bowel source of bleeding is suspected. The drawbacks of capsule endoscopy include the fact that real-time reading is not possible, accurate localization of findings is almost impossible, and no therapeutics can be administered. Actively bleeding sources identified in the small bowel have required surgery in the past, either for surgical resection, or for endoscopic therapy during intraoperative enteroscopy. More recently, newer endoscopic techniques such as double-balloon enteroscopy have been developed that allow reach of almost the entire small bowel for endoscopic therapy, but these may be associated with a higher degree of morbidity and complications compared with routine endoscopic procedures. These studies can be considered in refractory situations or in obscure gastrointestinal bleeding (Table 47.3).

Newer tests that have been studied include computed tomographic angiography, wherein arterial-phase images may demonstrate vascular abnormalities such as angiodysplasia, or may even demonstrate extravasation of contrast into the bowel lumen in patients with rapidly bleeding sources. Although computed tomographic angiography may provide a less invasive option compared with conventional angiography, this option has not been systematically studied as a diagnostic option in acute LGIB. Computed tomography and magnetic resonance enterography may allow detailed evaluation of the small bowel wall and mucosa for potential bleeding lesions and inflammation. These newer and advanced radiologic options can be considered in refractory situations and in obscure gastrointestinal bleeding (Table 47.3).

TABLE 47.3   **Obscure Lower Gastrointestinal Bleeding[a]**

Approach
Consider repeating endoscopic procedures: push enteroscopy, colonoscopy, capsule
    endoscopy
If bleeding is rapid and severe with hemodynamic compromise, repeat tagged RBC scan
Consider angiography
    During bleeding episode, to localize bleeding by demonstration of contrast extravasation
    During nonbleeding interval, to identify characteristic angiographic patterns of potential
        bleeding lesions such as angiodysplasia and neoplasia
    CT or MR angiography are options, but therapy (vasopressin infusion, embolization) is not
        possible
Consider CT or MR enterography to look for luminal or mural small bowel lesions
Consider double-balloon enteroscopy, a new technique that may allow visualization of the
    entire small bowel
Consider intraoperative enteroscopy:
    Healthy individuals with significant bleeding recurrences and a potential small bowel source
    Radiologic studies or advanced endoscopic studies demonstrating a potential small bowel
        source amenable to endoscopic therapy
    For localization of a likely small bowel source, for surgical resection
Provocative measures (administration of heparin, thrombolytic agents or vasodilators) are very
    rarely used, and should not be recommended except in very refractory situations, in patients
    without comorbidities, under very close observation by experienced personnel

RBC, red blood cell; CT, computed tomography; MR, magnetic resonance.
[a]Obscure LGIB consists of persistent or recurrent bleeding, with no bleeding source evident on conventional endoscopy.

TABLE 47.4	Management of Vascular Lesions[a]

Initial management
Endoscopic ablation when possible, using thermal cautery, argon plasma coagulation or laser:
   Lesions accessible with conventional endoscopy
   Double-balloon enteroscopy in specialized cases
   Numerous lesions may not be amenable to endoscopic therapy
Iron repletion
   Oral iron therapy, ferrous sulfate 325 mg tid or equivalent
   Intravenous or parenteral iron repletion when oral iron is not tolerated or inadequate
Intermittent blood transfusions
Surgery: rare, only for isolated, discrete, limited vascular lesions such as hamartoma or
   Dieulafoy lesion
Refractory situations
Continue above measures
Consider adding medications with anecdotal and limited evidence in decreasing blood loss:
   Epsilon-amino caproic acid
   Combination estrogen-progesterone hormone therapy
   Danazol
   Octreotide by subcutaneous injection

tid, three times daily.
[a]Vascular lesions include angiodysplasia, telangiectasia, hamartoma, arteriovenous malformation, nevus, Dieulafoy lesion.

Diverticulosis and angiodysplasia account for >50% of colonic bleeding sources. Diverticular bleeding is arterial bleeding, and therefore presents with clinically significant painless episodes of bright red blood in the stool. Bleeding spontaneously ceases in >80% of patients, but one-quarter may develop recurrent bleeding. Multiple recurrences of diverticular bleeding are an indication for resection of the offending segment of colon. Bleeding

TABLE 47.5	Levels of Diagnostic Certainty in Interpreting Test for Acute Lower Gastrointestinal Bleeding

Definitive evidence of a bleeding source
Active oozing or bleeding visualized at colonoscopy or angiography
Stigmata of recent bleeding (adherent clot, nonbleeding visible vessel) identified on colonoscopy
Positive tagged RBC scan associated with either of above
Circumstantial evidence of a bleeding source
Single potential bleeding source on colonoscopy with fresh blood in the same segment
Single potential bleeding source on colonoscopy or angiography in the same area as a positive
   tagged RBC scan
Bright or dark red blood on objective stool testing, single potential source (without endoscopic
   stigmata) on colonoscopy, negative upper endoscopy and capsule endoscopy
Bright or dark red blood, maroon stool, or melena on objective stool testing, single potential
   source (without endoscopic stigmata) on capsule endoscopy, negative upper endoscopy
   and colonoscopy
Equivocal evidence of a bleeding source
"Hematochezia" unconfirmed by objective testing, potential sources (without endoscopic
   stigmata) on colonoscopy or capsule endoscopy

RBC, red blood cell.

from angiodysplasia can be slow and more persistent, and may be associated with iron deficiency anemia. Endoscopic ablation of bleeding lesions may decrease the rate of bleeding, but patients typically require iron repletion and supplementation (Table 47.4). In refractory situations, medications with anecdotal or limited evidence can be considered, but these approaches can be associated with serious thrombotic complications. Hemorrhoids account for 5% to 10% of episodes of acute LGIB, and are the most common cause of bright red blood in the stool or toilet tissue in the ambulatory patient. Other causes are less common, and include neoplasia, colitis, Meckel diverticulum, and radiation proctopathy. Angiodysplasias are the most common small bowel cause of acute LGIB. Other small bowel causes include tumors, including stromal tumors, lymphoma, and, rarely, adenocarcinoma, inflammatory disorders including Crohn's disease, and ulcers/erosions from nonsteroidal anti-inflammatory drug use.

One of the dilemmas in patients with acute LGIB is making a clinical determination as to whether the lesion identified on diagnostic testing is indeed the source for the patient's bleeding episode. This is particularly important as active bleeding or stigmata of recent bleeding are not always identified on potential bleeding lesions. At times, more than one potential bleeding lesion may be identified. Criteria have been suggested to assess the level of diagnostic certainty in interpreting diagnostic tests in acute LGIB, which may help determine the nature of definitive management or follow-up needed, especially when surgery is recommended based on the results of diagnostic tests (Table 47.5).

Suggested Reading

Eisen GM, Dominitz JA, Faigel DO, et al., American Society for Gastrointestinal Endoscopy. Standards of Practice Committee.An annotated algorithmic approach to acute lower gastrointestinal bleeding. *Gastrointest Endosc.* 2001;53:859–863.

Green BT, Rockey DC. Lower gastrointestinal bleeding—management. *Gastrointest Clin North Am.* 2005;34:665–678.

Zuckerman GR, Prakash C. Acute lower gastrointestinal bleeding. Part 1: clinical presentation and diagnosis. *Gastrointest Endosc.* 1998;48:606–617.

Zuckerman GR, Prakash C. Acute lower gastrointestinal bleeding. Part 2: etiology, therapy and outcomes. *Gastrointest Endosc.* 1999;49:228–238.

Zuckerman GR, Prakash C, Askin MP, et al. AGA technical review on the evaluation and management of occult and obscure gastrointestinal bleeding. *Gastroenterology.* 2000;118:201–221.

ACUTE PANCREATITIS
Michael J. Hersh and
Sreenivasa S. Jonnalagadda

BACKGROUND

Acute pancreatitis is acute inflammation of the pancreas associated with pancreatic autodigestion, edema, necrosis, and hemorrhage of pancreatic tissue. The clinical course varies from mild, self-limited episodes to severe pancreatitis with associated multiorgan dysfunction or local complications such as infected peripancreatic fluid collections. Up to 20% of patients presenting with pancreatitis have a severe course.

Alcohol and gallstone disease account for nearly 75% of cases of acute pancreatitis in developed countries. Other less common causes include medications, malignancy (pancreatic or ampullary), pancreas divisum, hypercalcemia, endoscopic retrograde cholangiopancreatography, infection, trauma, surgery, hypertriglyceridemia, penetrating peptic ulcer disease, and sphincter of Oddi dysfunction (Table 48.1).

EVALUATION

Initial evaluation of a patient with suspected acute pancreatitis should include a detailed history with attention to alcohol intake, previous gallstone disease, medications, and hypertriglyceridemia. Patients with malignancy as the underlying cause are typically elderly and may have associated symptoms such as weight loss. Epigastric abdominal pain radiating to the back is a common complaint. Abdominal pain can be accompanied by nausea, vomiting, and/or abdominal distention. Although abdominal tenderness, particularly in the epigastrium, is common, other physical findings indicative of intra-abdominal hemorrhage such as ecchymoses of the flanks (Grey-Turner's sign) or of the periumbilical regions (Cullen's sign) rarely may be present. Guarding and rebound tenderness may be found in more severe cases. An ileus is common at the time of initial presentation. Hypotension, tachycardia, tachypnea, and fever could be indicative of extensive inflammation or a simultaneous infectious complication.

The diagnosis of pancreatitis is confirmed by elevated serum amylase and lipase levels (greater than three times normal) in the setting of typical abdominal pain. Serum amylase is less specific, and also originates from the small bowel, salivary glands, ovaries, fallopian tubes, lungs, tonsils, breast milk, malignant neoplasms, and can be elevated because of macroamylasemia. Lipase levels are more sensitive in the diagnosis of acute pancreatitis, and remain elevated for a longer period of time compared with serum amylase. In renal failure, however, both amylase and lipase levels may be artificially elevated. Mild elevations in liver enzymes and bilirubin could reflect compression of the common bile duct (CBD) by pancreatic edema or residual bile duct stones. The failure of an elevated bilirubin and transaminases to trend to normal during a 12- to 24-hour period is suggestive of residual stones in the CBD. Serum triglycerides should be checked at the time of initial evaluation as the levels rapidly decline once the patient is maintained without a diet. In rare instances, hypercalcemia may cause pancreatitis.

IMAGING STUDIES

Imaging studies are necessary to establish the cause of acute pancreatitis. Although operator-dependent, ultrasonography is the best noninvasive and cost-effective tool for the initial evaluation of a patient presenting with pancreatitis. If gallstones with or without choledocholithiasis are seen on abdominal ultrasonography, most patients with self-limited acute

TABLE 48.1	Causes of Acute Pancreatitis
Gallstones	Autoimmune pancreatitis
Alcohol	Sphincter of Oddi dysfunc-
Medications	tion
Iatrogenic (post-ERCP)	Hereditary
Hypertriglyceridemia	Scorpion bites
Hypercalcemia	Ischemia
Pancreatic neoplasm	Abdominal trauma
Ampullary neoplasm	Infections
Pancreas divisum	Idiopathic

ERCP, endoscopic retrograde cholangiopancreatography.

pancreatitis will not require further imaging. Dilation of the bile ducts could reflect a residual stone in the CBD, or CBD compression due to pancreatic edema or a malignancy. Visualization of a bile duct stone may be hampered by poor visualization of the distal bile duct. Abdominal computed tomography (CT) can be very specific at evaluating pancreatic inflammation, necrosis, and complications such as pseudocysts, but it may not contribute significantly to the initial management, particularly in those predicted to have a mild course; additionally, CT carries the additional risk of contrast nephropathy. Magnetic resonance imaging provides cross-sectional imaging similar to CT and does not carry the same associated risks, but it also is generally not used in the initial evaluation. If clinical suspicion exists, CT, magnetic resonance cholangiography, and endoscopic ultrasonography all provide high-resolution images that can identify pancreatic neoplasms.

ASSESSMENT OF SEVERITY

Despite advances in critical care medicine, the mortality rate from severe pancreatitis in the presence of infectious complications ranges from 10% to 30%. In contrast, mild pancreatitis has an excellent outcome. Early identification of patients at risk for severe pancreatitis allows for close monitoring and also helps keep patients informed of their individual prognosis. A number of systems have been developed to risk-stratify these patients. These include the Ranson criteria, Glasgow criteria, CT criteria, and the APACHE II (Acute Physiologic and Chronic Health Evaluation II) system. An elevated C-reactive protein and obesity with a body mass index >30 are also associated with a higher risk of severe pancreatitis (Tables 48.2 and 48.3).

MANAGEMENT

Patients with persistent or severe pain, vomiting, dehydration, and elevation of amylase and lipase should be hospitalized for observation. Poor urine output, tachycardia, tachypnea, hypoxemia, and hemoconcentration may indicate a severe course and mandate closer monitoring in the intensive care unit. Supportive care is the main goal of treatment in acute pancreatitis. Aggressive intravenous fluid volume resuscitation is necessary, with careful monitoring of fluid balance. Invasive hemodynamic monitoring may be required to provide optimal care for the critically ill patient. Careful attention should be paid to serum electrolytes, calcium, and glucose levels with repletion provided as needed. Narcotic analgesia by patient controlled anesthesia (PCA) or on-demand dosing should be provided for pain management. While narcotics are indispensable in the control of pain, occasionally they can contribute to ileus. Bowel rest should be maintained until pain and nausea have resolved. For patients with severe nausea and vomiting and those noted to have an ileus, low intermittent gastric decompression via a nasogastric tube suction may be helpful. Acid suppression for stress ulcer prophylaxis should be provided in the intensive care unit patient.

In gallstone pancreatitis, fever and/or chills, jaundice, and right upper quadrant pain (Charcot's triad) are indicative of cholangitis. Although treatment with antibiotics should

TABLE 48.2	Computed Tomography (CT) Grading of Acute Pancreatitis: CT Severity Index[a]	

Grade[b]	Findings	Score
A	Normal pancreas: normal size, sharply defined, smooth contour, homogeneous enhancement, retroperitoneal peripancreatic fat without enhancement	0
B	Focal or diffuse enlargement of the pancreas; contour may show irregularity, enhancement may be inhomogeneous but there is on peripancreatic inflammation	1
C	Peripancreatic inflammation with intrinsic pancreatic abnormalities	2
D	Intrapancreatic or extrapancreatic fluid collections	3
E	Two or more large collections of gas in the pancreas or retroperitoneum	4

Necrosis score based on contrast-enhanced CT

Necrosis (%)	Score
0	0
<33	2
33–50	4
≥50	6

[a]CT severity index equals unenhanced CT score plus necrosis score: maximum = 10, ≥6 = severe disease.
[b]Grading based on findings on unenhanced CT.

be promptly initiated when cholangitis is suspected, biliary decompression is pivotal to successful patient outcome. Gram-negative pathogens such as *Escherichia coli* are the typical biliary pathogens, and broad-spectrum Gram-negative and anaerobic coverage with piperacillin-tazobactam, fluoroquinolone plus metronidazole, third-generation cephalosporins, or carbapenems such as imipenem and meropenem is appropriate until the cultures and sensitivities are available to direct therapy.

At least three prospective studies have conclusively shown improved patient outcome with early (24 to 72 hours) endoscopic retrograde cholangiopancreatography in patients with suspected residual bile duct stones. A residual bile duct stone can cause persistently elevated transaminases, alkaline phosphatase, and bilirubin, as well as biliary colic, cholangitis, and a dilated biliary tree. Patients with a residual bile duct stone should undergo interval cholecystectomy with intraoperative cholangiography (Table 48.4).

Patients with severe pancreatitis are at risk for systemic complications such as respiratory and renal failure. The local complications include infections of the pancreas and peripancreatic fluid, inflammatory fluid collections, and abdominal fluid sequestration. Patients may develop worsening nausea, vomiting and/or abdominal pain, leukocytosis, bacteremia, and fever. In a patient with septic physiology, rising white blood cell count, fevers, and clinical deterioration, prophylactic use of antibiotics is recommended. There are data to support the use of imipenem for 1 to 2 weeks to reduce the occurrence of infectious complications. An increased incidence of fungal infections following antibiotic use in this patient population has not been conclusively established. If there is failure to clinically improve despite 2 to 3 days of conservative management, repeat imaging by dynamic CT or magnetic resonance imaging to evaluate for fluid collections and infected pancreatic necrosis should be performed. Potentially infected fluid collections can be percutaneously sampled and drained under ultrasound or CT guidance.

The other option for an infected fluid collection is exploratory laparotomy with debridement of necrotic or infected material and drain placement. However, surgery in

TABLE 48.3	Methods to Predict the Severity of Acute Pancreatitis

Ranson criteria[a]

	0 hours
Age	>55 years
White blood cell count	>16,000/mm^3
Blood glucose	>200 mg/dL (11.1 mmol/L)
Lactate dehydrogenase	>350 U/L
Aspartate aminotransferase	>250 U/L
	48 hours
Hematocrit	Fall by ≥10%
Blood urea nitrogen	Increase by ≥5 mg/dL (1.8 mmol/L) despite fluids
Serum calcium	<8 mg/dL (2 mmol/L)
po$_2$	<60 mm Hg
Base deficit	>4 mEq/L
Fluid sequestration	>6,000 mL

Glasgow system: poor prognostic factors[b]

White blood cell count	>15,000/mcL
Serum glucose concentration	>180 g/dL (10 mmol/L) with no history of diabetes
Blood urea nitrogen	>45 mg/dL (16 mmol/L) with no response to fluids
po$_2$	<60 mm Hg
Serum calcium concentration	<8 mg/dL (2 mmol/L)
Serum albumin concentration	<3.2 g/dL (32 g/L)
Lactate dehydrogenase	>600 U/L
Aspartate aminotransferase	>200 U/L

[a]The presence of one to three criteria represents mild pancreatitis; the mortality rate rises significantly with four or more criteria.
Ranson, JHC, Rifkind, KM, Roses, DF, et al. Prognostic signs and the role of operative management in acute pancreatitis. *Surg Gynecol Obstet.* 1974;139:69–81.
[b]The presence of three or more of these criteria within the first 48 hours is indicative of severe pancreatitis.
Corfield, AP, Williamson, RCN, McMahon, MJ, et al. Prediction of severity in acute pancreatitis: prospective comparison of three prognostic indices. *Lancet.* 1985;24:403–407.

these critically ill patients is associated with a significant morbidity and mortality and the presence of necrosis alone is not sufficient grounds for surgical intervention. There is evidence that delayed surgery in this setting is associated with a better prognosis. Minimally invasive approaches such as percutaneous drainage, laparoscopic retroperitoneal debridement, or endoscopic approaches may successfully bridge the patient to recovery or surgical exploration in a more stable clinical scenario. If the fluid is sterile, fevers and leukocytosis may reflect inflammation rather than infection. Antibiotic coverage should be optimized for any positive blood or fluid culture.

Patients with mild pancreatitis typically resume a normal diet within a few days. However, most patients with severe pancreatitis will have to abstain from oral intake until clinical improvement occurs. The ideal approach in this situation is enteral feeding via a nasojejunal tube. Enteral nutrition preserves the intestinal mucosa and has the added benefit of potentially reducing incidence of bacterial translocation from the gut. Outcome studies have shown that enteral nutrition is associated with reduced central line infections, reduced sepsis, less need for surgical intervention, decreased length of hospital stay, and lower cost. The incidence of multiorgan failure and mortality is no different between parenteral and enteral nutrition. Enteral nutrition should be the route of choice for nutrition unless it is not tolerated or if enteral access cannot be maintained. If enteral nutrition is poorly tolerated by the patient, total parenteral nutrition can be used.

ALGORITHM 48.1 | **Management of Pancreatic and Peripancreatic Fluid Collections in the Intensive Care Unit**

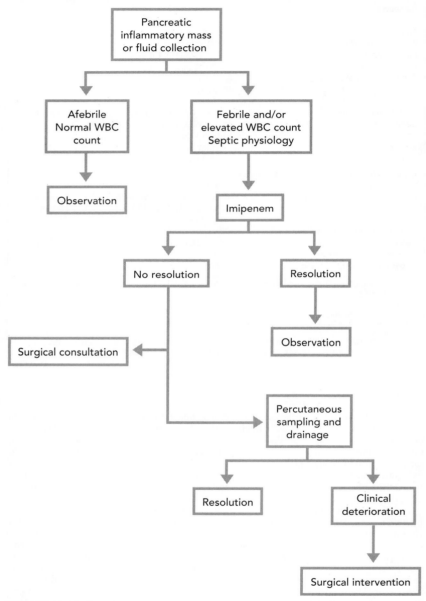

WBC, white blood cell

TABLE 48.4	Indications for Endoscopic Retrograde Cholangiopancreatography in Acute Biliary Pancreatitis

- Bilirubin and liver enzymes not trending to normal over during 12–24 hours
- Bile duct stone on ultrasonography
- Bile duct dilation on ultrasonography
- Obstructive jaundice
- Cholangitis
- Biliary colic
- Prohibitive risk for cholecystectomy

Suggested Reading

Lankisch PG, Lerch MM. The role of antibiotic prophylaxis in the treatment of acute pancreatitis. *J Clin Gastroenterol.* 2006;40:149–155.
   A review of antibiotics and their use in acute pancreatitis.
McClave SA, Chang WK, Dhaliwal R, et al. Nutrition support in acute pancreatitis: a systematic review of the literature. *JPEN J Parenter Enteral Nutr.* 2006;30:143–156.
   An excellent review on the role of nutrition in acute pancreatitis.
Tenner S. Initial management of acute pancreatitis: critical issues during the first 72 hours. *Am J Gastroenterol.* 2004;99:2489–2494.
   A review of early management of acute pancreatitis, including gallstone pancreatitis.
Whitcomb DC. Acute pancreatitis. *New Engl J Med.* 2006;354:2142–2150.
   A thorough, broad review of nutrition, antibiotics, grading systems and surgical management in acute pancreatitis.
Wyncoll DL. The management of severe acute necrotizing pancreatitis: an evidence based review of the literature. *Intensive Care Med.* 1999;25:146–156.
   A review of severe acute pancreatitis, grading systems and management.

XIV | Neurologic Disorders

49 | STATUS EPILEPTICUS
Manu S. Goyal and Yekaterina Axelrod

Status epilepticus (SE) is defined as a seizure lasting >30 minutes or two discrete seizures occurring without a return to consciousness. A seizure persisting beyond just a few minutes is more likely to be resistant to pharmacologic treatment, cause neuronal injury, and develop self-escalating behavior; therefore, seizures lasting >5 minutes may signal impending SE and warrant immediate and aggressive intervention. Mortality may be as high as 30% in adults, and even higher in the elderly or critically ill population.

The causes of SE include inadequate levels of anticonvulsants in patients with known epilepsy, cerebrovascular accidents, anoxic/ischemic brain injury, alcohol withdrawal, drugs, infections (particularly viral encephalitis), mass lesions, trauma or postoperative changes, and metabolic causes. Occasionally the cause may be reversible (e.g., isoniazid toxicity treated with intravenous administration of pyridoxine). The immediate treatment of SE remains the primary goal and is the same regardless of the cause, while determining the cause is a secondary aim.

SE can be divided into three types: generalized convulsive, focal motor, and nonconvulsive SE (Table 49.1). Generalized convulsive SE with impaired consciousness and continuous motor activity carries the highest morbidity and mortality risk. The treatment algorithm described here is designed for this condition. Beware of the diagnosis of nonconvulsive SE in patients with neuromuscular paralysis or myopathy as either condition may mask convulsive activity. As many as 8% of comatose patients without overt seizure activity may have nonconvulsive SE. Some subtle manifestations include lack of pupillary response, eyelid and eye twitching, and gaze deviation.

The principle of treatment is to terminate the seizure as rapidly as possible while preventing side effects from the anticonvulsants. Constant attention must be paid to airway protection, adequate cerebral oxygenation/perfusion, and bodily harm prevention. Vital signs and heart rhythm should be monitored repeatedly. Treatment begins with intravenous lorazepam and simultaneous intravenous loading with phenytoin at 20 mg/kg. A common pitfall is to administer too little phenytoin with failure to achieve a therapeutic level in the serum. Occasionally, additional phenytoin or valproic acid may be necessary. An initial treatment algorithm is provided in Algorithm 49.1.

TABLE 49.1	Types of Status Epilepticus		
Generalized convulsive	**Focal motor**	**Nonconvulsive**	
Impaired consciousness, motor activity frequently apparent High morbidity and mortality risk Initiate immediate and aggressive interventions Treat underlying cause	Intact consciousness, focal motor activity evident Variable prognosis depending on cause Oral or rectal benzodiazepines, oral antiepileptics Treat underlying cause	Impaired consciousness, no rhythmic motor activity apparent Frequently seen in an ICU setting Requires EEG confirmation	
ICU, intensive care unit; EEG, electroencephalogram.			

If this initial attempt fails to control seizures, continuous electroencephalogram (EEG) monitoring should begin. It is necessary to induce adequate neuronal suppression to prevent further injury from prolonged SE. The goal is to achieve seizure freedom, or in more refractory cases, induce a burst-suppression pattern on EEG pharmacologically (Fig. 49.1), thus allowing time to establish therapeutic levels of anticonvulsants and initiate treatment of potential causes or contributing factors (Alg. 49.2). Because respiratory drive inhibition and hypotension are common at this point, intubation, fluid resuscitation, and vasopressor administration should be considered.

Once burst-suppression pattern is achieved, it should be maintained for 24 to 48 hours. Keeping the patient in burst-suppression is associated with a range of potential complications. The entire organism is in a state of a very low metabolic rate ("shutdown") and, therefore, prone to cardiovascular depression (hypotension and bradycardia), pulmonary edema (ciliary inhibition), various infections, ileus, and thromboembolic complications. Each complication should be closely monitored for and aggressively addressed. Figure 49.2 provides information for the management of burst-suppression.

As a next step, the medication causing cortical inhibition is slowly weaned under close EEG monitoring. If breakthrough seizures occur, the infusion is restarted until burst-suppression is accomplished, and another attempt is made after 24 hours of seizure freedom. Further adjustments of antiepileptic medications may be necessary during that time.

Outcome of SE strongly depends on the response to the initial dose of the anticonvulsant and the presence of a structural lesion in the brain. Anoxic/ischemic injuries to the brain, encephalitis, diffuse axonal injury, SE lasting for more than an hour, and older age predict poor outcome.

ALGORITHM 49.1   **Initial Treatment of Status Epilepticus**

- Protect airway, administer oxygen
- Monitor vitals and ECG
- Ascertain adequate venous access
- Send labs: hemogram, chemistries, electrolytes, blood gases, anticonvulsant levels, toxicology, coagulation panel, liver profile

Initial antiepileptic treatment:

- Lorazepam 4 mg IV, may repeat 2 mg IV every 10 minutes not to exceed a total of 0.1 mg/kg AND
- Phenytoin/fosphenytoin IV load of 15–20 mg/kg at rate of 50 mg/min (phenytoin) or 150 PE/min (fosphenytoin)
- Consider dextrose (50 mL D50) and 100 mg of thiamine intravenously

Initial general management:

- Perform further diagnostic steps: head CT, lumbar puncture (new fever, altered mental status, recent brain surgery)
- Check phenytoin level, goal range, 15–25 mg/dL
- Supplement with additional phenytoin 5–10 mg/kg IV infusion
- Monitor for arrhythmias, hypotension, and respiratory failure
- Intubate if signs of aspiration or hypoxia are evident

ECG, electrocardiogram; IV, intravenous; D50, dextrose 50% in water; CT, computed tomography.

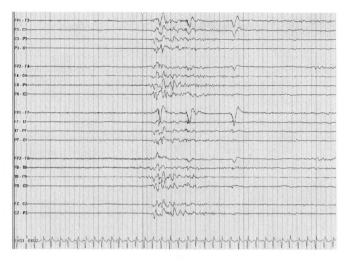

Figure 49.1 Burst-suppression pattern on electroencephalogram.

ALGORITHM 49.2   **Treatment of Refractory Status Epilepticus**

Seizure activity did not resolve with two anticonvulsants

Induce cerebral burst-suppression:

- Start the agent most readily available: Phenobarbital 20 mg/kg load at 75 mg/min
OR
    Midazolam 0.2 mg/kg IV bolus
- Start continuous infusion of: Pentobarbital 5 mg/kg load, 2–5 mg/kg/hr drip
OR
    Midazolam 0.2 mg/kg load, 0.1–2.0 mg/kg/hr drip
OR
    Propofol 1–2 mg/kg load, 2–10 mg/kg/hr drip;
- Titrate infusion until burst-suppression of cortical activity is seen on EEG

General management:

- Continuous EEG monitoring
- Consult Neurology
- Monitor vital signs closely
- Intubate patient if not done
- Treat hypotension with fluids and vasopressors
- Obtain detailed history, brain imaging, laboratory tests
- Maintain high serum level of the anticonvulsants

IV, intravenous; EEG, electroencephalogram.

While in burst-suppression

- Continuous EEG monitoring
- Continue infusion of the drug that induced burst-suppression for 24–48 hours
- Check for toxicity (daily anticonvulsant levels, blood cell count, liver function)
- Treat underlying cause of seizures (such as meningitis, cerebral edema)
- Monitor closely for:
  - o Infections, especially pneumonia
  - o Hypotension and bradycardia, pulmonary edema
  - o Ileus
- Use compression stockings and pneumatic devices to prevent thromboembolism
- Treat acidosis and fever

Weaning burst-suppression

- Slowly wean the infusion off during 6–12 hours, continue all other anticonvulsants
- Watch EEG for recurrence of seizures
- If breakthrough seizure occurs, resume infusion for 24 hours and retry

Figure 49.2 Maintenance of burst-suppression and weaning. EEG, electroencephalogram.

Suggested Reading

Bassin S, Smith TL, Bleck TP. Clinical review: status epilepticus. *Crit Care.* 2002;6:137–142.

A freely available full text document on the internet providing a concise practical overview on the mechanisms and treatment of status epilepticus.

Chen JW, Wasterlain CG. Status epilepticus: pathophysiology and management in adults. *Lancet Neurol.* 2006;5:246–256.

A review of the pathophysiological mechanisms and reasoning behind the current recommended management for convulsive status epilepticus. The authors also provide a very useful chart for organizing treatment in the acute phase.

Treiman DM, Meyers PD, Walton NY, et al. A comparison of four treatments for generalized convulsive status epilepticus. Veterans Affairs Status Epilepticus Cooperative Study Group. *N Engl J Med.* 1998;339:792–798.

A well-designed study comparing diazepam, phenytoin, lorazepam, and phenobarbital in the acute treatment of status epilepticus in terms of stopping seizure activity within 20 minutes. They conclusively demonstrate the usefulness of lorazepam for initial intravenous treatment when dosed adequately.

Walker M. Status epilepticus: an evidence based guide. *BMJ.* 2005;331:673–677.

A well-written review on the management of status epilepticus based on current evidence.

ACUTE ISCHEMIC STROKE

Manu S. Goyal and Yekaterina Axelrod

50

Stroke is the third leading cause of death in the United States. Approximately 85% of all strokes are ischemic. Several scenarios of acute ischemic stroke warrant intensive care. Patients who have undergone thrombolysis are usually admitted for monitoring for hemorrhagic complications and blood pressure (BP) management. Anatomically large strokes or infarctions affecting the brainstem require close neurologic monitoring in a critical care setting as well.

BASIC PRINCIPLES OF MANAGEMENT

Stroke is a sudden loss of adequate perfusion to a segment of the brain causing irreversible ischemic damage. Its presentation varies considerably and may be as subtle as minor sensory loss or as impressive as locked-in syndrome. Thalamic and brainstem infarctions may cause a nonspecific alteration of the mental state or coma that may be difficult to distinguish from encephalopathy because of metabolic derangements or infectious disorders. Clinical diagnosis is usually possible if the acute onset history and a pattern of deficits match a typical stroke syndrome. Intracranial hemorrhage should be ruled out by appropriate brain imaging, typically a noncontrast computed tomography scan. The differential diagnosis of stroke includes postictal paralysis, neoplastic or infectious processes, complicated migraine, and psychosomatic disorders. Meticulously obtained history helps differentiate these entities. Magnetic resonance imaging of the brain may be required to establish the diagnosis; bright lesions identified on diffusion-weighted images are usually consistent with stroke.

Aspirin should be given to ischemic stroke patients within 48 hours. For ischemic strokes <3 hours old, intravenous thrombolysis with tissue plasminogen activator (tPA) is the intervention of choice in select patients (Figure 50.1).

Stroke often causes reactive hypertension; it provides adequate cerebral perfusion to the areas at risk for hypoperfusion and further ischemic damage. High BP should not be treated unless there is ongoing end-organ damage (such as acute myocardial infarction, dissecting aneurysms, heart failure) or tPA was given. For the first 24 hours after thrombolysis, systolic BP is kept under 180 and diastolic BP under 110 mm Hg to avoid hemorrhagic complications. Labetalol, nicardipine, or hydralazine can be used; nitrates are avoided because of their potential for venous dilatation and thus intracranial pressure elevation.

Seizure prophylaxis is not indicated, but seizures should be treated properly. The use of anticoagulation for deep venous thrombosis prevention can be instituted 24 hours following the onset of stroke or tPA administration if no concern for hemorrhagic conversion exists. Low-molecular-weight heparin is the agent of choice. Fever and hyperglycemia worsen outcomes in patients with acute stroke and should be appropriately treated.

Determining the cause of stroke is necessary to guide therapy for secondary prevention. Telemetry, echocardiography, brain magnetic resonance imaging, carotid Doppler study, and various forms of angiography may be used. However, proper use and interpretation of these diagnostic tests is best reserved for stroke physicians, given the increasing complexity of stroke management. General methods of the past, such as universal anticoagulation and carotid endarterectomy, have changed to more complex algorithms and will likely evolve even further. Consultation with a stroke physician for all cases of acute ischemic stroke is advised.

Indications for tPA

- Acute onset of focal neurologic symptoms in a defined vascular territory, consistent with ischemic stroke
- **Clearly defined** onset of stroke <3 hours prior to planned start of treatment (if patient awakens with symptoms, onset is defined at "last seen normal")
- Age 18 or older
- No evidence of intracranial hemorrhage, nonvascular lesions (e.g., brain tumor, abscess) or signs of advanced cerebral infarction such as sulcal edema, hemispheric swelling, or large areas of low attenuation consistent with acute stroke on CT

Contraindications for tPA

- Onset of stroke >3 hours prior to planned start of treatment
- Rapidly improving symptoms
- Mild stroke symptoms/signs (relative)
- If MCA stroke, an obtunded or comatose state may be a relative contraindication
- Seizure at onset of stroke symptoms or within 3 hours prior to tPA administration
- Clinical presentation suggestive of subarachnoid hemorrhage regardless of CT result
- Hypertension: SBP >185 mm Hg or DBP >110 mm Hg. Hypertensive patients are excluded if BP remains elevated on consecutive measurements or aggressive treatment is required to lower BP into appropriate range.
- Minor ischemic stroke within 1 month or major ischemic stroke or head trauma within the last 3 months
- History of intracerebral or subarachnoid hemorrhage if recurrence risk is substantial
- Untreated cerebral aneurysm, arteriovenous malformation, or brain tumor
- Gastrointestinal or genitourinary hemorrhage within the last 21 days
- Arterial puncture at a noncompressible site within the last 7 days or lumbar puncture within the last 3 days
- Major surgery or major trauma within the last 14 days
- Clinical presentation suggestive of acute myocardial infarction or post-MI pericarditis
- Patient taking oral anticoagulants and INR >1.7
- Patient receiving heparin within the last 48 hours and having an elevated aPTT
- Patient receiving low-molecular-weight heparin within the last 24 hours
- Pregnant, or anticipated pregnant, female
- Known hemorrhagic diathesis or unsupported coagulation factor deficiency
- Received tPA <7 days previously
- Glucose <50 or >400 mg/dL
- Platelet count <100,000/mm^3
- INR >1.7 or elevated aPTT
- Positive pregnancy test

Figure 50.1 Indications and Contraindications for Thrombolysis. tPA, tissue plasminogen activator; CT, computed tomography; MCA, middle cerebral artery; SBP, systolic blood pressure; DBP, diastolic blood pressure; BP, blood pressure; MI, myocardial infarction; INR, international normalized ratio; aPTT, activated partial thromboplastin time.

ALGORITHM 50.1   **Management of Malignant Cerebral Edema Due to Stroke**

Determine level of care per family and patient's prior wishes

Stage 1: Initial intensive care and monitoring
- Monitoring of vitals and mental status at least every 2 hours
- Keep the head of bed at 30 degrees elevation or more
- Avoid jugular compression
- Treat fever
- Avoid enteral and intravenous hypotonic solutions
- Permissive hypertension, treat only SBP >220 or DBP >120
- Avoid thrombolytics
- Intubation for airway protection (GCS <9 or bulbar weakness)

Stage 2: Osmotic therapy for intracranial hypertension
- Avoid hypercarbia (ascertain adequate minute ventilation, treat fever)
- Give intravenous boluses of mannitol (see Chapter 52)
- Consider hypertonic saline if mannitol is unsuccessful or contraindicated

Stage 3: Surgery for cerebral edema (for patients under 60 years or with cerebellar lesions)
- Consult Neurosurgery for possible decompressive hemicraniectomy
- Discuss with family benefits and risks of the procedure
- Continue osmotic therapy and medical management

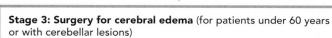

Stage 4: Experimental techniques (induced hypothermia)

SBP, systolic blood pressure; DBP, diastolic blood pressure; GCS, Glasgow Coma Scale.

CEREBRAL EDEMA

A large acute ischemic stroke typically causes cytotoxic edema. In younger patients with minimal or nonexistent cerebral atrophy, edema may have dire consequences requiring close monitoring and aggressive interventions. Some strokes may cause compression of the cerebral ventricular system and lead to obstructive hydrocephalus. Edema due to cerebellar infarctions may compress the fourth ventricle and result in herniation of the cerebellar tonsils. Simple measures such as keeping the head elevated at 30 or more degrees, avoiding hypotonic solutions, and careful monitoring may be sufficient. In more advanced cases, external ventricular drainage or decompressive posterior craniectomy may be necessary.

Large infarctions (middle cerebral artery territory or hemispheric lesions) often require more aggressive interventions. These strokes commonly cause significant cerebral edema resulting in tissue shifts and herniation. The peak effect typically occurs within 3 to 5 days, but in severe cases, rapid deterioration can occur within the first 2 days. The mortality rate is close to 80%. Risk factors for deterioration within the first day include patients of younger age, those with larger infarcts, or those treated with thrombolysis.

Interventions for cerebral edema range from medical methods to drastic surgical treatments. The intensivist must establish early a clear understanding of the patient's and family's wishes regarding the degree of interventions desired. Algorithm 50.1 demonstrates an algorithm for a stepwise approach to management of these patients beginning with intubation for airway protection, osmotic therapy, consideration for decompressive craniectomy, and lastly, with experimental techniques such as induced hypothermia to 33°C to 35°C.

Recent trials indicate that decompressive craniectomy may improve outcomes in younger patients (under age 60) with less comorbidity and substantially improves mortality in all stroke victims. Some argue that this treatment should be reserved for patients with nondominant hemisphere infarctions as those result in considerable morbidity because of language dysfunction; however, some studies find no significant differences in quality of life. Nevertheless, the procedure requires a consenting neurosurgeon, and early consultation helps avoid confusion and discontent. The ideal timing of surgery remains unclear.

Suggested Reading

Adams H, Adams R, Del Zoppo G, et al; Stroke Council of the American Heart Association; American Stroke Association. Guidelines for the early management of patients with ischemic stroke: 2005 guidelines update a scientific statement from the Stroke Council of the American Heart Association/American Stroke Association. *Stroke.* 2005;36:916–923.
An evidence based review and most up-to-date guidelines for the management of patients with acute ischemic stroke. Freely available on the internet

Andrews PJ. Critical care management of acute ischemic stroke. *Curr Opin Crit Care.* 2004;10:110–115.
A retrospective and prospective review on the management of acute stroke in the critical care setting

Gupta R, Connolly ES, Mayer S, et al. Hemicraniectomy for massive middle cerebral artery territory infarction: a systematic review. *Stroke.* 2004;35:539–543.
An excellent review of factors to account for when deciding whether to proceed with decompressive hemicraniectomy for hemispheric malignant infarction.

ELEVATED INTRACRANIAL PRESSURE

51

Manu S. Goyal and Yekaterina Axelrod

Elevated intracranial pressure (EICP) is commonly seen as a result of a variety of severe neurologic insults including intracranial hemorrhage, traumatic brain injury, brain tumors, and ischemic stroke. Regardless of its cause, EICP may interrupt the cerebral blood flow (CBF) precipitating ischemia and triggering herniation, leading to greater disability and even death. Because patients with EICP may rapidly progress to brain death, recognition of herniation syndromes is critical. Frequent neurologic examination permits fast and reliable detection of an impending catastrophe.

The brain is primarily composed of noncompressible tissue bathed and perfused by two noncompressible fluids, cerebrospinal fluid and blood, all contained within the rigid skull. When ICP rises acutely, the entire brain or one of its segments can be displaced. Masses or edema in a cerebral hemisphere cause contralateral and downward displacement of the midline structures (subfalcine and uncal herniation) manifesting with decreased level of consciousness, ipsilateral third cranial nerve palsy (ptosis and pupillary dilatation along with lateral and downward deviation of the eye), and contralateral hemiplegia. Lesions of the cerebral structures located in the posterior fossa may cause compression of the medulla, resulting in breathing abnormalities, decreased consciousness, hypertension, and bradycardia (Cushing's reflex, representing an attempt to improve cerebral perfusion when ICP is high). These patients are at risk of sudden respiratory or cardiac arrest; therefore, addressing the airway early is mandatory.

The cerebral perfusion pressure (CPP) is driven by the mean arterial pressure (MAP) and impeded by the pressure in the cerebral veins and subarachnoid space: CPP = MAP – ICP. Increases in MAP will increase CPP, whereas reductions will lower it. When CPP falls, the cerebral arterioles dilate to maintain CBF and delivery of oxygen and nutrients; when CPP rises, the vessels constrict keeping CBF stable, a process called *autoregulation*. In an injured brain this mechanism may be impaired; a fall in CPP below 60 mm Hg leads to ischemia. Thus, CPP is a useful surrogate of CBF; CPP monitoring requires an ICP monitor.

An algorithm for the treatment of EICP is shown in Algorithm 51.1. Simple initial steps include keeping the head of the patient elevated at 30 degrees with the neck straightened to avoid jugular compression. The essential concepts in ICP management are reviewed here.

AIRWAY

As in any emergency, the airway should be addressed first. Hypercapnia raises ICP by causing vasodilation. Noninvasive positive pressure ventilation may be a temporizing measure; however, patients with EICP as a rule are unable to protect the airway. If prolonged or traumatic intubation is anticipated, pretreating with 0.5 to 1 g/kg of mannitol is recommended. Every attempt should be made to prevent coughing, vomiting, and anxiety, as these factors may further elevate ICP. Lidocaine may be used for cough suppression. Succinylcholine is avoided during intubation as it may elevate ICP.

HYPERVENTILATION

Hyperventilation causes hypocarbia, leading to vasoconstriction and decreased ICP. However, vasoconstriction may lower CBF and worsen cerebral ischemia. Moreover, weaning patients off prolonged hyperventilation can cause rebound ICP elevation. Hyperventilation is used in an emergent setting *shortly* while other treatments take effect.

ALGORITHM 51.1 **Management of Elevated Intracranial Pressure (ICP)**

Immediate measures to lower ICP
- Elevate head of the bed to >30°
- Avoid jugular compression
- Address airway and avoid hypercapnia
- Avoid agitation/sedate to Ramsey 4 using benzodiazepines
- Mannitol IV bolus at 0.75–1.5 g/kg
- If renal failure, 30–60 mL of 23.4% saline IV via *central line*

↓

Ascertain patient's stability to undergo head CT

↓

Non-contrast head CT
- Hemorrhage, stroke, edema, hydrocephalus, mass
- Presence of midline shift
- Abnormal ventricular size (compressed or dilated)
- Invisibility of the gyri/sulci, grey/white matter difference

↓

Obtain Neurology or Neurosurgery consult for further management

IV, intravenous; CT, computed tomography.

HYPERTENSION

Unless a patient is experiencing end-organ damage (such as hypertensive encephalopathy, acute myocardial ischemia, aortic dissection, ongoing hemorrhage), lowering MAP may be detrimental to cerebral perfusion. It is safe to decrease the MAP by 10% to 15%. Short-acting medications are preferred; drugs of choice are beta-blockers and nicardipine. Nitrates should be avoided because of the risk of cerebral venous dilatation with subsequent ICP elevation.

OSMOTIC THERAPY

Mannitol, an osmotic agent, causes water to shift from the intracellular and interstitial spaces into the intravascular compartment, thus shrinking the cerebral tissue. Mannitol may produce hemodynamic changes mainly related to acute transient intravascular volume expansion, requiring close cardiac monitoring. Massive diuresis is seen after each dose with subsequent elevation of serum sodium and loss of magnesium, potassium, and phosphorus. Replacing urine output with normal saline to maintain euvolemia and prevent renal damage is essential. Electrolyte monitoring and proper replacement are necessary on a daily basis (Alg. 51.2).

In patients with contraindications to mannitol (renal failure), 23.4% saline can be used via a central venous catheter to acutely lower ICP and maintain high serum osmolality, targeting sodium levels of 150 to 160 mEq/L. In patients without central venous access, continuous infusions of hypertonic saline (1.25% to 3%) may help to keep serum osmolality elevated.

Caution should be exercised during osmotic therapy weaning because rapid normalization of elevated serum sodium may cause rebound swelling and thus EICP (Alg. 51.3). As a rule, 5 to 8 mEq in 24 hours appears to be safe. Close neurologic monitoring is essential during weaning.

CORTICOSTEROIDS

There is evidence against the use of corticosteroids in management of intracranial hemorrhage, ischemic stroke, and traumatic brain injury. These agents are reserved for management of vasogenic cerebral edema caused by neoplasms or certain central nervous system infections. Prophylaxis of gastric ulcers and hyperglycemia management while using high doses of steroids should be instituted.

FLUID MANAGEMENT

Free water intake should be strictly limited; hypotonic intravenous fluids must be avoided and tube feedings changed to a more concentrated formula. Other useful steps include using normal saline instead of water in flushes and changing or concentrating intravenous medications (antibiotics, vasopressors, sedative infusions).

SEDATION

Pain, discomfort, and Valsalva-like maneuvers should be strictly limited, as they may elevate ICP. Agitated or combative patients may be sedated with benzodiazepines. Fentanyl is used cautiously because it can elevate ICP in some patients. End-tidal CO_2 should be closely monitored to maintain normocarbia during sedation. Short-acting sedating agents are preferred to allow serial neurologic examinations. Barbiturates can be used as a *last resort* for refractory EICP management in head trauma patients. Neuromuscular paralysis, unless used for oxygenation purposes, should not be used routinely in patients with high ICP.

SURGICAL INTERVENTIONS

If EICP is due to a space-occupying lesion, neurosurgical consultation for possible resection should be obtained. In some instances, removing the skull and expanding the dura overlying

ALGORITHM 51.2 **Management of Osmotic Therapy**

Using mannitol

- Initial mannitol bolus of 0.75–1.5 g/kg, use peripheral venous access with caution
- Continue 0.5–1 g/kg q4–6h
- Monitor input and output closely
- Prevent hypovolemia; replace urine loss with isotonic fluids
- Correct potassium, magnesium, and phosphorus daily
- If acute renal failure, discontinue mannitol
- If ICP remains high and sodium is under 150 mmol/L, add hypertonic saline
- Closely monitor patients with very poor EF—may develop transient pulmonary edema

---

Mannitol clearance monitoring

- Check premannitol serum osmolality and BMP to calculate osmolal gap:
  $$2\ [Na] + BUN/2.8 + Glucose/18\ \textit{Measured Serum Osmolality}$$
- Calculate osmolal gap prior to every other dose of mannitol
- **If gap is above 18, hold a dose; recheck gap**

Osmolal gap 18 or above

- Stop mannitol
- If ICP remains elevated and sodium under 150 mmol/L, switch to hypertonic saline

Osmolal gap 12–18

- Continue same dose of mannitol or decrease by 25%
- Watch renal function and osmolal gap closely

Using hypertonic saline

- 23.4% saline given as IV boluses q3–6h for patients with refractory ICP elevation
- Dose is calculated as 2/3 of the mannitol dose (30–70 mL average)
- Can be alternated with mannitol or used exclusively **via central line**
- Check serum sodium prior to every other dose
- Target serum sodium level of 150–160 mmol/L
- Continuous intravenous infusion of 1.25%–3% saline is an alternative

EF, ejection fraction; BUN, blood urea nitrogen; IV, intravenous.

ALGORITHM 51.3   **Weaning Osmotic Therapy**

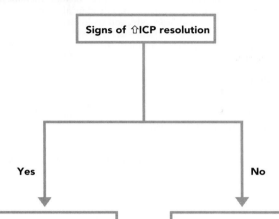

Signs of ⇧ICP resolution

Yes

No

Wean osmotic therapy

- Cut mannitol by 25 g/dose over 24-hour period
- For 23.4% saline, increase interval between doses or use as needed for ICP >25 for 5 minutes
- Allow slow decrease of sodium level (no more than 5–8 mEq/day) by changing tonicity of enteral fliuds
- Continue close neurological monitoring

Continue aggressive ICP management

- If hydrocephalus, place external ventricular drain to decompress ventricles
- Consider ICP monitoring
- If hemorrhage, consult Neurosurgery to consider evacuation
- If massive hemispheric edema, consult Neurosurgery for possible decompressive hemicraniectomy
- If cerebellar mass or edema, consult neurosurgery for the posterior fossa decompression
- Treat fever aggressively with antipyretics and cooling blankets

ICP, intracranial pressure; PRN,

the affected hemisphere can reduce ICP. By preventing herniation and cerebral ischemia, this procedure *reduces mortality* and may improve outcome. Posterior fossa craniectomy is performed for hemorrhages and ischemic strokes of the cerebellum when the clinical picture is suggestive of impending brainstem compression. The clinical signs include obtundation, changes in the respiratory pattern and heart rate, and wide variations in blood pressure. In patients with hydrocephalus, external ventricular cerebral spinal fluid drainage can be performed as a means of EICP management; this intervention can be used even in the absence of hydrocephalus.

Suggested Reading

Andrews PJ, Citerio G. Intracranial pressure. Part one: historical overview and basic concepts. *Intensive Care Med.* 2004;30:1730–1733.

Excellent well-written articles on the basic concepts, physiology, diagnostic monitoring, and management of elevated intracranial pressure.

Citerio G, Andrews PJ. Intracranial pressure. Part two: clinical applications and technology. *Intensive Care Med.* 2004;30:1882–1885.

Diringer MN, Zazulia AR. Osmotic therapy: fact and fiction. *Neurocrit Care.* 2004;1:219–233.

A detailed review of mechanism of action and practical aspects of osmotic therapy administration.

ANEURYSMAL SUBARACHNOID HEMORRHAGE

52

Manu S. Goyal and Yekaterina Axelrod

Aneurysmal subarachnoid hemorrhage (SAH) occurs because of a rupture of an aneurysm into the cerebrospinal fluid compartment; it accounts for approximately 80% of all cases of SAH. The causes of nonaneurysmal SAH include arteriovenous malformations, trauma, venous thrombosis, and blood dyscrasias. In the United States, approximately 30,000 people suffer from SAH each year. Risk factors include hypertension, cigarette smoking, heavy alcohol consumption, and a history of SAH in first-degree relatives. This condition imparts substantial mortality and morbidity on its victims. Ideally, patients with SAH should be treated at neurocritical care units with expertise in both neurologic monitoring and management of cerebral vasospasm.

The diagnosis of SAH is made based on a noncontrast computed tomography (CT) of the head or lumbar puncture in patients presenting with sudden onset of a severe headache (Alg. 52.1). Both CT and lumbar puncture have sensitivities exceeding 93%. The diagnosis of SAH should be pursued aggressively, as early treatment may prevent rebleeding and potential disability or death. Hydrocephalus, respiratory distress, and cardiac distress should be addressed in tandem, without delaying diagnostic measures. Once SAH is diagnosed or strongly suspected, angiography is performed. Digital subtraction angiography is considered the gold standard; it permits concurrent endovascular treatment ("coiling" of the aneurysm). Measures to prevent contrast-induced nephropathy should be instituted for those at risk.

The initial management focuses on stabilizing the patient and preventing rebleeding, which occurs at a rate of 20% without treatment and is often fatal. Patients who are somnolent or comatose at presentation may need to be intubated; they should be evaluated and, if needed, treated for hydrocephalus. Consultation with Neurosurgery is necessary to discuss further treatment options or place an external ventricular catheter for hydrocephalus. Early treatment of ruptured aneurysms substantially reduces the risk of rebleeding. Surgical clipping and endovascular coiling are two effective options. Prior to definitive treatment of the aneurysm, blood pressure should be aggressively controlled to help prevent rebleeding; as a rule, mean arterial pressure (MAP) is kept under 110 mm Hg. Short-acting antihypertensives and opioids are used; nitrates are best avoided.

Following "protection" of the aneurysm, frequent neurologic assessments, daily measurement of electrolytes and urine output, as well as continuous monitoring of blood pressure are required. A higher MAP is permitted at this point. Fluids and vasopressors (as needed) should be instituted to maintain euvolemia and adequate MAP. Situations causing sudden elevations in intracranial pressure should be prevented. Seizure prophylaxis, stool softeners and laxatives, cough suppressants (if on mechanical ventilation), narcotics, and benzodiazepines may be used.

Common early complications of SAH include hydrocephalus, rebleeding, hyponatremia, cardiac arrhythmias, and neurogenic pulmonary edema. Altered mental status should prompt immediate concern, as it may be a manifestation of hydrocephalus or rebleeding.

Hyponatremia after SAH may be due to the syndrome of inappropriate antidiuretic hormone secretion or cerebral salt wasting. Distinguishing between the two is important because therapeutic approaches oppose one another. In the syndrome of inappropriate antidiuretic hormone secretion, low urine output and hypervolemia direct treatment by lowering fluid intake; whereas in cerebral salt wasting, negative sodium balance, high urine output, and low central venous pressures suggest increased fluid intake and use of hypertonic saline to correct low serum sodium level.

Patient has subarachnoid hemorrhage
- Presents with sudden onset of the worst headache of his or her life with or without LOC
- Non-contrast head CT shows hyperdense signal around the brainstem, in the basal cisterns, Sylvian fissure, and sulci of the brain; blood may be present in the ventricles
- Lumbar puncture shows xanthochromia in a patient with negative head CT

- Bed rest, airway protection, maintain MAP <110 to prevent rebleeding, monitor vitals, frequent neurologic examinations
- Institute anticonvulsants, laxatives, pain and anxiety control
- Order immediate cerebral angiography or local equivalent (CTA or MRA)
- Transfer patient to intensive care unit, preferably specialized neurointensive care unit
- Place EVD if signs of hydrocephalus

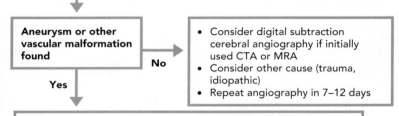

Aneurysm or other vascular malformation found

No →

- Consider digital subtraction cerebral angiography if initially used CTA or MRA
- Consider other cause (trauma, idiopathic)
- Repeat angiography in 7–12 days

Yes

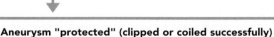

Treat vascular malformation to prevent rebleeding
- Consult Neurosurgery and Neurointerventionalist to determine optimal treatment plan (clipping vs. coiling of aneurysms, embolization and resection of AVM)
- Immediate treatment of aneurysms is strongly recommended
- Evacuation of hematoma if focal deficits consistent with herniation or increased ICP

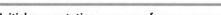

Aneurysm "protected" (clipped or coiled successfully)

Initial preventative measures for vasospasm
- Maintain euvolemia
- Permissive hypertension
- Nimodipine 60 mg orally or enterally every 4 hours

Monitor closely for common complications
- Frequent neurologic examination
- Monitoring of ICP if appropriate
- Frequent monitoring of vitals, CVP, heart rhythm, electrolytes
- Place Foley catheter to monitor input and output closely
- See Figure 52.2

LOC, loss of consciousness; CT, computed tomography; MAP, mean arterial pressure; CTA, CT angiography; MRA, magnetic resonance angiography; EVD, external ventricular drain; AVM, arteriovenous malformation; ICP, intracranial pressure; CVP, central venous pressure.

ALGORITHM 52.2   **Management of Complications of Subarachnoid Hemorrhage (SAH)**

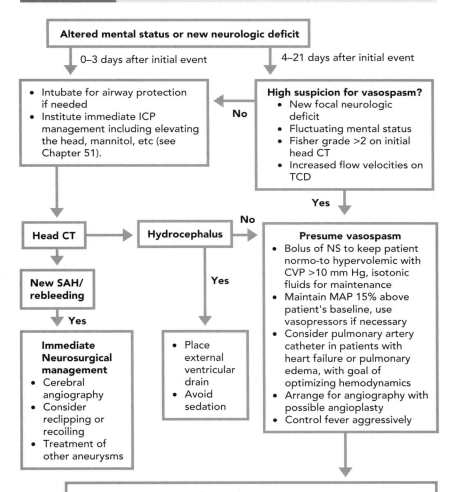

ICP, intracranial pressure; CT, computed tomography; TCD, transcranial Doppler; NS, normal saline; CVP, central venous pressure; MAP, mean arterial pressure.

SAH may cause *reversible* cardiac injury. Sympathetic hyperactivation may lead to arrhythmias, cardiac enzyme elevations, conduction block, transient myocardial stunning with pump failure, and pulmonary edema. Electrocardiography often shows broad, deeply inverted "cerebral" T waves, ST segment elevation/depression, and prolonged QT segments. Echocardiography helps to determine the extent of cardiac failure. A pulmonary artery catheter may aid in addressing intravascular volume status and cardiac function, which can be optimized as needed with inotropes.

CEREBRAL VASOSPASM

Starting 4 days following SAH and for the next 2 weeks, patients with SAH are at risk for cerebral vasospasm. In up to 40% of patients, vasospasm leads to delayed neurologic ischemic deficits (strokes). Vasospasm represents a combination of three factors: narrowing of the large cerebral vessels in response to surrounding blood products, hypovolemia, and loss of distal cerebral vascular autoregulation. During this time, any alteration in neurologic function warrants rapid assessment for this possibly devastating condition (Alg. 52.2). Fluctuating changes in mental status particularly may herald the onset of vasospasm.

Nimodipine, a calcium channel antagonist, is the only effective neuroprotective agent in SAH to date. It should be started at the diagnosis of SAH and given at a dose of 60 mg every 4 hours orally or via a nasogastric tube for 14 to 21 days. This dose can be reduced if MAP falls unacceptably low. Evacuation of blood from the cerebrospinal fluid via lumbar drainage during initial surgery may be helpful.

Once vasospasm is suspected, hemodynamic augmentation by aggressively maintaining normovolemia to hypervolemia and infusing vasopressors to increase MAP should be initiated. The goal is to improve cerebral perfusion and thus prevent strokes. In cases of pump failure, inotropic agents are used to augment cardiac function. The diagnosis of vasospasm is confirmed by angiography. Intra-arterial balloon angioplasty may be performed

TABLE 52.1	Commonly Used Scales for Subarachnoid Hemorrhage Grading

Grade	Criteria
	Hunt and Hess Grading System
1	Asymptomatic or mild headache
2	Moderate or severe headache, nuchal rigidity, or no neurologic deficit other than a cranial nerve palsy
3	Confusion, lethargy, and/or mild focal neurologic deficit
4	Stupor and/or hemiparesis
5	Comatose with or without decerebrate posturing
	World Federation of Neurological Surgeons Scale
I	GCS of 15 without any motor deficit
II	GCS of 13-14, without any motor deficit
III	GCS of 13-14 with motor deficit
IV	GCS of 7-12
V	GCS 3-6
	Fischer Scale
Scale	Appearance of CT scan 48 hours after symptom onset
I	No blood
II	Diffuse subarachnoid blood without clots or layers of blood >1 mm
III	Clots or layers of blood greater than 1 mm in thickness
IV	Intraventricular clots are present

GCS, Glasgow Coma Scale.

if vasospasm is detected in the proximal cerebral vessels. Investigative intra-arterial administration of various agents holds promise in further ameliorating vasospasm and should be considered when the measures previously mentioned fail to cause improvement. Hemodynamic augmentation should be continued for 3 to 5 days and slowly weaned if neurologic status of the patient remains stable. It must be recognized that high-dose vasopressors and hypervolemic therapy entail the risk of complications including arrhythmias and pulmonary edema.

CLINICAL GRADES AND PROGNOSIS

Three different scales are commonly used in patients with SAH (Table 52.1). The Hunt and Hess as well as World Federation of Neurological Surgeons scales are commonly used to predict perioperative mortality. The Fisher scale, addressing the amount of blood on initial CT, is predictive of vasospasm risk; those with Fisher grade 3 or above, have >30% risk.

Long-term prognosis of patients with aneurysmal SAH is poor; 12% to 25% die before receiving medical attention, 30-day mortality is up to 40%. Survival is inversely proportional to SAH grade on presentation: for Hunt and Hess grade 1, survival is approximately 70%; for grade 5, it is only 10%. Roughly one-third of survivors will have persistent neurologic deficits; most survivors will be left with a cognitive deficit. Mortality and morbidity are influenced by the magnitude of the hemorrhage (worse with higher Fisher grade), age, comorbidities, and the occurrence of medical complications.

Suggested Reading

Suarez JI, Tarr RW, Selman WR. Aneurysmal subarachnoid hemorrhage. *N Engl J Med.* 2006;354:387–396.
   Finely written review on the pathophysiology, diagnosis, and management of aneurysmal subarachnoid hemorrhage.
van Gijn J, Kerr RS, Rinkel GJ. Subarachnoid haemorrhage. *Lancet.* 2007;369:306–318.
   An updated review on the management of aneurysmal and non-aneurysmal SAH.

53

INTRACEREBRAL HEMORRHAGE
Yo-El Ju, R. Brian Sommerville, and Yekaterina Axelrod

Intracerebral hemorrhage (ICH), accounting for 10% to 15% of all strokes, is caused by a rupture of a vessel into the brain parenchyma. Patients with this condition usually present with headache, altered level of consciousness, and focal neurologic symptoms. ICH is diagnosed by noncontrast computed tomography; clinical differentiation between various types of stroke is difficult. There are several causes of ICH, including hypertension, trauma, bleeding disorders, amyloid angiopathy, drug abuse (e.g., amphetamines and cocaine), and vascular anomalies. Hypertensive bleeds are most frequently located in the deep gray matter (basal ganglia or thalamus), pons, or cerebellum. Amyloid angiopathy typically causes lobar hemorrhages in *nonhypertensive elderly* patients. ICH resulting from trauma usually presents as a parenchymal contusion; if associated with aneurysmal rupture, ICH is located near the circle of Willis. Anticoagulation raises the risk of ICH and rebleeding in any of these settings.

ICH may cause damage to the brain by several means. Hematoma interrupts the normal neuronal pathways; blood and its breakdown products are highly toxic, causing seizures, electrolyte derangements, fever, and autonomic changes. A recently ruptured vessel is prone to rebleeding. Lastly, elevated intracranial pressure (ICP) due to hematoma and the subsequent edema may endanger other portions of the brain. All these insults make ICH the subtype of stroke with the highest mortality (35% to 50% at 30 days) and morbidity.

Patients with ICH are at high risk for early deterioration and should initially be cared for in an intensive care setting (Alg. 53.1). Enlarging hematoma manifests with headache, vomiting, and a decreased level of consciousness as ICP rises or intracranial tissue shifts begin. Clinical symptoms usually worsen gradually during minutes to hours. Intubation is indicated in patients with signs of brainstem damage, bulbar weakness, signs of herniation (decreased level of consciousness with pupillary asymmetry), or low (<8) Glasgow Coma Scale score.

MAINTAINING BRAIN PERFUSION: BLOOD PRESSURE MANAGEMENT

High blood pressure (BP) was thought to contribute to rebleeding; however, there is no convincing evidence that lowering BP improves outcome. A higher BP may be necessary to provide adequate blood flow to the brain while ICP is elevated, particularly in chronically hypertensive patients with impaired autoregulation; aggressive BP management may cause hypoperfusion. Even in normotensive patients, ICH may lead to transient hypertension resolving during a few days spontaneously. A modest (approximately 15%) reduction in BP does not seem to worsen neurologic outcome. However, ongoing damage to other organs such as the heart or kidneys, is a compelling indication to treat elevated BP. If mean arterial pressure is above 130 to 140 mm Hg or end-organ damage is present, short-acting agents are used to gently lower BP. Nitrates are avoided because of the risk of cerebral vasodilatation with worsening edema. Addressing pain may also help control elevated BP (Table 53.1).

PREVENTION OF REBLEEDING

Even in the absence of coagulopathy, ICH is prone to recur, usually in the first 24 hours. All anticoagulants and antiplatelet agents should be stopped. Normal coagulation should be restored with vitamin K and fresh-frozen plasma (Table 53.2). Recombinant factor VIIa

ALGORITHM 53.1	**Blood Pressure Management after Intracerebral Hemorrhage**

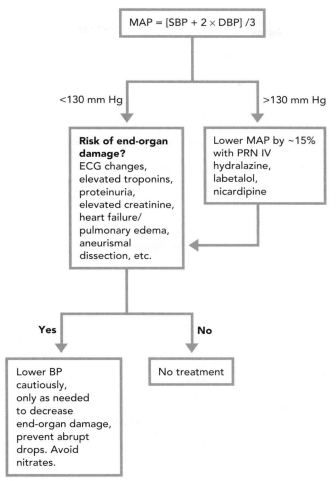

MAP, mean arterial pressure; SBP, systolic blood pressure; DBP, diastolic blood pressure; ECG, electrocardiogram; BP, blood pressure; PRN, as needed; IV, intravenous.

TABLE 53.1	Issues to Address During Management of Intracerebral Hemorrhage

- Blood pressure
- Coagulation status
- Cerebral edema
- Seizures
- Indications for neurosurgical intervention

(rFVIIa) or prothrombin complex concentrate may be used in those at risk of volume overload or lung injury. Of note, rFVIIa is expensive, requires frequent dosing, and may be contraindicated in patients at risk for thromboembolic disease, with artificial heart valves, or other situations in which hypercoagulable state may precipitate additional morbidity.

TREATMENT OF CEREBRAL EDEMA

Elevated ICP occurs at two different times after ICH. In the first 2 days, ICP relates to hematoma size and enlargement. A patient with ICH and signs of herniation at presentation should receive osmotic therapy immediately (see Chapter 51). The second phase ("late edema") occurs during days 9 to 21 after ICH; it should be treated with osmotic agents if it manifests with neurologic deterioration. Unless ICH is associated with intraventricular hemorrhage and hydrocephalus, ICP monitoring is not usually necessary.

SEIZURES

The primary neuronal damage and blood products increase seizure risk after ICH. Seizures occur in 5% to 15% of these patients, usually on day 1. Prophylactic anticonvulsants are not usually indicated; however, they decrease seizure incidence in *lobar* hemorrhages. The current recommendations are to use *prophylactic* anticonvulsants, if needed, for 1 month and taper if no seizures occur. Any patient who is actively seizing should be treated appropriately.

NEUROSURGICAL INTERVENTION

Surgical evacuation of the hematoma in ICH can be performed, however, hematoma evacuation does not improve outcome. Currently, surgical management is reserved for clots >3 cm located in the posterior fossa (cerebellum) or causing compression of the brainstem leading to rapid deterioration (e.g., temporal lobes). In cases of intraventricular hemorrhage and hydrocephalus, neurosurgical evaluation for external ventricular drain placement is reasonable. If edema causes tissue shifts and herniation, craniotomy may be considered (refer to Table 53.3 for guidelines on neurosurgical interventions).

TABLE 53.2	Stabilizing Coagulation Status after Intracerebral Hemorrhage

- Discontinue all antiplatelet and anticoagulant medications
- Reverse anticoagulation or correct coagulopathy:
  - ☐ Vitamin K 10 mg IV or enterally daily for 3 days
  - ☐ Fresh-frozen plasma 15–20 mL/kg
- Consider recombinant factor VIIa for coagulopathic patients needing an urgent surgical procedure or those at risk for volume overload.
- Follow coagulation panel frequently, keep corrected for 24–48 hours

TABLE 53.3	Indications for Neurosurgical Intervention after Intracerebral Hemorrhage (ICH)

- Posterior fossa or temporal lobe hemorrhage >3 cm
- ICH causing hydrocephalus or compressing the brainstem
- Hydrocephalus or intraventricular hemorrhage requiring EVD
- Location or appearance of ICH suggestive of an underlying vascular or mass lesion.
- Complicated cases requiring ICP monitoring

EVD, external ventricular drain; ICP, intracranial pressure.

GENERAL CARE

Patients with ICH , like all critically ill patients, are at risk for numerous complications including myocardial infarctions, congestive heart failure with pulmonary edema, deep vein thrombosis, aspiration pneumonia, urinary tract infections, pressure ulcers, and orthopaedic complications (such as contractures). Sequential compression devices should be used from admission, and deep vein thrombosis prophylaxis can be started after 48 hours with subcutaneous heparin or low-molecular weight heparin if there is no evidence of hematoma expansion. In patients for whom anticoagulation cannot be stopped for long periods (such as mechanical heart valve), it may be necessary to resume anticoagulation with a heparin drip with lower than usual partial thromboplastin time goals. Unfractionated heparin is preferred to low-molecular-weight heparin for therapeutic anti-coagulation because of the potential to reverse unfractionated heparin if necessary.

Suggested Reading

Mayer SA, Rincon F. Treatment of intracerebral haemorrhage. *Lancet Neurol.* 2005;4:662–720.

Qureshi AI, Tuhrim S, Broderick JP, et al. Spontaneous intracerebral hemorrhage. *N Engl J Med.* 2001;344:1450–1460.

54

COMA

Manu S. Goyal and Yekaterina Axelrod

Coma is a state of persistent unarousable unresponsiveness. It occurs because of a structural or general dysfunction of the brainstem, thalami, or both hemispheres. The underlying cause of coma may be immediately apparent on the basis of the initial history and examination; at times, the cause remains unknown for days. An extensive evaluation may result in finding the cause and providing the treatment for a remarkable recovery.

EVALUATION AND MANAGEMENT OF COMA

The mental states along the descent into coma have been described as stupor, lethargy, obtundation, and so forth. For practical purposes, a description of responses to various stimuli is more useful because of its sensitivity to changes over time. The Glasgow Coma Scale is used as a standard method to describe the depth of coma in a quick and concise manner (Table 54.1); it carries prognostic value for patients with traumatic brain injury. However, it is most helpful when health care team members simultaneously monitor and communicate the neurologic status of patients. New scales have been proposed, but await further validation.

Initial Evaluation and Stabilization

Prior to investigating the cause of coma, resuscitative measures should be provided. Intubation may be necessary for airway protection; fluids and/or vasopressors are instituted for hypotension; warming blankets may be required for hypothermia. Laboratory tests including a rapid blood glucose test, arterial blood gases, electrolyte panel, chemistries, blood counts, cultures, toxin screens, and thyroid and liver function tests should be ordered.

The examination first focuses on excluding conditions requiring immediate interventions. Pupillary and fundoscopic abnormalities may suggest an underlying intracranial structural lesion with elevated intracranial pressure; expedient head computed tomography and Neurosurgery consultation are warranted. The presence of fever, nuchal rigidity, or skin rash should prompt immediate lumbar puncture (head computed tomography is obtained first to rule out mass lesions) and antimicrobial therapy.

Many emergency departments employ a "coma cocktail," including intravenous administration of thiamine, glucose, and naloxone. Thiamine protects against the potentially fatal Wernicke encephalopathy; it should be given to all patients with unexplained coma or suspicion of malnourishment. Glucose is withheld until hypoglycemia is confirmed and thiamine has been given. Naloxone is useful as a therapeutic agent; it also can help rule out opiate toxicity.

General and Neurologic Examination

After the initial assessment and stabilization of the patient, a more thorough evaluation may proceed. History of present illness and recent past should be discussed with the caregivers or relatives. All clinical records should be reviewed with close attention to the vital signs dynamics. The cause may be apparent from the history; in some cases, a thorough physical examination may reveal subtle signs of underlying diseases (such as rashes, liver failure stigmata, murmurs).

The neurologic examination in patients with coma should assess level of consciousness, brainstem reflexes, motor function, and respiratory pattern. Consciousness is assessed by recording response to increasing intensities of stimuli. One begins with the

TABLE 54.1	Glasgow Coma Scale	
Best eye opening		
Spontaneous	4	
With voice only	3	
With pain only	2	
None at all	1	
Best verbal response		
Coherent speech	5	
Confused intelligible speech	4	
Inappropriate words	3	
Incomprehensible sounds	2	
No verbal output	1	
Best motor response		
Follows commands	6	
Localizes pain stimuli[a]	5	
Withdraws to pain stimuli	4	
Decorticate posturing	3	
Decerebrate posturing	2	
No movements at all	1	

[a]Localizing pain stimuli refers to gaze deviation, head turning, or hand movements toward the stimulus.

name softly, then loudly, then with a gentle shake. If these fail to arouse the patient, a painful stimulus (supraorbital pressure, sternal rub, or temporomandibular pressure) should be applied.

During the brainstem examination, most of the cranial nerves are assessed. The pupillary changes to light should be recorded in millimeters for each eye. Eye movements are examined by performing the oculocephalic maneuver by rapidly rotating the head in all directions and observing for contralateral deviation of the eyes. If cervical spine stability is in question, cold calorics (the oculovestibular reflex) should be tested instead (Alg. 54.1). For the corneal reflex, dripping sterile saline into each eye is preferred over cotton to avoid corneal damage. One can test the facial nerve by observing the grimace to a painful stimulus. The ninth and tenth nerves responsible for gag and cough are assessed during oral and endotracheal suctioning.

The motor system examination includes observation and description of spontaneous movements, movements to commands or noxious stimuli (deep nail bed pressure or a sharp proximal pinch). Such stimuli may elicit a posturing response. Decorticate (flexor) posturing, or reflexive elbow flexion with lower extremity extension, is typically less ominous than decerebrate (extensor) posturing, in which all extremities extend simultaneously. Spinal reflexes should not be confused with withdrawal or purposeful movements. The so-called triple flexion response refers to flexion at the hip, knee, and ankle in response to pain applied to the foot. Myoclonic jerks, often a sign of anoxic encephalopathy, suggest a poor outcome. Myoclonus, posturing, and spinal reflexes are often seen in coma. Subtle rhythmic motions may indicate ongoing seizures; urgent electroencephalography is warranted.

Various respiratory patterns depending on the cerebral structural damage and/or underlying metabolic abnormality may be exhibited; description of these is beyond the scope of this chapter. Close attention should be paid to the presence of a respiratory drive when pressure of carbon dioxide in blood is above normal.

Diagnostic Studies in Coma

A nonfocal neurologic examination should prompt investigation of toxic/metabolic or hypoxic/ischemic causes of coma; whereas any focality warrants brain imaging and/or

ALGORITHM 54.1   **Oculovestibular Testing (Cold Calorics)**

Inspect both ears and ascertain:

- Tympanic membranes are intact
- The EAC is not obstructed
- No blood, CSF, or brain tissue is in the EAC

↓

- Lift the head of the patient to 30°
- An assistant holds the eyelids of the patient open

↓

- Insert a soft catheter into the EAC
- Instill 30–50 mL of ice-cold water during 1 minute
- Observe for eye movements or nystagmus for 2–3 minutes after the instillation

↓

Eye movements present

- If intact, the eyes deviate toward cold water
- Wait for the eyes to return to midline ≈3 min
- Repeat on the other side

Eye movements absent

- Wait for 3 minutes
- Repeat on the other side

EAC, external auditory canal; CSF, cerebrospinal fluid.

TABLE 54.2	Common and Uncommon Causes of Coma

Drugs and toxins
Opiates, alcohol, sedatives, amphetamines, barbiturates, tranquilizers, bromides, salicylates, acetaminophen, lithium, anticholinergics, lead, methanol, ethylene glycol, carbon monoxide, arsenic

Metabolic and systemic
Anoxia or hypoxia, hypercapnia, hypotension, hypoglycemia, hyperglycemia, diabetic ketoacidosis, hypernatremia, hyponatremia, hypercalcemia, hypocalcemia, hypermagnesemia, hypothermia, hyperthermia, Wernicke's encephalopathy, hepatic failure, uremia, Addisonian crisis, myxedema

Infectious/inflammatory
Bacterial, viral, or fungal meningitis/meningoencephalitis, acute disseminated encephalomyelitis, syphilis, sepsis, malaria, Waterhouse-Friderichsen syndrome, typhoid fever

Structural brain lesions
Subarachnoid hemorrhage, intraparenchymal hemorrhage, ischemic infarctions, global cerebral hypoperfusion, cerebral venous sinus thrombosis, traumatic brain injury, hydrocephalus, basilar occlusion, central pontine myelinolysis, large hemispheric masses, pituitary apoplexy, cerebral abscess or multifocal infection, chemotherapy-induced leukoencephalopathy

Other
Nonconvulsive status epilepticus, locked-in syndrome, catatonia, hypertensive encephalopathy, heat stroke, psychogenic coma

cerebrospinal fluid studies. If the results of laboratory tests do not aid in determining the cause, electroencephalography should be considered. A list of common causes is presented in Table 54.2.

Ongoing Management of Patients in Coma

In addition to treating the underlying cause, several management principles should be initiated to maximize the chance of recovery. Mechanical ventilation with monitoring of arterial blood gases ensures adequate oxygenation and ventilation. Hypotension should be avoided; vasopressors are used as needed. Daily electrolyte replacement and steady normovolemia are important. Full nutrition, preferably by enteral feedings, should be instituted as soon as possible. Other essential steps in routine critical care including gastric ulcer prevention, thromboembolism prevention, skin care, and oral care cannot be underestimated.

Conditions That May Be Mistaken for Coma

There are a few conditions in which a patient may seem unarousable and unresponsive, but has an intact consciousness. Injury to certain parts of the pons may cause "locked-in syndrome;" patients cannot move any muscles, except for those controlling vertical gaze and blinking. Severe Guillain-Barré syndrome or parkinsonism may cause a similar scenario. Careful neurologic examination of the brainstem reflexes can help avoid mistaking these conditions for coma. Occasionally, patients may present with psychogenic unresponsiveness; they display resistance to eye-opening, purposeful eye movements, and/or nonepileptic seizures.

ASSESSING PROGNOSIS IN COMA

Prognosis is highly dependent on the underlying cause. Metabolic and toxic disturbances can often be reversed leading to a good prognosis despite a minimal Glasgow Coma Scale score. Comorbidities, age, the extent of the underlying disease, and depth and duration of coma may also contribute.

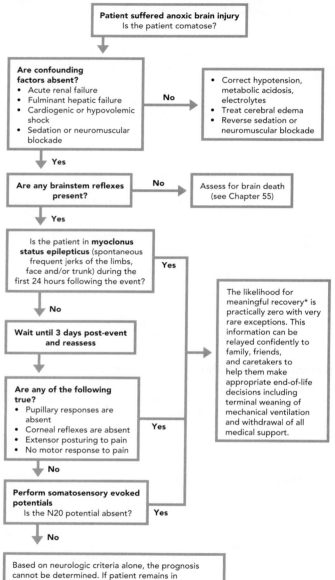

*Meaningful recovery is defined here as the absence of severe disability requiring constant nursing support, a vegetative state or death. Many patients, families, and caretakers may consider less severe forms of disability to be outside a desirable state of meaning recovery.

(Adapted from Wijdicks EF, Hijdra A, Young GB, et al. Quality Standards Subcommittee of the American Academy of Neurology. Practice parameter: prediction of outcome in comatose survivors after cardiopulmonary resuscitation (an evidence-based review): report of the Quality Standards Subcommittee of the American Academy of Neurology. *Neurology.* 2006;67:203–210, with permission.)

Prognosis in Coma Due to Anoxic Brain Injury

Anoxic brain injury following cardiac arrest, prolonged hypotension, or respiratory failure results in coma with a varying outcome. A panel of the American Academy of Neurology has issued guidelines on determining outcome following cerebral anoxia (Alg. 54.2); these guidelines do not apply to coma resulting from other reasons.

Prognosis in Patients with Prolonged Coma

Patients in a prolonged comatose state exhibit poorer outcomes. Often coma evolves into a "vegetative state" in which a patient may show normal sleep-awake cycles, but lacks overt signs of conscious awareness or responsiveness. If such state lasts for 12 months after brain trauma or 3 months in other cases, the chance for meaningful recovery is minimal. Neurologic consultation is necessary in most of these cases to help guide decision-making.

Suggested Reading

Wijdicks EF, Hijdra A, Young GB, et al. Quality Standards Subcommittee of the American Academy of Neurology. Practice parameter: prediction of outcome in comatose survivors after cardiopulmonary resuscitation (an evidence-based review): report of the Quality Standards Subcommittee of the American Academy of Neurology. *Neurology.* 2006;67:203–210.

55

DECLARATION OF BRAIN DEATH
Manu S. Goyal and Yekaterina Axelrod

Death by neurologic criteria (brain death) is defined by irreversible loss of all functions of the entire brain. The law or policy governing brain death varies among countries, states, and even different hospitals. Understanding the local law and policy for determining brain death is obligatory; we encourage physicians to make religious and ethnic considerations as they discuss their findings with families. The role of the intensivist in the management of a patient with brain death does not end at the diagnosis, as organ donation may proceed in suitable candidates. The health of organs with a potential for transplant must be maintained to maximize the chance of graft success. The United States and some other countries require physicians to contact local organ-procurement agencies once a patient is deemed to be a potential donor, even before the final confirmation of brain death.

DIAGNOSING BRAIN DEATH

By definition, diagnosing brain death requires evidence of coma and absent function of all parts of the brainstem, including the midbrain, pons, and medulla oblongata, following a catastrophic cerebral event. Brain death in adults most often results from traumatic brain injury and aneurysmal subarachnoid hemorrhage confirmed by imaging. Anoxic brain injury, large brain tumors, severe meningoencephalitis, or cerebral edema due to fulminant liver failure may also lead to brain death. Because various extreme states away from normal homeostasis may cause complete, but potentially reversible, brainstem failure, one must monitor and correct hypothermia, hypotension, hypoglycemia, severe electrolyte disturbances, and acid-base imbalance. Similarly, drug intoxication, poisoning, anesthesia, and neuromuscular blockade should be ruled out using appropriate screening tests as dictated by history. Locked-in states caused by lesions in the base of the pons or severe Guillain-Barré syndrome may mimic brain death. Careful history-taking helps avoid missing these cases; any suspicion or unclear aspects to the history should prompt ancillary tests to confirm brain death.

Once confounding factors have been eliminated, the process of determination of death by neurologic criteria may proceed (Alg. 55.1). It is important to ascertain and document normothermia (above 32°C) and normotension (systolic blood pressure above 90 mm Hg) during the examination. One must establish a comatose state by demonstrating lack of responsiveness to deep painful stimuli (supraorbital or nail bed pressure). Each section of the brainstem is tested for corresponding reflexes. Midbrain function is tested with pupillary reflexes to light; bilateral unresponsiveness proves lack of function. One should demonstrate loss of eye movements in oculovestibular (cold caloric) testing (see Chapter 54 for description). Absence of pontine function is further established by documenting loss of corneal reflexes. Lack of cough reflex, tested by moving the endotracheal tube and suctioning, suggests medullary failure. In order to confirm the absence of function of the whole brain, all aspects of the neurologic examination should be repeated in 1 to 24 hours, depending on the clinical situation.

Clinical confirmation of cerebral death requires proving absence of spontaneous respiratory function in the presence of hypercarbia (partial pressure of arterial carbon dioxide of at least 60 mm Hg) and respiratory acidosis. The apnea test is the most widely used method and is described in detail in Algorithm 55.1. If the patient is hemodynamically unstable, requiring high doses of vasopressors, or hypoxemic despite vigorous ventilator support, apnea testing should not be performed, and brain death may be confirmed with

ALGORITHM 55.1 Approach to Determination of Death by Neurologic Criteria

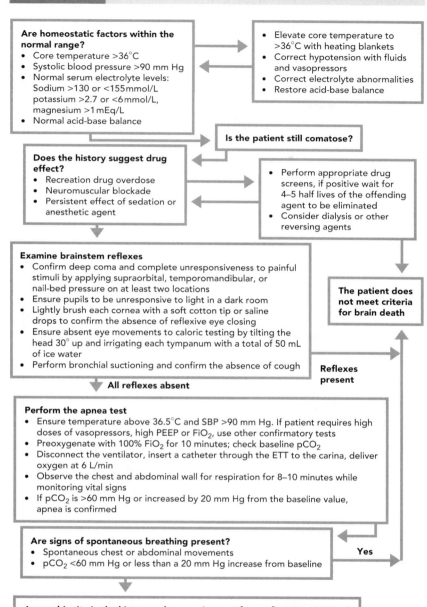

Are homeostatic factors within the normal range?
- Core temperature >36°C
- Systolic blood pressure >90 mm Hg
- Normal serum electrolyte levels: Sodium >130 or <155 mmol/L potassium >2.7 or <6 mmol/L, magnesium >1 mEq/L
- Normal acid-base balance

- Elevate core temperature to >36°C with heating blankets
- Correct hypotension with fluids and vasopressors
- Correct electrolyte abnormalities
- Restore acid-base balance

Is the patient still comatose?

Does the history suggest drug effect?
- Recreation drug overdose
- Neuromuscular blockade
- Persistent effect of sedation or anesthetic agent

- Perform appropriate drug screens, if positive wait for 4–5 half lives of the offending agent to be eliminated
- Consider dialysis or other reversing agents

Examine brainstem reflexes
- Confirm deep coma and complete unresponsiveness to painful stimuli by applying supraorbital, temporomandibular, or nail-bed pressure on at least two locations
- Ensure pupils to be unresponsive to light in a dark room
- Lightly brush each cornea with a soft cotton tip or saline drops to confirm the absence of reflexive eye closing
- Ensure absent eye movements to caloric testing by tilting the head 30° up and irrigating each tympanum with a total of 50 mL of ice water
- Perform bronchial suctioning and confirm the absence of cough

The patient does not meet criteria for brain death

Reflexes present

All reflexes absent

Perform the apnea test
- Ensure temperature above 36.5°C and SBP >90 mm Hg. If patient requires high doses of vasopressors, high PEEP or FiO_2, use other confirmatory tests
- Preoxygenate with 100% FiO_2 for 10 minutes; check baseline pCO_2
- Disconnect the ventilator, insert a catheter through the ETT to the carina, deliver oxygen at 6 L/min
- Observe the chest and abdominal wall for respiration for 8–10 minutes while monitoring vital signs
- If pCO_2 is >60 mm Hg or increased by 20 mm Hg from the baseline value, apnea is confirmed

Are signs of spontaneous breathing present?
- Spontaneous chest or abdominal movements
- pCO_2 <60 mm Hg or less than a 20 mm Hg increase from baseline

Yes

Any ambiguity in the history or law requirement for confirmatory testing?

No

Yes

- Patient meets standard clinical criteria for brain death
- Notify organ-procurement agency immediately

Perform confirmatory testing
- Use method required by law or hospital

SBP, systolic blood pressure; PEEP, positive end-expiratory pressure; ETT, endotracheal tube.

TABLE 55.1	Confirmatory Tests Used to Declare Brain Death by Neurologic Criteria

Method	Pros	Cons
Electroencephalography	• Safe • Can be done at bedside	• Prone to artifacts in the ICU • No confirmation of brainstem failure • Prone to confounding factors (false-negative in drug verdose)
Cerebral DSA	High sensitivity and specificity	• Requires transportation • Contrast injection
Cerebral scintigraphy	• Safe • Can be done at bedside • High sensitivity and specificity	
Cerebral TCD	• Safe • Can be done at bedside	• Operator-dependent results • Inability to assess posterior circulation • Repeat studies may be needed

ICU, intensive care unit; DSA, digital subtraction angiography; TCD, transcranial Doppler ultrasonography.

ancillary tests (see later discussion). Temperature of the patient during apnea testing should be ≥36.5°C. One must be prepared to address bradycardia and hypotension, which occasionally complicates this test, as hypoxemia and acidosis may develop.

If the clinical examination previously described confirms brain failure, a physician is permitted to pronounce brain death. In cases of historical ambiguity, significant family dissent, or substantial clinical instability for apnea testing, a confirmatory test may be required (Table 55.1). Cerebral scintigraphy showing lack of cerebral blood flow and metabolism is highly sensitive and specific and is used frequently. Isoelectric electroencephalography is perhaps the most validated method for establishing brain death, yet electroencephalography is prone to numerous artifacts and may be falsely negative in certain clinical scenarios. Cerebral angiography, perhaps the most expensive and cumbersome method, reveals absent flow in the intracranial vessels; it is associated with a risk of contrast injection and potentially dangerous for unstable patient transportation. The sensitivity of transcranial Doppler now exceeds 90% and it has a specificity of nearly 100% when used correctly; it is gaining wider use for this purpose despite some limitations.

Occasionally, body movements may be observed in patients who meet the criteria for brain death. These are due to spinal cord-mediated reflexes and can include triple flexion response of the lower extremities to painful stimuli, spontaneous rising of the arms, and even startling abdominal flexion that raises the upper half of the body completely off the bed. Confirmatory testing can be obtained in these situations, but is not necessary. Because of these phenomena, we encourage that the clinical examination be performed without family members present.

CARE FOR POTENTIAL ORGAN DONORS

A few important metabolic and hemodynamic derangements are uniformly seen as a result of brain death, including diabetes insipidus with hypovolemia and hypernatremia, hypotension, hyperglycemia, and hypothermia. All of these must be meticulously addressed to preserve organs suitable for donation (see Chapter 68 for details).

Desmopressin boluses (1 to 4 mg) are administered intravenously to treat diabetes insipidus; hypotonic fluids are given to correct elevated sodium levels. Because hypovolemia may be a contributing factor to hypotension, it must be properly treated; vasoactive agents and/or inotropes can be used to normalize blood pressure (goal systolic blood pressure above 90 mm Hg) and support cardiac function as needed. Respiratory acidosis developed during apnea testing should be corrected by appropriate ventilator setting changes to allow for normocarbia; adding sodium bicarbonate to infusing fluids may be necessary if metabolic acidosis is present. Hyperglycemia is best treated with continuous insulin infusions. Maintaining core temperature above 35°C is essential and may require several interventions including warming blankets, heated and humidified inhaled gases, and warmed replacement fluid. Blood products may be necessary to correct coagulopathy or maintain hematocrit above 30%.

Suggested Reading

Report of the Quality Standards Subcommittee of the American Academy of Neurology. Practice parameters: determining brain death in adults. Available at: http://www.aan.com/professionals/practice/pdfs/pdf_1995_thru_1998/1995.45.1012.pdf.
The professional standards for determining brain death in the United States.

Wijdicks EF. The diagnosis of brain death. *N Engl J Med.* 2001;344:1215–1221.
An excellent review of brain death: its mechanisms, the determination, pertinent testing, and clinical management.

Wood KE, Becker BN, McCartney JG, et al. Care of the potential organ donor. *N Engl J Med.* 2004;351:2730–2739.
A well-written review on caring for brain dead patients, and other patients who might become potential organ donors with detailed protocols.

56

DELIRIUM AND SEDATION
Yo-El Ju, R. Brian Sommerville, and Yekaterina Axelrod

Altered mental status is the most common neurologic problem among critically ill patients, with delirium as the most common treatable cause seen in up to 60% to 80% of this population. Delirium is associated with worse mortality, higher length of stay, and a risk of permanent cognitive disability or dementia; therefore, proper recognition and treatment of this potentially disabling disorder is essential.

Delirium is defined as an *acute* change in global cognitive function affecting attention, arousal, orientation, or perception. It has been described as "a syndrome of cerebral insufficiency" or end-organ dysfunction in the brain. There are two types of delirium, hypoactive and hyperactive. The course is usually fluctuating; cognitive function may vary from minute-to-minute with symptoms often worse at night ("sundowning"). Delirium must be distinguished from dementia (a chronic problem of impaired cognition) and neurologic emergencies (herniation) producing an acutely decreased level of alertness (Alg. 56.1). Patients with hyperactive delirium may be loud, agitated, and/or combative, eliciting a high degree of attention from staff. Even though hypoactive delirium is more common, particularly among the elderly, it tends to be overlooked. These patients may be quiet or sleepy, yet profoundly confused and disoriented. Monitoring for both types should be routine in all intensive care units (ICUs); the confusion assessment method may be used in identifying delirious patients (Fig. 56.1).

A useful conceptual model of delirium regards it as the product of two factors: *susceptibility* and *insults*. Susceptibility refers to underlying risk factors, such as age, history of dementia, sensory impairments, and so forth. (Table 56.1). Insults are new factors acutely worsening brain function, such as infections, organ dysfunction, and metabolic derangements. The sum of susceptibility and insults needs to cross a threshold to cause delirium. Of note, even after insult removal, a susceptible brain will take longer to return to its cognitive baseline. Demented elderly may take weeks to recover from even a minor infection.

WORKUP

The work-up of altered mental status in the ICU begins with a focused history, stressing the factors making the patient susceptible to delirium. It is essential to establish the baseline cognitive function eliciting history of dementia or psychiatric diseases. Patients should be assessed for pain and anxiety, which are frequent causes of abnormal behavior in the ICU.

The general and neurologic examinations guide the search for insults that cause delirium. Vital signs and oxygen saturation are checked, so obvious reasons for delirium like fever, hypoxemia, or hypotension are not overlooked. Hypoglycemia can present with focal symptoms mimicking stroke, and is easily corrected. The goal of the neurologic assessment is to identify focal signs inconsistent with delirium. Any asymmetry should raise concern for a focal lesion and may constitute an emergency. Subtle signs of seizure (eye or head deviation, rhythmic movements of the face or extremities) are sought.

The differential diagnosis of delirium is broad (Table 56.2). A careful examination, medication review, and basic laboratory studies will address most causes. Medications are among the most common insults to the brain in the ICU (Table 56.3). In addition to current medications potentially causing cognitive dysfunction, recently discontinued medicines with a withdrawal potential, new drug interactions or change in the metabolism of previously well-tolerated medications should be addressed. Liver and renal dysfunction may alter medication levels; elderly patients may become delirious even with "therapeutic" levels.

ALGORITHM 56.1   **Approach to Delirium**

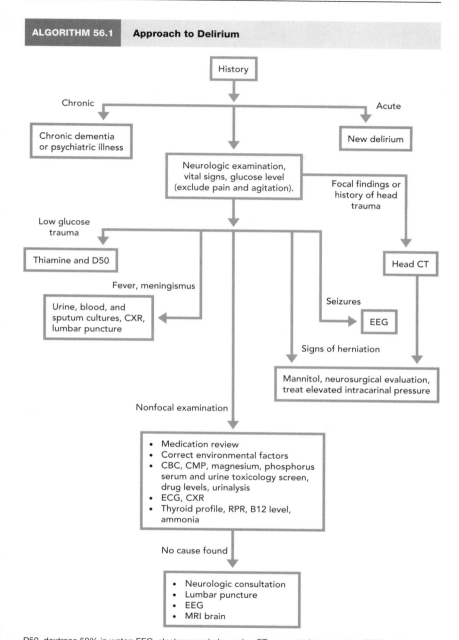

D50, dextrose 50% in water; EEG, electroencephalography; CT, computed tomography; CXR, chest x-ray; CBC, complete blood count; CMP, complete metabolic profile; ECG, electrocardiogram; RPR, rapid plasma reagin; MRI, magnetic resonance imaging.

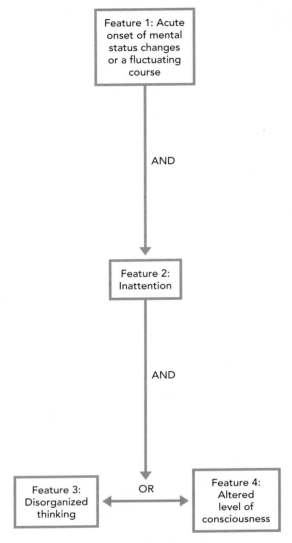

Figure 56.1. Definition of Delirium (Confusion assessment method for the intensive care unit)

Basic studies include chemistries, blood counts, electrolytes, urine and blood toxicology, ammonia, drug levels, urine analysis, electrocardiogram, and chest radiography. Thyroid testing, vitamin B_{12} level, and rapid plasma reagin are checked to look for reversible causes of dementia. Any suspicion for infection such as fever, meningismus, or leukocytosis should be pursued with blood cultures and lumbar puncture. Other causes of delirium (Table 56.4) should also be sought and corrected, if possible.

TABLE 56.1	Risk Factors for Delirium

Age
Baseline dementia or cognitive impairment
Psychiatric comorbidity
History of alcohol or drug abuse
Low albumin/malnutrition
Psychosocial stress (e.g., death of spouse)
Hearing or visual impairment
Sleep deprivation
Multiple medical problems

TABLE 56.2	Causes of Delirium

Vascular	Stroke, hemorrhage, reversible posterior leukoencephalopathy, vasospasm, migraine
Toxins	Medications, alcohol, illicit drugs, occupational exposures, withdrawal
Seizures	Aura, ictal state, nonconvulsive status epilepticus, postictal state
Other organs	Hepatic, uremia, cardiac disease, lung disease
Electrolytes	Hypoglycemia, hyponatremia, hypocalcemia, hypomagnesemia
Neoplastic	Primary tumor, metastases, carcinomatous meningitis, paraneoplastic syndromes
Infection	UTI, pneumonia, meningitis/encephalitis, sepsis, any other infection
Trauma	Direct trauma, edema, diffuse axonal injury, postconcussive syndrome
Autoimmune	Neuropsychiatric lupus, Hashimoto encephalopathy, CNS vasculitis, limbic encephalitis
Endocrine	Hypo/hyperthyroidism, hypopituitary state, hyper/hypoparathyroidism
Nutritional	Vitamin B_{12} deficiency, Wernicke encephalopathy (thiamine deficiency), Machiafava-Bignami

UTI, urinary tract infection.

TABLE 56.3	Medications That Can Cause Delirium

During use	Withdrawal
Anticholinergic agents	Appetite suppressants
Sedatives	Cough/cold remedies
Antiemetics	Alcohol (even without delirium tremens)
Antipsychotics	Selective serotonin reuptake inhibitors
Antispasmodics	Nicotine
Tricyclic antidepressants	Baclofen
Muscle relaxants	
Digoxin	
Cimetidine	
Anticonvulsants	
Corticosteroids	
Lithium	
Benzodiazepines	
Barbiturates	
Opioids	

TABLE 56.4	Nonmedication Causes of Delirium

Cause	Treatment
Disorientation	Frequent reorientation
Sleep cycle change	Provide stimulating activity, keep out of bed during day, no interruptions at night
Sensory deficits	Put on glasses, hearing aids
Poor communication	Communication devices
Catheters, restraints	Remove lines, tubes, and restraints as early as possible
Dehydration	Assess for dehydration and hydrate
Malnutrition	Feed, with parenteral nutrition if needed
Pain	Assess for and treat pain
Immobility	Remove restraints early, range of motion exercises, keep out of bed
Urinary retention	Place a bladder catheter or start scheduled catheterizations
Constipation	Disimpact if needed, start bowel routine
Fever	Antipyretics, scheduled if necessary
Infection	Search for and treat underlying infection
Hypoxemia, hypercarbia	Check arterial blood gases, ventilate or oxygenate as needed

If the cause of delirium is not found, neurologic consultation should be obtained. Serious conditions can exhibit subtle findings or even nonfocal examination. For instance, strokes in the nondominant hemisphere can cause delirium in the absence of hemiparesis, or fluent aphasia may be mistaken for delirium. Nonconvulsive status epilepticus may have no symptoms except delirium (see Chapter 49). Lumbar puncture, electroencephalography, brain imaging, and more specific laboratory studies are usually needed at this point.

TREATMENT OF DELIRIUM

A methodical and thorough approach will help identify the cause of delirium in most cases. Family members can be very helpful with familiar tools (glasses, hearing aids, clocks, calendars) and regular reorientation of the patient. The first step in treatment is to eliminate any potential inciting medications. If the offending drug cannot be eliminated, delirium may be treated pharmacologically. Even though no randomized controlled trials have been done to prove efficacy of any one agent for delirium, clinical experience has shown relative efficacy of antipsychotic medications. Although atypical antipsychotics are becoming more popular, haloperidol is still the most commonly used medication. It is given at 1 to 10 mg intravenously or intramuscularly repeated every 30 minutes until effect, and then continuing at 25% of the effective dose every 6 hours. A scheduled regimen is more effective than as needed dosing; elderly or small patients receive a smaller dose. Newer antipsychotics include quetiapine, risperidone, olanzapine, all of which are given orally or enterally, and ziprasidone, which is also available in an intramuscular form.

Patients treated with antipsychotics need to be carefully monitored for fever or rigidity (indicating neuroleptic malignant syndrome), extrapyramidal symptoms (tremors, stereotypic movements, dystonia), and QT interval prolongation, which can lead to fatal arrhythmias. All patients should have a baseline and daily electrocardiogram. Benzodiazepines mask symptoms by sedation and should not be used, with the one exception of withdrawal from chronic use of alcohol, benzodiazepines, or barbiturates. An unfortunately common habit in the ICU is to overmedicate patients with sedatives and analgesics while undertreating delirium. A more prudent approach is to evaluate for delirium, pain, and anxiety separately and treat each specifically.

TABLE 56.5	Modified Ramsay Sedation Scale

1 Patient anxious and agitated or restless or both
2 Patient cooperative, oriented, and tranquil
3 Patient responds to commands only
4 Asleep, brisk response to a light glabellar tap or loud auditory stimulus
5 A sluggish response to a light glabellar tap or loud auditory stimulus
6 No response to a light glabellar tap or loud auditory stimulus

SEDATION IN THE ICU

In critical care medicine, sicker patients are becoming more dependent on invasive devices, frequently necessitating pharmacologic sedation for patient comfort. Titrating to a predefined goal and avoiding oversedation is imperative. The risk of delirium after sedation is proportional to the amount of medications used. The modified Ramsay sedation scale (Table 56.5) is a commonly used tool in the ICU setting; another scale focusing more on agitation is the Riker sedation-agitation scale (Table 56.6). Having a sedation goal with frequent titration of medicines as part of institutional protocols eases communication between medical personnel, and helps to avoid under- or oversedation.

Usual sedation protocols combine benzodiazepines and opioids. Continuous infusions may be beneficial in avoiding oversedation and withdrawal, but may not be available in all situations. Propofol, with a very short half-life is advantageous in situations in which frequent neurologic examinations are needed. However, because of the lipid components of propofol formulation and subsequent infection risk, propofol should only be used for the short term. The central alpha-2 agonist dexmedetomidine (Precedex) allows for patients to be aroused for examinations, but otherwise keeps them comfortably sedated. Sedation protocols differ and should be targeted to the specific patient population (neurologic, medical, or surgical ICU), in addition to having a built-in sedation target with parameters for modification for each individual patient.

Sedation should be weaned as soon as possible. Daily weaning trials have been shown to decrease ventilation time; they also allow for better neurologic examinations. Ideally, in order to avoid withdrawal, patients should be switched to scheduled dosing of longer acting drugs prior to discontinuing continuous sedation, and should be slowly tapered thereafter.

TABLE 56.6	Riker Sedation-Agitation Scale

7 Dangerous agitation	Pulling at ETT, trying to remove catheters, climbing over bed rail, striking at staff, thrashing side-to-side
6 Very agitated	Does not calm despite frequent verbal reminding of limits, requires physical restraints, biting ETT
5 Agitated	Anxious or mildly agitated, attempting to sit up; calms down to verbal instructions
4 Calm and cooperative	Calm, awakens easily, follows commands
3 Sedated	Difficult to arouse, awakens to verbal stimuli or gentle shaking but drifts off again, follows simple commands
2 Very sedated	Arouses to physical stimuli but does not communicate or follow commands, may move spontaneously
1 Unarousable	Minimal or no response to noxious stimuli, does not communicate or follow commands

ETT, endotracheal tube.

Suggested Reading

Jacobi J, Frasier GL, Coursin DB, et al. Clinical practice guidelines for the sustained use of sedatives and analgesics in the critically ill adult. *Crit Care Med.* 2002;30:119–141.
Updated (original version published in 1995) practice guidelines for sedation of adult patients in the intensive care setting with comprehensive review of literature.

Lacasse H, Perreault MM, Williamson DR. Systematic review of antipsychotics for the treatment of hospital-associated delirium in medically or surgically ill patients. *Ann Pharmacother.* 2006;40:1966–1973.
Comprehensive review of data on available anipsychotics for the treatment of delirium.

ACUTE SPINAL CORD DISORDERS

Yekaterina Axelrod

57

Acute spinal cord injury (SCI) results from numerous traumatic and nontraumatic causes (Table 57.1). It may lead to immediate mortality as well as devastating life-long disability with major health, emotional, and financial impact. Certain types of myelopathy can be reversible if addressed in a timely fashion; therefore, prompt recognition of clinical symptoms cannot be underestimated. Detailed history in cases of nontraumatic myelopathy helps with differential diagnosis. The usual clinical presentation involves a triad of motor impairment (may be asymmetric), sensory loss, and sphincter dysfunction (urine retention, incontinence of stool and/or urine). Pain at the corresponding level of the spine is not always present. Algorithm 57.1 presents a detailed initial approach to this serious medical emergency.

TRAUMATIC SPINAL CORD INJURY

Cervical cord injury is the most common type of traumatic SCI. Traumatic brain injury is found in up to a half of these patients; just as many may have injuries to other organs. Almost 50% of victims of cord trauma will present in spinal shock with flaccid areflexic paralysis and lack of sensation in all modalities; it usually resolves within 48 hours. Cord stability (the ability of the spinal cord to endure physical movement without suffering further damage) should be assessed to help making decisions about surgical interventions as well as an approach to the airway management. Immobilization, performed to limit secondary cord damage due to improper positioning of the unstable spine, carries its own risks, including increased intracranial hypertension, airway compromise, diminished chest wall mobility, pressure sores, and pain. Neurosurgery consultation for further surgical management should be sought immediately.

Neuroprotection

For those patients who present within 3 hours of traumatic injury, methylprednisolone infusion for 24 hours may improve neurologic function; however, it does not always translate into better outcome. The infusion may be continued for 48 hours if the injury is 3 to 8 hours old; however, there is an increased risk of gastrointestinal bleeding associated with prolonged infusion.

Cardiovascular Management

Many patients with cervical or upper thoracic cord injury may develop neurogenic shock because of the lack of sympathetic innervation to the heart and blood vessels resulting in cardiovascular depression with bradycardia, hypotension, and low systemic vascular resistance. Hemodynamic monitoring is advised, as this population is prone to congestive heart failure with overzealous fluid resuscitation. Vasopressors with chronotropic features (norepinephrine, dopamine) are preferred to augment systolic function and address bradycardia. The optimal blood pressure goal is unclear; experimental data show that hypotension further worsens SCI due to hypoperfusion. We recommend targeting mean arterial pressure of 70 to 80 mm Hg as long as the interventions to achieve this goal do not harm other organs. Atropine should be kept at bedside; transcutaneous pacing may be needed in rare cases of symptomatic refractory bradycardia.

TABLE 57.1	Causes of Spinal Cord Injury

- Traumatic and degenerative (compression fractures, disc herniation)
- Vascular (infarcts, epidural hematoma, arteriovenous malformations)
- Infections (abscesses, myelitis, empyema, tuberculosis)
- Inflammatory/demyelinating (transverse myelitis, acute disseminating encephalomyelitis, multiple sclerosis)
- Neoplastic (tumors and metastases, postradiation)
- Other (vitamin B_{12} deficiency, syringomyelia, amyotrophic lateral sclerosis, spinal canal stenosis, spondylosis)—usually more chronic course

Airway and Breathing

Endotracheal intubation is recommended for those cord trauma victims who have associated traumatic brain injury with low Glasgow Coma Scale (see Chapter 59) or signs of elevated intracranial pressure. Any airway compromise due to focal edema, fractures, and/or hemorrhages of the neck may also require intubation. Only physicians with advanced airway skills should attempt intubation, especially in patients with an unstable spine; fiberoptic intubation is gaining popularity for its safety. Measures should be taken to avoid hypotension during intubation; succinylcholine is contraindicated in SCI of >24 hours. Neurosurgeons should be at bedside to help with immobilization of the spine.

Close respiratory monitoring in a critical care setting is necessary, as SCI victims encounter multiple pulmonary complications (neurogenic pulmonary edema, pneumonia, atelectasis, pleural effusions, pulmonary embolism) and are prone to respiratory failure even days after the initial injury. With lesions above C3 level, diaphragmatic function is lost often resulting in apnea and respiratory arrest; most patients need mechanical ventilation immediately. With lesions between C3 and C5, diaphragmatic function is partially preserved; however, the rest of the respiratory muscles are compromised, leading to diminished lung volumes and hypoventilation. Supine position may be beneficial for temporizing breathing problems in these patients, yet most will also require mechanical ventilation. With lower cervical and thoracic lesions, although diaphragmatic innervation is intact, paralysis of the intercostal or abdominal muscles can cause progressive atelectasis because of a poor cough.

Thromboembolism Prevention

The majority of patients with SCI eventually develop deep venous thromboses, with the highest risk in the first 3 months after the injury. Weekly surveillance Doppler studies are optional. Pneumatic compression devices and elastic stockings should be applied as soon as possible; adding pharmacologic means of prevention (low-molecular-weight heparin or adjusted dose unfractionated heparin) may be delayed until surgical plans are finalized and there is no risk of bleeding. Therapeutic anticoagulation should be withheld for 3 to 7 days after surgery or trauma; vena cava filter placement may be required.

Gastrointestinal Management

Acute gastroparesis, seen sometimes immediately after the injury, requires gastric suctioning and administration of prokinetic agents to avoid aspiration. Ileus and constipation commonly complicate the course in patients with SCI; bowel regimen (e.g., scheduled laxatives, suppositories every other day) should be instituted early to prevent fecal impaction. H_2-antagonists or proton pump inhibitors are given for stress ulcers and gastrointestinal bleeding prophylaxis.

Skin

Because this patient population is prone to skin problems, frequent turning in bed, pressure relief, and meticulous care are necessary. Low-air-loss suspension beds may diminish the incidence of decubitus ulcers and facilitate healing of existing ulcers.

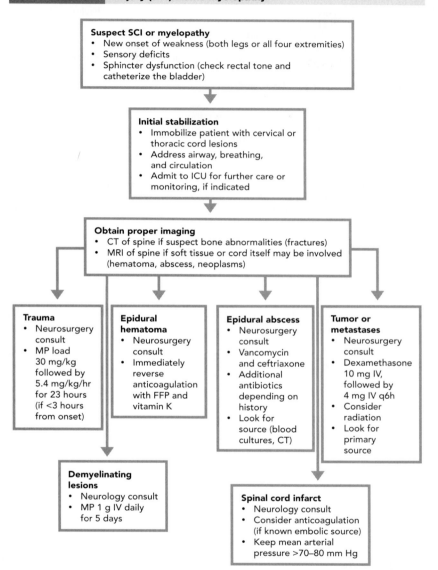

ALGORITHM 57.1 | **Initial Approach to a Patient with Suspected Spinal Cord Injury (SCI)/Acute Myelopathy**

Suspect SCI or myelopathy
- New onset of weakness (both legs or all four extremities)
- Sensory deficits
- Sphincter dysfunction (check rectal tone and catheterize the bladder)

Initial stabilization
- Immobilize patient with cervical or thoracic cord lesions
- Address airway, breathing, and circulation
- Admit to ICU for further care or monitoring, if indicated

Obtain proper imaging
- CT of spine if suspect bone abnormalities (fractures)
- MRI of spine if soft tissue or cord itself may be involved (hematoma, abscess, neoplasms)

Trauma
- Neurosurgery consult
- MP load 30 mg/kg followed by 5.4 mg/kg/hr for 23 hours (if <3 hours from onset)

Epidural hematoma
- Neurosurgery consult
- Immediately reverse anticoagulation with FFP and vitamin K

Epidural abscess
- Neurosurgery consult
- Vancomycin and ceftriaxone
- Additional antibiotics depending on history
- Look for source (blood cultures, CT)

Tumor or metastases
- Neurosurgery consult
- Dexamethasone 10 mg IV, followed by 4 mg IV q6h
- Consider radiation
- Look for primary source

Demyelinating lesions
- Neurology consult
- MP 1 g IV daily for 5 days

Spinal cord infarct
- Neurology consult
- Consider anticoagulation (if known embolic source)
- Keep mean arterial pressure >70–80 mm Hg

ICU, intensive care unit; CT, computed tomography; MRI, magnetic resonance imaging; MP, methyl-prednisolone; FFP, fresh-frozen plasma; IV, intravenous.

Other Issues

Spasticity and contractures become a major problem for these patients within weeks after the injury. Early physical and occupational therapy should be initiated; baclofen, diazepam, and dantrolene are useful agents for spasticity. Infections involving the pulmonary tree and bladder are common. Universal precautions for ventilator-associated pneumonia should be instituted. Urinary retention is seen almost universally; proper bladder care is important. Pain and depression are seen in most patients and should be addressed promptly.

NONTRAUMATIC MYELOPATHY

Most patients with nontraumatic SCI do not require an intensive care unit admission, unless the upper cord levels are involved. It is important to identify those at risk for respiratory failure or hemodynamic instability. Neurosurgery or Neurology consultation should be obtained early to institute proper surgical (e.g., hematoma, abscess) or conservative treatment for SCI.

Suggested Reading

Stevens RD, Bhardwaj A, Kirsch JR, et al. Critical care and perioperative management in traumatic spinal cord injury. *J Neurosurg Anesthesiol.* 2003;15:215–229.
   An excellent evidence-based review on multifaceted approach to patients with traumatic spinal cord injury.

NEUROMUSCULAR DISORDERS IN THE CRITICALLY ILL

58

Manu S. Goyal and Yekaterina Axelrod

Neuromuscular (NM) disorders are seen in the critically ill patients as a primary diagnosis or a complication of another illness. The most common neurologic conditions include Guillain-Barré syndrome (GBS), myasthenia gravis (MG), amyotrophic lateral sclerosis, myopathies, and neuropathies. Patients with severe sepsis and prolonged use of corticosteroids and/or NM blockade may develop critical illness polyneuropathy or myopathy (Table 58.1). Patients with the NM disorders are often admitted to the intensive care unit (ICU) for close observation as some may develop respiratory failure (RF), autonomic instability (as seen in GBS patients), or hypotension during plasmapheresis.

NEUROMUSCULAR RESPIRATORY FAILURE

The necessary NM components for a healthy respiration include the diaphragm and various accessory muscles of the face and chest, cranial, phrenic and intercostal nerves, anterior horn cells, tracts of the spinal cord, and the respiratory center in the medulla. Dysfunction of any of these components can lead to RF. Recognition of patients with NM disorders at risk for RF is important because signs of respiratory distress in this population may be underwhelming. Monitoring of clinical dynamics is preferred to checking blood gases; hypercarbia and hypoxemia are not seen in early RF.

Two bedside measurements of ventilatory reserve are most useful: negative inspiratory force (NIF) and forced vital capacity (FVC). The NIF is a maximum inspiratory effort produced after a forceful exhalation; it is measured with a mouthpiece attached to a pressure gauge. Healthy adults typically generate pressures of −50 to −70 cm H_2O; values close to −30 suggest impending RF. The FVC measures the amount of air exhaled with maximum speed and force. Normal FVC exceeds 3.5 liters; values below 30 mL/kg require close monitoring; however, very frequent checking may lead to excessive fatigue. Of note, weakness of the oropharyngeal muscles may prevent the patient from forming a tight seal around the mouthpiece; a facemask pressed tightly around the lips may help overcome this difficulty. Three repetitions help ensure accuracy. Following a *trend* of serial measurements of both parameters along with the clinical picture may be more useful than absolute values.

In the presence of impending RF, a trial of noninvasive positive pressure ventilation may be beneficial; however, endotracheal intubation is needed in those with poor cough and copious secretions (Alg. 58.1). Treatment of the underlying NM disorder should not be delayed; it expedites relief from respiratory weakness. Succinylcholine is avoided in patients for paralysis during intubation because of its potential to cause massive potassium release and cardiac arrest. Any mode of mechanical ventilation (MV) can be used; adequate pressure support helps to avoid fatigue and hypoventilation; hyperventilation is not advised. Weaning is started when the patient's condition has improved after proper treatment, and FVC and NIF exceed 10 mL/kg and −20 cm H_2O, respectively. Satisfactory oxygenation, ventilation, and hemodynamic stability are necessary. Daily trials of pressure support ventilation are used. Tracheostomy is postponed until 2 to 3 weeks, as only about one third of patients will need it.

DYSAUTONOMIA

Dysfunction of the autonomic nervous system is an important cause of morbidity and death in patients with severe GBS. Predictors of developing dysautonomia include tetraplegia, bulbar involvement, and RF. Wide fluctuations of blood pressure and heart rate are seen in

TABLE 58.1	Typical Causes of Neuromuscular Respiratory Failure

Peripheral neuropathies
   Guillain-Barré syndrome and chronic inflammatory demyelinating polyneuropathy
   Critical illness polyneuropathy
   Infectious (cytomegalovirus, West Nile virus, diphtheria)
Neuromuscular junction disorders
   Myasthenia gravis and Lambert-Eaton myasthenic syndrome
   Botulism
   Organophosphate poisoning
   Iatrogenic prolonged neuromuscular blockade
   Hypermagnesemia
   Puffer fish or shellfish toxicity
Myopathies
   Critical illness myopathy
   Rhabdomyolysis
   Polymyositis and dermatomyositis
   Muscular dystrophies
Myelopathies
   Traumatic cervical or thoracic spine injury
   Transverse myelitis
   Spinal cord infarction
   Neoplastic lesions
Anterior horn cell disorders
   Amyotrophic lateral sclerosis
   Infection (West Nile virus, poliomyelitis)

up to 20% of patients. Sinus bradycardia may be severe enough to lead to cardiac arrest; endotracheal suctioning and tracheostomy manipulations may provoke these episodes. Atropine always should be kept at bedside; temporary pacemaker may be needed in refractory cases. Blood pressure fluctuations may occur within minutes; therefore, they do not usually require interventions. Prolonged hypotension can be managed with Trendelenburg position and fluid boluses, short-acting alpha-agonists may rarely be needed; whereas hypertension, unless risk of end-organ damage, should not be treated pharmacologically. *Beta-blockers have been linked to cardiac arrest in this population.* Urinary retention and incontinence, gastroparesis, ileus, diarrhea, and constipation are seen commonly and should be addressed promptly.

MYASTHENIA GRAVIS

The hallmark of muscular weakness in MG is fatigability with repetitive movements. Oropharyngeal (bulbar) weakness is common; thus, RF is of significant concern. MG is an autoimmune process resulting in production of antibodies blocking the NM junction, thus preventing normal conduction. Diagnosis is clinical; detection of the antiacetylcholine receptor antibodies in the serum and electromyography confirm the diagnosis. The course is usually progressive; RF may develop suddenly during severe exacerbations.

    Myasthenic crisis is a life-threatening event requiring MV. Many factors may precipitate crisis, including subtle infections and a number of medications (Table 58.2). Treatment options for crisis include plasmapheresis or intravenous immunoglobulin G (IV IgG) infusions. Two to 4 liters of plasma are exchanged every other day to remove the antibodies during plasmapheresis. Hypotension and coagulopathies are common. IV IgG is given during 2 to 5 days in divided daily doses (a total dose of 2 g/kg); close monitoring for anaphylactic and hemolytic reactions as well as renal failure are advised.

ALGORITHM 58.1	Algorithm for Managing Neuromuscular Respiratory Failure

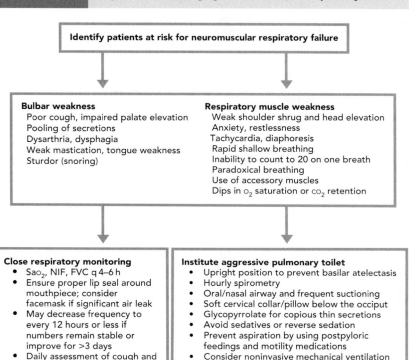

Identify patients at risk for neuromuscular respiratory failure

Bulbar weakness
Poor cough, impaired palate elevation
Pooling of secretions
Dysarthria, dysphagia
Weak mastication, tongue weakness
Sturdor (snoring)

Respiratory muscle weakness
Weak shoulder shrug and head elevation
Anxiety, restlessness
Tachycardia, diaphoresis
Rapid shallow breathing
Inability to count to 20 on one breath
Paradoxical breathing
Use of accessory muscles
Dips in O_2 saturation or CO_2 retention

Close respiratory monitoring
- Sao_2, NIF, FVC q 4–6 h
- Ensure proper lip seal around mouthpiece; consider facemask if significant air leak
- May decrease frequency to every 12 hours or less if numbers remain stable or improve for >3 days
- Daily assessment of cough and secretions

Institute aggressive pulmonary toilet
- Upright position to prevent basilar atelectasis
- Hourly spirometry
- Oral/nasal airway and frequent suctioning
- Soft cervical collar/pillow below the occiput
- Glycopyrrolate for copious thin secretions
- Avoid sedatives or reverse sedation
- Prevent aspiration by using postpyloric feedings and motility medications
- Consider noninvasive mechanical ventilation (exercise caution if patient is likely to vomit)

Signs of impeding respiratory failure
- FVC <15–20 mL/kg
- FVC falls from baseline by >30%
- NIF below –30 cm H_2O
- Hypoxemia pao_2 <70 mm Hg

Endotracheal intubation
- Avoid succinylcholine
- Limit use of neuromuscular blockers
- Optimal mode of ventilation based on comorbidities and severity of RF
- Wean when general condition is better by using daily spontaneous breathing trials
- Delay tracheostomy until 2–3 weeks

Treat underlying disorder if possible
- Plasmapheresis and/or IV IgG for GBS, MG
- Intravenous steroids for CIDP, inflammatory myopathies, tranverse myelitis
- Antibiotics for bacterial infections

NIF, negative inspiratory force; FVC, forced vital capacity; IV IgG, intravenous immunoglobulin G; GBS, Guillain-Barré syndrome; MG, myasthenia gravis; CIDP, chronic inflammatory demyelinating polyradiculoloneuropathy.

TABLE 58.2	Medications That Can Aggravate Weakness in Myasthenia Gravis

Antibiotics (aminoglycosides, ciprofloxacin, clindamycin, erythromycin, tetracyclines, polymixin B, colistin)
Antiarrhythmics (quinidine, procainamide, lidocaine, beta-blockers and calcium channel blockers)
Hormones (corticosteroids, thyroid, oral contraceptives)
NM blockers (succinylcholine, vecuronium, pancuronium, etc)
Others (phenytoin, lithium, quinine)

GUILLAIN-BARRÉ SYNDROME

GBS (acute inflammatory demyelinating polyradiculoneuropathy) is an autoimmune process leading to severe motor weakness, usually precipitated by an upper respiratory or gastrointestinal viral infection. The antibodies are directed against myelin; therefore, electrical conduction along the damaged nerves is diminished. The clinical picture includes ascending weakness/paralysis, hyporeflexia to areflexia, and autonomic disturbances. GBS is a clinical diagnosis; cerebrospinal fluid analysis and electromyography are confirmatory. Respiratory difficulties are more likely to occur in patients with rapid progression of symptoms, bulbar weakness, and dysautonomia. Treatment approach is similar to that of myasthenic crisis and consists of plasmapheresis or IV IgG infusions.

CRITICAL ILLNESS MYOPATHY AND POLYNEUROPATHY

In ICU patients, myopathy and polyneuropathy usually occur as a complication of critical illness. Severe sepsis, multiorgan failure with high systemic inflammatory response syndrome and Acute Physiology, Age and Chronic Health Evaluation (APACHE)-II scores, aggressive corticosteroid and aminoglycoside use, prolonged NM blockade, and disuse atrophy are among the risk factors for the critical illness myopathy/polyneuropathy. These entities are often suspected and diagnosed during attempts of weaning from MV; up to 30% to 35% of ICU patients are affected. Nonrespiratory manifestations include generalized weakness in mainly the lower extremities associated with hyporeflexia; cranial nerves may be spared.

Clinically, these disorders cannot be distinguished; electromyographic studies help differentiate nerve versus muscle involvement; biopsy offers definitive diagnosis. Aggressive and early treatment of multiorgan failure and sepsis may help prevent critical care-related NM disorders. Other prophylactic measurements include restricted use of the NM blocking agents to a minimum, with frequent monitoring of the depth of blockade, providing "drug holidays" and utilization of sedating agents instead. Early involvement of rehabilitation services may be beneficial. Most survivors will be left with residual weakness.

General ICU care of patients with NM weakness and paralysis should also include aggressive thromboembolism prophylaxis, pulmonary infection prevention, adequate nutrition, skin care, and early rehabilitation.

Suggested Reading

Chalela JA. Pearls and pitfalls in the intensive care management of Guillain-Barré syndrome. *Semin Neurol.* 2001;21:399–405.
An exceptionally well-written article detailing the management of Guillain-Barré syndrome and how to avoid dangerous situations given the myriad complications of this disorder.
De Jonghe B, Sharshar T, Hopkinson N, et al. Paresis following mechanical ventilation. *Curr Opin Crit Care.* 2004;10:47–52.
A review of neuromuscular weakness in patients with critical illness.
Richman DP, Agius MA. Treatment of autoimmune myasthenia gravis. *Neurology.* 2003; 61:1652–1661.
An updated evidence-based review of the treatment of myasthenia gravis, including associated respiratory failure.

TRAUMATIC BRAIN INJURY

Yekaterina Axelrod

59

Severe head trauma is a leading cause of death among young adults. Almost 1.5 million people sustain a traumatic brain injury (TBI) in the United States; of those, approximately 50,000 die and 200,000 to 250,000 are hospitalized. Approximately 25% of patients are not able to return to work after TBI.

The Glasgow Coma Scale (GCS) is widely used for classification and prognosis (Fig. 59.1). An assessment of eye opening/level of consciousness and motor and verbal responses is performed and recorded. According to this scale, head injuries are classified as mild (GCS 14-15), moderate (GCS 9-12), and severe (GCS 3-8).

Initial management focuses on the airway, breathing, and circulation. Those patients with GCS below 8 usually require endotracheal intubation and mechanical ventilation. In cases of ongoing bleeding and hypotension, fluid resuscitation, possible hemotransfusion, and/or vasopressors to maintain adequate perfusion should be initiated. Because almost 15% of patients with TBI have an associated spinal cord injury, an effort is made to stabilize and immobilize the spine.

Once the initial steps have been performed, a noncontrasted head computed tomography and plain films of spine to assess the magnitude and type of injury should be obtained. The range of head injuries extends from simple scalp lacerations, skull fractures, to contusions, hemorrhagic insults (epidural, subdural, intraparenchymal, subarachnoid hemorrhages), and diffuse axonal injury. Neurosurgery consultation should be sought emergently as certain types of TBI require immediate operative treatment.

Further management of head injury is based on prevention, recognition, and aggressive treatment of secondary insults to the brain, including hypoxia, hypotension, hypoperfusion, and elevated intracranial pressure (ICP).

MANAGEMENT OF PATIENTS WITH SEVERE TBI

Although every effort is made to control elevated ICP, maintenance of adequate cerebral perfusion is the main goal of treatment. Patients with severe TBI are admitted to the intensive care unit for ICP and cerebral perfusion pressure (CPP) monitoring (Fig. 59.2). The gold standard of ICP monitoring is cerebrospinal fluid (CSF) pressure measuring in the ventricular system via ventriculostomy, which allows CSF drainage in order to reduce ICP. Even though intraparenchymal ICP monitors (bolts) are widely used, they lack the ability to drain CSF.

ICP Control

Elevated ICP (above 20 mm Hg) after head injury is associated with more unfavorable outcome. In approximately half of those who die after severe TBI, raised ICP is the primary cause of death. For detailed discussion on management of elevated ICP, see Chapter 51. Hyperventilation is recommended only as a brief temporizing measure for symptoms of herniation. Barbiturates in high doses may be used in cases of elevated ICP that is refractory to conventional ICP-lowering strategies; however, one should recognize that prophylactic use of barbiturates for ICP lowering is not indicated (Alg. 59.1).

CPP Threshold

CPP is the difference between mean arterial pressure (MAP) and ICP. MAP is accurately measured by direct cannulation of one of the arteries (e.g., radial, femoral). Maintenance of

Best eye opening

Spontaneous	4
With voice only	3
With pain only	2
None at all	1

Best verbal response

Coherent speech	5
Confused intelligible speech	4
Inappropriate words	3
Incomprehensible sounds	2
No verbal output	1

Best motor response

Follows commands	6
*Localizes pain stimuli	5
Withdraws to pain stimuli	4
Decorticate posturing	3
Decerebrate posturing	2
No movements at all	1

*Localizing pain stimuli refers to gaze deviation, head turning, or hand movements toward the stimulus.

Figure 59.1. Glasgow Coma Scale.

CPP at 60 to 70 mm Hg is necessary to maintain constant cerebral blood flow; reduction below these level results in increased risk of ischemia. CPP may drop because of a decrease in MAP, an increase in ICP, or by a combination of these two mechanisms. Maintenance of CPP at 60 mm Hg is achieved by administering fluids to keep patients euvolemic and vasopressors to keep adequate for cerebral perfusion MAP (Fig. 59.3).

- Patients with GCS <9 and an abnormal CT scan (cerebral edema, contusions, hematoma)
- Patients with a normal CT scan and two of three features:
  - o Age >40
  - o Unilateral or bilateral motor posturing
  - o Systolic BP <90 mm Hg

Figure 59.2. Indications for intracranial pressure and cerebral perfusion pressure monitoring. GCS, Glasgow Coma Scale; CT, computed tomography; BP, blood pressure.

ALGORITHM 59.1   **Management of Elevated Intracranial Pressure (ICP)**

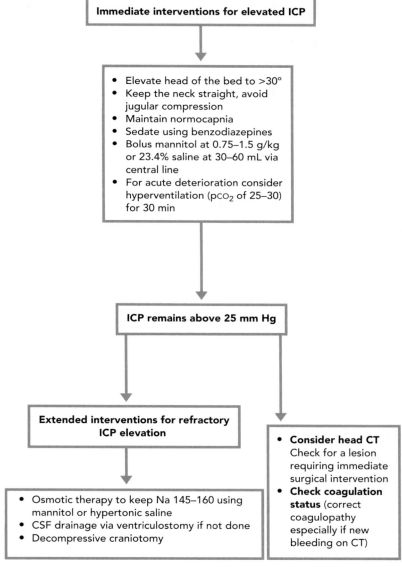

Immediate interventions for elevated ICP

- Elevate head of the bed to >30°
- Keep the neck straight, avoid jugular compression
- Maintain normocapnia
- Sedate using benzodiazepines
- Bolus mannitol at 0.75–1.5 g/kg or 23.4% saline at 30–60 mL via central line
- For acute deterioration consider hyperventilation (pco$_2$ of 25–30) for 30 min

ICP remains above 25 mm Hg

Extended interventions for refractory ICP elevation

- Osmotic therapy to keep Na 145–160 using mannitol or hypertonic saline
- CSF drainage via ventriculostomy if not done
- Decompressive craniotomy

- **Consider head CT** Check for a lesion requiring immediate surgical intervention
- **Check coagulation status** (correct coagulopathy especially if new bleeding on CT)

CSF, cerebrospinal fluid; CT, computed tomography.

> - Keep MAP above 80 mm Hg until CPP can be measured
> - Use normal saline boluses and vasopressors if needed
> - Once ICP monitor is inserted, CPP goal 60 mm Hg (CPP = MAP – ICP)
> - Control ICP; see Figure 59.3
> - Use vasopressors to keep CPP within goals while correcting hypovolemia

Figure 59.3. Cerebral perfusion pressure (CPP) management. MAP, mean arterial pressure; ICP, intracranial pressure.

General Care

Because metabolic expenditures are higher in patients with severe TBI, caloric intake should be adjusted to provide approximately 140% of expected requirements. At least 15% of calories should be supplied as protein. Early feeding (within 48 to 72 hours of insult) is important, resulting in a trend toward fewer infectious complications and lower mortality. The jejunal route is preferred.

Almost 25% of TBI patients will experience a posttraumatic seizure. Early seizures are associated with late epilepsy development in as many as 25% of cases. Seizure prevention with anticonvulsants is indicated for 7 days after TBI. Continuation of prophylaxis should not extend beyond 1 week as it does not affect the development of late epilepsy.

Suggested Reading

The Brain Trauma Foundation. The American Association of Neurological Surgeons. The Joint Section on Neurotrauma and Critical Care. Guidelines for cerebral perfusion pressure. *J Neurotrauma.* 2000;6/7:471–520.

Valadka AB, Andrews BT, eds. *Neurotrauma: Evidence-based Answers to Common Questions.* New York: Thieme Medical Publishers; 2005:88–90.
A good evidence-based review book in an easy-to-read format, it encompasses numerous common questions in management of patients with traumatic brain injury.

NEUROLOGIC APPROACH TO CENTRAL NERVOUS SYSTEM INFECTIONS

60

R. Brian Sommerville, Yo-El Ju, and Yekaterina Axelrod

The central nervous system (CNS) has a limited repertoire of responses to infection, and clinical suspicion for infection should be raised by any combination of altered mental status, headache, fever, meningismus, and focal neurologic signs; peripheral leukocytosis may not be present. In immunocompromised patients, the index of suspicion is even higher, as any one of these symptoms may be the sole manifestation of infection. Once the suspicion is raised, lumbar puncture (LP) should be performed immediately with measurement of an opening pressure. Prior brain imaging is required in immunocompromised patients and those with depressed level of consciousness, papilledema, or focal neurologic signs due to herniation potential (Table 60.1 presents LP contraindications). Blood products may be needed to correct coagulopathy.

Antimicrobials should not be delayed for LP, although blood cultures should be drawn prior to administration of antibiotics. After LP and blood cultures, empiric antibiotic treatment should be continued until the suspected infection has been either ruled out or further characterized (Alg. 60.1 for treatment algorithm). After the cell count, protein, and glucose are known, additional studies can be added to identify the organism. Table 60.2 lists the various cerebrospinal fluid (CSF) patterns according to cause. If suspicion is high enough to look for a certain organism in the CSF, antimicrobial coverage for that organism should be initiated (e.g., if sending herpes simplex virus [HSV] for polymerase chain reaction, start acyclovir). For further review of risk factors, pathogens, antimicrobial treatment, and duration, see Chapter 33.

MENINGITIS

Meningitis is the most common type of CNS infection, with mortality reaching 60%; delay in proper recognition and immediate treatment can be deadly.

Bacterial Meningitis

A preceding pneumonia, otitis media, or acute sinusitis is common. Bacterial meningitis carries a very high morbidity and mortality; patients should be monitored closely for complications including septic shock, cerebral edema, hydrocephalus, venous sinus thrombosis, seizures, disseminated intravascular coagulation, hearing loss, and syndrome of inappropriate antidiuretic hormone secretion. Patients with bacterial meningitis after head trauma may have a repairable dural sinus fistula; further imaging studies after treatment initiation and Neurosurgery consultation are advised.

Viral Meningitis

Most cases of viral meningitis are self-limiting and carry a favorable outcome. Of note, meningitides caused by HSV or varicella-zoster virus are treatable with acyclovir.

Noninfectious Aseptic Meningitis

If all microbiology tests have negative results, and there is no clinical improvement with antibiotics; consider noninfectious causes of meningitis (Table 60.3). CSF cytology with flow cytometry should be requested if malignancy is suspected.

TABLE 60.1	Contraindications to Lumbar Puncture

Absolute	Relative
Space-occupying lesion in the posterior fossa	International normalized ratio above 1.4
Presence of midline shift	Platelet count below 50,000/mcL
Effacement of the cisterns or fourth ventricle	
Skin infection in the area of puncture	
Lumbar epidural abscess or empyema	

ENCEPHALITIS

Encephalitis is an infection of the brain parenchyma. Encephalitis and meningitis are often two ends of a spectrum, sharing many of the same pathogens. As with viral meningitis, therapy is supportive in most cases.

Herpes-simplex Encephalitis

HSV encephalitis tends to present with focal neurologic findings such as hemiparesis, dysphasia, aphasia, ataxia, or focal seizures that are of generally short (under 1 week) duration. Xanthochromia may be present as a result of mild hemorrhage into the subarachnoid space; otherwise CSF findings are similar to those of viral meningitis. Characteristic findings on imaging include involvement of one or both temporal lobes. Prompt diagnosis and treatment of this infection is of paramount importance given its significant morbidity and mortality; acyclovir should be given intravenously for the entire duration of treatment. Because refractory seizures or status epilepticus are commonly seen, patients with altered mental status should undergo electroencephalography.

Arthropod-borne (Arboviral) Encephalitis

Encephalitides of the arthropod-borne type include St. Louis encephalitis, California encephalitis, Japanese B encephalitis, Eastern and Western equine encephalitis, and West Nile encephalitis. Treatment of these infections is generally supportive.

BRAIN ABSCESS

Brain abscess arises from one of three sources: direct spread (from an infected sinus), hematogenous spread from another source, or trauma. Neurosurgical patients are also at particular risk in the months or even years after a procedure. Most brain abscesses are bacterial and often polymicrobial, although fungal infections are also possible, especially in the immunocompromised patient. Common aerobes include *Streptococcus* species (including *viridans* in endocarditis patients), *Staphylococcus* species (especially after surgical procedures), *Pseudomonas* species, and *Enterobacter* species (otitis media). Anaerobic abscesses (*Bacteroides* and *Actinomyces* species) may arise from oral sources and abdominal or pelvic infections. Neutropenic patients and transplant recipients have a particular predilection for *Aspergillus* abscesses. Toxoplasmosis is the most common intracranial infection in patients with acquired immune deficiency syndrome (AIDS).

The presentation of a brain abscess typically involves headache lateralizing to the side of the abscess, accompanied by focal signs and, occasionally, meningismus. Evidence of elevated intracranial pressure (papilledema, vomiting, or depressed level of consciousness) may also be present; LP is contraindicated because of risk of herniation. Diagnosis of brain abscess relies primarily on neuroimaging with a contrast agent. The typical abscess appears as a ring-enhancing

ALGORITHM 60.1   **Approach to Treatment of Suspected Infection of the Central Nervous System**

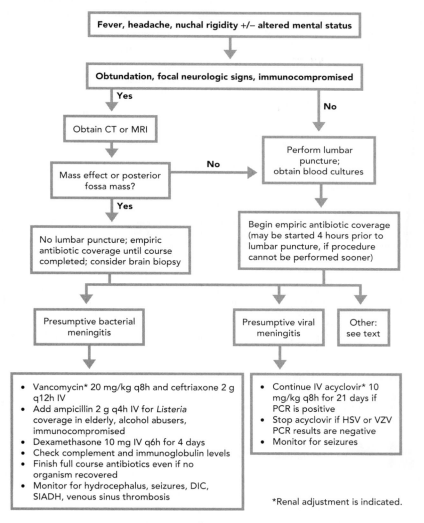

CT, computed tomography; MRI, magnetic resonance imaging; IV, intravenous; DIC, disseminated intravascular coagulation; SIADH, syndrome of inappropriate antidiuretic hormone secretion; PCR, polymerase chain reaction; HSV, herpes simplex virus; VZV, varicella-zoster virus.

TABLE 60.2	**Cerebrospinal Fluid (CSF) Findings Suggestive of Infection**		

CSF parameter	Bacterial meningitis	Viral meningitis	Fungal meningitis
Opening pressure (mm H_2O)	>180	Often normal	Variable
White cell count	1,000–10,000	<300	50–200
Percent neutrophils	>80	<20	Usually <50
Protein	100–500	Often normal	Variably elevated
Glucose	<40	>40	Usually <40
Gram stain (% positive)	60–90	0	0
Culture (% positive)	70–85	50	25–50

From Zunt JR, Marra CM. Cerebrospinal fluid testing for the diagnosis and central nervous system infection. *Neurol Clin.* 1999;17:675–689, with permission.

lesion with surrounding edema. Abscesses resulting from hematogenous spread (septic emboli due to endocarditis) may present as multiple lesions. Abscesses due to direct invasion from the facial sinuses or dental infections will typically affect the frontal lobes.

Workup entails a search for the source; blood and urine cultures, echocardiography, and possibly further body imaging are indicated. Toxoplasma titers are checked in immunocompromised patients. Definitive characterization may require stereotactic aspiration followed by empiric antibiotic coverage until specific organisms and sensitivities have been determined.

Antimicrobial coverage for brain abscesses varies with the presumptive source of infection. Empiric treatment for a hematogenous source includes vancomycin and metronidazole. Abscess originating from a sinus, otogenic, or oral source requires metronidazole and either penicillin G or ceftriaxone. Neurosurgical patients with postoperative abscess require vancomycin and ceftazidime. Immunocompromised hosts (including neutropenic and recent posttransplant patients) require amphotericin B for additional fungal coverage. A total course of 6 to 8 weeks is standard in all cases.

FUNGAL INFECTIONS

Fungal CNS infections (meningoencephalitis, brain abscess, or granuloma) are usually encountered as opportunistic infections in the immunosuppressed hosts. Amphotericin B

TABLE 60.3	**Noninfectious Causes of Meningitis**

- Medications and toxins
  - Nonsteroidal anti-inflammatory medications (ibuprofen, ketorolac)
  - Chemotherapy agents (especially intrathecal preparations)
  - Antibiotics (metronidazole, trimethoprim-sulfamethoxazole, isoniazid)
  - Vaccinations
  - Intravenous immunoglobulin G
  - Intravenous contrast
- Neoplastic (leptomeningeal metastases)
- Autoimmune or inflammatory disorders
  - Systemic lupus erythematosus
  - Sjögren syndrome
  - Primary central nervous system angiitis
  - Behçet disease

(1 mg/kg daily intravenously) is the first-line agent for most infections and because of poor CNS penetration, flucytosine (25 mg/kg every 6 hours orally) is added. Both medications require renal adjustment; patients should be closely monitored, as risk of side effects is high. After a 4- to 6-week course, a suppressive phase with a triazole is continued for at least 6 weeks. Infectious disease specialist consult is highly recommended.

INFECTIONS RELATED TO NEUROSURGERY

Infections following neurosurgery include meningitis, encephalitis, ventriculitis, abscess, and hardware infection. These typically occur within weeks of surgery, although vulnerability to infections remains for years. Ventriculoperitoneal shunt infections may present with symptoms of hydrocephalus (increasing headaches, vomiting, lethargy) and abdominal distention; otherwise, symptoms are similar to other types of CNS infections. Neurosurgical consultation is mandatory.

In addition to the usual workup, shunts are assessed with imaging to determine their functional status and tapped to identify the etiologic organism. Infected hardware must be removed if possible. The most common organisms causing postneurosurgical infection include *Staphylococcus* species and Gram-negative organisms.

THE IMMUNOCOMPROMISED PATIENT

The immunocompromised population includes patients with AIDS, solid-organ or bone marrow transplantation recipients, and those receiving chemotherapy or immunosuppressants for autoimmune conditions. Such patients are at high risk of opportunistic CNS infections; any one symptom of possible CNS infection should elicit brain imaging and LP. The most common infections include toxoplasmosis, cryptococcal meningitis or encephalitis, fungal abscess (*Aspergillus*), and progressive multifocal leukoencephalopathy (JC virus). Because most of these infections present with CNS mass lesions, imaging must always be performed prior to LP. Special CSF testing includes polymerase chain reaction testing for *Toxoplasma*, JC virus, Epstein-Barr virus, and cytomegalovirus, as well as *Cryptococcus* and *Histoplasma* antigen testing. The Venereal Disease Research Laboratory test should also be requested, given the higher incidence of neurosyphilis in AIDS patients. An infectious diseases consult is strongly recommended if CNS infection is suspected in an immunocompromised patient.

Suggested Reading

Pruitt AA. Infections of the nervous system. *Neurol Clin.* 1998;16:419–447.
> *An excellent review of comprehensive approach to infections of the central nervous system with special attention to the immunocompromised patients.*

Tunkel AR, Hartman BJ, Kaplan SL, et al. Practice guidelines for the management of bacterial meningitis. *Clin Infect Dis.* 2004;39:1267–1284.
> *Current recommendations for the diagnosis and management of bacterial meningitis representing data published through May 2004.*

Ziai WC, Lewin JJ 3rd. Advances in the management of central nervous system infections in the ICU. *Crit Care Clin.* 2006;22:661–694.
> *Most recent review of management of various acute central nervous system infections in the critical care setting.*

Zunt JR, Marra CM. Cerebrospinal fluid testing for the diagnosis and central nervous system infection. *Neurol Clin.* 1999;17:675–689.
> *A detailed review of various methods of testing cerebrospinal fluid for suspected infection of the central nervous system.*

XV Hematopoietic Disorders

61 THROMBOCYTOPENIA IN THE INTENSIVE CARE UNIT
Warren Isakow

Thrombocytopenia is a very common occurrence in the intensive care unit (ICU), occurring in as many as 60% of patients. The normal platelet count ranges between 150,000 and 450,000/mcL. In the ICU, it is important to recognize that the absolute platelet count is important, but trends in the platelet count, specifically a decline by more than one-half, may be evidence of a serious clinical problem such as heparin-induced thrombocytopenia, which requires urgent attention. A systematic approach to the diagnosis allows for the common causes to be detected early and enables rational use of platelet transfusions (Alg. 61.1). Platelet survival in the circulation is approximately 7 to 10 days, and one-third of the platelets are sequestered in the spleen under normal circumstances.

Recognition of thrombocytopenia normally occurs after a complete blood count is drawn, but it is important to remember that mucocutaneous bleeding is a classic sign of thrombocytopenia. Bleeding from thrombocytopenia normally occurs only once the platelet count is <50,000/mcL in postsurgical patients; spontaneous bleeding can occur with counts <5,000/mcL. The diagnostic approach starts with a thorough history and physical examination, followed by examination of the peripheral smear. A pathophysiologic approach to thrombocytopenia enables all common causes to be rapidly screened for and facilitates recognition of potential causes (Table 61.1). Careful attention should be paid to prescription and over-the-counter drugs (Table 61.2).

The common causes of thrombocytopenia in an ICU setting are as follows:

- Drug-induced (heparin, H_2-receptor blockers, GP2b3a inhibitors, antibiotics, alcohol)
- Sepsis
- Massive bleeding
- Thrombocytopenia with microangiopathic hemolytic anemia (thrombocytopenic thrombotic purpura [TTP], hemolytic uremic syndrome [HUS], disseminated intravascular coagulation [DIC]).

Clinical recognition of the cause is vital as the therapies differ considerably depending on the etiology. For example, a patient with thrombocytopenia secondary to bleeding

ALGORITHM 61.1   **Diagnostic Algorithm for Thrombocytopenia**

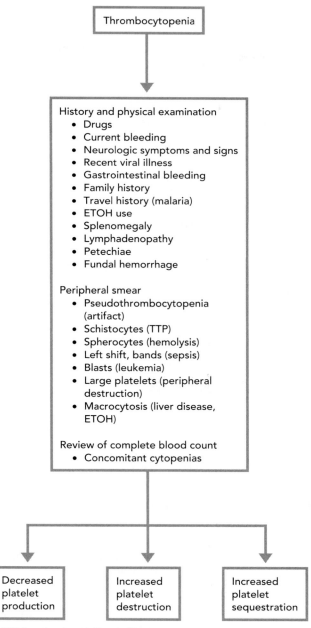

ETOH, alcohol; TTP, thrombocytopenic thrombotic purpura.

TABLE 61.1	Pathophysiologic Classification of Thrombocytopenia

Decreased production	Increased destruction	Increased sequestration
Aplastic anemia	Immunologic	Hypersplenism from any
Hematologic malignancies	ITP	cause:
Lymphoma	Heparin-induced (HIT)	Cirrhosis
Leukemia	Drug-induced (see Table 61.2)	Portal hypertension
Myelodysplasia	HIV	Congestive heart failure
Metastatic malignancy	Autoimmune disease	Hematologic malignancies
Nutritional (B_{12} and folate)	Infectious	Lipid storage disorders
Drugs (see Table 61.2)	Posttransfusion purpura	
Chemotherapy and radiation	Antiphospholipid antibody	
Alcohol	syndrome	
Viral infections	Nonimmunologic	
HIV	DIC	
Mumps	HUS/TTP	
Parvovirus	HELLP syndrome	
Varicella	Preeclampsia/eclampsia	
Rubella	Malignant HTN	
Ebstein-Barr	Sepsis	
Hepatitis C	Cardiac valves	
	Burns	
	Massive bleeding	

HIV, human immunodeficiency virus; ITP, immune thrombocytopenic purpura; HIT, heparin-induced; DIC, disseminated intravascular coagulation; HUS, hemolytic uremic syndrome; TTP, thrombocytopenic thrombotic purpura; HELLP, hemolysis, elevated liver enzyme levels and a low platelet count; HTN, hypertension.

should be treated with platelets, compared with a patient with TTP/HUS, in whom platelet transfusion is generally contraindicated. A few common conditions will be discussed and readers are encouraged to refer to the suggested reading for further details.

IMMUNE THROMBOCYTOPENIC PURPURA

Immune thrombocytopenic purpura (ITP) is a condition caused by autoantibodies directed against the platelets surface glycoproteins. Binding of the antibodies results in accelerated platelet removal by the spleen. *Evans syndrome* refers to ITP together with autoimmune hemolytic anemia. The diagnosis of ITP is made by exclusion; checking for antiplatelet antibodies has no role in the diagnosis. Treatment consists of corticosteroids, intravenous immunoglobulin, anti-RhD antibodies, rituximab, danazol, cyclophosphamide, azathioprine, or splenectomy.

HEPARIN-INDUCED THROMBOCYTOPENIA

Heparin-induced thrombocytopenia (HIT) is a very serious disorder that occurs when patients develop antibodies against the heparin-platelet factor-4 complex. It can be induced by exposure to unfractionated or low-molecular-weight heparins. Important clues to the diagnosis include a >50% decline in the platelet count 5 to 10 days after being exposed to heparin for the first time. A more rapid decline in platelet counts can occur with prior heparin exposures.

    The major clinical problem is that continued exposure to heparin will cause devastating thrombotic complications in up to 50% of patients. These thromboses can be venous or arterial and can result in life-threatening complications such as limb ischemia. When this diagnosis is suspected, all sources of heparin products should be immediately stopped, a

TABLE 61.2	Common Drugs Associated with Thrombocytopenia

Decreased production	Immune-mediated destruction
Chemotherapeutic agents	Abciximab
Daunorubicin	Amphotericin B
Cytosine arabinoside	Aspirin
Busulfan	Carbamazepine
Cyclophosphamide	Cimetidine
Methotrexate	Chloroquine
Vinca alkaloids	Digoxin
6-Mercaptopurine	Eptifibatide
Thiazide diuretics	Fluconazole
Ethanol	Heparin
Estrogens	Phenytoin
	Piperacillin
	Quinine
	Ranitidine
	Trimethoprim/sulfamethoxazole
	Valproic acid

serologic test for heparin-dependent antibodies should be requested, and the patient should be started on a direct thrombin inhibitor such as lepirudin (renally metabolized) or argatroban (hepatically metabolized). Platelets should not be given unless there is life-threatening bleeding.

SEPSIS-INDUCED THROMBOCYTOPENIA

Sepsis-induced thrombocytopenia is usually multifactorial and caused by marrow suppression, increased platelet destruction, drugs, and associated DIC. Treatment is supportive and possible offending drugs should be stopped. Specific infections tend to cause thrombocytopenia, and physicians should be aware of the common culprits, according to their geographic location. In Missouri, ehrlichiosis needs to be considered and travelers should be screened for malaria. DIC is recognized by the combination of microvascular thrombosis and bleeding, thrombocytopenia, coagulopathy, and low fibrinogen levels. Treatment for this complication is supportive with platelets, fresh-frozen plasma, and cryoprecipitate.

THROMBOTIC THROMBOCYTOPENIC PURPURA

The diagnostic pentad of TTP is:

- Microangiopathic hemolytic anemia
- Thrombocytopenia
- Renal failure
- Fever
- Altered mental status

However, all five criteria are met in <40% of patients. The major differential diagnosis is DIC (coagulopathy) and Evans syndrome (positive Coombs test). The peripheral smear will reveal schistocytes and the thrombocytopenia can be severe. Platelet transfusions in these patients are contraindicated in the absence of life-threatening bleeding as they can precipitate vasoocclusive crises of vital organs, such as the brain and myocardium. This disorder is caused by an acquired deficiency of ADAMTS13, which normally cleaves von Willebrand factor multimers. Absence of ADAMTS13 activity results in large circulating multimers of von Willebrand factor, which cause platelets to adhere to the endothelium with resultant thrombosis, thrombocytopenia, and shearing of red cells as they pass the thrombi, which causes a microangiopathic hemolytic anemia. The syndrome is most commonly precipitated by infections (*Escherichia coli* O157:H7 enteritis, human immunodeficiency virus) or drugs (ticlopidine, cyclosporine, tacrolimus, clopidogrel).Treatment consists of plasma exchange or fresh-frozen plasma/intravenous immunoglobulin if plasma exchange is not immediately available. The assay for ADAMTS13 plays no role in diagnosis in the acute setting.

PLATELET TRANSFUSIONS

The indications for transfusing platelets depend on the cause of the thrombocytopenia and the presence of bleeding. As previously noted, transfusions should be avoided in TTP and HIT unless the patient is experiencing life-threatening bleeding. For other causes, platelets should be transfused prophylactically when the platelet count is <10,000/mcL to prevent spontaneous intracranial bleeding. For major surgery, the counts should be >100,000/mcL; for minor procedures, the counts should be >50,000/mcL.

Suggested Reading

Akca S, Haji-Michael P, de Mendonca A, et al. Time course of platelet counts in critically ill patients. *Crit Care Med.* 2002;30:753–756.
This prospective, observational multicenter cohort study identified late thrombocytopenia (day 14) as being predictive of death and related changes in platelet count over time to patient outcome.

Arepally GM, Ortel TL. Clinical practice. Heparin-induced thrombocytopenia. *N Engl J Med.* 2006;355:809–817
An excellent recent review of the incidence, diagnostic algorithm and therapies available.

Cines DB, Bussel JB. How I treat idiopathic thrombocytopenic purpura. *Blood.* 2005;106:2244–2251.
A thorough review of the topic for clinicians.

George JN. Clinical practice. Thrombotic thrombocytopenic purpura. *N Engl J Med.* 2006;354:1927–1935.
An excellent review of the topic for clinicians.

Sekhon SS, Vivek R. Thrombocytopenia in adults: a practical approach to evaluation and management. *South Med J.* 2006;99:491–498.
A concise review for clinicians with relevant suggestions for daily clinical practice.

Strauss R, Wehler M, Mehler,K et al. Thrombocytopenia in patients in the medical intensive care unit: bleeding prevalence, transfusion requirements, and outcome. *Crit Care Med.* 2002;30:1765–1771.
Prospective observational study in a university hospital, found that 44% of patients developed ICU acquired thrombocytopenia. These patients had higher mortality, more bleeding and greater transfusion requirements.

Vanderschueren S, De Weerdt A, Malbrain M, et al. Thrombocytopenia and prognosis in intensive care. *Crit Care Med.* 2000;28:1871–1876.
Prospective observational cohort study which identified thrombocytopenia as a readily available risk marker for mortality, independent of severity of disease indices.

Vincent JL, Yagushi A, Pradier O. Platelet function in sepsis. *Crit Care Med.* 2002;30:S313–S317.
A review of the multifactorial etiology of thrombocytopenia in septic patients and the role of platelets in modulating sepsis.

ACUTE MANAGEMENT OF THE BLEEDING PATIENT/COAGULOPATHY

62

Mark A. Schroeder

Coagulopathies are commonly encountered in the intensive care unit (ICU). The acute management of the coagulopathic and bleeding patient through transfusion support requires an appropriate workup and diagnosis to prevent unnecessary exposures to blood products and/or worse outcomes.

ICU patients consume a large amount of blood products, and hemostatic defects contribute to this large demand. A prospective, observational study of an adult ICU determined the incidence and cause of coagulation problems within an ICU population. Laboratory evidence of coagulopathy was seen in 67% of patients, and 14% of patients had coagulation defects requiring transfusions. Of the identifiable causes of elevated international normalized ratio (INR), the most commonly reported, in descending order of incidence, were liver failure, disseminated intravascular coagulation (DIC), transfusion, warfarin, cardiopulmonary bypass, heparin, and vitamin K deficiency. Thrombocytopenia (platelets <100,000/mcL) was identified in 38% of patients; the most common causes were DIC, dilution following major transfusion with cardiopulmonary bypass, and liver failure. Excess bleeding resulted in the death of approximately 6% of patients.

Acute blood loss has a direct impact on blood volume and oxygen supply to tissues. Normal response to blood loss involves a cardiovascular response and erythropoietic response. Loss of blood volume up to 20% of total blood volume can be tolerated in a healthy individual by reflex venospasm and redistribution of the blood pool. When blood loss exceeds 20% (>1,000 mL in a 70-kg person) patients develop symptoms. Hypovolemic shock occurs at >40% volume loss. The marrow response is to rapidly increase red cell production, and this capacity depends on the level of erythropoietin stimulation, normal bone marrow, and adequate iron stores. Erythropoietin is increased at hemoglobin levels <11 g/dL by a healthy kidney in a matter or hours, but marrow production takes days to weeks. Red cell oxygen delivery is compensated for in the acidic environment of ischemic tissues, and oxygen is more readily dissociated (Bohr effect). During hours the amount of 2,3-diphosphoglycerate in the red cell increases to maintain a higher level of oxygen delivery. These compensatory mechanisms can only temporarily relieve the stress of an acute bleed, and without intervention to correct the hemorrhaging situation, patient death will ultimately occur.

Coagulopathies encountered in the ICU are most often acquired disorders and are rarely inherited. They result from a disruption of normal hemostasis, which involves primary and secondary events. Primary factors involve platelets, von Willebrand factor (vWF), and endothelium; secondary events involve the activation of the coagulation cascade and formation of the fibrin clot complex. A defect in primary or secondary hemostasis can result in hemorrhage. Signs of defective primary hemostasis include epistaxis, gum bleeding, hematochezia, melena, petechiae, or bruising. Secondary hemostasis disorders usually involve deeper structures, for example, hemarthroses or intramuscular hemorrhage.

This chapter will initially focus on the general evaluation and therapies of the acutely bleeding patient followed by a discussion of common acquired disease states encountered in the ICU, and, finally, a brief introduction to inherited disorders will be discussed.

INITIAL EVALUATION

The evaluation of a patient with anemia relies on the acuity of onset. Subacute to chronic anemia is usually insidious in onset and patients can present with hematocrits <20%

without significant symptoms. These chronic anemias are usually secondary to underproduction. Acute anemia usually presents with symptoms of hemodynamic instability (tachycardia, hypotension), light-headedness, dyspnea, and is a result of the rapid change in intravascular volume and oxygen-carrying capacity. Anemia that develops rapidly suggests bleeding or hemolysis.

Patients presenting with severe, ongoing hemorrhage are often easily identified at the bedside. Timing and location will determine the patient's symptoms, physical signs, and laboratory findings. For example, variceal bleeds in cirrhosis patients usually present with episodic large-volume bleeds with hematemesis and melena. The patient with peptic ulcer disease may present with hematemesis, melena, or both. If the blood loss into the gastrointestinal tract is >200 mL/day, this will result in an osmotic diarrhea and maroon stools or melena. In large-volume blood loss, the clinical presentation depends on the patient's underlying cardiovascular health and other systemic illnesses. Common symptoms are palpitations, shortness of breath, fatigue, light-headedness, difficulty concentrating, and headache. Signs include orthostatic hypotension, rapid thready pulse, cool, clammy skin, air hunger, and confusion. If volume loss exceeds 50%, heart failure and death will result unless volume expanders are administered. The cause, location, magnitude, and duration of blood loss all play a role in the clinical presentation.

The initial evaluation of the acutely bleeding patient involves a focused history and physical examination with attention to the following: a history of easy bruising or bleeding, a history of prolonged bleeding after prior challenges such as dental extraction procedures, gastrointestinal blood loss, symptoms of liver or renal disease, toxin exposures, a detailed medication list, a family history of inherited bleeding disorders, alcohol use, systemic symptoms of illness, history of autoimmune disorder, and B symptoms (weight loss, fevers, night sweats) to suggest an underlying malignancy. Physical examination findings such as tachycardia, hypotension, or obvious source of bleeding or evidence of coagulopathy (petechiae, purpura, ecchymoses, mucosal bleeding) can also help guide the initial assessment.

Initial laboratory evaluation of the acutely bleeding patient involves a complete blood count, type and screen, activated partial thromboplastin time (aPTT), and prothrombin time (PT). If coagulopathy is suspected, thrombin time (TT), fibrinogen, and review of the peripheral smear for evidence of microangiopathic hemolytic anemia are essential. Figure 62.1 reviews the pathways of coagulation and the factors that are involved in testing PT, aPTT, and TT. Table 62.1 illustrates testing used in the workup of the acutely bleeding and coagulopathic patient. Recall that the hemoglobin and hematocrit will change little immediately after an acute hemorrhage because they are reflective of volume ratios and will only be reflective 24 hours after the incident. Severe hemorrhage can also cause an increase in the granulocyte count to levels of 20,000/mcL or higher, and immature white cells can appear in the circulation because of the demargination of granulocytes from catecholamine release. Likewise, platelet counts can reach 1 million in the days after acute hemorrhage. Therefore, interpretation of laboratory studies depends on the timing of the bleeding episode.

ACUTE THERAPEUTIC INTERVENTIONS

Appropriate use of volume expanders and blood components is important in the management of the acutely bleeding patient. Table 62.2 presents a summary of infusional products.

First: Stabilize the Patient with the ABCs of First Aid

Control bleeding at any obvious bleeding sites. MAST (military antishock trousers) may be applied to provide an autotransfusion of 600 to 1,500 mL and to tamponade lower extremity bleeding.

Second: Establish Intravenous Access

Rapid infusion of blood products can be facilitated more quickly with a peripheral 16- to 18-gage intravenous (IV) catheter rather than a central triple-lumen catheter. If a central venous catheter is desired in the acutely bleeding patient, a large-bore Cordis catheter is preferred and can be placed at compressible sites (internal jugular or femoral) in the coagulopathic patient.

Intrinsic Pathway: aPTT

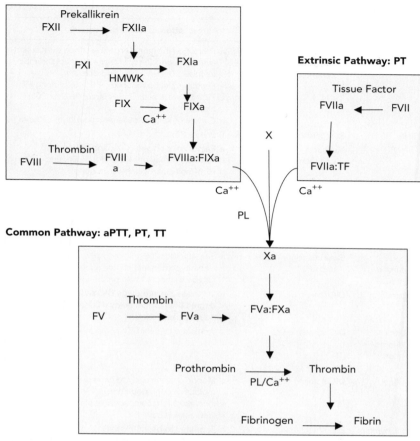

Figure 62.1. Coagulation Cascade: The normal coagulation cascade is split into the intrinsic, extrinsic, and common pathways. Activation of the intrinsic or extrinsic pathways leads to activation of factor (F) X to Xa. Disorders of the intrinsic pathway prolong only the activated partial thromboplastin time (aPTT), disorders of the extrinsic pathway prolong only prothrombin time (PT), and disorders of the common pathway will prolong aPTT, PT, and thrombin time (TT). (HMWK, high-molecular-weight kininogen; PL, phospholipids; Ca⁺⁺, calcium)

Third: Aggressive Fluid and Volume Expansion

Crystalloid and colloid solutions are readily available, but blood products will take time. Saline and lactated ringers can be used as volume expanders if used in sufficient quantities. Three to 4 liters must be infused to expand intravascular volume 1 liter. As a general rule, if >6 liters of crystalloid are required in the first 1 to 2 hours, it is unlikely the patient can be maintained without the infusion of colloid and red blood cells (RBCs) to prevent cardiovascular collapse. Elderly patients and patients with multiple medical comorbidities require more judicious fluid administration and transfusion of RBCs sooner. Colloid solutions can provide 1:1 volume expansion, and are preferable when large volumes must be replaced prior to the availability of

TABLE 62.1	Summary of Commonly used Laboratory Tests in Coagulopathy	

Test	Use	Interpretation of abnormal result
PT	Measure of extrinsic (tissue factor) and common pathways	■ Prolonged in vitamin K deficiency or antagonism (warfarin), deficiency of factor V, direct thrombin inhibitors or fibrinogen disorders ■ Factors must be reduced >50% to prolong PT ■ PT >2× normal indicates factor levels <20% normal ■ Can be prolonged by large amounts of heparin
INR	Standardizes PT	Same as PT
aPTT	Measures intrinsic and common pathways	■ Factor deficiencies IX, XI, and VIII ■ Total deficiency of FXII, prekallikrein, and high-molecular-weight kininogen ■ Deficiencies in common pathway factors ■ Acquired inhibitors or fibrinogen abnormality ■ Sensitive to heparin and lupus anticoagulant
TT	Evaluate last step in common pathway: fibrinogen to fibrin	■ Prolonged in hypo- and dysfibrinogenemia, DIC, and liver disease, monoclonal gammopathies, direct thrombin inhibitors, and heparin
50:50 Mixing study	Evaluate abnormal PT and aPTT	■ See Algorithm 62.1 ■ Heparin contamination can affect results but this can be eliminated with protamine
Fibrinogen	DIC screen	■ Decreased in late-stage DIC secondary to fibrin degradation products, dysfibrinogenemia ■ Acute-phase reactant
Fibrin degradation products	DIC screen	■ Increased in early DIC
D-Dimer	DIC screen	■ Monoclonal antibody to cross-linked D regions of degraded fibrin ■ Increased in hypercoaguable states ■ Increased in early DIC
Antithrombin III	DIC screen and hypercoaguable disorders	■ Expected to be <60% in DIC ■ Low in liver disease and inherited hypercoaguable disorders
Bleeding time	Evaluate platelet function (primary hemostasis)	■ Confounded by many variables such as medications, interoperator variability ■ In general, not clinically useful in the ICU

PT, prothrombin time; INR, international normalized ratio; aPTT, activated partial thromboplastin time; TT, thrombin time; DIC, disseminated intravascular coagulation; ICU, intensive care unit.

blood. When massive transfusion is needed (>5 L blood loss), volume expanders will need to be accompanied by RBCs, platelets, and coagulation factors to guarantee hemostasis. In general, four to six units of fresh-frozen plasma (FFP) are needed in the acutely bleeding patient to raise factor levels to the 30% level that is needed for normal hemostasis.

Fourth: Red Blood Cell Transfusion

The decision to transfuse needs to take into consideration the clinical status, including cardiovascular compensation, mentation, age, and complicating illness. Hypovolemic shock can

TABLE 62.2	Blood Products and Transfusion Adjuncts Guide

Product	Content	Use/Caution
Colloid solutions		Volume-for-volume expansion
■ 5% albumin	■ Purified 5% albumin in isotonic saline	■ Expensive and in short supply
■ Purified plasma protein fraction	■ 4% albumin + 1% other globulins in isotonic to hypotonic solution	■ Can cause hyponatremia
■ Hydroxyethyl starch solution (hetastarch)	■ 6% in isotonic saline	■ Can inhibit platelet function, lower factor VII and vWF levels, rapid removal from circulation
Fresh-frozen plasma	200 mL of plasma containing factors XI, IX, VIII, X, V, and VII	■ Each unit will increase factor levels by 5%–7% ■ Allergic response in up to 10%
Packed red blood cells (RBCs)	200 mL of RBCs suspended in 50–75 mL of plasma	■ Increases HgB by 1 g/dL per unit ■ Allergic response possible ■ Blood-borne infection risk
RhoGam	Anti-D antibody	■ Childbearing individuals who are Rh negative and received Rh positive blood ■ 20 mg/mL of transfused blood administered up to 3 days following RBC transfusion
Platelets	Pooled or single donor final volume ~250 mL Minimal content of platelets is 2×10^{11}	■ >5 units RBCs transfused consider platelet transfusion ■ Increment platelets 30,000–50,000/mcL/unit ■ Risk of alloimmunization ■ Risk of bacterial infection
Cryoprecipitate	Concentrated factors VIII and XIII, vWF, and fibrinogen	■ Consumptive coagulopathy and dysfibroginemia ■ 30–40 U/kg = 10 units IV TID to keep fibrinogen >100–200
Humate-P	Factor VIII + vWF concentrates	■ All types of vWD ■ Severe bleed: 40–75 IU/kg IV q day, adjust to vWF: Ag >50% ■ Mild bleed: 20–30 IU/kg one time
Recombinant factor VIII	Recombinant protein half-life = 8–12 hours	■ Hemophilia A ■ Load: 1 U/kg to increment 2% factor activity ■ Repeat infusion q12h at half-loading dose to maintain level >50%
Recombinant factor IX	Recombinant protein half-life = 24 hours	■ Hemophilia B ■ Load: 1 U/kg to increment 1% factor activity ■ Repeat infusion q18h at half-loading dose to maintain level >50%
Recombinant factor VIIa (NovoSeven)	Activated factor VII	■ CNS bleed ■ FVIII or IX inhibitor ■ 90–120 mcg/kg q 2–3 hours until hemostasis achieved

(continued)

TABLE 62.2	Blood Products and Transfusion Adjuncts Guide *(Continued)*	

Product	Content	Use/Caution
Epsilon-aminocaproic acid (Amicar)	Inhibits plasminogen activation to plasmin	■ Load 100–150 mg/kg IV then 10–15 mg/kg/hr ■ PO swish used for mucosal bleeds
DDAVP	Synthetic analog of antidiuretic hormone; stimulates release of vWF	■ Uremic patients and vWD (except 2B) ■ Increases factor VIII and vWF 3- to 5-fold ■ IV or SC 0.3 mcg/kg or intranasal 300 mcg/kg
Oxymetazoline (Afrin)	Alpha adrenergic agonist	■ Local vasoconstriction for epistaxis
Drotrecogin alfa	Activated protein C	■ Severe sepsis and APACHE II score ≥25 or two or more organ failures
Erythropoietin	Recombinant erythropoietin	■ No proven role in the ICU setting ■ 100–150 IU/kg twice weekly will produce 1.5–2 units RBCs in 3 wk
Iron	IV or PO formulation Sulfated or gluconated	■ Normal adult males will exhaust their iron stores when more than 1,000 mL of RBCs are lost, whereas the middle-aged woman may exhaust her stores with as little as 200–300 mL

vWF, von Willebrand factor; HgB, hemoglobin; vWD, von Willebrand disease; IV, intravenous; PO, orally; DDAVP, desmopressin; SC, subcutaneously; APACHE, Acute Physiology and Chronic Health Evaluation; ICU, intensive care unit.

result in a metabolic acidosis, which can be made worse by transfusion of RBC products more than 14 days old. If transfusion can be delayed 30 minutes or more, the ABO type should be determined and the patient's plasma screened for anti-red blood cell antibodies. Type-specific blood reduces risk of transfusion reaction. Type O (Rh negative) RBCs can be given in an emergent situation without risk of transfusion reaction, but supply is limited. Time may not allow for Rh-specific blood. In a patient past childbearing age, Rh positive RBCs into an Rh negative recipient is of little consequence. There is a 20% chance of sensitizing a patient, and this is most relevant in a patient of childbearing age in whom these antibodies may cross the placenta. Anti-D antibody (RhoGam) at 20 mg/mL of transfused blood administered up to 3 days following RBC transfusion eliminates this risk. Each unit of RBCs should increase the hemoglobin level by 1 g/dL (hematocrit by 3% to 4%) and provide 250 mg of iron.

Fifth: Correct Coagulopathy

Life-threatening bleeds in critically ill patients require prompt correction of coagulopathy, regardless of the underlying cause. Thrombocytopenia or platelet function defects are treated with platelet transfusion. Single-factor deficiency can be reversed by FFP or purified factor. Vitamin K and FFP can be used to correct coagulopathies resulting from multiple-factor deficiencies from warfarin or other causes. Long-term management can be considered when the patient is stabilized. Several questions should be considered. First, is there a problem with the patient's platelets? Second, does the patient have a single-factor deficiency or inherited coagulopathy? Third, does the patient have deficiency of vitamin K-dependent factors (II, VII, IX, X)? Fourth, does the patient have a circulating anticoagulant? Finally, does the patient have a consumptive coagulopathy? Algorithms 62.1 and 62.2 offer guidance into the evaluation and treatment of the coagulopathic patient.

ACQUIRED COAGULATION DISORDERS

Vitamin K Deficiency

Low vitamin K levels are common in ICU patients, with one series reporting a 43% incidence. Vitamin K is an essential cofactor for the carboxylation of coagulation factors II, VII, IX, and X, and anticoagulant proteins C and S. Without vitamin K, these proteins are unable to bind calcium ions and phospholipids, thus making them inactive. This manifests mainly in a prolonged PT/INR (which corrects with mixing) because of the short half-life of factor VII, but will eventually lead to elevation in the aPTT as well. The incidence of major bleeding resulting solely from vitamin K deficiency is rare. Nonetheless, vitamin K deficiency should be anticipated in the critically ill patient, and supplements provided to patients who are critically ill, malnourished, or receiving broad-spectrum antibiotics.

Vitamin K can be supplemented by mouth, intravenously, or subcutaneously. The oral form has excellent bioavailability and is the preferred route. Subcutaneous injection in critically ill patients may not be reliable when patients are edematous or on vasopressors. IV vitamin K carries the risk of anaphylactic reaction and is to be avoided if possible. However, in patients with malabsorption, IV may be the only feasible route of administration. If given IV, the infusion is given slowly by IV piggyback. One to 2 mg of vitamin K should be enough to correct minor coagulopathies (INR <5).

Correction of vitamin K-deficient coagulopathy should occur in 12 to 24 hours after dosing. If this does not occur, one should look for other causes of the coagulopathy or consider a different route of administration of vitamin K.

Liver Disease

Bleeding in the patient with liver disease is often multifactorial. The liver is responsible for the synthesis of all coagulation factors with the exception of vWF and factor VIII (FVIII). Liver dysfunction decreases factor synthesis and clearance of activated clotting factors, as well as results in abnormal fibrinogen and prothrombin. In the acutely ill patient with multisystem organ dysfunction from systemic inflammatory response syndrome, sepsis, DIC, or pre-existing cirrhosis, a coagulopathy is often present, reflected in an elevated PT, aPTT, and TT. This prolongation will correct with a 50:50 mixing assay. Patients with cirrhosis are at risk for portal hypertension, which results in esophageal varices and hemorrhoids, which are at risk of spontaneous rupture. Cirrhosis and portal hypertension also results in splenomegaly, which can cause sequestration of platelets and thrombocytopenia. Platelet function can also be affected by high levels of circulating fibrin degradation products. Coagulopathy in the cirrhotic patient is supportively managed. In general, FFP and platelets are reserved for the acutely bleeding patient. Vitamin K is usually ineffective in correcting the coagulopathy because of underlying synthetic dysfunction.

Goals of transfusion in the acutely bleeding patient are to keep platelets >100,000/mcL, fibrinogen >100 to 200 mg/dL, and intermittent transfusions of FFP to replace FVII (two units will increase factors by 5% to 10%). Prolonged PT and aPTT will persist and aggressive attempts to correct these will result in volume overload. Instead, focus on replacing platelets and fibrinogen (with intermittent administration of FFP) should be the goals of therapy. Antifibrinolytic therapy with epsilon-aminocaproic acid (Amicar) may be beneficial as well.

Renal Failure

Uremia causes platelet dysfunction and this correlates with the degree of uremia. Guanidinosuccinic acid is not cleared and acts as an inhibitor of platelet function by inducing endothelial nitric oxide release. Common sites of bleeding include sites of central venous lines, epistaxis, and mucosal bleeds. This condition is corrected by hemodialysis. Platelet function can be enhanced transiently by using desmopressin (DDAVP) and conjugated estrogens (0.6 mg/kg IV every day for 5 days), which may improve platelet function for up to 2 weeks.

ALGORITHM 62.1 Mixing Analysis of Prolonged Prothrombin Time (PT) and Activated Partial Thromboplastin Time (aPTT)

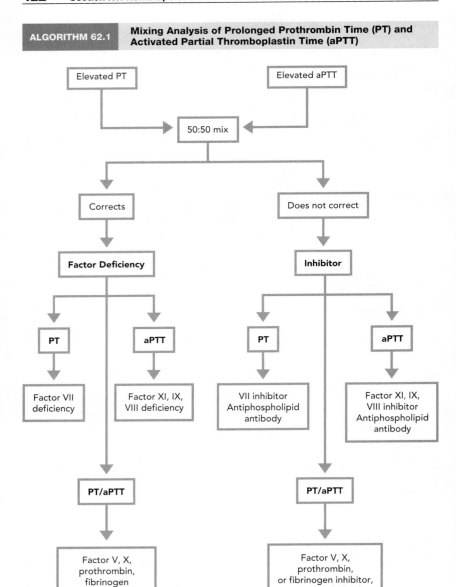

Patient's serum is mixed with equal amount of normal serum, and PT or aPTT is analyzed prior to mix and at 30- and 60-minute intervals. Correction of the time to normal or near normal indicates a factor deficiency, whereas no correction implies a factor inhibitor. Adding excess phospholipid can confirm antiphospholipid antibody, and adding protamine can confirm heparin contamination.

ALGORITHM 62.2   **Management of the Acutely Bleeding Patient**

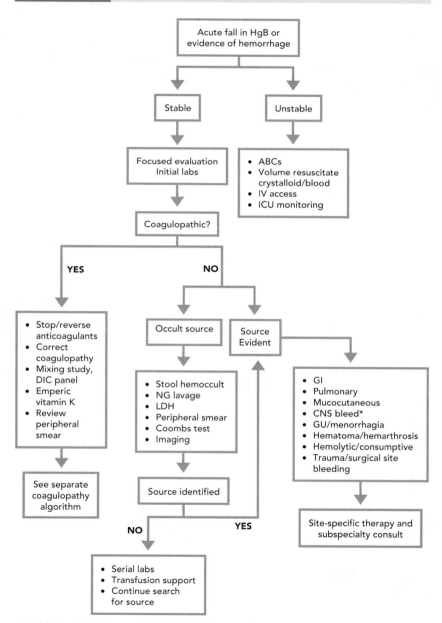

*CNS bleed unlikely to cause significant fall in hemoglobin.

HgB, hemoglobin; IV, intravenous; ICU, intensive care unit; DIC, disseminated intravascular coagulation; NG, nasogastric; LDH, lactate dehydrogenase; GI, gastrointestinal; GU, genitourinary.

Disseminated Intravascular Coagulation

DIC is a thrombohemorrhagic disorder that often occurs in critically ill patients and is always secondary to an underlying disorder. DIC is an independent predictor of mortality in patients with sepsis and severe trauma. The early recognition of DIC in critically ill patients impacts survival. DIC results in procoagulant activation, fibrinolytic activation, inhibitor consumption, and end-organ damage. The widespread activation of coagulation leads to vascular fibrin deposition. This ongoing activation combined with impaired synthesis and increased degradation causes depletion of coagulation factors, protease inhibitors, and platelets.

DIC presents in a spectrum from changes in routine coagulation tests or a small decrease in platelets, to widespread microvascular thrombosis and profuse bleeding. Patients may present with thromboembolic disease or microvascular thrombosis resulting in multiorgan dysfunction or severe bleeding. Often, simultaneous thrombosis and hemorrhage are present. Major bleeding occurs in only a minority of patients with DIC, and organ failure is the most common manifestation.

A screening DIC laboratory evaluation should include fibrin degradation products (FDPs), D-dimer, and antithrombin (AT). The diagnosis is confirmed by thrombocytopenia, prolonged PT/PTT, increased D-dimer, low fibrinogen, increased FDP, and low AT in combination with evidence of end-organ damage. FDP and D-dimer will detect the early procoagulant stage of DIC. AT is used to gage the severity of DIC and prognosis. A scoring system proposed for DIC is 93% sensitive and 98% specific for DIC when 5 or more points are scored.

The foundation of DIC treatment is to reverse the underlying disorder with specific and vigorous measures. Supportive measures are often necessary while treatment of the underlying disorder is taking effect. No therapy directed at DIC has been shown to change the severity of DIC or survival, except perhaps activated protein C in patients with sepsis. Plasma and platelet replacement therapy is indicated in the bleeding patient or patients requiring an invasive procedure. In addition, platelets should be maintained >10,000/mcL to decrease the risk of spontaneous bleeding. Goals of therapy in the bleeding patient should be to keep platelets >50,000/mcL (>100,000/mcL if a major procedure required or CNS bleed is present), fibrinogen >100 mg/dL, and to normalize PT/PTT.

Finally, there has been no proven benefit of anticoagulant therapy in DIC, but this can be considered in patients who present predominately with thrombosis. In addition, AT is consumed in DIC, and several randomized trials have evaluated the role of AT concentrate in DIC, but none have shown survival benefit.

MISCELLANEOUS ACQUIRED DISORDERS

Acquired inhibitors of coagulation factors may arise *de novo* or in patients exposed to recombinant factor, and are most commonly directed against FVIII. Treatment with high-dose factor can often overcome the inhibitor, or activated factor VIIa may also be considered. Disorders of fibrinogen are usually acquired and occur commonly in liver disease. Fibrinogen can be replaced with cryoprecipitate.

Chemotherapy patients are at increased risk for bleeding and from chemotherapy-induced cytopenias. Furthermore, chemotherapy can cause mucositis, which predisposes to mucosal bleeding. Topical epsilon-aminocaproic acid is a good adjunct to platelet transfusion to help promote hemostasis. These patients are also at risk for epistaxis, and oxymetazoline nasal spray can be used to provide local control. Menorrhagia can be a problem; it often responds to medroxyprogesterone, 10 mg per day, which can be increased to 20 mg per day. If bleeding persists, conjugated estrogen can be added initially at a low dose of 0.625 three to four times a day and titrated to effect to bridge the patient through her period of thrombocytopenia.

SELECTED INHERITED BLEEDING DISORDERS

Hemophilia A

Hemophilia A is an X-linked coagulation disorder caused by FVIII deficiency, which leads to impaired intrinsic pathway coagulation. Primary hemostasis is preserved in these patients but bleeding episodes may occur hours to days after trauma or surgery. The severity of the disease depends on the level of FVIII (6% to 30% mild, 2% to 5% moderate, <1% severe). Hemorrhage often occurs into deep structures such as joint spaces or muscles. Treatment depends on the severity of hemophilia and the extent of hemorrhage. DDAVP can be used in mild or moderate disease with minor bleeding. DDAVP increases FVIII levels by three to five times. Typical dosing is 0.3 mcg/kg IV or subcutaneously and will increase FVIII level for 5 to 8 hours. Patients with severe hemophilia and any bleeding require the replacement of FVIII.

FVIII concentrates come in two forms, purified from pooled plasma or recombinant form. Recombinant form eliminates the risk of blood-borne infections. FVIII is dosed in units, each unit per kilogram of actual body weight will increase the plasma level by 2%. FVIII level should be checked prior to transfusion to guide therapy. The goal factor level varies with the extent of bleeding: minor bleeding, 25% to 30%; moderate-to-severe bleeding, 50%; surgical procedures or life-threatening bleeding, 75% to 100%. FVIII has an 8-hour half-life. Levels should be monitored and factor redosed every 8 to 12 hours at half the initial dose. Treatment continues until bleeding is stabilized, and in postoperative patients for 10 to 14 days. It is not uncommon for hemophiliacs to develop inhibitors that will prevent FVIII concentrates from working. In these cases, bleeding patients are treated with recombinant factor VIIa at 90 mcg/kg every 2 hours until hemostasis is achieved. A trained hematologist should be consulted to assist with the management of these patients.

Hemophilia B

Hemophilia B is an X-linked coagulation disorder involving deficiency of factor IX. It is clinically indistinguishable from hemophilia A. Treatment involves factor IX concentrates or recombinant factor IX. Each unit per kilogram of actual body weight causes a 1% increment in factor level. Factor IX half-life is 24 hours; therefore, dosing is every 18 to 24 hours at half the initial loading dose. Goal factor levels are as for hemophilia A patients and should be monitored likewise. Inhibitors to factor IX may develop, and the treatment of the bleeding patient, as in hemophilia A, is with recombinant factor VIIa.

von Willebrand Disease

von Willebrand factor is a glycoprotein that is essential to platelet function, and therefore primary hemostasis, and also stabilizes and transports FVIII in the circulation. Von Willebrand disease results from a quantitative or qualitative defect in vWF resulting in mucocutaneous bleeding, which can be life-threatening in the severe form of the disease. There are three types of von Willebrand disease: type 1, partial quantitative; type 2, qualitative; and type 3, entire loss of vWF. All three types can be treated with cryoprecipitate, or preferably Humate-P, to treat bleeding episodes. Type 1 and certain type 2 patients may also respond to DDAVP.

Suggested Reading

Bernard GR, Vincent JL, Laterre PF, et al. Efficacy and safety of recombinant human activated protein C for severe sepsis. *N Engl J Med.* 2001;344:699–709.
   Phase III trial examining activated protein C in 1690 septic patients with DIC. The group receiving human activated protein C at 24 ug/kg/hr × 96 hrs had decreased mortality 24.7% vs 30.8% for placebo.
Chakraverty R, Davidson S, Peggs DK, et al. The incidence and cause of coagulopathies in an intensive care population. *Br J Haematol.* 1996;93:460–463.
   A retrospective review of 235 patients admitted to an adult ICU in England with attention to common etiologies of coagulopathy.
Drews, RE Critical issues in hematology: anemia, thrombocytopenia, coagulopathy, and blood product transfusions in critically ill patients. *Clin Chest Med.* 2003;24:607–622.
   Evidence based review of anemia, thrombocytopenia, and coagulopathies in ICU patients, with emphasis on diagnosis and transfusional therapies.
Hillman RS, Ault KA, Rinder HM. Blood loss anemia. In: *Hematology in Clinical Practice.* 4th ed. New York: McGraw-Hill Professional, 2002:122–134.
   Evidence based review of hemostatic defects observed in patients with end stage liver disease and discusses their management.

Kujovich J. Hemostatic defects in end stage liver disease. *Crit Care Clin.* 2005;21:563–587.

Levi M. Disseminated intravascular coagulation: what's new? *Crit Care Clin.* 2005;21: 449–467.

Evidence based review of DIC from pathophysiology to diagnosis and treatment.

Noris M, Remuzzi G. Uremic bleeding: closing the circle after 30 years of controversies. *Blood.* 1999;94:2569–2574.

Discusses the etiology of platelet dysfunction associated with uremia and reviews proposed mechanisms, implicating guanidosuccinate as the key mediator.

Taylor, FBJ, Toh CH, Hoots WK, et al. Towards definition, clinical and laboratory criteria, and a scoring system for disseminated intravascular coagulation. *Thromb Haemost.* 2001;86:1327–1330.

Validates a scoring system used in diagnosis of DIC.

TRANSFUSION PRACTICES

James C. Mosley, III and Morey A. Blinder

63

Anemia is a common problem in the intensive care unit (ICU) setting. In the critically ill patient, oxygen delivery and oxygen consumption may be impaired by factors such as decreased cardiac output, decreased red cell mass, decreased circulating blood volume from red blood cell (RBC) loss, and altered acid-base status. Causes of anemia in this setting are varied and include overt blood loss from bleeding or hemolysis, a functional decrease in usable iron, and decreased erythropoietin production.

Anemia is traditionally treated with infusions of RBCs in order to increase oxygen-carrying capacity and tissue delivery of oxygen. Various studies have estimated that more than 40% of all ICU patients receive blood transfusions and that more than 66% of these transfusions were not for replacement.

There is great variability in transfusion parameters and guidelines from center-to-center, and yet the optimal management of anemia in the ICU setting is not well defined. One approach compares a "transfusion-trigger" for a hemoglobin level <10 g/dL, a more "restrictive" pattern of transfusions for a hemoglobin value of <7 g/dL only. Although results vary, most studies have noted no increased mortality from the "restrictive" trans-fusion threshold of 7 g/dL, suggesting that hemoglobin levels of 7 to 9 g/dL are well tol-erated in the critically ill patient. Furthermore, a trend toward increasing morbidity and mortality in groups with the more aggressive transfusion threshold for hemoglobin levels <10 g/dL has been noted. However, under circumstances of acute coronary syndromes, a clear trend toward increased survival has been demonstrated with transfusions for hemo-globin levels <10g/dL. Nevertheless, transfusion practices must take into account sys-temic organ dysfunction that may affect oxygen delivery, anticipated blood losses, and overall patient morbidity, resulting in patient and situation-specific use of RBCs. It is cur-rently recommended that, except in the circumstance of an acute coronary syndrome, patients be transfused for hemoglobin values of <7 g/dL, with a goal of maintaining hemoglobin levels of 7 to 9 g/dL.

DOSING AND ADMINISTRATION

Each unit of packed RBCs is approximately 300 mL and is generally given during 2 to 3 hours. One unit of packed RBCs is expected to increase hemoglobin by approximately 1 g/dL and raise the hematocrit by approximately 3% in a healthy individual without ongoing blood loss or destruction. Prior to transfusions, the patients' blood should be tested for ABO status, but type O negative RBCs can be given in emergency situations.

TYPES OF RBC PRODUCTS

Table 63.1 presents some of the various blood products and their indications. Included in this section is further discussion of common products.

Whole Blood

Whole blood is currently used in autologous donation situations (prior to surgery, and so forth). Whole blood contains all normal constituents of human plasma, including RBCs, platelets, and plasma proteins.

TABLE 63.1	Blood Products	
Product	**Indications**	**Comments**
Packed red blood cells	■ Increase oxygen-carrying capacity in patients with anemia ■ Can be used to increase blood volume in acute loss	■ Transfusions to keep Hgb 7–9 g/dL in ICU setting ■ Data support higher levels in ACS
Platelets	■ Thrombocytopenia with high risk of bleeding ■ *NOT* indicated in presence of increased destruction without bleeding	■ Prophylactic transfusion only if platelet count <10,000/mcL. ■ Thresholds for procedures vary by institution
Fresh-frozen plasma	■ Bleeding in setting of factor deficiency or coagulopathy ■ Warfarin reversal ■ Severe DIC	■ Dosage ranges from 5–15 mL/kg, but generally start with 2 units and recheck PT/PTT
Cryoprecipitate	■ Fibrinogen deficiency	■ Contains fibrinogen as well as vWF, Factor VIII, and fibronectin
Humate-P	■ vWD types 2B, 2N, 3	■ A specific vWF-containing, Factor VIII concentrate
Factor VIII and IX concentrates	■ Hemophilia A and B treatment, respectively	■ Virally inactivated ■ Recombinant technologies have eliminated infectious risks
Recombinant Factor VIIa	■ Bleeding complications in acquired hemophilia A and B ■ Factor VII deficiency	■ Recombinant ■ Used for surgery and acute bleeding in hemophilia

Hgb, hemoglobin; ICU, intensive care unit; ACS, acute coronary syndrome; DIC, disseminated intravascular coagulation; PT/PTT, prothrombin time/partial thromboplastin time; vWF, von Willebrand factor; vWD, von Willebrand disease.

Packed RBCs

Packed RBCs contain approximately 200 mL of RBCs resuspended in a preservative solution. Each bag has a hematocrit of approximately 55% to 60% and approximately 200 mg of iron.

Gamma-irradiated

External-beam radiation is applied to the unit of blood to produce gamma-irradiated blood. This allows for destruction of donor T lymphocytes for prevention of graft-versus-host disease in stem cell transplant patients and severely immunocompromised patients.

Cytomegalovirus Antibody-negative

Cytomegalovirus (CMV) antibody-negative blood is used in patients who are known to be CMV-negative and at high risk for complications if infected with CMV (e.g., transplant patients and pregnant patients). Leukocyte reduction is also a relatively effective method for reducing risk of CMV infection. Leukocyte reduction is performed most often at the time of product collection.

Washed RBCs

The donor cells are processed with normal saline to remove as much of the donor serum as possible. This is most commonly used in patients who are immunoglobulin

A (IgA)-deficient and at a high risk for anaphylaxis during transfusions, as well as in paroxysmal nocturnal hemoglobinuria patients to deplete complement.

RISK OF TRANSFUSIONS

Transfusion of blood products carries risks. These risks can be divided based on whether the complication is short term (related to each unit that is transfused) or long term (proportional to the total number of units that a patient receives over his or her lifetime).

Short-term Transfusion Risks

Acute Hemolytic Reactions
The most serious and immediately life-threatening complication of transfusions is an acute hemolytic reaction. This is due to antibodies, usually immunoglobulin M, in the recipient's serum against major antigens present on the donor RBCs, and occurs with an estimated frequency of 1 in 250,000 to 1 in 1,000,000. This is initially manifested acutely as fever, dyspnea, tachycardia, back pain, hypotension, chills, and chest pain, within the first several minutes of the transfusion. If an acute hemolytic reaction is suspected, *the infusion should be stopped immediately,* and the blood bank notified. Algorithm 63.1 outlines management strategies for acute hemolytic reactions.

Delayed Hemolytic Reactions
Delayed hemolytic reactions usually occur more than 24 to 48 hours, and up to 7 to 10 days, after a transfusion. Delayed reactions result from antibodies in the recipient's serum that are directed toward minor antigens on the donor's RBCs, which are produced by an anamnestic response. This usually manifests as an asymptomatic but sudden decrease in hemoglobin concentration, with laboratory evidence of hemolysis, including a positive direct Coombs test and increased indirect bilirubin concentration.

Nonhemolytic Febrile Reactions
Nonhemolytic febrile reactions occur in approximately 1% of transfusions and are the result of antibodies in the recipient's serum against white blood cells in the donor's product. This manifests acutely as an increase in body temperature and is more common in patients who have been previously alloimmunized by numerous transfusions. This reaction is treated with antipyretic medications.

Allergic Reactions
Allergic reactions occur because of transfused allergens in the donor's product, with symptoms such as urticaria and bronchospasm; they occur in approximately 1 in 100 transfusions. This condition is treated with antihistamine medications. However, a potentially severe form may be encountered in IgA-deficient individuals who can have anaphylactic reactions to serum from non–IgA-deficient donors. This is best prevented with washed-RBCs, but can be treated with high-dose corticosteroids, airway protection, and antihistamines.

Transfusion-related Acute Lung Injury
Transfusion-related acute lung injury (TRALI) occurs by a poorly understood mechanism, but an immune antibody-mediated process has been established in a majority of cases. A nonimmune mechanism has been postulated as well. Data from animal models and recent clinical studies suggest that both processes occur and that TRALI may be the end result of diffuse neutrophil activation and capillary leak by these mechanisms. TRALI presents with diffuse capillary damage in the pulmonary vasculature with rapid-onset dyspnea, hypoxia, fever, and bilateral pulmonary infiltrates resembling acute respiratory distress syndrome, in the absence of volume overload or heart failure. Treatment is supportive as most cases are self-limiting, but patients may require mechanical ventilation.

Bacterial Infection
Blood units can be contaminated with bacterial agents, including cold-growing organisms such as *Yersinia enterocolitica*, as well as various Gram-negative organisms. Incidence of

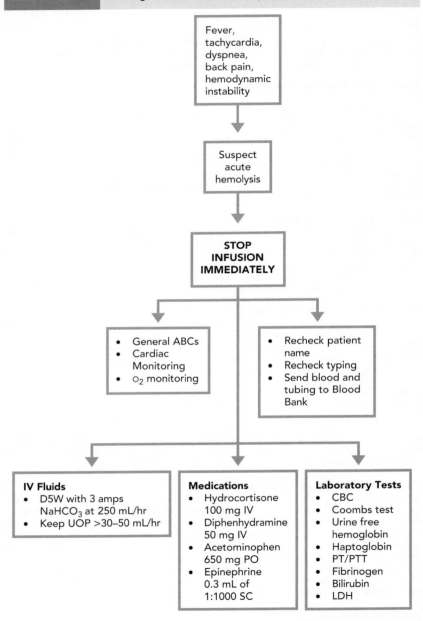

ALGORITHM 63.1 **Management of Acute Hemolytic Reaction**

Fever,
tachycardia,
dyspnea,
back pain,
hemodynamic
instability

↓

Suspect
acute
hemolysis

↓

**STOP
INFUSION
IMMEDIATELY**

- General ABCs
- Cardiac
  Monitoring
- O₂ monitoring

- Recheck patient
  name
- Recheck typing
- Send blood and
  tubing to Blood
  Bank

IV Fluids
- D5W with 3 amps
  NaHCO₃ at 250 mL/hr
- Keep UOP >30–50 mL/hr

Medications
- Hydrocortisone
  100 mg IV
- Diphenhydramine
  50 mg IV
- Acetaminophen
  650 mg PO
- Epinephrine
  0.3 mL of
  1:1000 SC

Laboratory Tests
- CBC
- Coombs test
- Urine free
  hemoglobin
- Haptoglobin
- PT/PTT
- Fibrinogen
- Bilirubin
- LDH

IV, intravenous; D5W, 5% dextrose in water; UOP, PO, orally; SC, subcutaneously; CBC, complete blood
count; PT/PTT, prothrombin time/partial thromboplastin time; LDH, lactate dehydrogenase.

TABLE 63.2	Transfusion-Associated Infections		
Virus	Risk factor (per million)	Estimated frequency (per unit)	No. of deaths (per million units)
Hepatitis A	1	1/1,000,000	0
Hepatitis B	7–32	1/30,000–1/250,000	0–0.14
Hepatitis C	4–36	1/30,000–1/150,000	0.5–17
HIV	0.4–5	1/200,000–1/2,000,000	0.5–5
HTLV I and II	0.5–4	1/250,000–1/2,000,000	0
Parvovirus B19	100	1/10,000	0

HIV, human immunodeficiency virus; HTLV, human T-lymphotropic virus.
Adapted from Goodnough LT, Brecher ME, Kanter MH, et al. Transfusion medicine: first of two parts, Blood transfusion. *N Engl J Med.* 1999;6:438–441, with permission.

bacterial infection has dramatically decreased since the introduction of disposable plastic blood bags.

Long-term Transfusion Risks

Viral Infections
Infectious complications of blood transfusions are located in Table 63.2. All blood products are currently screened for hepatitis B, hepatitis C, human immunodeficiency virus 1 and 2, and human T-lymphotropic virus I and II. Other infectious risks include viruses that are not screened for, such as CMV and parvovirus B19, and the prion transmitted Creutzfeldt-Jacob disease.

Iron Overload
Although not typically an issue in the ICU setting, secondary iron overload syndromes occur in proportion to the number of blood products a patient receives. Patients at highest risk include those with multiple transfusions over long periods of time (e.g., sickle-cell disease, thalassemias, myelodysplastic syndromes). Each milliliter of packed RBCs contains approximately 1 mg of iron. Patients who are repeatedly transfused in the absence of blood loss are at risk of overwhelming the body's ability to use iron with resultant deposition into tissues such as the myocardium, bone marrow, and liver.

Suggested Reading
Drews RE. Critical issues in hematology: anemia, thrombocytopenia, coagulopathy, and blood product transfusions in critically ill patients. *Clin Chest Med.* 2003;24:607–622.
   A systematic review of diagnosis, evaluation and treatment of blood and bleeding disorders commonly encountered in the critical care setting.
Goodnough LT, Brecher ME, Kanter MH, et al. Transfusion medicine: first of two parts. Blood transfusion. *N Engl J Med.* 1999;6:438–441.
   A review article on principles of basic transfusion medicine, including complications and indications for transfusion.
Herbert PC, Wells G, Blajchman MA, et al. A Multicenter, randomized, controlled clinical trial of transfusion requirement in critical care. *N Engl J Med.* 1999;6:409–417.
   A randomized trial of 838 ICU patients to receive transfusions for hemoglobin levels of less than 10 g/dL, or 7 g/dL. Overall 30-day mortality was similar in the two groups, but there was significantly less in-hospital mortality in patients transfused for hemoglobin levels less than 7 g/dL (22.2% versus 28.1%, p = 0.05), demonstrating that a "restrictive" transfusion strategy is well-tolerated and potentially superior to liberal transfusion strategies.

McLellan SA, McClelland DB, Walsh TS. Anaemia and red blood cell transfusion in the critically ill patient. *Blood Rev.* 2003;17:195–208.
A review of anemia and transfusion strategies in critically ill patients.
Pajoumand M, Erstad BL, Camamo JM. Use of Epoetin Alfa in critically ill patients. *Ann Pharmacother.* 2004;38:641–648.
A review of the use of Epoetin Alfa for reduction of red blood cell transfusions in critically ill patients with anemia.
Triulzi, DJ. Transfusion-related acute lung injury: an update. *Hematology Am Soc Hematol Educ Program.* 2006;497–501.
Review of current research and proposed mechanisms of TRALI.
Uy GL. Transfusion medicine. In: Lin TL, ed. *Hematology and Oncology Subspecialty Consult.* Baltimore: Lippincott, Williams & Wilkins; 2004:73–79.
Book chapter focusing on basic transfusion medicine and practical information about blood products and proper use.
Vincent JL, Baron JF, Reinhart K, et al. Anemia and blood transfusion in critically ill patients. *JAMA.* 2002;12:1499–1507.
A prospective observational study of patients in European ICUs evaluating the prevalence of anemia and transfusion use in this setting.

HYPERCOAGULABLE STATES

James C. Mosley, III

64

Hypercoagulable states are a heterogeneous group of inherited or acquired disorders that predispose individuals to the inappropriate formation of a clot in the venous or arterial circulation. The inappropriate formations of thrombi occur in the presence of Virchow's triad of hypercoagulability, stasis, and endothelial damage. Embolization of these clots can occur, resulting in pulmonary embolism (PE) in the case of venous embolic disease, or emboli to vital organs in the setting of arterial thrombosis.

Various manifestations of hypercoagulability are demonstrated in the intensive care unit (ICU) setting. Patients are at an increased risk of venous thromboembolic disease because of their prolonged immobilization, the numerous procedures that they are exposed to, and their underlying disease states. Patients in the ICU setting may have only transient risk factors for thromboembolic disease, or may also have underlying conditions that increase their risk. Listed in Table 64.1 are common causes of hypercoagulability.

DEEP VENOUS THROMBOSIS AND PULMONARY EMBOLISM

Deep venous thrombosis (DVT) and PE are very common in the ICU and are likely underdiagnosed. Some observational studies have demonstrated a 20% to 40% incidence of DVT in the ICU setting.

Diagnosis of DVT and PE in the ICU can be difficult (Algs. 64.1 and 64.2). Various studies have demonstrated that 10% to 100% of DVTs diagnosed by ultrasound in this setting were not found on physical examination. Furthermore, patients in the ICU setting have a number of factors confounding the diagnosis, including their numerous comorbid conditions, inability to communicate symptoms, numerous procedures and medications, and inability to undergo various diagnostic tests. Table 64.2 lists the diagnostic modalities for DVT and PE.

Treatment of DVT and PE should commence when clinically suspected. As previously mentioned, diagnosis can be difficult in the ICU setting, but delay in treatment can lead to increased morbidity and mortality. Clinically suspected DVT or PE should be treated with weight-based unfractionated heparin or with low-molecular-weight heparin. Dosing guidelines for unfractionated heparin and alternatives are listed in Tables 64.3 and 64.4.

DVT prophylaxis decreases the incidence of PE and venous thromboembolism in the ICU patient. In general, all patients in the ICU should receive DVT prophylaxis if no contraindication exists.

ARTERIAL THROMBOEMBOLISM

Acute arterial thrombosis can be secondary to embolization of material (e.g., from the atria in atrial fibrillation or from a proximal source secondary to a damaged artery), or an in situ formation of clot. Symptoms are generally related to the territory served by the artery that has thrombosed, and generally is noted as a painful, pale, and cool extremity, or an acute neurologic deficit in the case of a stroke. However, in the ICU setting, these symptoms may be masked by the patient's other comorbidities.

Clues from the physical examination can yield evidence as to the source of the thrombosis. Multiple sites of ischemia are typical of an embolic phenomenon (but can also be seen in the setting of vasculitis), whereas isolated ischemia is more typical of in situ thrombosis. Further evaluation of suspected arterial thrombosis can be performed with compression ultrasound, although computed tomography angiography is often more helpful.

TABLE 64.1	Causes of Hypercoagulability

Acquired causes	Inherited causes
Trauma/surgery	Factor V Leiden mutation
Malignancy	Prothrombin G20210A mutation
Immobilization	Protein C deficiency
Nephrotic syndrome	Protein S deficiency
Obesity	Antithrombin deficiency
Pregnancy	Increased factor VIII activity
Oral contraceptive use	
Congestive heart failure	
Myeloproliferative disorders	
Antiphospholipid antibodies	
Lupus anticoagulant	
Anticardiolipin antibodies	

Treatment of suspected arterial thrombosis should be instituted immediately, as delay in treatment can result irreversible damage due to ischemic tissue. Anticoagulation should be initiated as outlined in Tables 64.3 and 64.4, and surgical consultation should be sought for possible operative management.

HYPERCOAGULABILITY EVALUATION

Patients in the ICU have many transient risk factors for the development of thromboembolic disease. Because of this, most instances of thromboembolism do not warrant workup for an underlying hypercoagulable state. The optimal time for laboratory evaluation of hypercoagulable states is unclear, but is often undertaken approximately 6 weeks to 6 months after the event. Laboratory evaluation in the immediate days to weeks following a

TABLE 64.2	Diagnostic Tests for Deep Venous Thrombosis (DVT) and Pulmonary Embolism (PE) in the Intensive Care Unit Setting

Test	Indication for testing	Key points
Venous duplex ultrasound	Suspected DVT in extremities	■ Good sensitivity and specificity for proximal DVT
Spiral computed tomography	Suspected PE	■ Good sensitivity for large PEs ■ Contrast bolus predisposes to nephrotoxicity
Ventilation-perfusion scanning	Suspected PE	■ Good sensitivity for PEs ■ Difficult to interpret in setting of recent pneumonia or other infiltrative process
Computed tomography angiography/venography	Suspected DVT or PE	■ Not widely available ■ Large bolus of contrast used

Adapted from Cook D, Douketis J, Crowther MA, et al. The diagnosis of deep venous thrombosis and pulmonary embolism in medical-surgical intensive care unit patients. *J Crit Care.* 2005;25:314–319, with permission.

ALGORITHM 64.1   **Algorithm for Diagnosis of Deep Venous Thrombosis (DVT)**

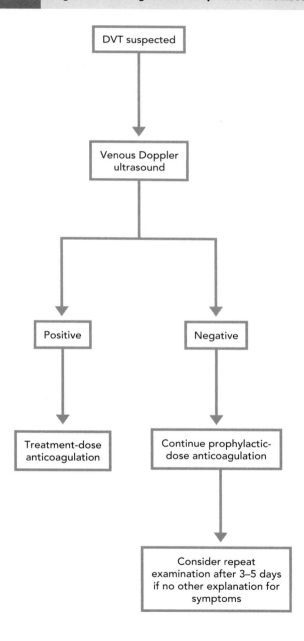

ALGORITHM 64.2 Algorithm for Diagnosis of Pulmonary Embolism (PE)

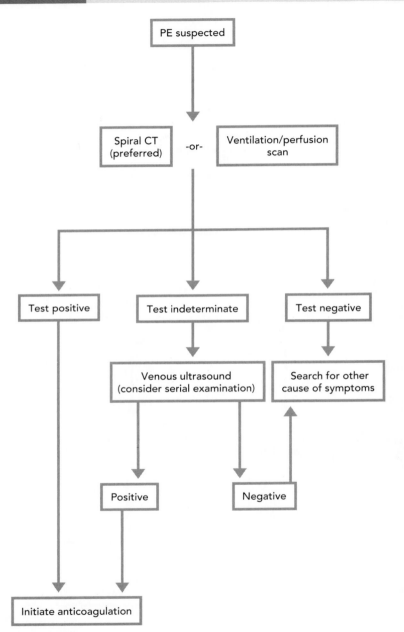

CT, computed tomography.

TABLE 64.3	Weight-Based Unfractionated Heparin Dosing

Initial Dose
Bolus 60–80 U/kg
Infusion 14–18 U/kg/hr

Adjustment: aPTT[a]

<40	2.000 units IV bolus and increase infusion rate by 2 U/kg/hr
40–44	Increase infusion rate by 1 U/kg/hr
45–70	No change
71–80	Decrease infusion by 1 U/kg/hr
81–90	Hold infusion for 30 min, decrease infusion rate by 2 U/kg/hr
>90	Hold infusion for 1 hour, decrease infusion rate by 3 U/kg/hr

IV, intravenous.
[a]aPTT should be drawn 6 hours after any adjustment to dose.

thrombosis can yield false results because of the increase in acute-phase reactants associated with acute clot formation, which can result in false-positive tests for hypercoagulable states. However, in the setting of recurrent thrombosis, cerebral vein or visceral vein thrombosis, and nonembolic arterial thrombosis, further evaluation is warranted. Minimal workup should include evaluation for lupus anticoagulant, anticardiolipin antibody, and fasting plasma homocysteine level. In cases marked by recurrent thrombosis or cerebral or visceral

TABLE 64.4	Alternative Anticoagulants

Drug	Mechanism of action	Use	Prophylaxis dosing	Therapeutic dosing
Enoxaparin	Inactivation of factor Xa	Prophylaxis and treatment of DVT/PE	40 mg SC q24h	1 mg/kg SC q12h OR 1.5 mg/kg SC q24h
Dalteparin	Inactivation of factor Xa	Prophylaxis and treatment of DVT/PE	5,000 U SC q24h	100 U/kg SC q12h OR 200 U/kg SC q24h
Fondaparinux	Inactivation of factor Xa	Prophylaxis and treatment of DVT/PE, HIT	2.5 mg SC q24h	7.5 mg SC q24h OR 10 mg SC q24h if >100 kg
Lepirudin	Direct thrombin inhibitor	HIT	0.1 mg/kg/hr IV	0.4 mg/kg IV bolus, then 0.15 mg/kg/hr IV
Argatroban	Direct thrombin inhibitor	Treatment of thrombosis in HIT	2 mcg/kg/min IV	

DVT, deep venous thrombosis; PE, pulmonary embolism; SQ, subcutaneously; HIT, heparin-induced thrombocytopenia; IV, intravenous.

vein thrombosis, further workup should include a prothrombin G20210A mutation analysis as well as a factor V Leiden mutation analysis. Hematology consultation should be obtained for further evaluation and long-term treatment planning.

CONDITIONS ASSOCIATED WITH DECREASED PLATELETS AND HYPERCOAGULABILITY

There are occasional conditions that present with thrombocytopenia as well as hypercoagulability. Heparin-induced thrombocytopenia is a serious condition manifested by the formation of antibodies to platelets in response to heparin administration. This condition can cause thrombosis in the setting of severe thrombocytopenia, and is discussed in detail in Chapter 61.

Thrombotic thrombocytopenia purpura is another condition associated with hypercoagulability and thrombocytopenia. This serious condition is the result of a deficiency of or inhibitor to the von Willebrand factor cleaving protease, ADAMTS 13. It is manifested by thrombocytopenia, microangiopathic changes on peripheral blood smear (schistocytes), fever, mental status changes, and varying degrees of renal insufficiency. Treatment is emergent and requires immediate hematology consultation and plasma exchange. This condition is discussed further in the Chapter 61.

Disseminated intravascular coagulation can also present with thrombocytopenia and coagulopathy in the setting of hypercoagulability. Underlying conditions such as sepsis, ischemia, acidosis, and multiorgan failure can induce a consumptive coagulopathy, resulting in the formation of diffuse thrombi as well as diffuse hemorrhage.

Suggested Reading

Cook D, Douketis J, Crowther MA, et al. The diagnosis of deep venous thrombosis and pulmonary embolism in medical-surgical intensive care unit patients. *J Crit Care.* 2005; 25:314–319.
Review of current data investigating diagnostic modalities for DVT and PE with focus on patients in the critical care setting.

Geerts WH. Prevention of venous thromboembolism in high-risk patients. In: *American Society of Hematology Education Program Book.* Washington, D.C.: American Society of Hematology; 2006:462–466.
Review of prophylactic modalities for DVT in patients in various clinical circumstances.

Levine JS, Branch DW, Rauch J. The antiphospholipid syndrome. *N Engl J Med.* 2002;10: 752–763.
A review of the pathogenesis, diagnosis, and treatment strategies of the Antiphospholipid Antibody Syndrome.

Nachman RL, Silverstein R. Hypercoagulable states. *Ann Intern Med.* 1993;8:819–827.
A review of the major pathophysiologic mechanisms underlying inherited and secondary hypercoagulable states and review of the frequency, natural history, diagnosis, and management of the disorders.

Peles S, Pillot, G. Thrombotic disease. In: Pillot G, Chantler M, Magiera H, et al, eds. *Hematology and Oncology Subspecialty Consult.* Baltimore: Lippincott, Williams & Wilkins, 2004:25–32.
Edited book chapter describing hypercoagulable disease states, with focus on diagnosis and treatment strategies.

Rosenberg RD, Aird W. Vascular-Bed specific hemostasis and hypercoagulable states. *N Engl J Med.* 1999;20:1555–1564.
A review of the pathophysiologic mechanisms underlying coagulation disorders on a cellular level, describing the interaction of coagulation factors with vascular-bed specific cellular signaling pathways.

Tabatabai, A. Disorders of hemostasis. In: Ahya SN, Flood K, Parajothi S, eds. *Washington Manual of Medical Therapeutics.* 30th ed. Baltimore: Lippincott, Williams & Wilkins, 2001:394–412.
Edited book chapter describing differential diagnosis, diagnostic strategies, and treatment modalities for hypercoagulable states, as well as bleeding disorders.

Pregnancy XVI

PREECLAMPSIA AND ECLAMPSIA
Tracy M. Tomlinson and Yoel Sadovsky   65

Preeclampsia is a hypertensive disorder of pregnancy that is associated with proteinuria. It occurs typically after the 20th gestational week or in the early postpartum period. Preeclampsia complicates up to 10% of all pregnancies and is one of the leading causes of maternal mortality worldwide. Women at risk for preeclampsia are typically those with a history of preeclampsia in a prior pregnancy, primigravidas, women younger than age 20 or older than age 35, and those carrying multifetal gestations. Diverse medical conditions predispose women to preeclampsia. Examples include chronic hypertension, obesity, diabetes, renal disease, connective tissue disease, and thrombophilic disorders. Although the cause of preeclampsia is currently unknown, this disease is associated with the presence of placental trophoblastic tissue and may occur even without a fetus, as seen in women with a hydatidiform mole. Placental factors, such as regulators of angiogenesis, growth factors, cytokines, and regulators of arterial tone are likely released into the maternal circulation and cause systemic endothelial cell dysfunction that may culminate in multisystem disease.

Mild preeclampsia is characterized by hypertension (blood pressure >140/90 mmHg but <170/110 mmHg) and proteinuria (>300 mg/day). Women with mild preeclampsia are usually asymptomatic or may complain of slight increase in peripheral edema and accelerated weight gain. The examination often confirms edema and may reveal hyperreflexia. A blood count may reveal hemoconcentration. Progression to severe preeclampsia is often rapid, and is defined by dysfunction of several target organ systems. These include renal failure, thrombocytopenia, hypofibrinogenemia, and right upper quadrant or epigastric pain with elevated hepatic transaminases. Involvement of the central nervous system presents as symptoms of occipital or frontal headaches, scotomata or blurred vision, and even altered mental status. These symptoms and signs likely reflect severe cerebral vasospasm and often precede the onset of eclampsia. Fetal involvement includes intrauterine growth restriction secondary to placental dysfunction, as well as a risk for placental abruption. These complications, as well as the maternal condition, frequently result in preterm delivery of a premature infant, which largely contributes to the neonatal morbidity and mortality that is attributed to preeclampsia.

TABLE 65.1	End-Stage Complications in Patients with Preeclampsia/Eclampsia

System	Complications
CNS	Seizures, cerebrovascular hemorrhage, temporary cortical blindness
Cardiopulmonary	Critical hypertension, heart failure, cardiopulmonary arrest, pulmonary edema
Renal	Acute renal failure
Hepatic	Subcapsular hematoma, hepatic rupture with hemorrhage
Hematologic	Disseminated intravascular coagulation, hemolysis
Fetal	Fetal demise, placental abruption, intrauterine growth restriction, preterm delivery

Preeclampsia/eclampsia is the third leading cause of maternal mortality, and accounts for nearly 20% of pregnancy-related maternal deaths. Severe, life-threatening complications are listed in Table 65.1. Eclampsia is defined as preeclampsia with generalized tonic-clonic seizures and/or coma. Approximately 50% of all cases of eclampsia are diagnosed during the antepartum period, 20% present with an intrapartum event, and the remaining 30% are diagnosed during the postpartum period. Even though most postpartum seizures occur in the first 48 hours, cases have been reported as late as 3 weeks after delivery. Notably, nearly 15% of women with eclampsia initially present without hypertension and another 15% may lack proteinuria. Furthermore, the severity of hypertension and proteinuria in a preeclamptic patient are poor predictors of progression to eclampsia.

The syndrome of hemolysis, elevated liver enzymes, and low platelets (HELLP syndrome) is a life-threatening variant of severe preeclampsia. Women with HELLP syndrome may present with vague epigastric discomfort or mild nausea and vomiting. Interestingly, HELLP can be found in patients with minimal or absent hypertension and proteinuria. The laboratory findings in HELLP syndrome overlap with other life-threatening complications of pregnancy, such as acute fatty liver of pregnancy and thrombotic thrombocytopenic purpura, which should be considered in the differential diagnosis. The main differential diagnosis of preeclampsia/eclampsia/HELLP syndrome is presented in Table 65.2, and several helpful laboratory tests are presented in Table 65.3.

TABLE 65.2	Key Differential Diagnosis of Severe Preeclampsia/Eclampsia/HELLP

1. CNS
   a. Seizure disorder
   b. Hypertensive encephalopathy
   c. Cerebrovascular
      i. Intraventricular-intracerebral hemorrhage
      ii. Arterial embolism or thrombosis
      iii. Hypoxic ischemic encephalopathy
      iv. Angioma, atrioventricular malformation or aneurism
   d. Reversible posterior leukoencephalopathy syndrome
   e. Tumors
   f. Cerebral vasculitis
2. Thrombotic thrombocytopenic purpura
3. Acute fatty liver of pregnancy
4. Metabolic disease
   a. Hypoglycemia
   b. Hyponatremia

HELLP, syndrome of hemolysis, elevated liver enzymes, and low platelets.
Modified from differential diagnosis figure. Sibai BM. Diagnosis, prevention, and management of eclampsia. *Obstet Gynecol.* 2005;105:402–410, with permission.

TABLE 65.3   **Imitators of Preeclampsia/HELLP: Laboratory Findings**

Laboratory finding	Normal pregnancy	Pre-eclampsia/HELLP	TTP	AFLP
Hematocrit	↓ 4%–7%	↑ with hemoconcentration ↓ with hemolysis	↓	↔
Platelet count	Slight ↓, but remains >150,000 mcL	↓	↓	↔ to slight ↓
Fibrinogen	↑ (nl >300 mg/dL)	↔ or may ↓ with thrombocytopenia, DIC	↔	↓
PT and PTT	↔	↔ except in DIC	↔	↑
Serum creatinine	↓	↑	↑	↑
Serum uric acid	↓ 33%	↑	↑	↑
Urine protein	↑ but remains <300 mg/day Protein/creatinine ratio <0.19[a]	↑ >300 mg/day Protein/creatinine ratio >0.19[a]	↔ to ↑	↔
Hepatic transaminases	↔	↑	↔ to ↑	↑
WBC	Slight ↑	↔	↑	↑
LDH	↔	↑	↑	↑
Glucose	↔	↔	↔	↓
Ammonia	↔	↔	↔	↑
Bilirubin	↔	↑	↑	↑ (>5 mg/dL)

HELLP, syndrome of hemolysis, elevated liver enzymes, and low platelets; TTP, thrombotic thrombocytopenic purpura; AFLP, acute fatty liver of pregnancy; DIC, disseminated intravascular coagulation; PT, prothrombin time; PTT, partial thromboplastin time; WBC, white blood cell; LDH, lactate dehydrogenase.
[a]Shown to correlate strongly with 24-hour urine protein quantity.
Modified from Sibai BM. Imitators of severe preeclampsia/eclampsia. *Clin Perinatol.* 2004;31:835–852, with permission.

The definitive treatment of severe preeclampsia, eclampsia, and HELLP syndrome is delivery. However, close attention should be initially paid to the medical stability of the mother, with consideration of specific target organs (Alg. 65.1). Once maternal stabilization is accomplished, the well-being of the fetus should be assessed using heart rate monitoring and ultrasound, as emergency cesarean delivery is often necessary when the fetal status worsens. This is particularly important during periods of maternal seizures, which may be associated with impaired fetal oxygenation. When the fetus is very immature (<32 weeks) and exhibits reassuring tests of well-being, maternal stabilization can be attempted with intensive monitoring of both mother and fetus. In these circumstances, deteriorating fetal well-being may dictate an urgent delivery. Although it is unusual for this therapy to result in prolongation of pregnancy more than 10 to 14 days, this interval may reduce neonatal complications and the need for a prolonged stay in the neonatal intensive care unit. When preeclampsia/eclampsia presents in the postpartum period or in association with molar pregnancy, uterine evacuation and curettage may be needed to remove retained placental fragments.

In addition to delivery, other medical approaches that are relatively specific to preeclampsia/eclampsia should be highlighted. The prevention and treatment of seizures are paramount. Magnesium sulfate is the preferred antiseizure drug in the setting of preeclampsia/eclampsia. It is provided as an initial intravenous load of 4 to 6 g over 20 minutes, followed by continuous infusion of 2 g/hr. During seizures, the patient's airway should be protected and adequate oxygenation ensured. If seizures recur while the patient is receiving magnesium, a repeat (4-g) bolus of magnesium may be given. Other alternatives include intravenous administration of amobarbital or benzodiazepines (lorazepam or diazepam). Because magnesium undergoes renal clearance, serum levels should be assessed in any woman with evidence of impaired renal function, and the dose adjusted as needed to sustain a blood level between 4 and 7 mEq/L (4.8 to 8.4 mg/dL, 2 to 4 mmol/L). Phenytoin may be used in women with impaired renal function or compromised cardiopulmonary function. Seizure prophylaxis should continue for 24 hours after delivery, and extended if the patient does not demonstrate evidence of improvement.

Unlike other hypertensive disorders, the course of preeclampsia/eclampsia is not influenced by antihypertensive therapy. Treatment with these medications is designed to prevent stroke and congestive heart failure. Furthermore, the preeclamptic patient is often edematous secondary to extravasation of fluid into the interstitial tissues in the setting of capillary leakiness and reduced oncotic pressure. This results in reduced intravascular volume despite the increase in total whole-body water that characterizes the disease. Therefore, vasodilatation should be performed carefully, as it may contribute to diminished organ perfusion, which may also impact uteroplacental perfusion and jeopardize the undelivered fetus. The use of furosemide should be reserved for the treatment of pulmonary edema. Antihypertensive drugs, including hydralazine, calcium channel blockers, or labetalol, are generally administered for the treatment of diastolic blood pressure levels of 110 mm Hg or higher or systolic blood pressure levels above 170 mm Hg. There is no clear evidence that one of these antihypertensive agents is superior to the others for improving maternal and/or fetal outcomes. Similarly, use of the pulmonary artery catheter in preeclamptic patients with severe hypertension, pulmonary edema, and oliguria has been recommended, but remains controversial.

Although not routinely indicated, head imaging using computed tomography or magnetic resonance imaging of preeclamptic women may reveal reversible posterior leukoencephalopathy. Conditions that may prompt providers to obtain central nervous system imaging studies in order to rule out cerebrovascular hemorrhage or other diseases include lateralizing signs, prolonged unconsciousness, papilledema, seizures while taking magnesium, delayed presentation more than 48 hours after delivery, or an uncertain diagnosis of eclampsia.

Most women with preeclampsia/eclampsia are expected to have a full recovery after delivery and removal of trophoblastic tissue. It is rare for patients to develop chronic renal failure or permanent neurologic deficits following preeclampsia. The recovery phase is heralded by the onset of increased diuresis, which can be expected within 24 hours after delivery, but in rare cases can be delayed up to 1 week postpartum. Seizure prophylaxis can be usually discontinued once diuresis begins and the neurologic symptoms have resolved.

ALGORITHM 65.1   Treatment Guidelines for Patients with Severe Preeclampsia/eclampsia

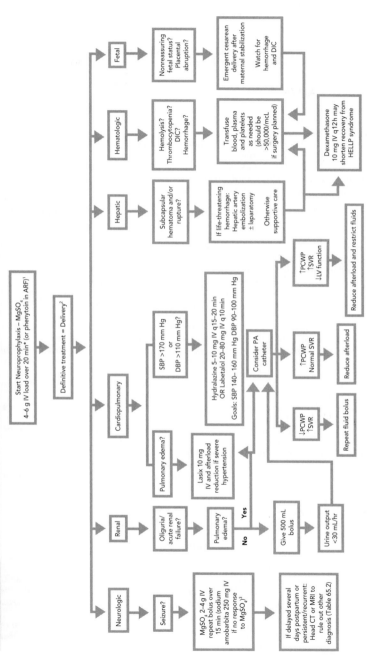

[1]The loading dose of magnesium is followed by MgSO$_4$ 2 g/hr with adjustment for therapeutic magnesium levels (4–7 mEq/L, 4.8–8.4 mg/dL).
[2]See exception in the text for a very preterm fetus (<32 weeks) in a stable preeclamptic patient.
[3]Consider lorazepam or diazepam IV with careful attention to respiratory depression.

ARF, acute renal failure; SBP, systolic blood pressure; DBP, diastolic blood pressure; DIC, disseminated intravascular coagulation; IV, intravenous; CT, computed tomography; MRI, magnetic resonance imaging; PA, pulmonary artery; PCWP, pulmonary capillary wedge pressure; SVR, systemic vascular resistance; LV, left ventricle; HELLP, hemolysis, elevated liver enzymes, and low platelets.

Lastly, high-dose corticosteroids postpartum may facilitate the recovery from HELLP syndrome, but should not be considered a part of the definitive treatment.

Because of the high incidence of preeclampsia in pregnancy, the severe sequelae of the disease are among the most common indications for admission of a pregnant or postpartum patient to an intensive care unit. Through prompt and coordinated care by perinatal and critical care specialists, most patients will recover from preeclampsia/eclampsia without residual disease.

Suggested Reading

Baxter JK, Weinstein L. HELLP syndrome: the state of the art. *Obstet Gynecol Surv.* 2004;59:838–845.
Review of the history, pathophysiology, clinical presentation, differential diagnosis, and management of HELLP syndrome.

Bolte AC, van Geijn HP, Dekker GA. Management and monitoring of severe preeclampsia. *Eur J Obstet Gynecol Reprod Biol.* 2001;96:8–20.
An overview of current developments in management and monitoring of severe preeclampsia, eclampsia, and HELLP syndrome.

Dekker G, Sibai B. Primary, secondary, and tertiary prevention of preeclampsia. *Lancet.* 2001;357:209–215.
Review of risk factors for preeclampsia, methods of early detection, and the failure of primary and secondary prevention of the disease, highlighting the need for proper antenatal care and timed delivery in tertiary prevention.

Duley L, Henderson-Smart DJ, Meher S. Drugs for treatment of very high blood pressure during pregnancy. *Cochrane Database Syst Rev.* 2006;3:CD001449.
A review of 24 trials of medications used in the treatment of severe hypertension in pregnancy, demonstrating that hydralazine, labetalol, and calcium channel blockers are acceptable options.

Isler CM, Barrilleaux PS, Rinehart BK, et al. Postpartum seizure prophylaxis: using maternal clinical parameters to guide therapy. *Obstet Gynecol.* 2003;101:66–69.
Prospective clinical study demonstrating that clinical criteria could be used successfully to shorten the duration of postpartum magnesium sulfate administration for seizure prophylaxis in preeclamptic patients.

Lucas MJ, Leveno KJ, Cunningham FG. A comparison of magnesium sulfate with phenytoin for the prevention of eclampsia. *N Engl J Med.* 1995;333:201–205.
A randomized clinical trial demonstrating the superiority of magnesium to phenytoin in the prevention of eclampsia.

Mabie WC. Management of acute severe hypertension and encephalopathy. *Clin Obstet Gynecol.* 1999;42:519–531.
Review of the pathophysiology and management of preeclampsia, briefly discussing the similarities and differences between eclampsia and hypertensive encephalopathy.

Redman CW, Sargent IL. Preeclampsia, the placenta and the maternal systemic inflammatory response–a review. *Placenta.* 2003;24:S21–27.
Review of the evidence that preeclampsia is caused by a maternal systemic inflammatory response which, in mild from, accompanies normal third trimester pregnancy.

Sibai BM. Diagnosis, prevention, and management of eclampsia. *Obstet Gynecol.* 2005;105:402–410.
Comprehensive review of eclampsia—timing of onset, cerebral pathology associated with the disease, differential diagnosis, maternal and perinatal outcomes, prevention, and management.

Sibai BM. Imitators of severe preeclampsia/eclampsia. *Clin Perinatol.* 2004;31:835–852.
Review of disorders which should be included in the differential diagnosis of severe preeclampsia, focusing on acute fatty liver of pregnancy and thrombotic microangiopathies.

Sibai BM, Mercer BM, Schiff E, et al. Aggressive versus expectant management of severe preeclampsia at 28 to 32 weeks gestation: a randomized controlled trial. *Am J Obstet Gynecol.* 1994;171:818–822.

A randomized trial demonstrating maternal and fetal safety with expectant management of severe preeclampsia less than 32 weeks, resulting in decreased neonatal morbidity.

Walker JJ. Preeclampsia. *Lancet.* 2000;356:1260–1265.

Review of the pathophysiology, diagnosis, management, morbidity and mortality associated with preeclampsia.

Zeeman GG. Obstetric critical care: A blueprint for improved outcomes. Crit Care Med 2006;34:S208–214.

Review of critical care issues in the obstetric patient and treatment options for preeclampsia and massive obstetric hemorrhage.

XVII

Surgical Problems

66 TRAUMA CARE FOR THE INTENSIVE CARE UNIT
Douglas J.E. Schuerer

Care of the traumatically injured patient is a complex issue, given the multiple potential systems that are injured. This chapter reviews the initial evaluation and treatment of the trauma patient, then proceeds with those injuries that are most likely to cause early intensive care unit (ICU) death in this population. In addition, we review the management of the most likely problems that will result in an ICU admission. Any critical care of the trauma patient must be in conjunction with the various specialists that are needed for this population, including general surgery, neurosurgery, orthopaedic surgery, facial surgery, hand surgery, and rehabilitation medicine. This team approach is essential to ensure positive outcomes in the acutely injured patient. Another important factor in trauma care is that the trauma patient is often younger than the normal ICU population, and despite frequently initially becoming extremely ill, all have a high potential for recovery. Because of the brevity of this guide, in cannot be a thorough review of all traumatic injuries, but instead focuses on the most life-threatening ones that are related to eventual ICU care.

TRAUMA EVALUATION

The basic tenets of the initial resuscitation and management of the injured patient are described in the advanced trauma life support course. The course was designed to teach all physicians the basics of trauma care to better standardize and improve early interventions. Most trauma patients are initially evaluated in an emergency department, but transfers and other reasons may place a nonevaluated trauma patient directly in the ICU.

Primary Survey

The first phase of evaluation is the primary survey. The primary survey is the portion of care that is commonly remembered by the ABCs of trauma. It is performed rapidly but completely and in order. Systematic consistency is paramount to avoid missing injuries.

Airway

Assess for:

1. Obstruction, including foreign bodies, facial fractures, or bleeding. Begin measures to remove obstruction and establish airway.
2. Patency, which may be compromised because of head injury, intoxication, or swelling Note: Patients who are verbal without hoarseness or stridor usually have a patent airway, but this does not rule out future airway compromise. Maneuvers to obtain a definitive airway should begin immediately on recognition of the problem and before other lifesaving interventions.

Potential problems:

1. Swelling leading to delayed airway collapse.
2. Inability to obtain airway in a paralyzed patient; surgical airway a must.
3. Unknown laryngeal or tracheal disruption.

Breathing and Ventilation

Assess for:

1. Adequate chest wall excursion not limited by mental status, rib fractures, or pain.
2. Loss of or diminished breath sounds on either side from pneumothorax, hemothorax, pulmonary contusion or other lung pathology.
3. Evidence of bruising or laceration to the chest.
4. Deviated trachea from tension pneumothorax or neck hematoma.

Potential problems:

1. Airway compromise and ventilation failure may be difficult to discern from one another.
2. Massive pulmonary injuries may falsely seem to be airway-related because of severe dyspnea.
3. Airway placement may worsen some pulmonary issues because of positive pressure ventilation (worsening pneumothorax).

Circulation with Hemorrhage Control

Assess for:

1. Blood volume and cardiac output
   a. Mental status deteriorates with increasing amounts of blood loss and progression of hemorrhagic shock.
   b. Ashen gray skin and poor capillary refill both imply poor circulation.
   c. Pulses are a marker of perfusion in the younger patient without vascular disease. Full and regular pulses are positive. Fast, thready, or diminished pulses likely delineate poor global flow or decreased flow to the affected extremity. Irregular pulses may indicate blunt cardiac injury.
2. Bleeding
   a. External blood loss is recognized readily and is best stopped by direct pressure. Multiple layers of gauze make tamponade more difficult. Tourniquets should not be used except in unusual circumstances.
   b. Occult bleeding from internal hemorrhage should be expected if patient has signs of shock.
   c. Potential sources are:
      i. Abdomen: bruising, tenderness, or distension.
      ii. Chest: decreased breath sounds, evidence rib fractures.
      iii. Pelvis: unstable pelvis, pelvic bony pain.
      iv. Legs: femur fracture may have up to two units of blood in thigh.

Potential problems:

1. Patients on beta-blockade may not get tachycardic as a response to bleeding or anemia.
2. Elderly patients have less reserve and may decompensate quickly.
3. Children have more reserve and will not show signs of shock until severely volume-depleted.
4. Multiple occult sources for blood loss may exist in any one patient.

Disability or Neurologic Status

Rapid neurologic examination:

1. Glasgow Coma Score total score (3–15)
   a. Eye opening (1–4)
   b. Motor response (1–6)
   c. Verbal response (1–5)
2. Pupillary size and reactivity
3. Lateralizing signs
4. Spinal injury level

Potential problems:

1. Intoxication masking or reproducing a closed head injury.
2. Lucid intervals can be seen before compromise from intracranial lesions.

Exposure/Environmental Control

1. All clothing and dressings need to be removed to inspect for injuries and examination.
2. After assessment, patient should be covered as quickly as possible and warmth maintained. Hypothermia worsens bleeding and outcomes in trauma.

Resuscitation: During and continuing after the primary survey, resuscitation should be performed while completing each portion of the survey.

1. Airway: A definitive airway should be established if there is loss of the airway for any reason. If there is doubt or worsening of swelling, the airway should always be obtained early when it is safest.
2. Breathing and ventilation
   a. Add high-flow oxygen to all patients.
   b. If airway obtained, ensure continued ventilation with hand-bagging or a ventilator.
   c. Pneumothoraces and hemothoraces need to be released to permit adequate ventilation.
3. Circulation:
   a. Two large-bore intravenous (IV) lines should be obtained. If no peripheral IV access, consider a large-bore (not triple-lumen) catheter into a major vein.
   b. Adult interosseous needles are now available as well.
   c. Consider area of injury before placing IV access.

Adjuncts to the primary survey: Certain interventions are important in the resuscitation of the trauma patient. These are normally performed during the primary survey or immediately afterward.

1. Electrocardiographic monitoring: usually continuous on a monitor. Formal electrocardiogram may be needed if arrhythmias or possible ST segment changes present.
2. Pulse oximetry: helpful in assessing perfusion status and blood oxygenation trends.
3. Urinary catheter: assesses for blood and follows urine output. Risk of problems without assessing for signs of urethral injury first (bruising at perineum, blood at meatus, high-riding prostate.)
4. Gastric catheter: assesses stomach contents for blood and evacuates stomach to lessen the risk of aspiration. Risk of cranial injuries with nasogastric tube and facial injuries.
5. Continuous blood pressure monitoring: may need arterial line if critically unstable, but this should not delay definitive care.
6. Chest plain films if major blunt or penetrating trauma; pelvic films if blunt trauma or penetrating wound to abdomen. Other films are determined after the secondary survey.

Secondary survey: The secondary survey is a thorough examination and assessment of the entire patient after the primary survey is complete and resuscitation is started. The following list is not exhaustive, but shows an example of what each body areas examination should include.

1. History
   a. AMPLE History
      i. A – allergies
      ii. M – medications
      iii. P – past illness/pregnancy

  iv. L – last meal
  v. E – events of the injury
 b. Should include accident details or type of gun or knife used
2. Head: lacerations, bruises, eye injuries, vision
3. Maxillofacial: facial stepoffs, facial nerve injuries, intraoral mandible fractures
4. Neck: spine tenderness, trachea midline, hematomas
5. Chest: bruises, tenderness, change in breath sounds, crepitus, uneven chest excursion
6. Abdomen: bruising, tenderness, distention, evisceration of bowel or omentum.
7. Perineum: vaginal tears, rectal tone, hematomas, blood at meatus, rectal bleeding, and pregnancy test in female patients.
8. Limbs: distal pulses and capillary refill, tenderness, crepitus with movement, deformity of the limb.
9. Neurologic: detailed neurologic examination, especially levels of injury if paralysis.

Tertiary survey: Often patients admitted to the ICU have not been able to be fully assessed in the emergency department because of intoxication, head injury, or hemodynamic instability. It is therefore crucial that the ICU staff helps to perform a continual reassessment similar to the secondary survey of potential injuries as the patient stabilizes and is able to respond to the examiner. The tertiary survey must be done systematically and can often lead to undiagnosed fractures or other injuries.

Major Immediate Life-Threatening Conditions

After initial resuscitation, several immediately life-threatening conditions may be present, but may not be diagnosed of present at that time. These may become clinically apparent once the patient has arrived in the ICU for continued care.

Tension Pneumothorax
Tension pneumothorax often presents in delayed fashion, especially if patient is on positive pressure ventilation. This diagnosis should be clinical in most cases. Blunt or penetrating injury to the chest, or line insertion during resuscitation should make this possible.
  Diagnosis:

    Hypotension
    Distended neck veins
    Decreased breath sounds on one side
    Chest x-ray (only if stable)

  Treatment:

    Needle decompression if unstable
    Chest tube with closed suction drainage after needle decompression

Cardiac Tamponade
Cardiac tamponade most often is seen after penetrating injury to the heart, but can also develop from blunt injury from direct cardiac injury or broken ribs or sternum.
  Diagnosis:

    Hypotension
    Distended neck veins
    Equalization of pressures, if pulmonary artery catheter present
    Diminished heart sounds
    Echocardiography, if stable

  Treatment:

    Pericardiocentesis—may be repeated
    Surgery is the definitive treatment

Blunt Cardiac Injury
Blunt cardiac injury includes several different cardiac problems that all arise from blunt injury to the heart, including cardiac contusion, coronary artery dissection or transaction, valve injury, chordae tendinae rupture, septal defects, and pericardial tamponade.

Diagnosis:

Arrhythmias
Unexplained hypotension despite adequate resuscitation
Echocardiography
Cardiac enzymes (creatine phosphokinase, troponin) have *no* proven benefit in the diagnosis or treatment of blunt cardiac injury.

Treatment:

Inotropic agents
Supportive care
Surgery
Cardiac catheterization if coronary dissection

Massive Hemothorax

A massive hemothorax is a large collection of blood in the chest that causes problems from hemorrhagic shock as well as a tensionlike physiology in the chest. It can be due to major pulmonary vascular injury or blunt aortic rupture.
Diagnosis:

Hypotension
Decreased breath sounds
Chest x-ray
Computed tomography (CT) scan of the chest with IV contrast if hemodynamically stable.

Treatment:

Chest tube
Resuscitation
Surgery

OTHER INJURIES REQUIRING ICU CARE

Hemorrhagic Shock

Hemorrhagic shock can quickly arise in the traumatically injured patient. A patient may have one bleeding focus or many. Differentiating this from distributive or spinal shock is also necessary, but shock secondary to continued bleeding should always be considered and treated first.
Major causes:

Liver or spleen injuries
Massive hemothorax
Exsanguinating peripheral arterial injuries
Pelvic fractures
Long-bone fractures
Retroperitoneal hematomas

Diagnosis:

Known or suspected bleeding diathesis
Anemia
Tamponade and tension pneumothorax ruled out

Treatment:

Rapid transfusion of blood and products as needed
Control of bleeding through surgery, splinting, or embolization

Distributive (Spinal) Shock

This type of shock develops after spinal cord injury and is due to loss of sympathetic innervation to the heart and distal vessels. It must be a diagnosis of exclusion after hemorrhagic and cardiogenic causes are ruled out.

Diagnosis:

Known spinal cord injury
Hypotension unresponsive to appropriate fluid resuscitation
Treatment:
Vasopressors and inotropes as needed

Flail Chest

Flail chest is secondary to massive blunt injury to the chest causing fracture of at least three contiguous ribs in two or more places. It results in paradoxical movement of the chest wall during inspiration. Pulmonary contusions are often underlying the injury.
Diagnosis:

Chest x-ray
CT scan of the chest
Physical examination (paradoxical motion an extreme tenderness)

Treatment:

Pain control
Pulmonary toilet
Intubation and ventilation if needed
Surgical stabilization may be helpful if slow improvement

Pulmonary Contusion

Pulmonary contusion is common finding in the ICU trauma patient and ranges from mild to severe. Treatment is supportive as the lung heals. Pulmonary contusions usually worsen during 48 hours before improving, and that time lag is important when making future treatment decisions regarding the pulmonary system. Although the trauma patient often has massive needs for resuscitation, in patients with isolated pulmonary contusion, care should be taken not to overload fluid.
Diagnosis:

Chest x-ray
CT scan of the chest

Treatment:

Pulmonary toilet
Oxygen
Positive pressure ventilation if severe
Intubation if needed
Protective lung ventilation similar to patients with acute respiratory distress syndrome
Oscillatory ventilation
Consider placing affected side down if significant pulmonary hemorrhage

Spleen and Liver Injuries, Pelvic Hematomas

These are included together given the similarity of approach in these patients. For this group, the diagnosis is often known prior to ICU admission. The worst of these injuries that rendered the patient hemodynamically unstable have likely already been stabilized with packing or resection in the operative theater. Further management includes:

1. Serial assessment of blood counts and bleeding parameters
2. Continued resuscitation with appropriate fluids or products
3. If further bleeding continues, the patient likely requires further intervention with interventional radiology or surgery.
4. Need for pelvic stabilization to reduce venous bleeding in pelvic fractures

Head Injury

Often patients with multiple injuries also have head injuries. Intracranial injury care is reviewed elsewhere, but treatment strategies for the multiply injured patient are often different than those for isolated head injuries. The care of these patients must involve all of the specialty teams in the medical decision-making.

LATER COMPLICATIONS

Although the traumatically injured ICU patient is apt to develop any of the common ICU complications, pulmonary emboli and fat emboli are more common in this population. Careful thromboembolic prophylaxis must be initiated as soon as possible with careful screening for deep venous thrombosis throughout the hospital course. Fat emboli are associated with long-bone fractures, usually after repair, and can cause severe lung disease, but are treated as most respiratory distress patients with supportive care.

CONCLUSION

The traumatically injured patient often requires ICU care and monitoring. Recognizing the most common life-threatening concerns quickly is important in the care of these patients. The initial survey is important to systematically identify and treat those conditions as rapidly as possible. Continuous resuscitation is key to the survival and ultimate recovery of these patients, as well as following and recognizing the endpoints of that resuscitation.

Suggested Reading

American College of Surgeons, Committee on Trauma. *Advanced Trauma Life Support for Doctors.* 7th ed. Chicago: American College of Surgeons; 2004.

Dunham CM, Barraco RD, Clark DE, et al. Guideline for emergency tracheal intubation immediately after traumatic injury. *J Trauma.* 2003;54:391–416.

Pasquale M, Fabian T. Practice management guidelines of the screening of blunt cardiac injury. *J Trauma.* 1998;44:941–956.

Practice management guidelines for hemorrhage in pelvic fracture. Available at: http://www.east.org/tpg/pelvis.pdf. Accessed March 1, 2007.

Practice management guidelines for the nonoperative management of blunt injury to the liver and spleen. Available at: http://www.east.org/tpg/livspleen.pdf. Accessed March 1, 2007.

Practice management guidelines for *Pulmonary Contusion—Flail Chest.* Available at: http://www.east.org/tpg/pulmcontflailchest.pdf. Accessed March 1, 2007.

Schuerer DJ, Whinney RR, Freeman BD, et al. Evaluation of the applicability, efficacy, and safety of a thromboembolic event prophylaxis guideline designed for quality improvement of the traumatically injured patient. *J Trauma.* 2005;58:731–739.

Simon BJ, Cushman J, Barraco RD, et al. Pain management guidelines for blunt thoracic trauma. *J Trauma.* 2005;59:1256–1257.

Tishermam SA, Barie P, Bokhari F, et al. Clinical practice guideline: endpoints of resuscitation. *J Trauma.* 2004;57:898–912.

THE ACUTE ABDOMEN

Jennifer Gnerlich and Robb R. Whinney

67

Acute abdominal pathology is a common event in the intensive care unit (ICU) setting, but the diagnosis is often delayed because of the absence of typical signs and symptoms of peritonitis. Physical examination signs that define an acute abdomen, such as global tenderness, rigidity, rebound, and guarding, are not always obvious in the ICU setting when a patient has multiple ongoing medical issues. A retrospective cohort study of medical ICU patients with abdominal pathology found surgical delay was more likely to occur in patients with altered mental states, absence of peritoneal signs, previous opioid analgesia, antibiotics, and mechanical ventilation. The delay in diagnosis and management of an acute abdomen is associated with increased morality rates. Therefore, learning to identify an acute abdomen in a critically ill patient with masked physical symptoms is a life-saving skill.

PATIENT HISTORY

Obtaining a history from a patient in the ICU is frequently complicated by an altered mental state, chemical sedation, or intubation. A careful review of the patient's medical history, surgical history, allergies, medications, and family history can provide a possible cause of the abdominal pathology. If the patient is alert, the description of the pain, including quality and radiation, may help to focus the differential diagnosis. Most often, a patient is not alert and important medical history must be obtained from family members. One of the most important pieces of information influencing the differential diagnosis is whether or not the patient has recently had an operation. For example, a patient who recently underwent abdominal surgery (<3 days) is at greater risk for bleeding and anastomotic leaks, and a patient a week out from surgery is more likely to have an intra-abdominal abscess.

LABORATORY HISTORY

Laboratory tests are important adjuncts in the critical care setting, where most patients cannot provide an accurate history or description of their current physical symptoms. Following laboratory value trends can provide insight into an ongoing abdominal process. An increasing trend in the white blood cell (WBC) count is usually a signal of infection or inflammation but is fairly nonspecific after a recent surgical procedure or in a patient receiving steroids. Conversely, an extreme WBC (35,000 to 40,000 cells/mcL) can indicate a more severe infection, such as *Clostridium difficle* colitis, and the workup should be done accordingly. A normal or decreasing WBC count can be misleading; thus, it is important to obtain a differential cell count and evaluate for a left shift. A decreasing WBC to leukopenic levels with a large left shift is concerning for overwhelming sepsis.

Abnormal liver function tests including fractionated bilirubin, alkaline phosphatase, and transaminase levels may localize the pathology to the gallbladder, biliary system, or liver, but are rarely diagnostic. Instead, they help guide further diagnostic strategies like appropriate imaging. Of note, in the critically ill patient, an acute increase in bilirubin may signify acalculous cholecystitis. Elevated amylase and lipase levels hone the diagnosis to pancreatitis, whereas an isolated amylase elevation may indicate a perforated viscus or ischemic bowel. Concomitant increase in both bilirubin and amylase suggests obstruction at the distal common bile duct or pancreatic duct. An elevated lactate level (>4 mmol/L) may signal the emergent condition of mesenteric ischemia with necrotic bowel or, less specifically, is the result of acidemia, hypoxia, hypovolemia, anemia, or renal or liver failure. Arterial blood gas should be obtained to determine if acidosis or hypoxemia is present and to quantify the base deficit. Abdominal compartment syndrome should be suspected when acidosis, hypoxemia, oliguria, and a distended abdomen are present. Bladder pressure can be transduced; a pressure >30 mm Hg may require emergent surgical decompression. Urine analysis is not specific, but microscopic hematuria or pyuria can suggest a urinary tract infection or a lower abdomen/pelvic infection.

PHYSICAL EXAMINATION

The physical examination is less reliable in a patient receiving analgesics, sedatives, or steroids and must focus more on changing physical examination signs rather than the traditional signs of peritonitis. In a patient whose clinical course is declining, it is important that the abdominal examination is performed serially and a digital rectal examination is completed.

Because abdominal pain may be difficult to elucidate in the critically ill patient, nonspecific signs such as tachycardia, hypotension, and fever raise concern for occult abdominal pathology. A sudden change in ventilatory settings, overbreathing the ventilator, or increasing airway pressures may signal a patient's attempt to compensate for a metabolic acidosis or indicate an elevation in intra-abdominal compartment pressure. An increase in nasogastric output, abdominal distention, absence of bowel movements, or abrupt intolerance of enteral feeds is concerning for a bowel obstruction, mesenteric ischemia, or an acute ileus due to an intra-abdominal infection. Because the nursing staff spends more extended periods of time with the patient, it is important to communicate with them about changes in the patient's condition, including the quantity and quality of bowel movements (*C. difficile* colitis or intestinal ischemia), drain output (abdominal sepsis, leak, or fistula), and wound drainage (intra-abdominal abscess or wound dehiscence). For a patient who has recently undergone an abdominal procedure, these nonspecific signs would be concerning for some type of anastomotic leak (intestinal, biliary, pancreatic). For a patient who is about a week out of surgery, intra-abdominal sepsis, ischemia, or abscess should be considered.

An acute abdomen in the ICU setting may be of medical or surgical consequence, although there are some diagnoses that overlap (Table 67.1). To assist in differentiating abdominal pain in the critically ill patient in the ICU, the abdomen is best divided into six regions to help evaluate the source of the abdominal pathology (Table 67.2).

The actual explanation of all possible acute abdominal emergencies and their diagnosis and treatment is beyond the scope of this chapter. An algorithm is provided to help guide management decisions for those patients in the ICU who may be experiencing intra-abdominal pathology (Alg. 67.1).

RADIOGRAPHIC EXAMINATION

Imaging the abdomen helps to confirm or exclude intra-abdominal catastrophe. Initially, three plain film views of the abdomen (kidney/ureter/bladder, upright chest, and lateral decubitus) should be obtained. Air in the biliary tree or intestines, known as *pneumatosis*, suggests necrotic bowel and indicates the need for an emergent surgical consultation. Free air in the peritoneum and retroperitoneum suggests an intestinal or gastric perforation. However, in a patient who has recently undergone laparotomy, free air should be interpreted with caution as it may be the result of the procedure itself.

Abdominal ultrasound is noninvasive and is the imaging modality of choice for a patient with right upper quadrant symptoms or concerning liver function tests. Ultrasound can elucidate gallbladder pathology by demonstrating pericholecystic fluid, wall thickening, gallstones, ductal dilatation, or a distended gallbladder, indicating calculous or acalculous cholecystitis. If the concern for acalculous cholecystitis is high, then a hepatobiliary iminodiacetic acid scan will confirm the diagnosis. Abdominal ultrasound can also identify fluid in other areas, particularly around the pancreas or in the pelvis. Although nonspecific, fluid in the pelvis can indicate an intra-abdominal pathology or be a consequence of aggressive resuscitative efforts.

| TABLE 67.1 | Medical versus Surgical Causes of Acute Abdominal Pathology in the Intensive Care Unit |

Medical	Workup
Acute renal failure (uremia)	↓UOP, UA (casts), ↑ BUN and Cr, FeNa, renal ultrasound
Sickle cell crisis	↓Hematocrit, peripheral blood smear
Adrenal insufficiency/Addisonian crisis	BMP (↑ K^+, ↓ Na^+, ↓ glucose), plasma cortisol and ACTH, cosyntropin stimulation test
Spontaneous bacterial peritonitis	Ultrasound, paracentesis with Gram stain and culture
Diabetic ketoacidosis	Glucose, UA, BMP (Na^+ and K^+ levels), ABG (acidosis)
Gastroenteritis/enterocolitis	WBC,[a] stool ova/parasites
Esophagitis	EGD, barium swallow, pH monitoring
Hepatitis	LFTs, hepatitis panel (A, B, and C)
Peptic ulcer disease/gastritis	EGD, barium swallow, pH monitoring, manometry
Nephrolithiasis/pyelonephritis	UA (pyuria, hematuria), renal ultrasound
Myocardial infarction	ECG, troponins
Pneumonia	Chest x-ray, sputum sample, WBC
Urinary tract infection	UA (bacteria, leukocyte esterase, nitrites)
Gynecologic disease	Pelvic examination, gonorrhea/chlamydia, ultrasound

Medical and Surgical	Workup
Diverticulitis/IBD	WBC, CT scan,[b] flexible sigmoidoscopy/ colonoscopy
Clostridium difficile colitis	Stool toxin assay × 3, severely elevated WBC
Pancreatitis/pancreatic abscess	Amylase, lipase, ultrasound, CT scan to r/o necrosis
Intra-abdominal abscess	WBC, CT scan
Small/large bowel obstruction	WBC, lactate, plain film x-rays, CT scan
Choledocholithiasis	LFTs, RUQ ultrasound
Cholangitis	LFTs, WBC, RUQ ultrasound
Mallory-Weiss tear	EGD, hematocrit, coagulation studies

Surgical	Workup
Acute cholecystitis	WBC, LFTs, RUQ ultrasound
Acalculous cholecystitis	WBC, LFTs, RUQ ultrasound, HIDA scan
Perforated peptic or duodenal ulcer	Plain film x-rays (free air), upper GI series, CT scan
Acute appendicitis	WBC, CT scan with rectal contrast, ultrasound to r/o other pathology
Mesenteric ischemia and necrotic bowel	WBC, lactate, ABG (acidosis), CT scan
Colonic perforation	WBC, plain film x-rays (free air), CT scan
Ruptured or leaking abdominal aortic aneurysm	Hematocrit, coagulation studies, CT angio (only need IV contrast)
Toxic megacolon	C. difficile stool toxin assay × 3, WBC, plain film x-rays, CT scan
Sigmoid or cecal volvulus	Plain film x-rays, CT scan
Boerhaave syndrome	Plain film x-rays, gastrografin swallow
Wound dehiscence	WBC, wound culture, ultrasound, CT scan
Anastomotic leak (intestinal, biliary, pancreatic)	WBC, CT scan (if patient had a recent surgical procedure)
Abdominal compartment syndrome	↓UOP, WBC, lactate, ABG (acidosis), bladder pressures

UOP, urine output; UA, urinalysis; BUN, blood urea nitrogen; Cr, creatine; BMP, blood metabolic profile; ACTH, corticotropin; ABG, arterial blood gas; WBC, white blood cell; EGD, esophagogastroduodenoscopy; ECG, electrocardiogram; CT, computed tomography; r/o, rule out; RUQ, right upper quadrant; HIDA, hepatobiliary iminodiacetic acid; GI, gastrointestinal; IV, intravenous.
[a] WBC should always be obtained with a differential cell count.
[b] CT scan should always be obtained with IV & oral contrast unless contraindicaton exists, i.e., abnormal renal function.

TABLE 67.2 Cause of Abdominal Pathology Based on Location

I. Right upper quadrant
Acute cholecystitis
Acalculous cholecystitis
Hepatitis
Choledocholithiasis
Cholangitis
Hepatic abscess
Pancreatitis
Peptic ulcer disease/gastritis
Nephrolithiasis/pyelonephritis
Appendicitis (women in pregnancy)
Myocardial infarction
Pneumonia

II. Epigastrium
Pancreatitis
Peptic ulcer disease/gastritis
Perforated peptic or duodenal ulcer
Mallory-Weiss tear
Boerhaave syndrome
Esophagitis
Gastroenteritis
Myocardial infarction
Pneumonia

III. Left upper quadrant
Splenic hemorrhage or abscess
Peptic ulcer disease
Perforated peptic or duodenal ulcer
Pancreatitis
Pancreatic pseudocyst or abscess
Nephrolithiasis/pyleonephritis
Pneumonia (left lower lobe)

IV. Right lower quadrant
Acute appendicitis
Small/large bowel obstruction
Cecal perforation
Cecal volvulus
Cecal diverticulitis
Enterocolitis
Inflammatory bowel disease
Nephrolithiasis
Urinary tract infection
Gynecologic disease

V. Periumbilical/nonspecific
Small/large bowel obstruction
Mesenteric artery ischemia or occlusion
Ruptured or leaking abdominal aortic aneurysm
Early appendicitis
Clostridium difficle colitis or toxic megacolon
Wound dehiscence
Abdominal compartment syndrome
Intra-abdominal abscess
Anastomotic leak (intestinal, biliary, pancreatic)

VI. Left lower quadrant
Sigmoid diverticulitis
Sigmoid volvulus
Colonic perforation
Small/large bowel obstruction
Enterocolitis
Inflammatory bowel disease
Nephrolithiasis
Urinary tract infection
Gynecologic disease

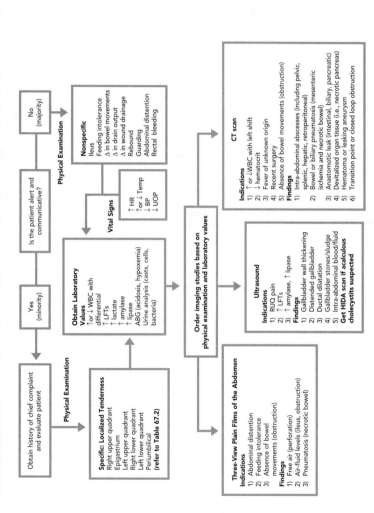

ALGORITHM 67.1   Diagnosis and Management of Acute Abdominal Pathology in the Intensive Care Unit

Obtain history of chief complaint and evaluate patient

Is the patient alert and communicative?

Yes (minority)

No (majority)

Physical Examination

Specific: Localized Tenderness
Right upper quadrant
Epigastrium
Left upper quadrant
Right lower quadrant
Left lower quadrant
Periumbilical
(refer to Table 67.2)

Physical Examination

Nonspecific
Ileus
Feeding intolerance
Δ in bowel movements
Δ in drain output
Δ in wound drainage
Rebound
Guarding
Abdominal distention
Rectal bleeding

Vital Signs
↑ HR
↑ or ↓ Temp
↓ BP
↓ UOP

Obtain Laboratory Values
↑ or ↓ WBC with differential
↑ LFTs
↑ lactate
↑ amylase
↑ lipase
ABG (acidosis, hypoxemia)
Urine analysis (casts, cells, bacteria)

Order imaging studies based on physical examination and laboratory values

Three-View Plain Films of the Abdomen
Indications
1) Abdominal distention
2) Feeding intolerance
3) Absence of bowel movements (obstruction)
Findings
1) Free air (perforation)
2) Air-fluid levels (ileus, obstruction)
3) Pneumatosis (necrotic bowel)

Ultrasound
Indications
1) RUQ pain
2) ↑ LFTs
3) ↑ amylase, ↑ lipase
Findings
1) Gallbladder wall thickening
2) Distended gallbladder
3) Ductal dilatation
4) Gallbladder stones/sludge
5) Intra-abdominal blood/fluid
Get HIDA scan if acalculous cholecystits suspected

CT scan
Indications
1) ↑ or ↓ WBC with left shift
2) ↓ hematocrit
3) Fever of unknown origin
4) Recent surgery
5) Absence of bowel movements (obstruction)
Findings
1) Intra-abdominal abscesses (including pelvic, splenic, hepatic, retroperitoneal)
2) Bowel or biliary pneumatosis (mesenteric ischemia and necrotic bowel)
3) Anastomotic leak (intestinal, biliary, pancreatic)
4) Devitalized organ tissue (i.e., necrotic pancreas)
5) Hematoma or leaking aneurysm
6) Transition point or closed loop obstruction

HR, heart rate; BP, blood pressure; UOP, urine output; WBC, white blood cell; LFT, liver function test; ABG, arterial blood gas; RUQ, right upper quadrant; HIDA, hepatobiliary iminodiacetic acid.

Computed tomographic scanning (CT scan) with contrast is useful in identifying bowel thickening secondary to edema, dilated and fluid-filled intestines, fat stranding, and pneumatosis, all imaging signs concerning for necrotic bowel and requiring immediate surgical evaluation. CT scan can also demonstrate a transition point in a bowel obstruction for easier surgical management. In a recent surgical patient with sudden clinical deterioration and a drop in hematocrit, a CT scan can reveal an evolving hematoma or an acute bleed. Finally, CT scan is useful in identifying the location and size of intra-abdominal abscesses and in guiding management by either percutaneous drainage or laparotomy and washout.

Suggested Reading

Fink MP. Acute abdominal pain. In: Kruse JA, Fink MP, Carlson RW, eds. *Saunders Manual of Critical Care*. Philadelphia: Elsevier Science; 2003:439–445.
   Short review of important physical exam findings, laboratory values, and imaging studies for the most common causes of an acute abdomen.

Gajic O, Urrutia LE, et al. Acute abdomen in the medical intensive care unit. *Crit Care Med.* 2002;30:1187–1190.
   Retrospective cohort study in a tertiary care center's medical intensive care unit that evaluated predictors of surgical delay for patients with an acute abdomen and the association between surgical delay and increased mortality in those patients.

Martin RF, Rossi RL. The acute abdomen: an overview and algorithms. *Surg Clin North Am.* 1997;77:1227–1243.
   Basic overview of managing a patient with an acute abdomen.

Martin RF, Flynn P. The acute abdomen in the critically ill patient. *Surg Clin North Am.* 1997;77:1455–1464.
   Overview of the diagnostic difficulties encontered in critically ill patient with an acute abdomen in the ICU and possible management strategies.

Sosa JL, Reines HD. Evaluating the acute abdomen. In: Civetta JM, Taylor RW, Kirby RR, eds. *Critical Care.* 3rd ed. Philadelphia: Lippincott, Williams & Wilkins; 1997:1099–1108.
   Textbook chapter reviewing the general approach to a patient with as acute abdomen in the ICU.

MANAGEMENT OF THE ORGAN DONOR
68

Ryan C. Fields and Bryan F. Meyers

Since 1998, the Health Care Financing Administration of the Department of Health and Human Services has required hospitals to contact the local organ-procurement organization when a patient is identified for whom death is imminent. In consultation with the intensive care unit (ICU) team, the organ-procurement organization establishes the criteria of donor suitability. Table 68.1 summarizes various criteria for establishing the suitability for organ donation.

Two cardinal rules should be followed by caring physicians when considering a patient for organ donation: (a) Blood testing to determine if a patient is a candidate for organ transplantation may be done after the family gives consent; however, (b) invasive procedures to determine if a patient is suitable for organ donation should not be performed prior to the patient being declared dead. A summary of the process of obtaining consent for organ donation is summarized in Table 68.2. Of note, the establishment of brain death should be performed by two clinical examinations, apnea tests, and laboratory confirmation 24 to 48 hours apart by physicians trained in this area. (The specifics of the criteria for brain death are covered in Chapter 55.)

Once a patient has been found to be a suitable candidate for organ transplantation and has been declared brain-dead, the goals of ICU care are to maintain end-organ function and viability. Increasingly, the transplant community has been considering organ transplants using organs donated after cardiac death in the absence of brain death. Several clinical problems apply both to the after-cardiac-death donors and to those with brain death, and these are discussed in the following sections and summarized in Algorithm 68.1.

ESTABLISH NORMOTHERMIA

The hypothalamus controls thermoregulation in healthy individuals. With traumatic injury, loss of regulation can lead to severe poikilothermia. Further, passive heat loss can contribute to sever hypothermia, which can lead to dramatic alterations in cellular metabolism and end-organ function. Measures that can be undertaken in the ICU to ensure normothermia include maintaining room temperatures above 75°F, keeping patients covered with blankets (including passive air-warming blankets), warming all intravenous fluids, and using heated and humidified air in the ventilator circuit.

NORMALIZE BLOOD PRESSURE

It is rare to encounter significant hypertension in brain-dead patients. If present, it is often related to brainstem herniation. Diastolic blood pressures >100 mm Hg should be treated to avoid arrhythmias. Sodium nitroprusside is the treatment of choice. Prolonged nitroprusside treatment should be avoided because of cyanide toxicity.

Hypotension, defined as a systolic blood pressure <90 mm Hg, is more frequently encountered in brain-dead patients. This has been attributed to the systemic inflammatory response that occurs with polytrauma and brain death, leading to peripheral vasodilation with an increase in the intravascular space, which leads to relative hypovolemia and hypotension. Even subtle and brief episodes of hypotension can lead to decreased end-organ perfusion and damage; thus, hypotension is treated aggressively. Most cases of hypotension can be treated with volume expansion to a central venous pressure of >12 mm Hg.

TABLE 68.1	Criteria for Organ Donation

- Donor age
  - Absolute contraindication → age >80
  - Organ-specific contraindication → lungs, kidneys <60
- Lack of significant past medical history
  - No malignancy with high potential for recurrent or metastatic disease
  - No significant system-specific disease (e.g., cardiac, pulmonary, liver)
  - No primary brain tumors
  - No significant infectious disease, including HIV, hepatitis, syphilis, toxoplasma. Routine serologic testing includes HIV, HTLV, hepatitis B, hepatitis C, CMV, syphilis, and toxoplasma.
  - No donor sepsis
  - Cause of death not due to massive poisoning, with potential for transplanted organ nonfunction (acetaminophen, tricyclic antidepressants, carbon monoxide, cyanide, ethanol)

HIV, human immunodeficiency virus; HTLV, human T-cell leukemia virus; CMV, cytomegalovirus.

Excessive volume losses due to hemorrhage is common in trauma victims. Crystalloid and colloid solutions, as well as blood products (packed red blood cells, fresh-frozen plasma) may be required initially to establish normovolemia. If this initial effort does not result in normalization of blood pressure, a pulmonary artery catheter (or other equivalent noninvasive monitor of cardiac function) should be placed to determine cardiac output and systemic vascular resistance.

Some donors will continue to be hypotensive in the setting of a central venous pressure >12. Often this is the result of a low systemic vascular resistance (<400 dynes/sec/cm) in the setting of neurogenic vasodilatation in the setting of a systemic inflammatory response. The use of vasoactive agents, namely dopamine, at a continuous infusion of 5 to 10 mcg/kg/min or norepinephrine, 2 to 12 mcg/min, may be necessary. Continued hypotension after the institution of these agents should raise the suspicion of donor sepsis.

Some donors may also exhibit depressed cardiac function for a number of reasons (following cardiac arrest, blunt cardiac trauma, or brainstem herniation). Brain death also directly leads to decreased ventricular function because of cardiac beta-receptor desensitization. The use of inotropic and chronotropic agents may be necessary to augment cardiac function to keep cardiac index >2 L/min/m². Agents of choice include continuous infusions of dopamine (as mentioned previously) or dobutamine (at 2 to 5 mcg/kg/min). Also, thyroid hormone replacement has been used to improve myocardial function, but its efficacy remains controversial.

TABLE 68.2	Obtaining Consent for Organ Donation

- Contact local organ-procurement organization (OPO)
- In conjunction with OPO, obtain verbal consent to perform non-invasive testing (blood sampling, ECG, radiology studies) to determine suitability for organ donation
- Establish the diagnosis of brain death (See Chapter 55)
- After brain death has been declared and in conjunction with OPO, obtain written family consent for donation.
- In the absence of brain death, consider the option of "Donation after Cardiac Death" or the so-called "Non-heartbeating Donor."

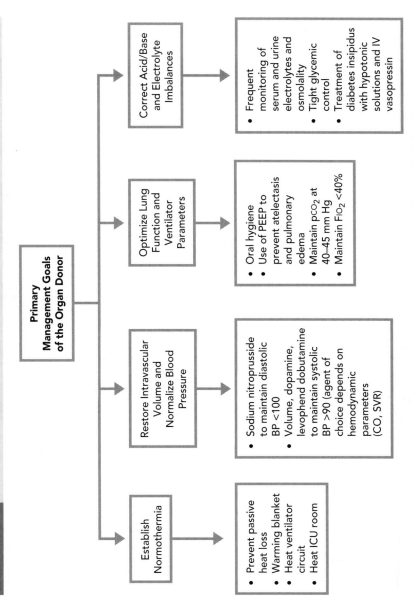

ALGORITHM 68.1   Management Goals of Organ Donor Patients

Primary Management Goals of the Organ Donor

Establish Normothermia
- Prevent passive heat loss
- Warming blanket
- Heat ventilator circuit
- Heat ICU room

Restore Intravascular Volume and Normalize Blood Pressure
- Sodium nitroprusside to maintain diastolic BP <100
- Volume, dopamine, levophend dobutamine to maintain systolic BP >90 (agent of choice depends on hemodynamic parameters (CO, SVR)

Optimize Lung Function and Ventilator Parameters
- Oral hygiene
- Use of PEEP to prevent atelectasis and pulmonary edema
- Maintain pCO_2 at 40–45 mm Hg
- Maintain FiO_2 <40%

Correct Acid/Base and Electrolyte Imbalances
- Frequent monitoring of serum and urine electrolytes and osmolality
- Tight glycemic control
- Treatment of diabetes insipidus with hypotonic solutions and IV vasopressin

ICU, intensive care unit; BP, blood pressure; CO, cardiac output; SVR, systemic vascular resistance; PEEP, positive end-expiratory pressure; IV, intravenous.

PREVENT RESPIRATORY INSUFFICIENCY

Maintenance of pulmonary function using mechanical ventilation must be tailored to prevent partial lung collapse or atelectasis, development of pneumonia, pulmonary edema, and hypoxia or hypercapnia. Good oral hygiene can prevent ventilator-associated pneumonias. Brain-dead patients often develop otherwise unexplained pulmonary edema, also attributed to systemic inflammatory and neurogenic responses. The use of positive end-expiratory pressure of 5 to 10 cm H_2O can offset this increased capillary permeability and maintain alveolar expansion. However, positive end-expiratory pressure levels >10 cm H_2O can impair venous return and negatively impact cardiac output. Ventilator settings should be optimized to maintain arterial PCO_2 at 40 to 45 mm Hg and, whenever possible, at a fraction of inspired oxygen at ≤40% to prevent oxygen toxicity.

CORRECT ACID-BASE AND ELECTROLYTE DISTURBANCES

Brain-dead patients often develop polyuria, with urine outputs in excess of 500 mL/hr. This can be attributed to physiologic, osmotic, chemical (furosemide) and hypothermic diuresis, central diabetes insipidus, or combinations of these. This can lead to profound hypernatremia, hypokalemia, and hyperosmolality. Frequent monitoring of serum and urine osmolality and electrolytes with correction to normal ranges is essential to prevent cardiac dysfunction. Tight control of blood sugars should also be instituted to prevent significant hyperglycemia-related osmotic diuresis.

When other causes of polyuria have been excluded, the diagnosis of diabetes insipidus (DI) can be established by measuring urine output, urine-specific gravity, urine and serum electrolytes, and osmolality. DI is established by three of the following criteria: urine output >500 mL/hr, serum sodium >155 mEq/L, urine-specific gravity <1.005, and serum osmolality >305 mOsm/L. When identified, DI should be treated by replacing 50% of the free water deficit rapidly with hypotonic saline or 5% dextrose in water. Frequent electrolyte and hemodynamic monitoring is essential to correct further imbalances. Refractory cases can be treated with intravenous vasopressin at an initial dose of 10 Units with titration to maintain urine output of 150 to 300 mL/hr. This can decrease plasma hyperosmolality, increase blood pressure, decrease inotrope use, and maintain cardiac output.

SUMMARY

In summary, the management of a patient determined suitable for organ donation focuses on preservation of end-organ function and viability. After the necessary steps are performed to select and consent a patient for donation, the ICU team is responsible for maintenance of normothermia, normalization of blood pressure, optimization of lung function, restoration of intravascular volume, and correction of acid-base and electrolyte disorders. This approach minimizes the effects of brain death on organs suitable for transplant and has the potential to improve long-term allograft function. Many of the steps are also suitable in preserving the viability of organs procured from donation after cardiac death in the absence of brain death.

Suggested Reading

Arbour R. Clinical management of the organ donor. *AACN Clin Issues.* 2005;16:551–580.
  An expanded and detailed guide to the topic of this chaper.
Kutsogiannis DJ, Pagliarello G, Doig C, et al. Medical management to optimize donor organ potential: review of the literature. *Can J Anaesth.* 2006;53:820–830.
  A lengthy review article discussing the evidence supporting management strategies for potential organ donors.
Pratschke J., Wilhelm MJ, Kusaka M, et al. Brain death and its influence on donor organ quality and outcome after transplantation. *Transplantation.* 1999;67:343–348.
  A study that evaluates the influence of the duration of brain death on the eventual outcome of the transplantation procedure.
Whiting JF, Delmonico F, Morrissey P, et al. Clinical results of an organ procurement organization effort to increase utilization of donors after cardiac death. *Transplantation.* 2006;81:1368–1371.
  Randomized study of 186 femoral or radial artery catheters which found similarly low rates of infection between the two sites.

XVIII

NUTRITION IN THE INTENSIVE CARE UNIT
Beth E. Taylor and G. Lee Collins

69

The metabolic response to critical illness is characterized by changes in carbohydrate, fat, and amino acid metabolism. These metabolic changes cause an important shift from an anabolic state to a catabolic state characterized by severe macromolecular breakdown of essential proteins, fats, and carbohydrates. The malnutrition associated with critical illness can have a negative impact on multiple organ systems. This may lead to increased length of stay, increased susceptibility to infection, impairment in respiratory function, ventilator dependence, and overall increase in morbidity and mortality.

The goals of nutrition support in the intensive care unit (ICU) patient are to provide adequate calories and protein to keep up with ongoing losses, prevent or correct nutrient deficiencies, support wound healing, and promote immune function. It is essential when determining the nutritional needs of critically ill patients that one incorporates the severity of disease, organ system involvement, metabolic derangements, gastrointestinal function, and impact of different therapeutic procedures to gain an overall assessment of each individual's need.

In addition to the patient's present status, other components of the nutrition assessment should include preadmission dietary history (specifically, recent intake), recent antecedent weight loss, functional status, alcohol intake, and body mass index (BMI). The patient's BMI may be calculated using either pounds or kilograms (Table 69.1).

Several studies support the use of early feeding in the ICU patient with premorbid malnutrition based on admission BMI (<18.5) or weight loss of >10% during the previous 6 months. Some evidence suggests, if enteral nutrition is to be used early, initiation of feeds within 48 hours of admission may lead to better wound healing and lower infection rates. Otherwise, initiation of nutrition support is indicated in the critically ill patient who is not expected to resume an oral diet in 7 to 10 days (Alg. 69.1). It is important to understand the potential consequences of initiating feeds in patients who have been starved for a period of time. The addition of a large glucose load can cause a massive shift of intracellular electrolytes, specifically potassium, magnesium, and phosphorus. This shift places the patient at risk of the sequelae associated with low serum levels of these electrolytes. This phenomenon is known as *refeeding syndrome* and may lead to serious consequences, including death.

TABLE 69.1	Body Mass Index Calculation

Weight (lbs) × 704/inches² or weight (kg)/m²

70-kg 5'6'' patient	70-kg 5'6'' patient
(70 × 2.2) × 704/(66)²	5'6'' = 66 × 2.54 = 167.64 cm
154 × 704/4356	167.64/100 = 1.67 meters
108416/4356	70/1.67²
24.88	70/2.78
	25.10

A nutrition-focused physical examination should consist of a review of oral health, skin turgor, and assessment for loss of muscle mass in the temporal, deltoid, and quadriceps muscle groups. Initial laboratory assessment should include a basic metabolic profile, magnesium, phosphate (for renal function and risk of refeeding syndrome), hepatic panel, and complete blood count.

Plasma albumin and prealbumin have a low sensitivity and specificity to changes in nutrition intake in the hospitalized patient. Both are affected by a plethora of factors. Levels are increased by corticosteroids, insulin, thyroid hormone, and dehydration. In contrast, levels are decreased by inflammatory mediators, severe liver and renal disease, malabsorption, and intravascular volume overload. In short, albumin and prealbumin levels in the critically ill patient reflect changes in protein synthesis, degradation, and distributive losses that are reflective of critical illness, not nutritional status.

Several equations exist to determine resting energy requirements in humans. The most commonly used is the Harris-Benedict equation (Table 69.2). The American Dietetics Association studied the reliability and validity of several predictive equations in a variety of hospitalized patients. These equations generate values within 10% of measured values in healthy subjects when compared with indirect calorimetry. However, they are much less accurate in persons who are at extremes in weight or who are critically ill. Only the Ireton-Jones equation is designed for use in the critically ill patient; however, it is cumbersome to complete (Table 69.3).

A more simple method for estimating caloric requirements in hospitalized patients has been developed using BMI (Table 69.4). The lower range in each category should be considered for initiation of nutrition support in insulin-resistant critically ill patients to decrease the risk of hyperglycemia and infection associated with overfeeding.

In general, protein needs are based on kilograms of ideal body weight, which can be determined using the Hamwi method (Table 69.5). The increased metabolic rate associated with critical illness along with several other potential factors including renal failure, extent of injury, presence of significant burns, and sepsis may significantly increase the requirements for protein (Table 69.6).

Once the decision to begin nutrition support has been made, the optimal delivery route needs to be determined and feeding initiated (Alg. 69.2). At present, the general consensus is to feed enterally whenever possible.

TABLE 69.2	Harris-Benedict Equation

Men
66 + (13.7 × W) + (5 × H) − (6.8 × A)
Women
665 + (9.6 × W) + (1.8 × H) − (4.7 × A)

W, weight in kilograms; H, height in centimeters; A, age in years.

ALGORITHM 69.1   **Timing of Nutrition Support (Assessment Should Begin within 48 Hours of Admission to the Intensive Care Unit)**

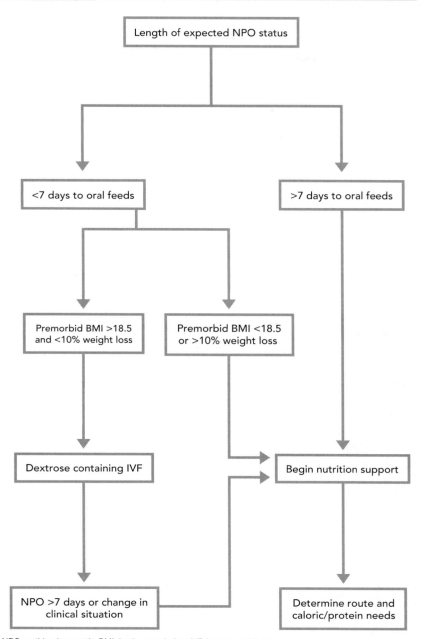

NPO, nothing by mouth; BMI, body mass index; IVF, intravenous fluids.

TABLE 69.3	Ireton-Jones Equation

Ventilator-Dependent patients
1784 − 11(A) + 5(W) + 244(S) + 239(T) + 804(B)

Spontaneously breathing patients
629 − 11(A) + 25(W) − 609(O)

A, age in years; W, weight in kilograms; S, sex (male = 1, female = 0);
T, trauma (present = 1, absent = 0); B, burn (present = 1, absent = 0);
O, obesity—body mass index >27 (present = 1, absent = 0).

TABLE 69.4	Needs Estimated on Body Mass Index (BMI)

BMI	Energy (Kcal/Kg/day)
<15	35–40
15–19	30–35
20–25	20–25
26–29	15–17
>29	15[a]

[a]Do not exceed 2,000 calories per day for obese patients, allowing for mobilization of adipose stores for energy.

TABLE 69.5	Hamwi Method to Determine Ideal Body Weight

Calculate ideal body weight[a]:
Men: 106 pounds for first 5 feet plus 6 pounds for each inch above 5 feet
Women: 100 pounds for the first 5 feet plus 5 pounds for each inch above 5 feet

[a]Conversion from pounds to kilograms: pounds ÷ 2.2.

TABLE 69.6	Recommended Daily Protein Intake[a]

Clinical condition	Protein needs (g/kg IBW/day)[b]
Normal (nonstressed)	0.75
Critical illness/injury	1.00–1.50
Acute renal failure (undialyzed)	0.80–1.00
Acute renal failure (dialyzed)	1.20–1.40
Peritoneal dialysis	1.30–1.50
Burn/sepsis	1.50–2.00
CVVHD	1.70–2.50

IBW, ideal body weight; CVVHD, continuous venovenous hemodialysis.
[a]Clinical conditions are not additive; to calculate needs, use value that prescribes the highest protein needs.
[b]Lower protein requirements may be necessary in hepatic encephalopathy.

ALGORITHM 69.2   **Determination of Route and Initiation of Feeding**

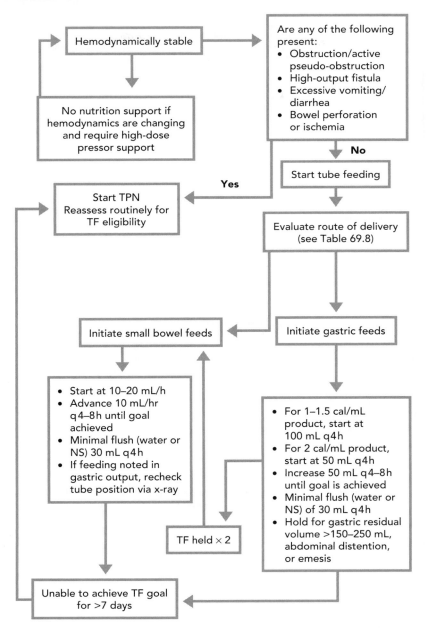

TPN, total parenteral feeding; TF, tube feeding; NS, normal saline.

TABLE 69.7	Advantages and Disadvantages of Enteral and Parenteral Nutrition	

Type of feeding	Advantages	Disadvantages
Enteral nutrition	Preserves gut mucosal integrity Less costly than TPN May blunt hypermetabolic response Less infectious complications	Requires functional GI tract More time to reach goal calories Multiple contraindications (e.g., obstruction, fistula)
Parenteral nutrition	Does not require functioning GI tract Full support in <24 hours	Intestinal atrophy Requires central IV access Increased rate of infectious complications

TPN, total parenteral nutrition; GI, gastrointestinal; IV, intravenous.

Enteral nutrition may be beneficial in protecting gut mucosal integrity Nutrients in the intestinal lumen may limit the migration of bacteria to the portal and systemic circulation, thereby decreasing the risk of sepsis. However, these data are more convincing in the animal model than in humans. Regardless, each route has advantages and disadvantages and conditions in which it is contraindicated (Table 69.7).

In critically ill patients, delivery of enteral feeding into the small bowel has been recommended as a strategy to reduce the risk of aspiration. Randomized controlled studies of gastric versus small bowel feeding in ICU patients have been inconclusive. However, patients who had significant risk factors for aspiration or who had gastric feeding intolerance were excluded from these studies. These patients may benefit from placement of a postpyloric feeding tube (Table 69.8). Whether the tube feeding is provided pre- or postpyloric, other than increased gastric residual volume, the recommendations to troubleshoot complications are the same (Table 69.9).

The appropriate type of tube feeding formula to use in the critically ill patient continues to be debated. Based on the current evidence, whole-protein formulas are recommended unless symptoms of malabsorption are present, then a peptide-based product should be

TABLE 69.8	Gastric and Small Bowel Feeding Indications

Gastric feeding	Small bowel feeding
▪ Majority of ICU patients ▪ Short gut (to maximize surface area fed) ▪ Total laryngectomies (cannot aspirate)	▪ Delayed gastric emptying ▪ Postoperative gastric ileus ▪ Severe gastroesophageal reflux disease ▪ Severe pancreatitis (unable to resume PO in 5–7 days) ▪ Proximal gastrointestinal fistula ▪ Intolerance to gastric feeds (despite prokinetic use); high gastric residual volumes, emesis ▪ Supine positioning ▪ Patients unable to protect their airway secondary to heavy sedation (Ramsey >5)

ICU, intensive care unit; PO, by mouth.

TABLE 69.9	Troubleshooting Tube Feeding Complications

Residuals: Gastric residual volume of 150 mL or more on more than one consecutive reading.
- Clinically examine for signs of intolerance: abdominal distention, fullness, discomfort, or presence of emesis.
- Start a prokinetic agent: IV metoclopramide 10 mg q 6 hours (if no renal failure present).
- Change to a more calorically dense product to decrease total volume infused.
- If a *Moss tube* is present, normal gastric output may reach 2 L/day because of drainage of proximal duodenum.
- Presence of a small amount of tube feeding from the gastric port is normal.
- A large amount of feedings may indicate malabsorption or incorrect positioning of the Moss tube.
- Order a small bowel feeding tube.

Diarrhea: Quantify amount of stool. It is normal for a patient on tube feedings to have four to five soft formed stools per day.
- Review medications. Diarrhea may be secondary to an enteral medication. Try changing medication route to IV.
- Rule out the presence of *Clostridium difficile*.
- Try adding a soluble fiber to feeds (Benefiber 1 Tbsp TID).
- Once infectious cause is ruled out, use an antidiarrheal agent (loperamide 2–4 mg q6h)
- KEEP FEEDING

Constipation: Difficulty passing or no bowel movement >3 days after feedings are at goal.
- Check for signs of dehydration, such as hypernatremia, prerenal azotemia, oliguria, low skin turgor, orthostatic hypotension
- Increase amount of free water.
- Rectal examination with disimpaction.
- Order KUB to rule out obstruction
- Once obstruction is ruled out, start bisacodyl suppository and/or enemas PRN.
- Start bowel regimen (docusate, 100 mg BID, and/or senna syrup, 5 mL BID).

IV, intravenous; TID, three times a day; KUB, kidney/ureter/bladder x-ray; PRN, as needed; BID, two times a day.

initiated. Studies using immune-modulating formulas (those enriched with glutamine, arginine, omega-3 fatty acids, antioxidants, or nucleotides) have been found to be positive in elective upper gastrointestinal surgical patients and trauma patients. Strong evidence supports the use of enteral glutamine in burn patients. No benefit of immune-modulating formulas has been established in patients with severe sepsis; in fact. products containing arginine may be harmful in these patients. Advantage has been shown with the use of formulas containing antioxidants and omega-3 fatty acids for patients with pulmonary capillary leak syndromes (acute respiratory distress syndrome or acute lung injury). At this point, there is no standard of care, and immune-modulating formulas continue to be controversial in the literature.

Critically ill patients presenting with injuries (traumatic brain injury) or conditions (severe dysphagia due to cerebral vascular accident) that will require >4 weeks of enteral support benefit from early placement of long-term feeding access. For conditions requiring <4 weeks of therapy, placement of short-term feeding access via the nose or mouth should be instituted. Several options of both short- and long-term access and their associated risks are reviewed in Table 69.10.

Total parenteral nutrition (TPN) must be administered via a designated port of a central venous catheter to avoid potential complications associated with incompatibilities with intravenous medication administration. Parenteral nutrition via a peripheral intravenous line is not appropriate for the critically ill patient. Subclavian lines are preferred because of the ease in maintaining an occlusive dressing and the lower rate of infectious. The least

TABLE 69.10	Short- and Long-Term Enteral Feeding Access

- **Salem Sump Nasogastric or Orogastric:** a short-term feeding tube generally placed by the bedside nurse for decompression that may be used for feeding. The patient must have a functioning GI tract, adequate gastric-emptying, and low risk of aspiration. Nasally placed tubes carry the risk of sinusitis and nasal necrosis.
- **Nasoenteric feeding tube** for gastric or small bowel placement: a short-term, softer, more flexible tube with less risk of causing sinusitis or nasal necrosis, this tube may also be placed orally. Generally placed in patients for comfort. Small bowel tubes are placed in patients with poor gastric-emptying and have a high risk of reflux.
- **G-tube**[a] for surgical or percutaneous endoscopic gastrostomy: a long-term feeding tube for patients with a functioning GI tract and adequate gastric-emptying. G-tubes have a lower risk of aspiration when compared with above-the-diaphragm feeding access.
- **J-tube**[a] for surgical or percutaneous endoscopic jejunostomy: a long-term feeding tube indicated for patients with a functioning GI tract, poor gastric-emptying, and a high risk for reflux and aspiration.
- **G-J tube**[a]: a long-term feeding tube placed at time of laparotomy in patients for feeding into the distal duodenum with a gastric port for decompression.

GI, gastrointestinal.
[a]All tubes that transverse the two epithelial barriers of the skin and mucosa of the GI tract carry the risk of hemorrhage and infection at the incision site as well as peritonitis and risk of dislodgment.

desirable is a femoral line that has been associated with a higher incidence of venous thrombosis. The choice of catheter type depends on the reason for TPN, expected duration of TPN, and the patient's overall status (Table 69.11).

When TPN is provided, the practitioner must be knowledgeable regarding the form in which electrolytes are provided, the normal amount recommended, and what conditions should precipitate an alteration in the amount provided (Table 69.12). One must be vigilant when prescribing the various electrolytes that are provided in TPN as there are inherent

TABLE 69.11	Catheter Selection for Total Parenteral Nutrition (TPN)

- **Triple/quad lumen catheter:** used for in-hospital patients on TPN. The distal port is preferred for the infusion of TPN solution to maintain sterility and avoid contamination. Blood is drawn through the medial port and other infusions are performed through the proximal port(s).
- **PICC (peripheral inserted central catheter):** PICC lines are placed via the brachiocephalic vein. PICC lines have a long catheter (60 cm) with the tip positioned in the superior vena cava.
- **Tunneled catheter:** This is a silastic catheter (single-, double-, or triple-lumen) that is tunneled subcutaneously several centimeters from the insertion site before exiting the skin. If no infection is present, these catheters can stay in place indefinitely.
- **Hohn:** A percutaneously placed catheter used for patients requiring 6 months or less of TPN or IV medication. The distal port (red) is preferred for the infusion of TPN solution to maintain sterility and avoid contamination.
- **Implanted venous access device:** This is a subcutaneously implanted chamber attached to a silastic central venous catheter, either single- or double-lumen. Because the reservoir is implanted in the SQ, it must be accessed with a needle for drawing blood or administering TPN or other IV infusions. These catheters are generally reserved for patients receiving chemotherapy who require periodic infusions.

IV, intravenous.

TABLE 69.12	Electrolytes Administered Via the Total Parenteral Nutrition Solution	
Suggested electrolytes (per liter)	Conditions that may require alteration of amount provided	Electrolyte carriers
Sodium 60–150 mEq	■ Renal function ■ Fluid status ■ GI losses ■ Traumatic brain injury	NaCl Na acetate NaPO$_4$
Potassium 40–120 mEq	■ Renal function ■ GI losses ■ Metabolic acidosis ■ Refeeding	KCl K acetate KPO$_4$
Phosphate 10–30 mM	■ Renal function ■ Refeeding ■ Bone disease ■ Hypercalcemia ■ Rapid healing[a] ■ Hepatic function	NaPO$_4$ KPO$_4$
Chloride 60–120 mEq	■ Renal function ■ GI losses (gastric) ■ Acid-base status	NaCl KCl
Acetate 10–40 mEq	■ Renal function ■ GI losses (small bowel) ■ Acid-base status ■ Hepatic function	NaAcetate KAcetate
Calcium 4.5–.2 mEq	■ Hyperparathyroidism ■ Malignancy ■ Bone disease ■ Immobilization ■ Acute pancreatitis ■ Renal function	Ca Gluconate CaCl$_2$
Magnesium 8.1–24.3 mEq	■ Renal function ■ Refeeding ■ Hypokalemia	Mg sulfate

GI, gastrointestinal.
[a]Rapid healing examples are burn, and young trauma patients who have rapid tissue generation.

risks associated with its administration. This is balanced with the need to avoid exceeding amounts, which may lead to precipitation with the TPN solution itself.

Clinicians often underestimate the importance of nutrition support in the ICU patient population. Early intervention by a nutrition support specialist as part of the multidisciplinary team is imperative to ensure that appropriate access is obtained and substrates provided. Understanding the massive catabolic state that exists with critical illness underscores the need for early and precise nutritional support. Early replacement of ongoing losses of micro- and macronutrients will aid in the patient's recovery once the critical illness has resolved and the anabolic building phase has commenced.

Suggested Reading
ASPEN Board of Directors and the Clinical Guidelines Task Force. Guidelines for the use of parenteral and enteral nutrition in adult and pediatric patients. *J Parenter Enter Nutr.* 2002;26[Suppl]:1–138.

American Society of Parenteral and Enteral Nutrition clinical guideline task force from 2002 which reviewed the literature and made recommendation based on the evidenced for nutritional support in the clinically ill.

Dabrowski GP, Rombeau JL. Practical nutritional management in the trauma intensive care unit. *Surg Clin North Am.* 2000;80:921–932.

A practical overview of nutritional management of the trauma patient.

Heyland DK, Dhaliwal R, Drover JW, et al. Canadian clinical practice guidelines for nutritional support in mechanically ventilated, critically ill adult patients. *J Parenter Enter Nutr.* 2003;27:355–373.

Canadian evidence-based practice guidelines for nutrition support in mechanically ventilated patients.

Heyland DK, Novak F, Drover JW, et al. Should immunonutrition become routine in critically ill patients? A systemic review of the evidence. *JAMA.* 2001;286:944–953.

In elective surgery patients immunonutrition is associated with a reduction in infectious complication rates and a shorter LOS. However, there was not a mortality advantage.

Kreymann KG, Berger MM, Deutz NE, et al. ESPEN guidelines on enteral nutrition: intensive care. *Clin Nutr.* 2006;25:210–223.

Consensus guidelines based on review of the literature since 1985 for enteral nutrition support in the critically ill with at least one organ failure.

Kudsk KA. Effect of route and type of nutrition on intestine-derived inflammatory responses. *Am J Surg.* 2003;185:16–21.

This review article looked at the effects on the gastrointestinal from lack of feeding. Findings included an increase in proinflammatory markers and showed that the addition of glutamine reverses many of the defects seen in starvation in the critically ill.

Pontes-Arruda Alessandro, Aragao AM, Albuquerque JP, et al. Effects of enteral feeding with eicosapentaenoic acid, γ-linolenic acid, and antioxidants in mechanically ventilated patients with severe sepsis and septic shock. *Crit Care Med.* 2006;34:2325–2333.

This study showed that in patients with severe septic shock requiring mechanical ventilation who were tolerating enteral feeding, a diet rich in EPA, GLA, and antioxidants imparted improved ICU and hospital outcomes and was associated with decrease mortality.

ARTERIAL CATHETERIZATION
Timothy J. Bedient
70

Arterial catheterization is the second most frequently performed invasive procedure in the intensive care unit after central venous catheterization. Indications for placing an arterial line include (a) frequent arterial blood gas measurements in patients with respiratory insufficiency, (b) direct arterial hemodynamic monitoring in patients on vasopressor or inotropic support, and (b) less commonly, for placement of an intra-aortic balloon pump or direct arterial administration of drugs (e.g., thrombolytics). Noninvasive arterial oxygen saturation is insufficient in unstable patients, and frequent direct measurement of the arterial pH, bicarbonate, and partial pressure of oxygen and carbon dioxide is often needed in patients on ventilator support or with suspected impending respiratory collapse. In unstable patients, noninvasive blood pressure monitors can be inaccurate, significantly underestimating blood pressure, necessitating the use of arterial lines for accurate hemodynamic monitoring.

Equipment required for catheterization includes (a) an intravascular catheter, (b) noncompliant tubing, (c) flush device with pressurized flush solution, (d) transducer, and (e) electronic monitoring equipment including a connecting cable and a monitor with an amplifier and display screen. Catheter sizes vary on the basis of arterial site (see following discussion) and, once inserted, are connected to the tubing The tubing is connected to the transducer, which in turn is connected to the electronic monitor via a connecting cable. The noncompliant tubing transmits the pressure waveform from the artery to the transducer, which converts the pressure waveform to an electrical waveform. The electric waveform is amplified and displayed on the oscilloscope screen. The flush device allows continuous fluid infusion to prevent thrombus formation and is pressurized to prevent backup of high-pressure arterial blood into the tubing.

The most common site selected for arterial catheterization is the radial artery, followed by the femoral artery. Less common sites include the dorsalis pedis, brachial, and axillary arteries. Although both radial and femoral sites are acceptable and have a similar complication profile, the radial site is generally attempted first.

The radial and ulnar arteries are the distal branches of the brachial artery and are located on the lateral and medial sides of the wrists in anatomic position, respectively. They

473

are connected to one another by the deep and superficial palmar arches in the hand. These arterial anastomoses are taken into consideration when a radial line is placed, as a potential complication of radial artery catheterization is thrombosis. If thrombosis occurs, collateral circulation from the ulnar artery through the palmar arches typically ensures adequate blood flow to the hand. Peripheral vascular disease that occludes the palmar arches could interrupt blood flow to the hand if radial artery thrombus occurs.

The modified Allen test is used in an attempt to identify patients who have compromised collateral palmar circulation. The test is performed by raising the patients arm to 45 degrees, with the examiner compressing the radial and ulnar arteries with both hands. The patient is asked to repeatedly open and close the hand to drain the blood from it. When pallor develops, one artery is released and the time to palmar flushing is timed. Less than 7 seconds is considered positive, 8 to 14 seconds is equivocal, and 15 or more seconds is considered a negative test and evidence for a lack of adequate collateral circulation. The test is repeated with the other artery.

One study compared Allen test to Doppler ultrasound examination. The study found the test had a sensitivity of 87%, meaning that patients who had a positive Allen test also had ultrasound documentation of collateral flow 87% of the time. However, the negative predictive value was only 18%, meaning that only 18% of patients who had a negative Allen test had documented lack of collateral circulation by ultrasound. In addition, many patients in whom arterial lines are placed have decreased mental status and cannot participate in the test. Results may also be difficult to interpret for patients on vasopressor support. Thus, many centers have now abandoned the routine performance of the Allen test.

Two types of arterial catheters are commonly in use. The most basic is a catheter-over-needle apparatus. The other is also a catheter-over-needle, but with the addition of a guidewire. Peripheral sites, including the radial artery, are generally cannulated with a 20-gage Teflon catheter. Larger vessels such as the femoral artery are cannulated with an 18-gage Teflon catheter kit containing introducer needles and guide wire.

STEPS FOR RADIAL ARTERY CANNULATION

1. Position the supine patient's hand with 30 to 60 degrees of extension by propping the dorsal wrist surface on a rolled towel or other supporting structure with the ventral surface up.
2. Remove all objects from the wrist and cleanse the wrist's ventral surface with an antiseptic solution such as chlorhexidine or Betadine.
3. Drape the wrist in a sterile fashion and with sterile technique including sterile drapes, gloves, gown, and a mask (a reasonable rule is to gown and mask when placing objects in a patient that will remain in place and be a potential source of infection).
4. Palpate the radial artery on the patient's ventral wrist with the first two fingers of the nondominant hand 3 to 4 cm proximal to the crease at the base of the thenar eminence.
5. With the dominant hand, hold the catheter like a pencil between the first and second fingers.
6. While palpating gently with the nondominant hand, enter the skin at a 30- to 45-degree angle with the catheter tip just distal (relative to the patient) to the fingertips of the nondominant hand (Fig. 70.1). Pressing too firmly on the radial artery can occlude flow and make cannulation difficult.
7. Advance the catheter toward the artery until a flash of blood enters the catheter tip.
8. If using a simple catheter-over-needle configuration, advance the tip of the needle slightly further into the artery to ensure that the tip of the catheter is in the arterial lumen (note: go to step 12 if using a device with a wire).
9. Drop the needle and catheter so that they lie flat on the skin (instead of at a 30- to 45-degree angle).
10. While holding the needle steady with the nondominant hand, advance the catheter gently forward into the artery lumen with a slight twisting motion.
11. Remove the needle; correct placement should result in pulsatile blood flow (if using a catheter without a wire go to step 15).
12. If using a catheter with a wire, when the flash of blood occurs, hold the catheter and needle steady and advance the wire into the arterial lumen, which should meet little resistance.

13. Now advance the catheter over the wire and into the arterial lumen.
14. Remove the needle and wire; correct placement should result in pulsatile blood flow.
15. Connect the catheter to the transducer tubing and flush device.
16. Secure the catheter securely to the skin, usually with suture or noninvasive device.
17. Cleanse the skin and catheter with antiseptic solution and cover with sterile dressing.

TIPS

If the initial attempt is unsuccessful, reposition the catheter and try again. A less steep angle may decrease your chance of traversing the artery. If further attempts are unsuccessful, try advancing the needle through the artery when the initial flash of blood is seen in the catheter tip. Then slowly withdraw the catheter until a flash of blood again occurs and attempt to advance the catheter into the arterial lumen. Deliberate palpation of the artery and focused technique will aid in a successful result. The artery often is transfixed initially with no blood flow. Thus, the catheter should always be withdrawn slowly as success is often achieved while withdrawing the catheter.

For *femoral artery cannulation,* a kit identical to the central venous catheterization kit is often used. The femoral artery lies in the femoral triangle bordered superiorly by the inguinal ligament, laterally by the sartorius muscle, and medially by the adductor longus muscle. From the lateral to medial positions in the triangle lie the femoral nerve, femoral artery, and femoral vein. The site should be cleaned and prepared in a sterile fashion. Similar to the radial artery, the femoral artery is palpated with the nondominant hand. Cannulation of the artery is performed in the same manner as venous cannulation (see Chapter 71), but when blood returns into the syringe and it is disconnected from the needle, pulsatile blood confirms arterial placement (although it may be nonpulsatile during cardiac arrest).

Complications of arterial line placement are listed in Table 70.1. The incidence of clinically significant complications is <5% at most centers. Thrombosis is the most common complication. The Thunder Project in 1993 by the American Association of Critical Care Nurses randomized 5,193 patients with arterial lines to heparinized and nonheparinized flush solutions and followed catheter patency for up to 72 hours. The study found that arterial lines maintained with heparin had a greater probability of remaining patent than lines maintained without heparin. Multiple meta-analyses have confirmed lower thrombosis rates when lines are maintained with a continuous infusion of heparin, generally at a heparin concentration of 1 U/mL and a rate of 3 mL/hr. For patients with contraindications to heparin, a continuous infusion with sodium citrate or saline should be used.

Infection also occurs with arterial line placement, and its incidence can be minimized with careful sterile technique during catheter placement and routine catheter care. Catheter dressings should be changed approximately every 48 hours. Careful sterile technique should be used when drawing blood samples from the catheter. The incidence of catheter-related infections for arterial lines does not differ based on site (i.e., radial vs. femoral) if sterile technique is used. Also, catheters kept in place longer than 7 days have not demonstrated

TABLE 70.1	Complications of Arterial Cannulation
Thrombosis	
Local or systemic infection	
Hematoma	
Pseudoaneurysm	
Hemorrhage	
Significant blood loss from frequent blood testing	
Heparin-induced thrombocytopenia (for heparin-flushed lines)	
Retroperitoneal hematoma (femoral lines)	
Limb ischemia	
Peripheral neuropathy	
Insertion site pain	

significantly higher rates of serious infections. In part due to higher pressure blood flow, arterial lines are less likely to become infected than central venous lines. For febrile patients, arterial lines do not necessarily need to be removed unless no other infectious source is identified. When catheters do become infected, the most common pathogen is *Staphylococcus epidermidis*. Catheters should be removed as soon as they are no longer needed.

Suggested Reading

American Association of Critical-Care Nurses. Evaluation of the effects of heparinized and nonheparinized flush solutions on the patency of arterial pressure monitoring lines: the AACN Thunder Project. *Am J Crit Care.* 1993;1:3–15.

Randomized trial of 5139 patients with arterial lines assigned to heparinized and nonheparinized flush solutions and followed for up to 72 hours, showing lines maintained with heparin had a significantly greater probability of remaining patent over time than lines maintained with nonheparinized solutions.

Glavin RJ, Jones HM. Assessing collateral circulation in the hand: four methods compared. *Anesthesia.* 1989;44:594–595.

Study comparing the Allen=s test, ultrasound, pulse monitor, and pulse oximeter to detect collateral circulation in the hand, showing that none, when compared with ultrasound, reliably documented adequate ulnar collateral circulation.

Thomas F, Burke JP, Parker J, et al. The risk of infection related to radial vs. femoral sites for arterial catheterization. *Crit Care Med.* 1983;10:807–812.

Randomized study of 186 femoral or radial artery catheters which found similarly low rates of infection between the two sites.

CENTRAL VENOUS CATHETERIZATION

Chad A. Witt

71

Central venous catheterization is commonly performed in the intensive care unit. Indications for central venous catheterization include administration of vasoactive medications, total parenteral nutrition, or other agents necessitating central venous access, central venous pressure monitoring, rapid large-volume fluid or blood product administration, and emergency venous access. Contraindications for central venous catheterization include known thrombosis of the target vessel and infection over the site of entry. There is no definitive cut-off for the performance of central venous catheterization in coagulopathic or thrombocytopenic patients, although the use of a micropuncture kit and/or correction with fresh-frozen plasma and/or platelet transfusion may be pertinent in this population prior to the procedure.

The most common complications of central venous catheterization include arterial puncture, pneumothorax, hydrothorax, hemothorax, air embolus, retroperitoneal hemorrhage, infections (central venous catheter-associated bacteremia, local site infection/cellulitis), and thromboembolic disease. Overall, the complication rate is related to the site of insertion, with the subclavian vein being less than the internal jugular vein, which is less than the femoral vein. The use of ultrasound guidance to aid in the placement of central venous catheters, especially in the internal jugular position, has been shown to decrease complication rates, decrease the number of attempts necessary to cannulate the vein, and decrease the amount of time necessary to perform the procedure.

Before performing central venous catheterization, obtain informed consent based on the policies of each institution. All present must agree on the patient identification, the procedure being performed, and the site of the procedure. Sterile precautions must be observed, including hand hygiene with alcohol foam/gel or antimicrobial soap, full sterile drape, sterile gloves, sterile gown, mask with face shield, and hair coverage. All persons present in the room should wear masks and hair coverage. It is helpful to have a nonsterile assistant present during the procedure.

The following guidelines are for the placement of central venous catheters using commercially available kits via Seldinger's (over guidewire) technique.

SUBCLAVIAN CENTRAL VENOUS CATHETER PLACEMENT

1. Place the patient in Trendelenburg position, and place a towel roll between the scapulae. Turn the head opposite from the side of line placement.
2. Don sterile gown, sterile gloves, mask with face shield, and hair cover.
3. Prepare with antiseptic solution (e.g., chlorhexidine or Betadine).
4. Use a sterile full-body drape and a sterile drape with a site hole or surgical towels to cover the body, head, and face, exposing only the necessary skin.
5. Flush all ports of the catheter to ensure appropriate functioning.
6. Place the index finger of the nondominant hand at the sternal notch and the thumb of the same hand on the clavicle where it bends over the first rib (approximately where the lateral third and medial two-thirds of the clavicle meet). The subclavian vein should traverse a line between the index finger and the thumb (Fig. 71.1).
7. Anesthetize the skin and subcutaneous tissue just inferior to the clavicle and lateral to the thumb.

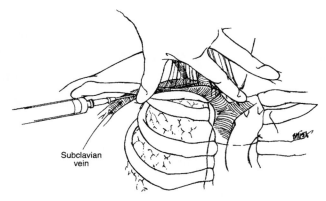

Subclavian
vein

Figure 71.1. Subclavian vein anatomy and cannulation. (From Lin TL, Mohart JM, Sakurai KA. *The Washington Manual Internship Survival Guide,* 2e. Philadelphia: Lippincott Williams & Wilkins; 2001:195.)

8. With the introducer needle, bevel up, enter the skin lateral to the thumb, inferior to the clavicle (approximately 2 cm inferior and 2 cm lateral to the bend in the clavicle). Aim at the index finger (sternal notch), aspirating while advancing. It is imperative to keep the needle parallel to the floor during advancement. If the clavicle is contacted, depress the entire needle with the thumb until it passes under the clavicle, rather than changing the angle of approach. Dark blood will enter the syringe when the vein is cannulated. If there is no blood return after advancing the needle 5 cm, withdraw the needle while continuing to aspirate (frequently the vein has been pierced, and successful blood flow will be obtained during withdrawal). Redirect the needle more cephalad, and try again. Multiple repeated attempts are not recommended (Fig. 71.1). Once appropriate venous return is noted, rotate the bevel of the needle inferior.

9. Securely hold the needle, remove the syringe (always place a finger over the needle hub to reduce the risk of air embolism), and insert the guidewire. The guidewire should advance with little resistance. If resistance is met, remove the guidewire, withdraw blood with the syringe to ensure that the needle is still in the vein, and advance the guidewire again. Leave enough of the guidewire outside the body to account for the catheter length.

10. While holding the guidewire *(NEVER LET GO OF THE GUIDEWIRE),* remove the introducer needle. Once the introducer needle is outside the patient's skin, hold the guidewire at the entry site and slide the needle off the guidewire.

11. Using a scalpel, make a small nick in the skin at the entry site. Ensure that the cutting edge of the scalpel is facing away from the guidewire and make a stabbing in-out motion to make the nick.

12. Pass the dilator over the guidewire, dilate the tract, and remove the dilator.

13. Ensure that the distal port of the catheter is open. Pass the catheter over the guidewire. When the catheter is near the entry site, feed the guidewire out until it emerges from the distal port on the catheter. Grasp the guidewire distally, and insert the catheter to the desired depth.

14. Hold the catheter in place, and withdraw the guidewire.

15. Flush all ports to ensure that they are functioning properly.

16. Secure the catheter with suture or a commercially available sutureless kit.

17. Cleanse the site with antiseptic solution and place a sterile dressing.

18. Obtain a stat chest radiograph for placement. The tip of the catheter should reside in the superior vena cava.

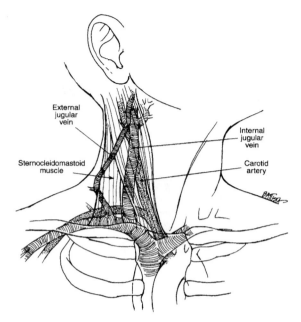

Figure 71.2. Internal jugular vein anatomy. (From Lin TL, Mohart JM, Sakurai KA. *The Washington Manual Internship Survival Guide,* 2e. Philadelphia: Lippincott Williams & Wilkins; 2001:191.)

INTERNAL JUGULAR CENTRAL VENOUS CATHETER PLACEMENT

(Note: ultrasound guidance is preferable, if available.)

1. Place the patient in Trendelenburg position, and have the patient turn his or her head 45 degrees to the direction opposite the site of catheter placement.
2. Don sterile gown, sterile gloves, mask with face shield, and hair cover.
3. Prepare the skin with antiseptic solution (e.g., chlorhexidine or Betadine).
4. Use a sterile full-body drape and a sterile drape with a site hole or surgical towels to cover the body, head, and face, exposing only the necessary skin.
5. Flush all ports of the catheter to ensure appropriate functioning.
6. Identify the triangle formed by the two heads of the sternocleidomastoid muscle and the sternum, and palpate the carotid pulse (Fig. 71.2).
7. Anesthetize the skin and subcutaneous tissue.
8. Palpate the carotid pulse. Lateral to the carotid pulse, advance the 22-gage needle (finder needle), bevel up, at a 30- to 45-degree angle to the patient, directed at the ipsilateral nipple while aspirating. If no venous blood return is noted, withdraw the needle and change the angle to a more lateral and then more medial position. Maintain palpation of the carotid pulse. When venous blood is aspirated, make note of the angle and depth of the finder needle, and remove the finder needle. *If the carotid artery is entered (bright red and/or pulsatile blood), remove the needle and hold pressure for 10 to 15 minutes.*
9. At the same site and angle as the internal jugular vein was entered with the finder needle, insert the introducer needle until free flow of dark venous blood is noted (Fig. 71.3).
10. Follow steps 10 through 19 for subclavian central venous catheter placement.

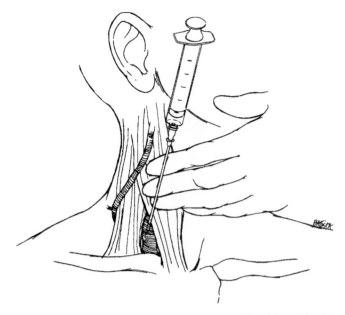

Figure 71.3. Cannulation of the internal jugular vein. (From Lin TL, Mohart JM, Sakurai KA. *The Washington Manual Internship Survival Guide,* 2e. Philadelphia: Lippincott Williams & Wilkins; 2001:192.)

FEMORAL CENTRAL VENOUS CATHETER PLACEMENT

1. Place the patient in the supine position, with the ipsilateral thigh slightly abducted and externally rotated.
2. Don sterile gown, sterile gloves, mask with face shield, and hair cover.
3. Prepare the skin with antiseptic solution (e.g., chlorhexidine or Betadine).
4. Use a sterile full-body drape and a sterile drape with a site hole or surgical towels to cover the body and legs, exposing only the necessary skin.
5. Flush all ports of the catheter to ensure appropriate functioning.
6. Palpate the femoral arterial pulse inferior to the inguinal ligament. The femoral vein is medial to the femoral artery (Fig. 71.4).
7. Anesthetize the skin and subcutaneous tissues, aspirating prior to injecting anesthetic.
8. Palpate the femoral pulse. With the introducer needle bevel up, enter the skin 1 cm medial to the pulse, inferior to the inguinal ligament, at a 30- to 45-degree angle (Fig. 71.5). Continue to aspirate as the needle is advanced until the return of venous blood. If the needle is advanced 5 cm with no return of venous blood, withdraw while continuing to aspirate, angle more medially, and try again. *If the femoral artery is entered (bright red and/or pulsatile blood), hold pressure for 10 to 15 minutes.*
9. Follow steps 10 through 18 for subclavian central ve catheter placement.

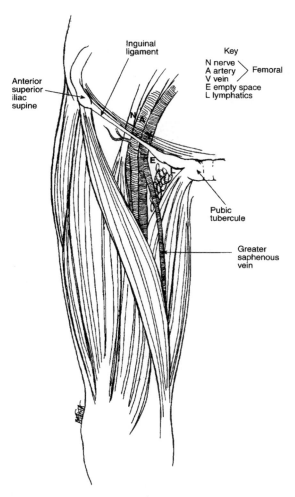

Figure 71.4. Femoral vein anatomy. (From Lin TL, Mohart JM, Sakurai KA. *The Washington Manual Internship Survival Guide,* 2e. Philadelphia: Lippincott Williams & Wilkins; 2001:183.)

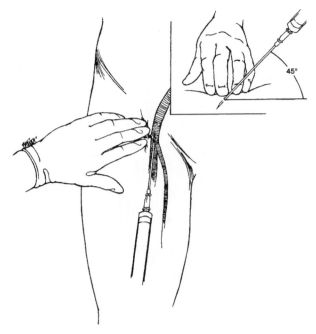

Figure 71.5. Femoral vein cannulation. (From Lin TL, Mohart JM, Sakurai KA. *The Washington Manual Internship Survival Guide,* 2e. Philadelphia: Lippincott Williams & Wilkins; 2001:197.)

Suggested Reading

Hind D, Calvert N, McWilliams R, et al. Ultrasonic locating devices for central venous cannulation: meta-analysis. *BMJ.* 2003;327:361.
Meta-analysis examining the utility and benefit of two dimensional ultrasound and doppler guidance for central venous catheter placement.
Lin TL, Mohart JM, Sakurai KA. *The Washington Manual Internship Survival Guide,* 2e. Philadelphia: Lippincott Williams & Wilkins; 2001:157–164.
Concise instructions on the indications, complications, and placement of central venous catheters.
McGee DC, Gould MK. Preventing complications of central venous catheterization. *N Engl J Med.* 2003;348:1123–1133.
Review of central venous catheter placement, and the various intervention and practice techniques available to reduce and/or prevent complications of central venous catheterization.

ENDOTRACHEAL INTUBATION

Michael Lippman

72

Endotracheal intubation maintains airway patency, assures delivery of preset tidal volume breaths from mechanical ventilators, facilitates pulmonary toilet, and helps prevent aspiration. Indications for endotracheal intubation include acute airway obstruction from trauma, infection, laryngeal edema or spasm or tumor; inability to protect the upper airway because of altered mental status from trauma, drug overdose, or cerebrovascular accident; respiratory failure and cardiopulmonary arrest (Table 72.1).

Risks include trauma to the oropharynx, hypoxemia from prolonged attempts, and unrecognized misplacement of the endotracheal tube. The incidence of complications markedly increases when intubation is attempted by inadequately trained or inexperienced providers. These providers should attempt to achieve adequate ventilation and oxygenation using bag-valve-mask devices or other advanced airway devices that do not require visualization of the vocal cords to place.

Assessment of the upper airway anatomy facilitates recognition of potentially difficult intubations allowing practitioners formulate alternative plans and to assemble necessary equipment. An abbreviated assessment should be performed even in emergent cases. Clinicians should pay particular attention to dentition and the presence of dental appliances, the mobility of the tongue and its size relative to the oropharynx (Mallampati classification; Fig. 72.1), range of extension and flexion of the cervical spine, mobility of the jaw, and presence of stridor. Difficult intubation may be anticipated in patients with thick or fat necks, narrow mouth openings, large tongues, and limited motion of the cervical spine.

All necessary equipment should be immediately available prior to intubation attempts. Necessary equipment includes a bag-valve-mask device, high-flow oxygen source, suction equipment, functioning laryngoscope handles and blades, appropriate-sized endotracheal tube (7.5 to 8.5 cm for most adults), stylet, syringe for endotracheal balloon inflation, medications for induction (if indicated), tape or other mechanism for securing the endotracheal tube, and a device to confirm placement of the tube in the trachea.

Successful intubation requires overcoming the normal barriers to objects entering the trachea. These include reflexes arising from laryngeal stimulation, the malalignment of the major axes of the upper airway, and the anatomic barriers of the tongue and epiglottis. Endotracheal intubation is an extremely uncomfortable procedure and even patients with decreased mental status may cough and actively resist attempts at intubation. Additionally, laryngeal stimulation increases sympathetic tone, with consequent increases in blood pressure, heart rate, and intracranial pressure.

Judicious use of appropriate medications can blunt the potential adverse physiologic effects and provide sedation and amnesia. Lidocaine given as a 1.5- to 2-mg/kg bolus at least 2 minutes prior to intubation can blunt increases in intracranial pressures and is used in patients with head trauma. Agents producing sedation and anesthesia include opioids, benzodiazepines, barbiturates, etomidate, and ketamine. Decisions regarding use of specific agents are based on knowledge of their advantages and disadvantages relative to the patient's clinical status and comorbidities (Table 72.2). Paralytic agents should be used only by practitioners who are highly skilled in endotracheal intubation.

The "sniffing" position helps align the oral, laryngeal, and pharyngeal axes (Fig. 72.2). This position is attained by flexing the neck approximately 30 degrees and extending the

TABLE 72.1	Indications for Endotracheal Intubation

- Acute airway obstruction
- Inability to protect the airway
- Respiratory failure
- Cardiopulmonary arrest

head at the atlanto-occipital joint to 20 degrees. Placement of a towel under the occiput facilitates maintenance of this position.

The laryngoscope is used to displace the tongue and lift the epiglottis away from the glottic opening. Laryngoscope blades vary in size and shape. Blade sizes range from 0 to 4, with higher the number corresponding to larger blades. The curved (MacIntosh) blade has broad, flat surface and tall flange. Straight blades include Miller, Wisconsin, and Phillips. The straight blades vary with regard to their width, presence and size of flange, and shape of distal end. Curved blades apply upward traction to the base of the tongue at the vallecula, indirectly lifting the epiglottis (Fig. 72.3) and straight blades lift the epiglottis directly (Fig. 72.4). Choice of specific equipment should be left to the individual practitioner. In general, straight blades allow visualization of a larger portion of the vocal cords as the epiglottis is removed from the field of view. It may be difficult to control a large tongue with a Miller blade, which is relatively narrow.

All equipment must be immediately available prior to intubation attempts. With the patient in the sniffing position, the laryngoscope is held in the left hand and the blade is inserted into the right side of the mouth to the base of the tongue. The blade is then moved to the midline, sweeping the tongue to the left. The laryngoscope handle and blade should align with the nasal septum. The tip of straight blades is advanced to the tip of the epiglottis, and the tip of curved blades is placed in the vallecula.

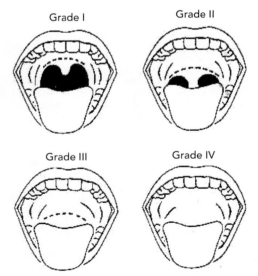

Grade I Grade II Grade III Grade IV

Figure 72.1. Mallampati classification for predicting ease of intubation. (From WK Health, with permission.)

TABLE 72.2	Agents Used for Intubation		
Agent	**Action**	**Advantages**	**Disadvantages**
Lidocaine	Blunts intubation-induced increases in ICP	May also decrease arrhythmias and blunt hemodynamic response	—
Fentanyl	Opioid; provides rapid onset of sedation and anesthesia	Also blocks rise in blood pressure	Increases ICP; may cause hypotension and apnea
Midazolam	Sedative-hypnotic benzodiazepine	Rapid acting with relatively short action	Negative inotrope
Thiopental	Sedative-hypnotic barbiturate	Cerebroprotective (decreases CNS metabolism)	Negative inotrope and vasodilator; bronchospasm from histamine release
Etomidate	Sedative-hypnotic carboxylated imidazole	Rapid onset of action with brief duration; cerebroprotective	Transient adrenocortical dysfunction

ICP, intracranial pressure; CNS, central nervous system.

The vocal cords are exposed by elevating the epiglottis through a lifting motion using the arm and shoulder in a plane 45 degrees from the horizontal. The wrist must be kept stiff to avoid a prying motion that uses the teeth as a fulcrum. When the vocal cords are visualized, the endotracheal tube is advanced from the right side of the mouth with the tip directed so that it intersects the tip of the laryngoscope blade at the level of the glottis, allowing the operator to view the entry of the tube into the trachea (Fig. 72.5). The tube is advanced through the vocal cords until the cuff disappears. The cuff is then inflated with sufficient air to prevent leakage during ventilation with a bag valve. The endotracheal tube must be held firmly in place at all times to prevent displacement.

Correct tube placement is established through visualization of chest expansion and auscultation over the epigastrium and lung fields during positive pressure ventilation, and confirmed using end-tidal CO_2 detection devices. On confirmation of placement, the endotracheal tube is secured firmly in place with either tape or a commercial device.

Cricoid pressure (Sellick maneuver) decreases the risk of aspiration by compressing the esophagus between the cricoid cartilage and the vertebral column. Pressure should be applied prior to intubation attempts and maintained until confirmation of correct endotracheal tube placement.

Attempts at intubation should not take longer than 1 minute. In patients in whom there is difficulty intubating the trachea, repeated attempts increase the risk of trauma and hypoxemia. Alternate approaches to endotracheal intubation via direct laryngoscopy include laryngeal mask airways, laryngeal tube airways, flexible fiberoptic scopes, and percutaneous tracheostomy.

Correct placement of the endotracheal tube is verified clinically visually by observing chest expansion and by auscultation over the abdomen and chest. Correct placement is further assured using an end-tidal CO_2 or esophageal detection device. Following confirmation, the tube can be secured in place using tape or a commercial device.

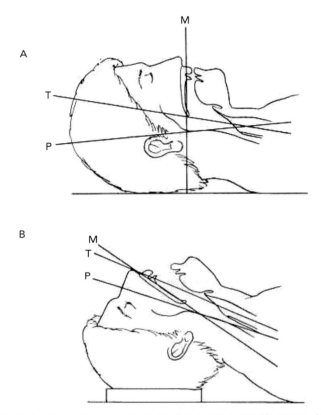

Figure 72.2. Anatomic axes for endotracheal intubation. **A:** With the head in the neutral position, the axis of the mouth (M), the axis of the trachea (T), and the axis of the pharynx (P) are not aligned with one another. **B:** If the head is extended at the atlanto-occipital joints, the axis of the mouth is correctly placed. If the back of the head is raised off the table with a pillow, thus flexing the cervical vertebral column, the axes of the trachea and pharynx are brought in line with the axis of the mouth. (From Snell RS. *Clinical Anatomy.* 7th ed. Philadelphia: Lippincott Williams & Wilkins; 2003, with permission.)

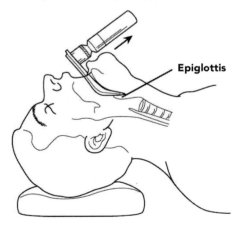

Epiglottis

Figure 72.3. Intubation with a Macintosh blade. Blade is used anterior to the epiglottis. (From Blackbourne LH. *Advanced Surgical Recall.* 2nd ed. Philadelphia: Lippincott Williams & Wilkins; 2004.)

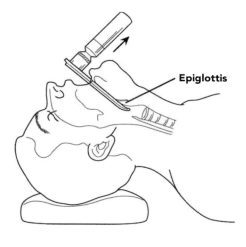

Epiglottis

Figure 72.4. Intubation with a Miller blade. Blade is used to hold the epiglottic (posterior to the epiglottis). (From Blackbourne LH. *Advanced Surgical Recall.* 2nd ed. Philadelphia: Lippincott Williams & Wilkins; 2004, with permission.)

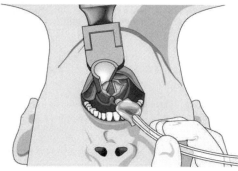

Figure 72.5. Endotracheal intubation-intubating. Illustration showing correct method for intubating victim during endotracheal intubation. (With permission from LifeART image, 2007. Lippincott Williams & Wilkins. All rights reserved.)

Suggested Reading

Blanda M, Gallo U. Emergency airway management. *Emerg Med Clin North Am.* 2003;21: 1–26.
Overview of techniques for endotracheal intubation.
Butler K, Clyne B. Management of the difficult airway: alternative techniques and adjuncts. *Emerg Med Clin North Am.* 2003;21:259–289.
How to recognize patients at high risk for difficult tracheal intubation and alternative techniques available to the practitioner.

73

PERCUTANEOUS TRACHEOSTOMY

Stephen C. Ryan and Martin L. Mayse

Tracheostomy is a technique for creating an artificial airway between the neck surface and cervical trachea. There are two main tracheostomy techniques. The surgical approach uses surgical dissection to form the tract between the neck surface and the trachea. More recently, a percutaneous approach has been developed. Variations on this approach use the Seldinger technique to form the tract between the neck surface and the trachea. Although not suitable for all patients, the percutaneous approach has potential advantages over the surgical approach in appropriately selected intensive care unit (ICU) patients. A meta-analysis showed a lower rate of peristomal bleeding and postoperative infection with percutaneous tracheostomy. In addition, because percutaneous tracheostomies are commonly performed in the patient's ICU room, the risk of adverse events associated with transporting critically ill patients is reduced, and scheduling flexibility is increased. Lastly, some research supports percutaneous tracheostomies as the more cost-effective tracheostomy approach for ICU patients.

The remainder of this chapter will focus on percutaneous tracheostomies.

INDICATIONS

1. Upper airway obstruction. A surgical approach is often more appropriate for upper airway obstruction due to tumor.
2. Need for long-term mechanical ventilation.
3. Access for frequent suctioning and other airway care.
4. Treatment of severe obstructive sleep apnea when continuous positive airway pressure is ineffective or not tolerated.

CONTRAINDICATIONS

Contraindications unique to the percutaneous approach include difficult-to-palpate neck anatomy or history of prior neck surgery or radiation. Patients with high ventilatory and oxygenation requirements may be better served by a surgical approach because of the reduced ability to ventilate around the bronchoscope and likelihood of greater positive end-expiratory pressure loss during the procedure. Coagulopathies should be corrected prior to proceeding, although there are no well-validated thresholds. One center described a low rate of complications for percutaneous tracheostomy in the setting of significant thrombocytopenia as long as platelets were administered before the procedure. Hypotension can be worsened because of the significant amount of sedatives commonly needed to perform the procedure, making hypovolemia and hypotension relative contraindications.

TIMING OF TRACHEOSTOMY PROCEDURE IN CRITICALLY ILL PATIENTS

Most patients receive tracheostomies in the ICU because of difficulty weaning from the ventilator or because they cannot protect and clear their own airways. Potential advantages of tracheostomy over prolonged endotracheal intubation include greater comfort, decreased sedation requirements, enhanced ability to participate in rehabilitation, and facilitated weaning. Optimal timing for tracheostomy in ICU patients is controversial. If prolonged intubation is predicted at admission, a tracheostomy on day 1 or 2 may be appropriate. In most patients, a tracheostomy is considered after 1 to 2 weeks of endotracheal intubation. A recent editorial argues that the preponderance of evidence supports earlier tracheostomy over prolonged endotracheal intubation, although the authors recognize that there are significant design shortcomings in the studies supporting this strategy.

PROCEDURE FOR PERCUTANEOUS TRACHEOSTOMY

Approaches differ slightly on the basis of operator preferences and the particular brand of percutaneous tracheostomy kit used. The following description describes the Ciaglia technique modified by the use of a single dilator with a hydrophilic coating.

1. Explain procedure including risks and benefits. Obtain consent.
2. A team approach makes the procedure more efficient and optimizes patient safety. The bronchoscopist is responsible for bronchoscopic guidance and maintenance of the airway. The bronchoscopist should be skilled in airway management in case of accidental extubation during the procedure. Video bronchoscopy is advantageous because it allows the operator to see the interior of the trachea continuously during the procedure. The nurse assists with intravenous anesthesia during the procedure. A respiratory therapist makes appropriate changes to the ventilator throughout the procedure. The operator performs the procedure and communicates to other members of the team to ensure coordination.
3. Increase FIO_2 to 100%.
4. Monitor blood pressure every 3 to 5 minutes; monitor other variables, including heart rate, pulse oximetry, and airway pressure, continuously.
5. A variety of anesthetic regimens can be used, although combinations of a benzodiazepine and short-acting narcotic or propofol work well. Traditionally, after deep sedation is achieved, a paralytic is administered to prevent coughing. Currently, we perform most of our procedures without a paralytic and have not had significant problems with this approach.
6. A small pad is placed under the shoulders to slightly extend the neck. The neck is prepared with chlorhexidine and a large surgical drape is used to completely cover the patient, with a small opening at the neck. The operator scrubs and dons a hat, protective eyewear, a mask, and sterile gloves and gown.
7. The operator selects the appropriate incision site by palpating the thyroid and cricoid cartilages and the sternal notch. Typically, the space between the first and second, or second and third cartilaginous rings can be approached with an incision halfway between the cricoid cartilage and the sternal notch.
8. After creating a skin wheal with lidocaine, the needle is raised to form a 90-degree angle with the trachea. The tract is anesthetized and the needle is advanced slowly while continuously aspirating. Air bubbles will appear when the needle penetrates the trachea.
9. A 1.5- to 2-cm incision through the skin and superficial subcutaneous tissue is made either horizontally or vertically.
10. A small, curved Kelley clamp is used to dissect a tract down to the trachea.
11. The bronchoscopist carefully withdraws the endotracheal tube over the bronchoscope until the tip lies just below the vocal cords and the tracheal lumen is visible. Firm pressure is applied to the trachea with the Kelly clamp to confirm placement between the appropriate cartilaginous rings.
12. Under continuous bronchoscopic visualization, the catheter-over-needle apparatus is advanced through the skin incision, between the selected tracheal rings, and into the trachea. The catheter is advanced off the needle into the trachea while the needle is withdrawn.
13. The guidewire is threaded through the catheter toward the carina.
14. The catheter is removed, leaving the guidewire in place.
15. A punch dilator is advanced through the trachea and then removed.
16. Next, the curved dilator is inserted over the wire into the trachea. Remove dilator.
17. Load tracheostomy tube onto dilator and advance over guidewire. Percutaneous tracheostomy tubes have tapered ends that allow for easier tracheal insertion.

18. Next, the bronchoscopist removes the bronchoscope from the endotracheal tube and quickly inspects through the tracheostomy tube to ensure proper placement. The patient is reconnected to mechanical ventilation through the tracheostomy tube.

19. The bronchoscopist can inspect the trachea above the tracheostomy tube to rule out active bleeding and to suction blood and secretions, and then completely remove the endotracheal tube.

20. The tracheostomy tube is sewed into place, secured with tracheostomy ties, and dressed appropriately.

21. The tracheostomy tube is changed on day 10 to 14.

COMPLICATIONS

Percutaneous tracheostomy complications are typically divided into early and late categories. More common early complications include transient hypotension and minor bleeding during the procedure. Massive hemorrhage from damage to the innominate vessels has been described but is exceedingly rare. Pneumothoraces and cardiac arrests are uncommon early complications. Fractured tracheal rings occur frequently, although the clinical significance of this complication is unknown. Late complications include stomal infections, bleeding, accidental decannulation, and tracheal stenosis. Bronchoscopic visualization reduces, although does not eliminate, older described complications such as posterior tracheal perforation. Tracheal stenosis rates vary widely in the literature, with some reports finding them to be rare and others finding them to be more common in patients undergoing percutaneous tracheostomies compared with those who undergo surgical tracheostomies.

The use of different techniques and study population selection may explain some of the discrepancies in the literature. When stenosis develops in patients who have undergone percutaneous tracheostomy, they tend to be subglottic in location and may be more challenging to correct surgically.

Suggested Reading

Ahrens T, Kollef MH. Early tracheostomy. Has its time arrived? *Crit Care Med.* 2004;32:1796–1797.
Discusses controversies surrounding timing of tracheostomies.

Barba CA, Angood PB, Kauder DR, et al. Bronchoscopic guidance makes percutaneous tracheostomy a safe, cost-effective, and easy-to-tech procedure. *Surgery.* 1995;118:879–883
Experience comparing percutaneous and surgical tracheostomies in 48 trauma patients. Percutaneous approach found to be easy to learn and perform and to be cost-effective.

Beiderlinden M, Walz MK, Sander A, et al. Complications of bronchoscopically guided percutaneous dilational tracheostomy: beyond the learning curve. *Intensive Care Med.* 2002; 28:59–62.
Reviews complications in 136 percutaneous tracheostomies in a mixed surgical and medical ICU setting. Other than clinically relevant bleeding episodes in 2.9% of patients complications were rare.

Ciaglia P, Firsching R, Syniec C. Elective percutaneous dilational tracheostomy—a simple bedside procedure; a preliminary report. *Chest.* 1985;87:715–719.
Description of percutaneous technique in 134 patients.

Freeman BD, Isabella K, Lin N, et al. A meta-analysis of prospective trials comparing percutaneous and surgical tracheostomy in critically ill patents. *Chest.* 2000;118:1412–1418.
Meta-analysis reviewing studies which compared surgical to percutaneous tracheostomies. It found a lower incidence of peristomal infection, postoperative bleeding, and overall postoperative complication rate with the percutaneous compared with the surgical approach.

Raghuraman G, Rajan S, Marzouk JK, et al. Is tracheal stenosis caused by percutaneous tracheostomy different from that by surgical tracheostomy? *Chest.* 2005;127:879–885.
A small study comparing the details of tracheal stenosis in percuatneous versus surgical tracheostomies.

DEFINITION

Thoracostomy refers to the insertion of a hollow, flexible tube into the pleural space.

INDICATIONS

1. Drainage of air or fluid from the pleural space.
2. Administration of therapeutic pleural agents such as sclerosants.

CONTRAINDICATIONS

1. Bleeding diatheses (prothrombin time or partial thromboplastin time greater than two times normal, platelets <50,000, or creatine level >6) should be corrected in nonemergent settings.
2. Caution is required when there is a history of thoracic surgery or pleurodesis on the side of proposed chest tube insertion. Lung tissue can adhere to the chest wall in these instances, resulting in lung injury during insertion. Image guidance or operating room placement may be required.

IMAGING

Confirmation of the suspected pleural process prior to tube placement is imperative. On standard radiographs, large bullae can mimic pneumothoraces and combinations of tumor and atelectasis can be mistaken for pleural effusions. Attempted chest tube placement can cause significant morbidity in these situations. Lateral decubitus films may help confirm the existence of free-flowing air or fluid. In difficult cases, chest computed tomography or ultrasound imaging may be needed.

SITE SELECTION

1. Physical examination findings consistent with a pleural effusion include decreased breath sounds on auscultation, dullness to percussion, and loss of tactile fremitus. Physical examination findings consistent with pneumothoraces include hyperresonance and decreased breath sounds. In tension pneumothoraces, shift of mediastinal structures may be observed.
2. For free-flowing air or fluid, chest tubes are traditionally placed in the fourth to sixth rib interspaces between the middle and anterior axillary lines. Alternatively, the second interspace in the midclavicular line can be used for drainage of pneumothoraces with small, percutaneous catheters.
3. Loculated air or fluid collections often require image guidance by ultrasound or fluoroscopy for optimal tube placement. A good understanding of the overlying anatomy is required in this situation to prevent damage to anatomic structures during tube insertion.

CHOOSING THE OPTIMAL APPROACH

The surgical and guidewire methods are the two most commonly used techniques for tube thoracostomy. Different indications dictate the appropriate approach. Loculated fluid collections are often more readily approached by a guidewire method. In these cases, small pockets of fluid can be safely entered with real-time visualization of a guidewire using ultrasound, fluoroscopy, or computed tomography. Small tubes ranging from 8 to 12 French have been successfully used to drain thick fluid collections, including empyemas. Hemothoraces or large bronchopleural fistulas often require the placement of a larger tube (32 French or greater) by the surgical approach to achieve adequate drainage.

Procedure Steps

Surgical Approach

1. Explain benefits, risks, alternatives and obtain consent.
2. Gather equipment including sterile towels, antiseptic, lidocaine, needles for local anesthesia, silk sutures, large Kelly clamps, scalpel, gauze pads, chest tube, and chest tube drainage system, as well as mask, hat, and sterile gown. Kits prepared ahead of time can simplify this process.
3. Typically, the patient is placed in a semirecumbent position with the head and shoulders about 30 degrees off the bed. The ipsilateral arm is placed above the head for exposure of the axilla and to increase the distance between ribs.
4. Clean the area with antiseptic and sterilely drape.
5. Anesthesia is primarily delivered locally, although intravenous narcotics such as fentanyl or morphine can increase patient comfort when appropriate monitoring is available. After rib identification, infiltrate subcutaneous tissue with lidocaine (Fig. 74.1). Next, inject local anesthesia down to the appropriate rib. Move needle over rib and continue to inject anesthesia. Confirm entry into air or fluid by aspirating the syringe as it is advanced. Generously anesthetize the parietal pleura. Typically, the equivalent of 25 to 40 mL of 1% lidocaine local anesthetic should achieve adequate local anesthesia.
6. Make a skin incision through the subcutaneous tissue that is wide enough to insert a finger.

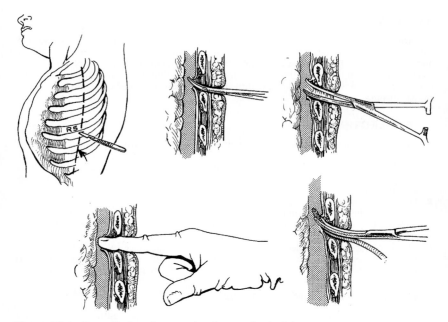

Figure 74.1. Chest tube insertion procedure (see text for details).

7. Using medium-sized Kelly clamps, bluntly dissect to the top of the selected rib. This is done by applying forward pressure with the clamps while opening, relaxing forward pressure while closing, and repeating as necessary. Once the rib is reached, continue with blunt dissection over the top of the rib. A rush of air or fluid signals entry into the pleural space. As the clamps enter into the pleural space, caution is needed not to push too far, so as to prevent lung injury.

8. Place finger through tract into the pleural space. Sweep around the entry site to confirm the lack of adherent lung in the direction of chest tube placement.

9. Clamp the end of the chest tube with a Kelly clamp and guide into the pleural space. Direction is generally anteroapical for drainage of air and inferoposterior for drainage of fluid.

10. Attach external end of tube to the drainage system. Drainage of air or fluid as well as evidence of respiratory variation suggest proper placement into the pleural space.

11. Securely suture tube to prevent dislodgment. Some operators place a mattress suture at the time of the insertion, leaving the ends loose, which they use to close the incision at the time of tube removal.

12. Using occlusive gauze to seal the skin around the tube is controversial. Some authors argue that this leads to skin breakdown.

13. Dress area with a generous amount of gauze and tape.

14. Check chest x-ray for proper placement.

15. Check on chest tube output, signs of respiratory variation, and the presence of air leaks at least daily. Evaluate site for bleeding or signs of infection.

16. Remove tube when drainage is no longer indicated.

Guidewire Approach

Note: this approach may vary slightly, depending on kit used.

1. Obtain consent, position patient, and prepare area as for surgical approach.

2. Anesthetize rib and pleural space in the selected interspace.

3. Insert the introducer needle just superior to the appropriate rib. Stop just past the point where fluid or air is aspirated.

4. Remove syringe and cover needle opening with finger to prevent excessive air entry. Introduce wire into pleural space. Remove needle from pleural space.

5. Make a small skin nick at the wire entry site to allow introduction of dilators and chest tube.

6. Using sequential dilators, dilate tract into pleural space.

7. Introduce chest tube over the wire into the pleural space. Confirm that all openings are in the pleural space. Remove wire.

8. Connect chest tube to drainage system.

9. Suture tube in place and dress with gauze and tape.

10. Check chest x ray for proper placement.

DRAINAGE SYSTEMS

The most common drainage system for hospitalized patient is the three-bottle drainage system. The functions of the three-bottle system are most commonly incorporated into one container today. The first column serves as a drainage repository, collecting fluid that drains from the pleural space. The second column serves as a water seal, which prevents retrograde air entry into the pleural space. The third column allows for adjustment of the negative pressure applied to the pleural space.

GUIDELINES FOR CHEST TUBE REMOVAL

There is considerable practice variation involved in chest tube removal. The most important requirement is for the resolution of the initial indication for placement. For pneumothoraces, this generally means a fully expanded lung with resolution of the air leak, and for pleural fluid, this implies a maximum drainage of 100 to 150 mL/day. There are arguments for pulling at end-expiration or end-inspiration as well as arguments in favor and against tube clamping, placing on water seal, or keeping on suction prior to removal.

Our approach is to place on water seal 12 to 24 hours with a follow-up chest x-ray. If there is no significant air leak or reaccumulation of air or fluid, the tube is removed. In difficult cases, the tube can be clamped for 2 to 4 hours, with careful monitoring and a repeat chest x-ray to confirm stability. Patients can be given a small amount of narcotic prior to removal. Remove sutures. Have patient make a full inspiration and pull tube out quickly while occluding the track with your other hand. Approximate the incision either by tying a previously placed mattress suture or by placing new suture. A follow-up chest x-ray should be taken 12 to 24 hours later (or sooner, if clinically indicated) to rule out recurrence of pneumothorax or pleural fluid.

COMPLICATIONS

Complications from chest tube placement are less well studied than complications associated with other common thoracic procedures. The site of placement (emergency department, intensive care unit, floor, or operating room) and circumstances of placement (emergent or elective) are undoubtedly important. One study looked at complications from chest tubes inserted by pulmonary fellows with attending supervision. Many, although not all, of the patients were in the intensive care unit. The largest number of chest tube placements in the study were for ventilator-associated or iatrogenic pneumothoraces. Problems were stratified as early (first 24 hours) or late and by size of the chest tube placed (less than or equal to 14 French or larger). Early complications included the tube not being placed in the pleural space, nonfunctional tubes, and laceration of the lung. Late complications included nonfunctional tubes, a site infection, and a leak around tube. All complications were more common with small tubes (36%) versus larger tubes (9%).

Other possible complications include hemothoraces from intercostal vessel injury or intra-abdominal placement. Infections associated with tube placement are uncommon. Prophylactic antibiotic use is supported by one meta-analysis in trauma patients, but is probably not justified in other clinical situations.

Suggested Reading

Bell RL, Ovandia P, Abdullah F, et al. Chest tube removal: end-inspiration or end-expiration? *J Trauma.* 2001;50:674–677.
Patients randomized to end-inspiration or end-expiration removal of tube. No significant difference in outcomes found.

Collop NA, Kim S, Sahn SA. Analysis of tube thoracostomy performed by pulmonologists at a teaching hospital. *Chest.* 1997;112:709–713.
Study of 126 tube thoracostomies performed by a pulmonary division at an academic medical center. Reviews indications and complications.

Fallon WF, Wears RL. Prophylactic antibiotics for the prevention of infectious complications including empyema following tube thoracoscopy for trauma: results of a meta-analysis. *J Trauma.* 1992;33:110–117.
Showed a benefit for prophylactic antibiotics in trauma patients requiring chest tube placement.

Martino K, Merrit S, Boyakye K, et al. Prospective randomized trial of thoracostomy removal algorithms. *J Trauma* 1999;46:369–371.
205 patients requiring chest tube insertion for blunt and penetrating trauma. When removal of the chest tube was indicated, patients were randomized to a water seal waiting period or to immediate removal of the chest tube. It appeared that a short period of time on water seal might allow for the detection of occult air leaks.

McVay PA, Toy PTCY. Lack of increased bleeding after paracentesis and thoracentesis in patients with mild coagulation abnormalities. *Transfusion.* 1991;31:164–171.
Retrospective study of 608 patients undergoing thoracentesis or paracentesis. Argues that prophylactic plasma and platelet transfusions are unnecessary for patients with mild to moderate coagulopathies.

Silverman SG, Mueller PR, Saini S, et al. Thoracic empyema: management with image-guided catheter drainage. *Radiology.* 1988;169:5–9.
43 patients treated with imaged guided catheters for empyemas. Proved successful by pre-defined criteria in 72% of patients.

Paracentesis is a procedure frequently performed in the intensive care unit for diagnostic and therapeutic purposes. Diagnostic paracentesis should be performed in patients with suspected spontaneous bacterial peritonitis or ascites of unknown cause. In patients with significant shortness of breath and/or abdominal discomfort, therapeutic paracentesis frequently alleviates symptoms. Complications include bleeding from the paracentesis site, fluid leak, bowel or bladder perforation, and the introduction of infection.

Many patients undergoing paracentesis (especially those with underlying liver disease) are coagulopathic and/or thrombocytopenic at the time of the procedure. It has been shown in such patients that there is no need to correct the coagulopathy or transfuse platelets prior to the procedure. Paracentesis should not be performed in patients with disseminated intravascular coagulation. Additionally, in patients with small bowel obstruction, a nasogastric tube should be placed prior to the procedure. Patients with urinary retention should undergo bladder catheterization prior to paracentesis. In patients who have had multiple abdominal operations, who do not have a large amount of ascites, have pronounced organomegaly, or those who have undergone failed conventional paracentesis, performing the procedure with ultrasound guidance may be necessary.

The most common sites of paracentesis are the left lower quadrant, suprapubic, or right lower quadrant areas of the abdomen. Physical examination, particularly percussion and examining for shifting dullness, can help determine the ideal site. In patients with loculated ascites, ultrasound can aid in performing the procedure at the site with greatest yield. When performing a paracentesis, the catheter should not be inserted through infected/inflamed skin or tissue or hematomas.

Once the site of the procedure has been determined and all present agree on the identification of the patient, the site, and the procedure being performed, one can proceed with paracentesis.

PERFORMANCE OF PARACENTESIS

1. Sterile gloves and a mask with face shield are worn.
2. The patient should be placed supine with the head of the bed slightly elevated.
3. The site is prepared with antiseptic solution (e.g., chlorhexidine or Betadine), and a sterile drape is placed.
4. Using a 22- or 25-gage needle, local anesthesia with 1% lidocaine is performed, starting with a subcutaneous wheel followed by deeper anesthesia. While injecting the deeper tissues, maintain continuous negative pressure on the syringe, and inject lidocaine periodically. Maintain an angle of entry perpendicular to the abdominal wall.
5. When ascitic fluid is obtained, inject lidocaine around the peritoneum.
6. Ideally, a needle/catheter specifically designed for paracentesis (e.g., Caldwell needle) should be used, although a large-bore intravenous catheter may be used. Attach a 10-mL syringe to the catheter.
7. Using a scalpel, make a small nick in the skin at the insertion site to facilitate insertion of the paracentesis catheter.
8. Using the Z-tract technique, pull the skin 2 cm caudad prior to inserting the catheter (this theoretically causes the tract to close, and thus reduces the rate of leakage when the catheter is withdrawn).

TABLE 75.1	Common Clinical Situations and Pertinent Studies for Ascitic Fluid		
Clinical situation	**Studies**	**Comments**	
Concern for SBP	▪ Cell count ▪ Culture (blood culture bottles inoculated at bedside)	▪ >250 cells/mm^3 consistent with SBP ▪ Culture definitive for diagnosis. ▪ Treat with third-generation cephalosporin or fluoroquinolone	
Determining if ascites is secondary to portal hypertension	▪ Serum albumin ▪ Ascites albumin	▪ SAAG ≥1.1 g/dL (portal hypertension) possibilities include cirrhosis, alcohol hepatitis, cardiac ascites, portal-vein thrombosis, Budd-Chiari syndrome, liver metastases ▪ SAAG <1.1 g/dL possibilities include peritoneal carcinomatosis, tuberculous peritonitis, pancreatic ascites, nephrotic syndrome, serositis	
Concern for malignant ascites	▪ Cytology	▪ Sensitivity can be increased by sending three samples, and examining samples promptly	

SBP, spontaneous bacterial peritonitis; SAAG, serum ascites albumin gradient = serum albumin − ascites albumin.

9. Insert the catheter slowly, with continued negative pressure on the syringe. When ascitic fluid is obtained, stop advancing the catheter, advance the plastic portion of the catheter over the needle, and remove the needle.
10. Obtain an adequate amount of ascitic fluid for diagnostic studies (culture bottles should be inoculated at the bedside).
11. If a therapeutic paracentesis is being performed, tubing should be connected from the catheter to the vacuum bottle.

DIAGNOSTIC CONSIDERATIONS

Diagnostic studies performed on ascitic fluid are determined by the clinical situation (Table 75.1). Other less common diagnostic studies include triglycerides (concern for chylous ascites), amylase (concern for pancreatic ascites), mycobacterial culture (concern for tuberculous ascites), and carcinoembryonic antigen and/or alkaline phosphatase (concern for hollow viscous perforation). If there is concern for spontaneous bacterial peritonitis (SBP), fluid should be sent for cell count and culture. As previously mentioned, culture bottles should be inoculated at the bedside to improve yield. Cell count showing >250 polymorphonuclear cells/mm^3 without secondary source of infection (e.g., perforated viscous) or a grossly bloody tap suggests SBP. The definitive diagnosis is based on positive culture results. In patients with findings suggestive or diagnostic of SBP, treatment should be initiated with a third-generation cephalosporin (ceftriaxone or cefotaxime) or a fluoroquinolone (ciprofloxacin or levofloxacin).

The use of albumin infusion after large-volume paracentesis (5 liters or more) to combat circulatory dysfunction and potential precipitation of hepatorenal syndrome remains controversial. If used, the dose of albumin is 6 to 8 g/L of fluid removed to be administered after the procedure.

Suggested Reading

Runyon BA. Management of adult patients with ascites. *Hepatology.* 2004;39;841–856.
> *An evidence based review of the diagnostic studies and their indications in patients with ascites, as well as a discussion of the treatment of several diagnoses, including refractory ascites, the hepatorenal syndrome, and SBP.*

Thomsen TW, Shaffer RW, White B, et al. Paracentesis. *N Engl J Med.* 2006;355:e21.
> *An excellent review of the indications, risks, performance of, studies to be sent, and complications of parencenteses.*

LUMBAR PUNCTURE

Manu S. Goyal

The lumbar puncture (LP) is commonly performed in the intensive care unit to obtain cerebrospinal fluid (CSF) for diagnostic purposes. This chapter will discuss the indications, technique, complications, and common pitfalls of performing an LP in adults.

INDICATIONS AND CONTRAINDICATIONS

It is useful to remember the old adage, "If you consider an LP, you should do it." Delay in diagnosis of meningitis may lead to inappropriate treatment and difficulty in establishing the diagnosis later when the patient fails to improve. Delay in the diagnosis of subarachnoid hemorrhage can prevent early treatment of aneurysms and prevention of rebleeding. Table 76.1 lists common indications for LP.

There are few contraindications to LP. Coagulopathy is an important contraindication because an LP may cause an epidural hematoma leading to compression of the cauda equina. No studies have established useful cutoffs, but an international normalized ratio >1.4, partial thromboplastin time >50, and/or platelet count <100,000/mm^3 are commonly corrected with fresh-frozen plasma and/or platelet transfusions prior to an LP. In the setting of altered mental status, papilledema, focal neurologic deficit, or suspicion for subarachnoid hemorrhage, a head computed tomography scan should be obtained prior to LP. Signs of herniation and large posterior fossa masses preclude an LP because the pressure drop following CSF removal can precipitate tonsillar herniation.

Other contraindications to LP include local skin infections, known spinal cord tumors, and very recent surgical instrumentation. Prior to performing an LP, informed consent must be obtained according to the policy at each institution.

TECHNIQUE

1. Collect the Supplies

Gather the following: sterile 20-gauge or smaller spinal needle with a stylet, a sterile 25-gauge needle and syringe for local anesthesia, topical antiseptic, sterile drape and gauze, 1% to 2% lidocaine solution, a sterile manometer, sterile surgical gloves, and tubes for collection of the fluid. With more experience, a smaller gauge spinal needle, preferably a Sprott needle, helps reduce post-LP headaches. In morbidly obese patients, a needle longer than the standard 3.5 inches may be necessary.

2. Position the Patient

Lateral decubitus positioning is required to accurately measure the intracranial CSF pressure. The patient is positioned such that the hips and shoulders are squarely above one another, the back is parallel to the wall, and the patient is curled up with the knees and chin tucked deeply into the torso (Fig. 76.1). In other cases, a sitting position aids in determining the midline of the spine, increases the space between spinous processes, and may increase filling of the lumbar cistern, thus improving the chance of successful LP. In this position, the patient is positioned such that the back is straight and arched outward, with

TABLE 76.1	Common Indications for Lumbar Puncture

- Diagnosis of bacterial, viral, fungal, parasitic, or mycobacterial meningitis
- Diagnosis of carcinomatosis meningitis
- Diagnosis of subarachnoid hemorrhage
- Assessing central nervous system and meningeal inflammation for diagnosis of conditions including multiple sclerosis, Devic disease, and neurosarcoidosis
- Measuring CSF protein levels for the diagnosis of Guillain-Barré syndrome
- Measuring intracranial pressure for diagnosis of pseudotumor cerebri
- Removing CSF for treatment of pseudotumor cerebri or normal-pressure hydrocephalus

CSF, cerebrospinal fluid.

the chin tucked deeply into the chest. Ultimately, the choice of positioning should be determined by the indications for the LP, patient comfort, and operator experience.

3. Find the L4-5 Space

In most adults, the spinal cord ends at L1 and in a few adults it ends at L2. Therefore, the L3-4, L4-5, and L5-S1 spaces represent safe and effective locations to insert a spinal needle. In most adults, a line (Tuffier line) drawn across the tops of both iliac crests crosses the L4 spinous process or the L4-5 space. Use the spinous space on or immediately below the Tuffier line. Attention to superficial anatomy helps ensure appropriate placement of the spinal needle.

4. Scrub and Anesthetize the Space

Scrub the location with antiseptic solution (e.g., chlorhexidine or Betadine). Using sterile gloves, place a sterile drape at the selected location with the lumbar space above it exposed. Lidocaine is injected subcutaneously and about 2 cm deep along the expected track of the spinal needle.

5. Insert the Spinal Needle

The spinal needle with its stylet in place should then be introduced through the skin in a tract that is angled toward the navel or about 15 degrees cephalad. The needle must be

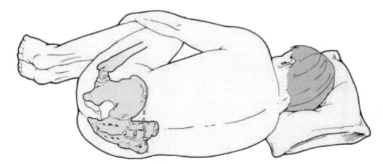

Figure 76.1. Positioning the patient. Tuffier line is indicated by the *dashed line*. (From Taylor C, Lillis CA, LeMone P. *Fundamentals of Nursing.* 2nd ed. Philadelphia: JB Lippincott; 1993:543, with permission.)

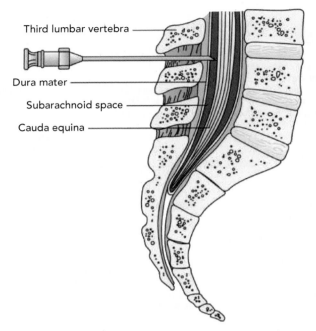

Third lumbar vertebra

Dura mater

Subarachnoid space

Cauda equina

Figure 76.2. The ideal tract of the spinal needle. (From Taylor C, Lillis CA, LeMone P. *Fundamentals of Nursing.* 2nd ed. Philadelphia: JB Lippincott; 1993:543, with permission.)

entered at midline and orthogonal to the plane of the back. The bevel should initially be perpendicular to the long axis of the body to minimize tearing of the dura and the subsequent post-LP headaches.

6. Advance the Spinal Needle

After penetrating the skin and subcutaneous fat, the needle should traverse the supraspinatus ligament, the interspinous ligaments, the ligamentum flavum, the epidural space, and finally the dura (Fig. 76.2). Severe pain may indicate being away from the midline. Once the needle has been inserted about 3 to 4 cm, or if a "pop" or sudden loss of resistance is experienced, remove the stylet to check for CSF. If no CSF is obtained, replace the stylet and advance the needle another 2 to 3 mm and remove the stylet again to check for CSF. Once the lumbar cistern has been entered, CSF should flow freely through the spinal needle, and the stylet can be replaced to limit CSF leakage until it can be collected or a manometer can be attached to measure CSF pressure. Hitting bone while inserting the needle indicates either incorrect angling of the needle or the skin has been entered away from the midline. When this occurs, retract the needle to the subcutaneous tissue, reposition its angle so that it is closer to being 15 degrees or less cephalad and more directed toward the midline, and then enter again. This procedure can be repeated a few times until a tract free of bone is achieved. After several attempts at the first lumbar space, using the L3-4 space (the space immediately above the Tuffier line) is permissible, but using any higher spaces risks inserting the needle into the tip of the spinal cord.

On occasion, the LP needle is inserted to the hub without obtaining CSF. This problem can be avoided by using a needle that is sufficiently long, ensuring a correct entry point and angle, and occasionally by sitting up the patient. Fluoroscopic guidance may be necessary in obese or uncooperative patients.

TABLE 76.2	Common Tests for Cerebrospinal Fluid (CSF) Analysis (to be Ordered Based on Clinical Concern)

- Complete cell count and differential
- CSF glucose and protein levels
- Gram stain and bacterial, fungal, and mycobacterial cultures
- Cytology and wet mount inspection
- Spectrophotometer analysis for xanthochromia
- IgG and albumin levels, serum IgG and albumin levels to determine the IgG index: $(CSF-IgG/CSF-albumin)/(Serum-IgG/Serum-albumin)$
- Oligoclonal bands
- PCR tests for a variety of pathogens including HSV, VZV, EBV, CMV, enteroviruses, TB, arboviruses, and toxoplasmosis
- Other tests for pathogens including syphilis (VDRL or FTA-ABS), cysticercosis, histoplasmosis, coccidiodpmycosis, and malaria

IgG, immunoglobulin G; PCR, polymerase chain reaction; HSV, herpes simplex virus; VZV, varicella-zoster virus; EBV, Epstein-Barr virus; CMV, cytomegalovirus; TB, tuberculosis; VDRL, Venereal Disease Research Laboratory; FTA-ABS, fluorescent treponemal antibody-absorption.

7. Measure CSF Pressure and Collect Fluid

Once the needle has entered the lumbar cistern, a manometer can be used to measure "opening" CSF pressure. This measurement is accurate only when the patient is in the lateral decubitus position and relaxed enough to allow visible respiratory excursions of the CSF in the manometer. Normal pressure is 8 to 22 cm H_2O, although it can be slightly higher in normal obese patients. The fluid in the manometer should be collected for CSF analysis. Sufficient CSF should be collected for all of the necessary tests, and additional fluid should be collected and saved in case further testing is desired. If the opening pressure is >50 cm H_2O, the minimum amount of fluid necessary should be collected. Fluid analyses are listed in Table 76.2. If the CSF appears bloody initially and later the clears, this suggests a "traumatic" tap, whereby the needle had punctured a vein en route to the lumbar cistern. Xanthochromia, or a yellowish tint to the fluid, indicates either blood products >12 to 24 hours old in the subarachnoid space or greatly elevated protein levels. Careful replacement of the stylet before and after collection helps avoid excessive CSF leak. After CSF collection, a closing pressure can be measured if necessary. Replace the stylet before removing the needle.

COMPLICATIONS

Immediately after a LP, the patient should be placed in the supine position for 1 hour. This procedure helps reduce headaches immediately following LP, but probably does not prevent post-LP headaches that occur because of a tear in the dura and persistent CSF leakage. The latter can be reduced by appropriate spinal needle selection and proper technique. Fluids, caffeine, acetaminophen, and nonsteroidal anti-inflammatory drugs are effective in most cases of post-LP headaches. Characteristically, the headache worsens with sitting up or standing and resolves when lying down. If the headaches persist longer than 5 or more days, a blood patch may be necessary.

Rarely, the patient may complain of paresthesias or pain referred to one leg. During the procedure, this indicates impingement of a nerve root, and the spinal needle should be retracted, repositioned further toward the midline, and then reinserted. Careful controlled insertion of the needle helps avoid such nerve damage. When these symptoms or symptoms of cord compression occur following the procedure, there is concern for an intraspinal epidermoid tumor or an epidural hematoma. In both cases, obtaining a magnetic resonance image or computed tomography is mandatory, and neurosurgical consultation is warranted if any such mass is discovered.

Other complications, including herniation syndromes and spontaneous rupture of a subarachnoid arterial aneurysm, are very rare and can be avoided by careful physical examination and, when indicated, brain imaging prior to the LP.

Suggested Reading

Boon JM, Abrahams PH, Meiring JH, et al. Lumbar puncture: anatomical review of a clinical skill. *Clin Anat.* 2004;17:544–553.

This comprehensive article reviews the relevant anatomy for peforming a lumber puncture. It is well written and is advised particularly when one is having trouble successfully performing the procedure.

Ellenby MS, Tegtmeyer K, Lai S, et al. Lumbar puncture. *N Engl J Med.* 2006; 355:e12.

A video and accompanying article that demonstrates the proper method of performing a lumber puncture. This is highly recommended to everyone who has never performed this procedure before.

Stephen C. Ryan and Martin L. Mayse

DEFINITION

Thoracentesis is a procedure in which a needle is inserted between the ribs into the pleural space for aspiration of air or fluid.

INDICATIONS

1. Evaluation of pleural effusions of unknown cause.
2. To exclude empyema or complicated parapneumonic effusions in patients with fever and pleural effusions.
3. Therapeutic removal of air or fluid from the pleural space.

RELATIVE CONTRAINDICATIONS

1. Uncooperative patient.
2. Cutaneous abnormality such as an infection at the proposed sampling site.
3. Uncorrectable bleeding diathesis that includes a prothrombin time or partial thromboplastin time greater than two times normal, platelets <50,000, or a creatine level >6. The diagnostic benefits of excluding empyema or hemothorax may outweigh bleeding risks if these are diagnostic considerations.

HISTORY

1. Patients with risk factors or a history suggestive of bleeding problems should have coagulation factors measured.
2. Screen for allergies to local anesthetics.

SITE SELECTION

1. Physical examination findings consistent with pleural effusions include decreased breath sounds, dullness to percussion, and loss of tactile fremitus.
2. A lateral decubitus film, ultrasound, or computed tomography scan of the chest can exclude other entities that mimic pleural fluid on standard chest films.
3. At least 1 cm of fluid should layer out on a lateral decubitus film in order to safely sample an effusion without ultrasound guidance.
4. Using ultrasound for site selection for all thoracenteses is controversial. If readily available, potential benefit from its routine use has been found in some studies. On the other hand, experienced operators can perform thoracentesis with a low complication rate without ultrasound. If two attempts at blind thoracentesis fail to sample fluid, the use of ultrasound guidance can improve the yield for obtaining fluid. Ultrasound-guided thoracentesis can be performed safely in patients on mechanical ventilation.

PROCEDURE

1. Explain benefits, risks, answer questions, and obtain consent.
2. A number of companies offer helpful prepackaged procedure kits that simplify the gathering of needed equipment.

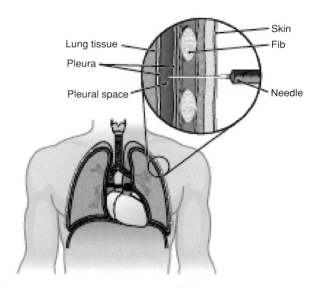

Figure 77.1. Schematic illustrating appropriate needle location for sampling & pleural effusion.

3. Sit patient straight up to maximize the amount of fluid in the posterior gutter.
4. The preferred site for needle insertion is generally midway between the spine and posterior axillary line. Percuss down the chest until an area of dullness is reached. Go one interspace below the area of dullness. Avoid the paraspinal area and do not go below the ninth rib interspace. If performed with ultrasound, site selection is directed by the ultrasound image.
5. Wear a mask and sterile gloves.
6. Clean area with chlorhexidine or other appropriate antiseptic.
7. Cover surrounding area with sterile drape or towels.
8. Using a 25-gauge needle filled with lidocaine, create a small skin wheal over the top of the appropriate rib.
9. Using a 22-gauge needle, go through the wheal, anesthetizing deeper levels of tissue as you go. The skin surface, top of the rib, and parietal pleura require the most anesthetic. Advance until fluid is aspirated. (Figure 75.1)
10. If using a needle without a catheter device, insert needle into previously anesthetized tract until fluid is aspirated. Collect fluid for studies.
11. If using a needle with a catheter device, first make a skin nick with a scalpel. Insert the needle and catheter device through the skin nick and advance while aspirating. After fluid is aspirated, advance needle and catheter 2 to 3 mm further into the pleural space and then advance the catheter off the needle into the pleural space while preventing the needle from advancing further. Remove the needle.
12. Using a large syringe, remove fluid for studies. Samples for chemical evaluation are typically sent in a mint green top blood tube, and cell counts in a lavender top blood tube. Cytology and microbiology samples for study can be sent in small, sterile containers. Although submission of large amounts of cytology fluid is commonly advocated, the yield for diagnosis appears to be independent of the fluid amount submitted. Fluid can be instilled in blood culture bottles in an effort to improve the yield of cultures, but this requires the submission of a separate sample to obtain a Gram stain. (See Chapter 15, "Pleural Effusion," for further guidance on fluid analysis.)

TABLE 77.1	Common Complications in Thoracentesis		
Complication	Overall no. (%)	Inexperienced no. (%)	Experienced no. (%)
Pain	77 (25)	64 (25)	13 (26)
Cough	37 (12)	25 (10)	12 (24)
Dry tap	33 (11)	32 (13)	1 (2)
Pneumothorax	31 (10)	29 (11)	2 (4)
Vasovagal	7 (2)	6 (2)	1 (2)
Worsened dyspnea	4 (1)	0	4 (8)

13. If performing a therapeutic procedure, connect the catheter to a syringe and collection bag system or directly to a vacuum bottle. It is generally recommended that the procedure be stopped after 1,200 to 1,500 mL if pleural fluid is removed or if the patient develops symptoms of cough or chest discomfort to avoid re-expansion pulmonary edema. Alternatively, one can monitor pleural manometry and keep pleural pressures less than −20 cm H_2O.
14. Remove the catheter while the patient exhales to avoid entrainment of air.
15. Chest x-rays are commonly performed to exclude pneumothorax, but are probably not needed unless there are concerning symptoms or problems with the procedure that suggests that the lung may have been punctured.

COMPLICATIONS

Complications can be separated into major complications, such as pneumothorax or significant bleeding, and minor complications, such as pain or dry taps. Table 77.1 summarizes common complications.

Operator experience plays a significant role in the risk of complications, emphasizing the importance of having the proper background knowledge and experience in the performance of the procedure.

Re-expansion pulmonary edema is a feared but uncommon complication of thoracentesis. The pathophysiology is unclear, but traditionally has been attributed to excessive negative pressure in the pleural space during pleural drainage procedures.

Suggested Reading

Bartter T, Mayo PD, Pratter, MR, et al. Lower risk and higher yield for thoracentesis when performed by experienced operators. *Chest.* 1993; 103:1873–1876.
   Prospective study involving 50 consecutive thoracentesis performed by pulmonary fellows or attendings. Showed significantly lower rates of major complications compared to similar studies of procedure performed by non-pulmonary housestaff.
Collins TR, Sahn SA. Thoracentesis: clinical value, complications, technical problems, and patient experience. *Chest.* 1987;91:817–822.
   Prospective study of 129 thoracenteses primarily performed by medical housestaff and students.
Jones PW, Moyers JP, Rogers JT, et al. Ultrasound-guided thoracentesis: is it a safer method? *Chest.* 2003;123:418–423.
   Prospective, descriptive study of 941 thoracenteses in 605 patients. Showed a low rate of complications when thoracentesis was performed under ultrasound by experienced operators. Also showed a low incidence of re-expansion pulmonary edema regardless of the amount of fluid removed.
McVay PA, Toy PTCY. Lack of increased bleeding after paracentesis and thoracentesis in patients with mild coagulation abnormalities. *Transfusion.* 1991;31:164–171.

Retrospective study of 608 patients undergoing thoracentesis or paracentesis. Argues that prophylactic plasma and platelet transfusions are unnecessary for patients with mild to moderate coagulopathies.

Petersen WG, Zimmerman R. Limited utility of chest radiograph after thoracentesis. *Chest.* 2000;117:1038–1042.

Prospective, cohort involving 251 thoracenteses. Showed that clinically significant pneumothoraces were always associated with symptoms or aspiration of air.

Seneff MG, Corwin RW, Gold LH, et al. Complications associated with thoracentesis. *Chest.* 1986;90:97–100.

Prospective study of 125 procedures primarily performed by housestaff.

PULMONARY ARTERY CATHETERIZATION

78

Warren Isakow

Since its inception in the 1970s, the clinical use of the pulmonary artery catheter (PAC) has been controversial. The PAC provides direct pressure measurements from the right atrium (RA), right ventricle (RV), pulmonary arteries (PAs), and pulmonary capillary wedge pressure as well as a means of measuring cardiac output by thermodilution. PAC rapidly gained favor when it was recognized how inaccurate were physician assessments of these parameters. Use of the catheter became widespread, and bedside management was often influenced by the hemodynamic parameters; however, no clinical validation of the benefit of this approach had been performed.

A number of subsequent trials in different patient populations, including surgical patients, patients with acute myocardial infarction, congestive heart failure, and acute lung injury, have shown no benefits, and possibly increased risk, from use of a PAC. A recent study by the acute respiratory distress syndrome clinical trials network found no differences in outcomes of patients with this syndrome who had their fluid balance guided by use of a central line with central venous pressure monitoring or use of a PAC. Routine use of the PAC should be avoided, but it still has a role in patients with pulmonary arterial hypertension and congenital heart disease, and in patients with complex fluid management issues. In addition, as new therapies emerge, information on treatment benefits may require invasive assessment of hemodynamic parameters.

Newer, noninvasive techniques to assess hemodynamic parameters are being refined and are reducing dependence on the PAC. The clinician using the PAC needs to ask how the information obtained from a PAC will change management of a specific patient, and be alert to possibly the greatest danger of the device: misinterpretation of its hemodynamic measurements. The PAC should be used for the shortest time possible and with the understanding that it is unlikely to alter the clinical course of a patient with multiple complex medical problems (Table 78.1).

PROCEDURE TECHNIQUE

The easiest insertion sites are normally the right internal jugular vein or the left subclavian vein; however, femoral or even brachial vein sites can be used. Prior to starting the procedure, an evaluation of any contraindications to the procedure should be made. In cases with suspected RV dysfunction, pulmonary artery hypertension, tricuspid regurgitation, or RA enlargement, consideration should be given to placing the PAC with fluoroscopy guidance, as direct visualization enhances ability to pass the PAC in difficult cases.

The intravenous lines, pressure bags, transducers, and zeroing apparatus should all be assembled and ready prior to the sterile insertion of the PAC. It is useful to have an assistant or nurse available for the procedure. A sterile procedural field should be used, with strict attention to handwashing, mask and cap usage, sterile glove and gown use, as well as full-length drapes. The introducer catheter is inserted in a similar manner to a central venous catheter using the Seldinger technique. The introducer catheter is slightly different in that the dilator is advanced through the introducer rather than as a separate piece of equipment, as occurs with a regular central venous catheter insertion. Additionally, the guidewire and dilator are removed together at the conclusion of the introducer insertion, which leaves the introducer alone in the vessel.

TABLE 78.1	Contraindications to, Indications for, and Complications of Pulmonary Artery Catheter Placement

Relative contraindications	Complications
Left bundle branch block Severe coagulopathy	Complications related to introducer placement: ■ Pneumothorax ■ Hemothorax ■ Hematoma at site of insertion ■ Infection at insertion site

Indications (controversial)
Diagnosis and management of
  shock states
Oliguric acute renal failure
Assessment of volume status
Titration of therapy for cardiogenic
  shock
Diagnosis of PAH
Vasodilator testing in PAH
Diagnosis of multiple cardiac
  disorders including pericardial
  constriction, VSD, RV infarction
Perioperative management of major
  procedures
	Complications related to PAC use:
	■ Arrhythmias
	■ Right bundle branch block
	■ Complete heart block (pre-existing left heart block)
	■ Catheter thrombosis
	■ Pulmonary embolism
	■ Pulmonary infarct
	■ Line sepsis
	■ Pulmonary artery rupture
	■ Pulmonary artery pseudoaneurysm
	■ Valvular damage
	■ Cardiac perforation
	■ Catheter kinking

PAC, pulmonary artery catheter; PAH, pulmonary arterial hypertension; VSD, ventricular septal defect; RV, right ventricle.

The PAC should have all ports flushed and the balloon checked for leaks prior to insertion. In addition, the operator should check that the balloon tip does not protrude beyond the inflated balloon as this can increase the risk of vascular rupture. All ports of the PAC should be attached to the pressure transducers and flushed prior to insertion. Waving of the catheter tip prior to insertion with verification of a waveform on the monitor confirms that the catheter ports are correctly attached. Prior to starting the procedure, a final check to verify that the protective catheter sheath has been inserted over the catheter should be performed. The catheter should be oriented prior to insertion to match the natural curve in the catheter to the projected course through the vasculature.

The PAC is advanced through the introducer, and when the catheter tip is in the RA, the balloon should be inflated gently (Fig. 78.1). The distance from the insertion site to the RA will vary depending on site, but is usually 15 to 20 cm from the right internal jugular (RIJ) or left subclavian sites. Once the balloon is inflated and the lock on the inflating syringe has been activated, the catheter is advanced and the waveforms on the monitor are inspected. The RA waveform will increase in amplitude as the RV is entered, which normally occurs at approximately 30 cm (from a RIJ approach). The passage of the catheter through the RV is arrhythmogenic and should not be of prolonged duration. Conversion of the RV waveform to a PA waveform, as the catheter tip traverses the pulmonary valve, is identified by an increase in the diastolic pressure and the development of a dicrotic notch in the tracing (often at 40 cm). Difficulty in traversing the pulmonary valve is not uncommon in patients with pulmonary arterial hypertension from any cause and, if excessive, catheter length has been advanced without this transition occurring; the most likely explanation is that the catheter is coiled in the enlarged RV. If this occurs, the balloon should be deflated and the catheter should be withdrawn until an RA tracing is obtained, after which the balloon should be inflated and the procedure attempted again. The pulmonary capillary wedge pressure tracing is identified by loss of the arterial tracing to a flatter tracing of lower amplitude than the PA diastolic pressure (often at 50 cm).

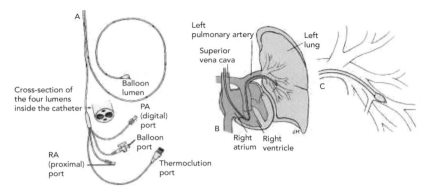

Figure 78.1. A: Swan-Ganz catheter. **B and C:** Location of the Swan-Ganz catheter within the heart and pulmonary vasculature. PA, pulmonary artery; RA, right atrium. (From Nettina SM, *The Lippincott Manual of Nursing Practice*. 7th ed.Baltimore: Lippincott Williams & Wilkins; 2001, with permission.)

At this point, the balloon should be deflated and the PA waveform should be observed. Gentle reinflation of the balloon while feeling for increased resistance and monitoring the waveform for overwedging is crucial. The 1.5-mL balloon should be fully inflated when a wedge tracing is obtained. If a wedge tracing is obtained and the balloon is only partially inflated, this signifies that the catheter tip is too distal and increases the risk of PA rupture by full inflation of the balloon. With this scenario, the catheter should be gently withdrawn 1 to 2 cm with the balloon deflated, and the balloon inflation procedure performed again to obtain a wedge tracing optimally at full balloon inflation. If there is no wedge tracing

TABLE 78.2	Examples of Hemodynamic Parameters Obtained by a Pulmonary Artery Catheter in Different Clinical Situations					
CVP (mm Hg)	RV pressures (mm Hg)	PA pressures (mm Hg)	PAOP (mm Hg)	CO (L/min)	SVR (dynes/ sec/cm^{-5})	Diagnosis
4	17–30/0–6	15–30/5–13	2–12	3–7	900–1,200	Normal
10	48/12	48/30	28	2.2	3,200	Cardiogenic shock
4	26/4	26/8	6	7	700	Sepsis
14	26/14	26/14	14	3.0	3,000	Cardiac tamponade
16	80/30	80/40	8	3.5	1,400	Pulmonary arterial hypertension
14	38/12	38/18	6	3	2,800	Pulmonary embolism (acute)
2	30/2	30/12	3	2.5	2,500	Hypovolemic shock

CVP, central venous pressure; RV, right ventricle; PA, pulmonary artery; PAOP, pulmonary arterial occlusion pressure; CO, cardiac output; SVR, systemic vascular resistance.

obtained with full inflation of the balloon, the catheter should be advanced with the balloon inflated till a wedge tracing is obtained. The catheter should never be withdrawn with the balloon inflated and should never be advanced without the balloon inflated, as this can result in perforation of the heart or a PA.

Once insertion is completed, the distance of insertion from the introducer site should be noted and recorded as a reference point. The catheter should be secured with tape and a sterile dressing and a chest x-ray should be obtained to verify catheter course, tip position, and to rule out any complications from the procedure, such as a pneumothorax. As the catheter warms up in the patient's body, it tends to soften and migrate distally, which increases the risk of overwedging, pulmonary infarction, and PA rupture with balloon inflation, so this should be re-evaluated with a daily chest x-ray as well as bedside by cautious inflation of the balloon and inspection of the waveforms (Table 78.2).

Suggested Reading

Binanay C, Califf RM, Hasselblad V, et al. Evaluation study of congestive heart failure and pulmonary artery catheterization effectiveness: the ESCAPE trial. *JAMA.* 2005;294: 1625–1633.
  Randomized controlled trial in 433 patients with severe symptomatic heart failure where therapy guided by a PAC did not affect mortality or hospitalization but did increase adverse events.
Cohen MG, Kelly RV, Kong DF, et al. Pulmonary artery catheterization in acute coronary syndromes: insights from the GUSTO 2b and GUSTO 3 trials. *Am J Med.* 2005;118: 482–488.
  Retrospective study of 26,437 patients experiencing acute coronary syndromes. 735 patients had PAC inserted and these patients had higher mortality even after adjustments for baseline patients differences. This did not apply to patients who were in cardiogenic shock.
Connors AF Jr, Speroff T, Dawson NV, et al. The effectiveness of right heart catheterization in the initial care of critically ill patients. *JAMA.* 1996;276:889–897.
  Observational study of 5735 critically ill patients, were after adjustment for treatment selection bias, PAC uses was associated with increased mortality and increased resource utilization.
Eisenberg PR, Jaffe AS, Schuster DP. Clinical evaluation compared to pulmonary artery catheterization in the hemodynamic assessment of critically ill patients. *Crit Care Med.* 1984;12:549–553.
  Prospective study in 103 patients which emphasized the difficulty of accurately predicting hemodynamics based on clinical evaluation. The study found that planned therapy was changed in 58% of the cases after insertion of a PAC, with unanticipated therapy added in 30% of the cases.
Harvey S, Harrison DA, Singer M, et al. Assessment of the clinical effectiveness of pulmonary artery catheters in management of patients in intensive care (PAC-Man): a randomized controlled trial. *Lancet.* 2005;366:472–477.
  Large multi-center randomized controlled study in UK ICU's which noted no difference in outcomes when a PAC was used to manage critically ill patients. 46 of 486 patients had a complication from PAC insertion, none of which were fatal.
Rhodes A, Cusack RJ, Newman PJ, et al. A randomized, controlled trial of the pulmonary artery catheter in critically ill patients. *Intensive Care Med.* 2002;28:256–264.
  Single center randomized trial in 201 critically ill patients did not show a mortality difference between the PAC and control groups.
Richard C, Warsjawski J, Anguel N, et al. Early use of the pulmonary artery catheter and outcomes in patients with shock and acute respiratory distress syndrome: a randomized controlled trial. *JAMA.* 2003;290:2713–2720.
  Multicenter randomized study of 676 patients with septic shock, ARDS or both, where clinical management with a PAC did not affect morbidity or mortality.
Sandham JD, Hull RD, Brant RF, et al. A randomized, controlled trial of the use of pulmonary artery catheters in high-risk surgical patients. *N Engl J Med.* 2003;348:5–14.
  Randomized trial in 1,994 elderly, high risk surgical patients, found no benefit to PAC

directed therapy over standard care and a higher rate of pulmonary embolism in the PAC group.

Steingrub JS, Celoria G, Vickers-Lahti M, et al. Therapeutic impact of pulmonary artery catheterization in a medical/surgical ICU. *Chest.* 1991;99:1451–1455.

An expert panel rated the performance of housestaff/attending interpretation of hemodynamic data in 154 medical/surgical patients. Most housestaff/attending performance was judged appropriate and the study suggested that information derived from a PAC was instrumental in managing patients who were unresponsive to initial therapy.

Swan HJ, Ganz W, Forrester J, et al. Catheterization of the heart in man with use of a flow-directed balloon-tipped catheter. *N Engl J Med.* 1970;283:447–451.

The landmark initial description of the technique.

The National Heart, Lung, and Blood Institute Acute Respiratory Distress Syndrome (ARDS) Clinical Trials Network. Pulmonary-artery versus central venous catheter to guide treatment of acute lung injury. *N Engl J Med.* 2006;354:2213–2224.

Randomized multi-center trial in 1000 patients with acute lung injury which had an explicit fluid management algorithm. PAC use did not improve survival or organ function and was associated with more complications than therapy guided by a regular central line.

79 PERICARDIOCENTESIS
Timothy J. Bedient

Pericardiocentesis is a procedure involving fluid removal from the pericardial space and can be a lifesaving procedure in patients with cardiac tamponade. This chapter discusses rational use of pericardiocentesis in the critical care setting and the steps required for pericardiocentesis; it is not intended as a complete review of pericardial disease and tamponade. Tamponade is also discussed in Chapter 4.

Tamponade occurs when inappropriate fluid in the pericardial space raises the intrapericardial pressure, compressing the heart and decreasing cardiac output. The size of the pericardial effusion required for tamponade varies widely. Effusions that collect during minutes to hours, such as occur with traumatic hemopericardium, can cause hemodynamic compromise with as little as 200 mL of fluid, and effusions that collect during days to weeks, such as occur in patients with malignant effusions, allow the pericardium to expand and can exceed 2,000 mL before tamponade occurs. Once the pericardium is no longer able to accommodate increasing amounts of fluid, any additional fluid will compress the heart and decrease cardiac output, resulting in tamponade.

Causes of pericardial effusions are listed in Table 79.1. Cardiac tamponade diagnosis is supported by (a) physical examination with hypotension, pulsus paradoxus (inspiratory systolic blood pressure decrease >10 mm Hg), muffled heart sounds, and prominent jugular venous distention; (b) electrocardiogram showing electrical alternans, low voltage, and tachycardia; (c) chest radiograph showing a globular or enlarged cardiac silhouette; and (d) hemodynamic instability in a patient with a known pericardial effusion or recent event known to cause a pericardial effusion (Table 79.1).

Although tamponade is a clinical diagnosis, it is a class I recommendation from the ACC/AHA/ASE (American College of Cardiology American Heart Association, American Society of Echocardiography) that patients with documented or suspected tamponade be urgently evaluated with transthoracic echocardiography to verify a pericardial effusion and to look for echocardiographic evidence of tamponade such as diastolic collapse of the right atrium and ventricle, respiratory variation in mitral and tricuspid flow velocities, and ventricular interdependence. Effusions can be graded on the basis of echo-free space during diastole as small (<10 mm), medium (10 to 20 mm), large (>20 mm), and very large (>>20 mm) with marked compression of the heart. An echocardiogram should also be used to look for aortic dissection, which is a major contraindication to pericardiocentesis (see Chapter 20 for the diagnosis and treatment of aortic dissection). Relative contraindications to pericardiocentesis include small, posterior, and loculated effusions, coagulopathy, and platelets <50,000/mm³. Surgical drainage is preferred for patient with hemopericardium and purulent pericarditis.

When tamponade is identified, patients should be treated as outlined in Chapter 4, including aggressive administration of intravenous fluid, and avoidance of diuretics. Vasopressors and inotropes are generally ineffective. Intubation should be avoided if possible as it increases intrathoracic pressure and may worsen cardiac output. Patients who have surgical indications for drainage should be taken to the operating room. Patients who respond to treatment and have minimal tamponade may be closely monitored with serial physical examinations and echocardiograms. However, patients with overt hemodynamic compromise should undergo emergent pericardiocentesis.

At most centers, including Washington University, pericardiocentesis is performed by an interventional cardiologist in the cardiac catheterization laboratory or the cardiac intensive care unit under echocardiographic or fluoroscopic guidance, often with the needle

TABLE 79.1	Causes of Pericardial Effusion

Neoplasm
Infectious pericarditis (viral, bacterial, tubercular, parasitic)
Uremia
Postmyocardial infarction pericarditis (Dressler syndrome)
Postcatheter-based procedure and cardiothoracic surgery
Traumatic hemopericardium
Systemic autoimmune diseases (SLE, RA)
Drugs (e.g., chemotherapeutic agents, anticoagulants)
Postradiation
Aortic dissection
Idiopathic

SLE, systemic lupus erythematosus; RA, rheumatoid arthritis.

attached to an electrocardiogram lead. Pericardiocentesis may also be performed at the bedside, and it is a current class IIa recommendation by the ACC/AHA/ASE to use echocardiography to guide and monitor pericardiocentesis when available. Blind pericardiocentesis should be performed only in patients with cardiac tamponade undergoing cardiac arrest or in patients with overt tamponade in which image guidance is not available. If time permits, coagulopathies should be reversed prior to pericardiocentesis. The following steps are used for pericardiocentesis with or without image guidance;

STEPS FOR BEDSIDE PERICARDIOCENTESIS

1. Gather the necessary equipment, which is available at most centers in a prepackaged pericardiocentesis kit. At Washington University, our pericardiocentesis kits contain an 18-gage needle with inner cannula, but other options include a 3.5-inch, 18-gage spinal needle, or equivalent, procedure needle. In patients with cardiac arrest, sterile technique is not always possible. Equipment includes, but is not limited to:
   18-gauge needle
   20- and 50-mL syringe
   Scalpel with number 11 blade
   10 to 20 mL of 1% lidocaine
   Antiseptic (Betadine or chlorhexidine gluconate)
   Sterile gown and gloves, face shield, and cap
   Additional equipment as listed below if a pericardial drain is placed
2. Position the head of the patient's bed at a 30- to 45-degree angle to cause fluid to collect inferiorly in the pericardial space.
3. Locate the patient's xiphoid process and left costal margin by palpation.
4. The needle insertion site is identified by moving 0.5 to 1 cm to the (patient's) left of the xiphoid process, and 0.5 cm (in thin patients) to 1.5 cm (in obese patients) caudal to the costal margin.
5. If time permits, prepare this area with antiseptic solution, sterile drapes, and local anesthetic with 1% lidocaine.
6. Make a small incision at the needle insertion site with the scalpel blade to assist in inserting the needle.
7. Two options exist for needle insertion into the pericardial space:
   An 18-gauge needle with inner cannula (go to step 9)
   An18-gauge needle attached to a 20-mL syringe (preferred in patients undergoing pericardiocentesis during cardiac arrest; go to step 8).
   The needle-with-cannula method is slower and relies on the passive flow of fluid when the cannula is removed to verify entry into the pericardial effusion. The inner cannula prevents tissue from clogging the syringe as it is advanced.

When the needle is attached to a syringe, constant suction is kept on the syring and the needle can be advanced more rapidly, with entry into the pericardial space verified by fluid flowing into the syringe. Thus, a needle attached to a syringe is preferred when performing pericardiocentesis during cardiac arrest. Needles with an inner cannula can be attached to a syringe when the cannula is removed.

8. If an 18-gage needle with syringe is used, fill the 20-mL syringe with 10 mL of lidocaine, evacuate the air, and attach to the needle.

Lidocaine is used for patient comfort and can be omitted in patients undergoing emergent pericardiocentesis during cardiac arrest.

Following the steps below, alternate between aspiration and lidocaine injection as the needle is inserted toward the pericardial space. Constant suction should be maintained on the syringe plunger at all times while it is being advanced (go to step 10).

9. If a needle with cannula is used, the needle is advanced towards the pericardial space, and the cannula is removed for 2 to 5 seconds every 0.5 to 1 cm to check for fluid flow.

10. Place the needle in the nondominant hand and place the needle tip in the incision site. The other hand should be on the syringe or inner cannula, depending on the method.

11. Position the needle at 45-degree angle from the skin surface with the needle directed toward the left shoulder (acromioclavicular joint).

12. Advance the needle until the needle tip is felt to be past the posterior border of the ribs.

13. Once past the posterior border of the ribs, reduce the needle angle to 15 degrees between the needle and the skin, and advance the needle toward the pericardial space.

14. A "give" or "pop" may be felt because of a decrease in resistance as the needle enters the pericardial effusion, but fluid flow from the syringe, or passive fluid flow from the needle, verifies placement.

15. If electrocardiogram monitoring is used during the procedure, ST segment elevation or premature ventricular contractions signify that the needle tip is in contact with the pericardium.

16. For procedures done under echocardiographic guidance, agitated saline injected into the syringe can be used as echocardiographic contrast to verify that the needle tip is in the effusion.

17. Vasovagal reactions are common when the needle enters the pericardial space, and atropine should be readily available.

18. Fluid can be removed by exchanging the 20-mL syringe for a 50-mL syringe and aspirating fluid. This is the easiest method to use during cardiac arrest, and removal of as little as 50 mL of fluid can rapidly improve cardiac output.

19. In most instances, a pericardial drain is placed for at least 24 to 48 hours to allow drainage of the effusion until decisions on definitive therapy have been addressed.

20. To place a pericardial drain, insert the guidewire through the blunt-tipped needle and into the pericardial space.

21. Remove the blunt-tipped needle over the wire and, while holding the wire steady, dilate the tract with a 6 to 8 French dilator.

An additional skin incision may have to be made where the wire enters the skin to facilitate dilator advancement.

22. Remove the dilator, keeping the wire in place, then advance the drainage catheter over the guidewire and into the pericardial space.

23. Remove the guidewire.

24. Attach the catheter to the tubing with three-way stopcock and attach the tubing to the drainage bag.

25. Suture the catheter to the skin and cover with a sterile dressing.

26. Fluid can be removed through the three-way stop-cock until hemodynamic improvement is achieved.

27. Further drainage occurs passively, but catheter patency needs to be maintained by one of three methods:

Placing the tubing on continuous suction via a suction bulb.

Flushing the tubing with small volumes of normal saline every 1 to 2 hours.

Some authors recommend alternatively filling the tubing and catheter with urokinase, and opening the catheter every 2 to 4 hours to drain for 1 hour.

TABLE 79.2	Complications of Pericardiocentesis	
Tachycardia and bradycardia arrhythmias		Pneumothorax
Cardiac arrest		Abdominal viscera trauma
Cardiac puncture or laceration		Coronary artery laceration
Hemopericardium		Infection
Pulmonary edema		Vasovagal reaction

28. Diagnostic studies should be requested and may include cell count and differential, glucose, protein, Gram stain and culture (aerobic, anaerobic, tubercular), hematocrit, lactate dehydrogenase, cytology and tumor markers, hematocrit, rheumatoid factor (RF), and antinuclear antibody. Additional studies depend on clinical suspicion.

Table 79.2 lists complications associated with pericardiocentesis. The complication rate varies depending on user experience, effusion size, acuity, and use of image guidance. In a review of 1,127 echocardiographically guided procedures performed at the Mayo Institute during a 21-year period, the major complication rate was 1.2%, which is consistent with other recent large studies. Pericardial drains are generally removed after 24 to 48 hours because of the risk of infection in the pericardial space. However, drains may be kept in place indefinitely in select situations, with rates of catheter obstruction and infection increasing with time. For effusions that are expected to recur, long-term surgical drainage may be required via pericardial window or pericardiectomy.

Suggested Reading

Chietlin MD, Armstrong WF, Aurigemma GP, et al. ACC/AHA/ASE 2003 Guideline update for the clinical application of echocardiography. *Circulation.* 2003;108:1146–1162.
Evidence-based guidelines for the rational use of echocardiography in the diagnosis and management of disease.
Little CL, Freeman GL. Pericardial disease. *Circulation.* 2006;113:1622–1632.
Concise review of pericardial disease including acute pericarditis, cardiac tamponade, and pericardial restriction.
Maisch B, Seferovic PM, Ristic AD, et al, for the Task Force on the Diagnosis and Management of Pericardial Diseases of the European Society of Cardiology. Guidelines on the diagnosis and management of pericardial diseases: executive summary. *Eur Heart J.* 2004;25:587–610.
Summary review og the current literature on the causes, diagnosis, and management or pericardial diseases, including cardiac tamponade.
Tsang TSM, Enriquez-Sarano M, Freeman WK, et al. Consecutive 1127 therapeutic echocardiographically guided pericardiocentesis: clinical profile, practice patterns, and outcomes spanning 21 years. *Mayo Clin Proc* 2002;77:429–436.
Registry review of echocardiographically guided pericardiocentesis from 1979 through 2000, highlighting causes of pericardial effusions in 3 to 7 year periods, and a high success and safety rate.

XX *End-of-Life Issues*

80 END-OF-LIFE CARE IN THE INTENSIVE CARE UNIT
Jonathan M. Green

Despite individuals' stated preference to die at home, the majority of persons die in institutions. In 2001, only 20% to 25% of U.S. deaths were at home, with the remaining in hospitals (approximately 50% to 60%) and nursing homes (20% to 25%). Of hospital deaths, almost half occurred in the intensive care units (ICUs). In 1995, the SUPPORT trial documented a number of deficiencies in end-of-life care in ICUs, including poor communication between physician and patient about preferences for cardiopulmonary resuscitation, failure to write do not resuscitate orders for patients who desire them, and inadequately treated pain and discomfort during the final days of life. Thus, it is critical that the ICU physician develop the skills and techniques appropriate to managing the dying patient. In this chapter I will discuss issues common to providing good end-of-life care to all patients, as well as those issues unique to the ICU patient population.

ESTABLISHING GOALS OF CARE

Patients admitted to ICUs are at an increased risk of death and also face the prospect of being subjected to invasive procedures and treatments. Studies have demonstrated that as the potential for good outcome declines, so does willingness to undergo highly burdensome treatment regimens. However, in one study, 26% of those surveyed stated they strongly agreed with receiving ICU care despite an outcome predicted to be a persistent vegetative state or terminal illness. Conversely, between 1% and 2% of patients did not wish to undergo ICU care, even if they were to be returned to a fully functional health status. Given these disparities in individual patient preferences, it is essential to establish appropriate goals of care either prior to admission or early in the course of an ICU stay.

On admission to the ICU, the staff should ascertain whether a patient has previously appointed a durable power of attorney for health care and/or completed an advance directive. If so, these documents should be obtained and, if possible, the contents of them should be discussed with the patient. However, the majority of patients have neither document, and despite the presence of life-limiting illness, many will have not discussed end-of-life care with either their personal physician or family members. Thus, it may be that these discussions are occurring in the ICU setting for the first time. If the patient is capable of participating, discussions to establish goals of care should be held directly with him or her. The outcome of these discussions should then be shared by the patient and physician together with the patient's family and loved ones, as directed by the patient. If the patient is not decisional either because of the acute condition or previous underlying disease, the discussion should be held with an appropriate surrogate (see "Surrogate Decision-making").

The purpose of the goals of care discussion is to ascertain what the patient and family's expectations are for the hospitalization. In addition, the physician should elicit the values, preferences, and wishes of the patient with respect to what the patient views as an acceptable outcome for the ICU stay. This may range from hope for cure to a desire for a painfree death, or anywhere in between. Patients often have multiple seemingly contradictory goals, in which case the physician should help in clarification and prioritization. It is equally important for the physician to provide prognostic information and advise the patient and family as to what can reasonably be expected during the hospitalization. Disparities between the patient's and physician's goals are frequent sources of conflict in the ICU. If significant differences are identified, ongoing discussions to identify reasons for the disagreement and reach a consensus are crucial. Possible reasons may include misunderstandings on the part of the patient or family as to nature of the disease or treatment options, or failure of the physician to appreciate cultural differences or other values inherent to the individual patient. It is also important to recognize that the goals may shift during the course of an acute illness. Therefore, as the clinical scenario changes, ongoing discussions to re-evaluate the goals of care are necessary.

SURROGATE DECISION-MAKING

Patients in the ICU are often unable to participate in decision-making because of either their acute illness or underlying disease process. In these instances, appropriate surrogates must be identified. Many, but not all, states have a legal order of surrogacy established. It is important to be familiar with the relevant laws in the state in which you practice. For the purposes of this discussion, a valid surrogate can be defined as an individual who can faithfully represent the goals, values, and wishes of the patient, and act accordingly and in the patient's best interest. Typically, it is presumed that family members are best able to fill this role; however, persons not related to the patient may also be able to serve as a valid surrogate. As implied by the definition, the role of the surrogate is to represent the patient's wishes. However, this is often a difficult task, and is almost always colored by the surrogate's own values and preferences. Studies of surrogate decision-making have shown that surrogates accurately represent the patient only 50% to 70% of the time.

There are often multiple individuals who could be considered a valid surrogate. The family may choose to appoint one person as spokesperson, or may prefer to decide as a group. Not infrequently, there is disagreement among them as to what the patient's wishes would be. If the patient has appointed a specific individual as durable power of attorney for health care, then in the absence of specific evidence that he or she is not acting in good faith, that individual should serve as primary decision-maker. Most often, there is no one individual specified. It is important that the critical care physician work to guide the family and help them reach consensus. Typically, a series of family meetings in which the disputed issues are explored will lead to consensus and resolution. It is often helpful to include nurses, social workers, chaplains, and other team members in these discussions.

The standards for surrogate decision-making are (a) substituted judgment and (b) best interest. The substituted judgment standard asks the surrogate to guide the team as to what decision the patient would make in this circumstance, essentially asking if the patient could speak for himself or herself, what he or she would say. If the patient and surrogate have had specific discussions that inform this decision, then this approach may be reasonable. Often, however, no such discussion has taken place, leaving the surrogate to speculate. The best interest standard asks the surrogate to help the physician determine whether the proposed treatment is in the best interest of the patient, weighing the potential benefits and burdens of the treatment with what is known about the goals and values of the patient. This standard can also be problematic because in the absence of specific information, it is difficult to determine what an acceptable outcome is and what level of treatment burden the patient would tolerate for that outcome. Typically, both surrogates and caregivers underestimate the willingness of patients to undergo aggressive interventions and the quality of life that patients deem to be acceptable.

WITHDRAWING AND WITHHOLDING LIFE-SUSTAINING TREATMENTS

Critical care physicians are often faced with decisions to limit life-sustaining treatment. In one large study of 851 patients admitted to a medical ICU requiring mechanical ventilation, almost 20% had ventilatory support withdrawn. These decisions can be a source of distress and conflict for health care providers as well as patients and families. The ethical basis for withdrawal of life-sustaining treatment stems directly from the principle of respect for autonomy. It is well accepted by the medical profession and society at large that a patient, and therefore by extension the surrogate, may make an informed decision to refuse any proposed treatment, even if the physician believes that such a decision is not in their best interest. From this, it follows directly that patients may opt to discontinue any treatment once initiated. If this were not the case, many patients might be reluctant to initiate potentially beneficial therapies for fear they would not be permitted to stop at a later time. Conflicts may arise when the health care provider believes that discontinuation of life-sustaining interventions violates the principles of beneficence and nonmaleficence, or because they think such actions are in opposition to their own conscience. Alternatively, surrogates may wish to continue aggressive care despite the recommendation of the team that such treatments are only prolonging an inevitable death (see "Futility").

Most commonly, withdrawal of life-sustaining treatments is equated with discontinuation of mechanical ventilation. However, discontinuation of hemodynamic support, hemodialysis, transfusions, or other interventions also may be considered in this context. The decision to withdraw life-sustaining treatments should be approached in a manner similar to all other treatment decisions. Although ultimate responsibility lies with the attending physician, it is particularly important in this circumstance that opinions of other health care providers are given voice and considered. The goal of withdrawal of life-sustaining interventions is to remove treatments that are no longer congruent with the patient's goals and are therefore no longer appropriate. If the patient is not decisional, it is essential that there has been prior discussion with the surrogate(s) and that they are in agreement with the proposed plan. This should be documented in the medical record.

Attention to the patient's comfort is paramount throughout the patient's ICU stay, but assumes particular importance during the process of withdrawal of life-sustaining treatments. Reluctance to administer adequate doses of analgesics and sedatives can result in undue and unacceptable levels of suffering to both the patient and surviving family members. There is ethical and legal consensus that although respiratory depression or hypotension may be a foreseeable consequence of these medications, if the intent is to relieve specific symptoms such as pain or dyspnea, it is essential to treat in adequate doses despite the possibility that death may be hastened. Ethically, the justification for this has been termed *the rule of double effect* (Table 80.1). Doses of medication vary considerably depending on

TABLE 80.1	The Rule of Double Effect

An action with two possible consequences, one good and one bad, is morally permissible if the action:

1. Is not in itself immoral.
2. Is undertaken only with the intention of achieving the possible good effect, without intending the possible bad effect, even though the bad effect may be foreseen.
3. The action does not bring about the good effect solely by means of the bad effect.
4. Is undertaken for a proportionately grave reason.

the patient. Most commonly, narcotics such as morphine or fentanyl are given in combination with a benzodiazepine, typically either midazolam or lorazepam. The medications should be administered initially as a bolus followed by continuous infusion. Each increase in infusion rate should be preceded by an appropriate bolus to allow for a rapid achievement of steady-state levels. Individual patients may have greatly differing medication requirements, depending on their illness and previous exposure to the drugs. Therefore, the dosage needs to be titrated to individual patient needs. Neuromuscular blocking agents should not be used as they do not provide any palliative effect to the patient and make assessment of comfort impossible.

If mechanical ventilation is to be discontinued, paralytic agents should be discontinued and their effect allowed to wear off. The patient is first placed on continuous positive airway pressure/peak systolic velocity settings of 5/5 mm Hg, adequate sedation is administered to minimize dyspnea and the patient is then extubated. There should be frequent assessment by the nursing and medical staff for comfort. Family members are given the option of being present during the extubation, depending solely on their personal preferences. If possible, the monitor screen in the patient's room should be turned off to allow the family to focus on the patient without distraction.

FUTILITY

The issue of medical futility has been a subject of prolonged and intense controversy. Typically, futility debates arise in the ICU when the health care team believes that continued aggressive interventions are highly unlikely to lead to patient survival, yet the patient's surrogate insists that all measures continue. Frustration on the part of the physicians and other team members results in the declaration that further treatment is futile, in an attempt to rationalize discontinuation of treatment without the consent of the surrogate. However, this is ethically problematic, and there remains no clear consensus on an approach to futility. Moreover, most clinical situations in which these conflicts arise can be favorably resolved by improved communication between the physician and family.

Bernard Lo provides three specific conditions that define interventions that are futile in the strict sense. (a) The intervention has no pathophysiologic rationale. An example of this would be the treatment of a Gram-negative infection with an antibiotic such as vancomycin. (b) Cardiac arrest occurs as a result of refractory hypotension or hypoxemia despite maximal supportive therapy. Performance of cardiopulmonary resuscitation in such a circumstance will be ineffective in restoring circulation. (c) The intervention has been tried and already failed in the patient. Treatments that meet these strict criteria do not need to be provided. However, these are clearly the minority of clinical situations in which futility is discussed. Many other looser futility criteria have been proposed, but these are problematic. Most of these rely on subjective determinations of what is an acceptable probability of a favorable outcome, or on determinations of quality of life.

Some groups have developed policies on futility that focus on process and conflict resolution rather than on absolute definitions. The advantage of these is that a defined series of steps are taken that result in enhanced communication. Ultimately, it is the process of increased communication between the health care providers and family members that leads to the satisfactory resolution of these difficult situations. Unilateral decision-making with regard to limiting life-sustaining care for critically ill patients using futility as a rationale is highly discouraged for several reasons. First, the criteria are often incorrectly and inconsistently applied, and perhaps most importantly, such action can lead to extreme distress and anger among the surviving family members. This is not to imply that physicians need to be held hostage to unreasonable demands of unrealistic families, but that the focus should be on continued communication to reach a plan of care that is acceptable to all involved parties.

DETERMINATION OF DEATH BY WHOLE-BRAIN CRITERIA

In 1981, the President's Commission for the Study of Ethical Problems in Medicine and Biomedical and Behavioral Research recommended a uniform standard for the determination of death. This stated that "An individual who has sustained either 1) irreversible

TABLE 80.2	Whole-Brain Criteria for Death

An individual with irreversible cessation of all functions of the entire brain, including the brainstem is dead.

1. Cerebral functions are absent.
   Presence of deep coma, cerebral unreceptivity and unresponsiveness.
2. Brainstem functions are absent.
   Absence of pupillary, corneal, oculocephalic, oculovestibular, oropharyngeal, and respiratory reflexes.
3. Irreversibility is recognized by:
   The cause of coma is established and is sufficient to account for the loss of brain function.
   The possibility of recovery of any brain function is excluded.
   The cessation of all brain functions persists for an appropriate period of observation and/or trial of therapy.

cessation of circulatory and respiratory functions, or 2) irreversible cessation of all functions of the entire brain, including the brainstem, is dead. A determination of death must be made in accordance with accepted medical standards." Although death by cardiopulmonary criteria is understood and well accepted by physicians and lay people alike, declaration of death by whole-brain criteria can be more problematic. Many families and religious groups are reluctant to accept this determination.

Determination of death by whole-brain criteria requires examination by an experienced physician. Essential elements include that the patient is in deep coma, that brainstem function is documented to be absent, the cause of coma is established and sufficient to account for the loss of brainstem function, that the possibility of recovery of any brain function is excluded, and that cessation of all brain function persists for an appropriate period of observation and/or trial of therapy (Table 80.2). Implicit in this is that reversible causes such as drug intoxications, severe metabolic disturbances, and hypothermia have been excluded as causes for the coma. The definition does not require the use of specialized testing, but in some instances cerebral perfusion scanning or electroencephalography testing may be helpful to document the absence of cerebral blood flow or electrical activity.

After the determination of death, the family should not be told the patient is "brain-dead," as this terminology is confusing to many. Instead, they should be informed that the patient has been pronounced dead by neurologic or whole-brain criteria. All previously initiated life-sustaining treatments, such as mechanical ventilation and pressor support, should be withdrawn. In some circumstances, the clinician may elect to continue these for a limited time to allow family members to come to the bedside or for arrangements to be made for organ donation. It is not necessary to provide sedation or analgesia to the patient at this time.

CONCLUSION

Physicians caring for the critically ill will continue to face challenges in providing appropriate care for the dying patient. Many factors, including increases in technology and an aging population, will almost certainly lead to greater numbers of patients dying in ICUs. Enhanced communication between care providers, patients, and families at all stages of the illness is key to assuring that a satisfactory outcome is achieved.

Suggested Reading

Angus DC, Barnato AE, Linde-Zwirble WT, et al.Use of intensive care at the end of life in the United States: an epidemiologic study. *Crit Care Med.* 2004;32:638–643.

Cook D, Rocker G, Marshall J, et al. Withdrawal of mechanical ventilation in anticipation of death in the intensive care unit. *N Engl J Med.* 2003;349:1123–1132.

Elpern EH, Patterson PA, Gloskey D, et al Patients' preferences for intensive care. *Crit Care Med.* 1992;20:43–47.
This study interviewed patients that had been in an ICU, and determined whether they would undergo ICU level care again given four specific outcome scenarios.

Fried TR, Bradley EH, Towle VR, et al Understanding the treatment preferences of seriously ill patients. *N Engl J Med.* 2002;346:1061–1066.
This study documents how patients modify their preferences in response to specific treatment strategies, weighing treatment burden against possible outcomes.

Halevy A, Brody BA.A multi-institution collaborative policy on medical futility. *JAMA.* 1996;276:571–574.

Lo B. *Resolving Ethical Dilemmas: A Guide for Clinicians.* Philadelphia: Lippincott Williams & Wilkins, 2005.
This is an outstanding text examining contemporary medical ethical issues in a practical way.

Murphy DJ, Barbour E. GUIDe (Guidelines for the Use of Intensive Care in Denver): a community effort to define futile and inappropriate care. *New Horiz.* 1994;2:326–331.

The Presidents Commission for the Study of Ethical Problems in Medicine and Biomedical and Behavioral Research. *Defining Death: Medical, Legal, and Ethical Issues in the Definition of Death.* Washington, DC: US Government Printing Office; 1981:159–166.

Shalowitz DI, Garrett-Mayer E, Wendler D. The accuracy of surrogate decision makers: a systematic review. *Arch Intern Med.* 2006;166:493–497.
This study is a meta analysis demonstrating the difficulty in relying on surrogate decision makers to guide treatment plans.

Support Principal Investigators. A controlled trial to improve care for seriously ill hospitalized patients. The study to understand prognoses and preferences for outcomes and risks of treatments (SUPPORT). *JAMA.* 1995;274:1591–1598.
This large multicenter trial demonstrated significant gaps in communication about critical end of life issues in intensive care units. However, in a second, intervention phase, implementation of enhanced communication strategies failed to improve outcomes.

Teno J. Facts on Dying, March 19, 2004. Center for Gerontology and Health Care Research, Brown University. Available at: http://www.chcr.brown.edu/dying/2001DATA.HTM. Accessed October 2, 2006.

XXI *Appendices*

81 COMMON EQUATIONS AND RULES OF THUMB IN THE INTENSIVE CARE UNIT
Warren Isakow

PULMONARY EQUATIONS

Alveolar Gas Equation

$$PA_{O_2} = FI_{O_2}\,(PB - PH_2O) - \frac{Pa_{CO_2}}{R}$$

Where PA_{O_2} = alveolar partial pressure of oxygen,
FI_{O_2} = fraction of inspired oxygen,
PB = barometric pressure (760 mm Hg at sea level),
PH_2O = water vapor pressure,
Pa_{CO_2} = partial pressure of carbon dioxide in the blood,
R = respiratory quotient, assumed to be 0.8.

Alveolar-arterial Oxygen Gradient

$$PA_{O_2} - Pa_{O_2}$$

Normal value is between 3 and 15 mm Hg, and is influenced by age. In a healthy 60-year-old person, it may be as high as 28 mm Hg.
For FI_{O_2} = 21%, should be 5 to 25 mm Hg
For FI_{O_2} = 100%, should be <150 mm Hg

Partial Pressure of Arterial Carbon Dioxide

$$Pa_{CO_2} = K \times \frac{V_{CO_2}}{(1 - Vd/Vt) \times VA}$$

Where Pa_{CO_2} = the partial pressure of carbon dioxide in the blood,
K = constant,
V_{CO_2} = carbon dioxide production,
Vd/Vt = dead space ratio of each tidal volume breath,
VA = minute ventilation.

Lung Compliance

$$\text{Compliance}_{\text{static}} = \frac{\text{Tidal Volume}}{\text{Plateau Pressure} - \text{PEEP (positive end-expiratory pressure)}}$$

Normal compliance in an intubated patient = 0.05 to 0.07 L/cm H_2O

Airway Resistance

$$\text{Airway Resistance} = \frac{\text{(Peak Inspiratory Pressure} - \text{Plateau Pressure)}}{\text{Peak Inspiratory Flow}}$$

Normal resistance in an intubated patient is 4 to 6 cm $H_2O.L^{-1}.sec^{-2}$.

ACID-BASE EQUATIONS

Acute Respiratory Acidosis or Respiratory Alkalosis

$$\Delta pH = 0.008 \times \Delta Pa_{CO_2} \text{ (from 40)}$$

Chronic Respiratory Acidosis or Respiratory Alkalosis

$$\Delta pH = 0.003 \times \Delta Pa_{CO_2} \text{ (from 40)}$$

Metabolic Acidosis

$$\text{Predicted } Pa_{CO_2} = 1.5 \times [HCO_3^-] + 8 \, (\pm 2)$$
$$\text{Bicarbonate deficit (mEq/L)} = [0.5 \times \text{body weight (kg)} \times (24 - [HCO_3^-])]$$

Metabolic Alkalosis

$$\text{Predicted } Pa_{CO_2} = 0.7 \times [HCO_3^-] + 21 \, (\pm 1.5) \text{ (when } [HCO_3^-] \text{ is } <40 \text{ mEq/L)}$$
$$\text{Predicted } Pa_{CO_2} = 0.75 \times [HCO_3^-] + 19 \, (\pm 7.5) \text{ (when } [HCO_3^-] \text{ is } >40 \text{ mEq/L)}$$
$$\text{Bicarbonate excess} = [0.4 \times \text{body weight (kg)} \times ([HCO_3^-] - 24)]$$

Validity of the Data, Henderson's Equation for Concentration of H^+

$$[H^+] = 24 \times \frac{Pa_{CO_2}}{HCO_3^-}$$

pH	$[H^+]$ (mmol/L)
7.60	25
7.55	28
7.50	32
7.45	35
7.40	40
7.35	45
7.30	50
7.25	56
7.20	63
7.15	71

Anion Gap

$$\text{Anion Gap} = [Na^+] - ([CL^-] + [HCO_3^-]) = 10 \pm 4$$

The anion gap should be corrected for albumin, and for every decrease of 1 g/dL in albumin, a decrease of 2.5 mmol in the anion gap will occur.

Delta Gap

$$\Delta gap = (AG - 12) - (24 - [HCO_3^-])$$
$$= 0 \pm 6$$

Positive delta gap signifies a concomitant metabolic alkalosis or respiratory acidosis. Negative delta gap signifies a concomitant normal anion gap metabolic acidosis or chronic respiratory alkalosis.

RENAL EQUATIONS

Calculated Osmolarity

$$\text{Osmolarity (mM)} = 2 \times [Na^+] + \frac{\text{BUN (mg/dL)}}{2.8} + \frac{\text{Glucose (mg/dL)}}{18} + \frac{\text{ETOH}}{4.8}$$

Where ETOH = alcohol.

Osmolar Gap

Osmolar gap = Measured osmolarity − calculated osmolarity. (Normal is <10 mOsm.)

Estimated Creatinine Clearance

$$\text{Creatinine Clearance} = \frac{140 - \text{Age (years)}}{\text{Serum creatinine (mg/dL)} \times 72} \times \text{weight (kg)} (\times 0.85 \text{ in females})$$

Creatinine Clearance

$$\text{Creatinine Clearance} = \frac{[\text{Urine Creatinine (mg/dL)}] \times [\text{urine volume (mL/day)}]}{[\text{Plasma Creatinine (mg/dL)}] \times [1,440 \text{ min/day})]}$$

Fractional Excretion of Sodium (FENa+)

$$FENa^+ = \frac{[\text{Urine Na}^+] \times [\text{Plasma Creatinine}]}{[\text{Urine Creatinine}] \times [\text{Plasma Na}^+]}$$

Fractional Excretion of Urea (FE urea)

$$FE\ Urea = \frac{[\text{Urine Urea}] \times [\text{Plasma Creatinine}]}{[\text{BUN}] \times [\text{Urine Creatinine}]}$$

Correcting Sodium for Hyperglycemia

$$\text{Corrected Na}^+ = 0.016 (\text{Measured Glucose} - 100) + \text{Measured Na}$$

Free Water Deficit

$$\text{Free Water Deficit} = 0.4 \times \text{Lean Body Weight} \times \left[\frac{\text{Plasma [Na}^+]}{140} - 1 \right]$$

Formula for Correcting Hyponatremia

$$\text{Sodium deficit} = (\text{desired [Na}^+] - \text{current [Na}^+]) \times 0.6 \times \text{body weight (kg)}$$

HEMODYNAMIC EQUATIONS

Mean Arterial Pressure (MAP) (70–100 mm Hg)

$$MAP = 1/3 (\text{Pulse Pressure}) + \text{Diastolic BP (blood pressure)}$$

Where pulse pressure = systolic BP − diastolic BP

Arterial Oxygen Content (Cao₂) (18 to 21 mL o₂/dL)

$$CaO_2 = \{1.39 \times [Hb\ (g/dl)] \times SaO_2\} + 0.003 \times PaO_2$$

Mixed Venous Oxygen Content (Cvo₂)(14.5 to 15.5 mL o₂/dL)

$$CvO_2 = \{1.39 \times [Hb\ (g/dL)] \times SvO_2\} + 0.003 \times MvO_2$$

Arterial-mixed Venous Oxygen Content Difference (3.5 to 5.5 mL o₂/dL)

$$avDo_2 = CaO_2 - CvO_2$$

Cardiac Output (CO) (4 to 7 L/min)

1.
$$CO = \text{heart rate} \times \text{stroke volume}$$

2.
$$CO\ (\text{Fick principle}) = \frac{\text{Oxygen Consumption} \times 10}{CaO_2 - CvO_2}$$

Cardiac Index (CI) (2.5 to 4 L/min/m²)

$$CI = CO/BSA$$

Where Body Surface Area (BSA, in m²) = $[\text{height (cm)}]^{0.718} \times [\text{weight (kg)}]^{0.427} \times 0.007449.$

Stroke Volume (SV) (50 to 120 mL per contraction)

Stroke Volume Index (SVI) (35 to 50 mL/m²)

$$SVI = SV/BSA$$

Oxygen Delivery (mL/min) (1,000 mL/min)

$$O_2\ \text{delivery} = CO \times CaO_2 \times 10$$

Systemic Vascular Resistance (SVR) (800 to 1,200 dyne.s.cm⁻⁵)

$$SVR\ (\text{dyne.s.cm}^{-5}) = 80 \times \frac{MAP - CVP}{CO}$$

Pulmonary Vascular Resistance (PVR) (120 to 220 dyne.s.cm⁻⁵)

$$PVR\ (\text{dyne.s.cm}^{-5}) = 80 \times \frac{\text{Mean PAP} - PAOP}{CO}$$

82 DRUG-DRUG INTERACTIONS
Jamie M. Rosini and Scott T. Micek

TABLE 82.1 | **Cytochrome P450 Enzyme Family Substrates, Inhibitors, and Inducers**

Isoenzyme				
1A2	**2C9**	**2C19**	**2D6**	**3A4**
Substrates				
Acetaminophen	Celecoxib	Amitriptyline	Amitriptyline	Alprazolam
Cyclobenzaprine	Ibuprofen	Citalopram	Carvedilol	Buspirone
Imipramine	Irbesartan	Diazepam	Codeine	Calcium Channel
Mexiletine	Losartan	Imipramine	Dextromethorphan	Blockers
Olanzapine	Phenytoin	Phenytoin	Haloperidol	Carbamazepine
Theophylline	Torsemide	Proton pump	Imipramine	Conivaptan
	Warfarin	inhibitors	Lidocaine	Cyclosporine
			Metoprolol	Diazepam
			Mexiletine	Fentanyl
			Ondansetron	Hydrocortisone
			Paroxetine	Lidocaine
			Propafenone	Midazolam
			Propranolol	Protease Inhibitors
			Risperidone	Sildenafil
			Tramadol	Sirolimus
			Venlafaxine	Statins (except
				pravastatin)
				Tacrolimus
Inhibitors				
(Increase the serum and tissue concentration of substrates)				
Cimetidine	Amiodarone	Cimetidine	Amiodarone	Amiodarone
Ciprofloxacin	Fluconazole	Fluoxetine	Cimetidine	Cimetidine
Clarithromycin	Isoniazid	Ketoconazole	Fluoxetine	Clarithromycin
	Metronidazole	Lansoprazole	Haloperidol	Conivaptan
	Sulfamethoxazole	Omeprazole	Methadone	Diltiazem
	Voriconazole	Voriconazole	Paroxetine	Erythromycin
			Quinidine	Itraconazole
			Ritonavir	Ketoconazole
				Protease Inhibitors
				Quinupristin-
				dalfopristin
				Verapamil
				Voriconazole
Inducers				
(Decrease the serum and tissue concentration of substrates)				
Carbamazepine	Bosentan	Bosentan		Bosentan
Rifampin	Phenobarbital	Carbamazepine		Carbamazepine
Tobacco	Rifampin	Rifampin		Phenobarbital
				Phenytoin
				Rifabutin
				Rifampin
				St. John's wort

From Mann HJ. Drug-associated disease:cytochrome P450 interactions. *Crit Care Clin.* 2006;22:329–345, with permission.

TABLE 82.2	Frequent Drug-Drug Interactions in Critically III Patients

Medication	Interacting drug	Effect [a]
Cardiac		
Amiodarone	2C9, 2D6, 3A4 Substrates (Table 82.1)	↑ Substrate
		↑ Digoxin
	Digoxin	
Beta-blockers	2D6 Inhibitors (Table 82.1)	↑ Beta-blocker
(2D6 substrates)	Carbamazepine	↓ Beta-blocker
Carvedilol	Phenytoin	↓ Beta-blocker
Metoprolol	Rifampin	↓ Beta-blocker
Propranolol		
Digoxin	Amiodarone	↑ Digoxin
	Clarithromycin	↑ Digoxin
	Erythromycin	↑ Digoxin
	Esomeprazole	↓ Digoxin
	Quinidine	↑ Digoxin
	Verapamil	↑ Digoxin
Diltiazem/verapamil (3A4 inhibitors)	3A4 Substrates (Table 82.1)	↑ Substrate
Lidocaine	Amiodarone	↑ Lidocaine
Antiepileptics		
Carbamazepine	1A2, 2C19, 3A4 Substrates	↓ Substrate
(enzyme inducer,	(Table 82.1)	↑ Carbamazepine
3A4 substrate)	Clarithromycin	↑ Carbamazepine
	Diltiazem	↑ Carbamazepine
	Erythromycin	↑ Carbamazepine
	Quinupristin-dalfopristin	↑ Carbamazepine
	Verapamil	
Oxcarbamazepine	Phenytoin	↑ Phenytoin
	Verapamil	↓ Oxcarbamazepine
Phenytoin (enzyme inducer)	3A4 Substrates (Table 82.1)	↓ Substrate
Antimicrobials		
Azithromycin	Antacids	↓ Azithromycin
	Cyclosporine	↑ Cyclosporine
	Digoxin	↑ Digoxin
	Tacrolimus	↑ Tacrolimus
Carbapenems	Valproic acid	↓ Valproic acid
Clindamycin	Aminoglycosides	↑ Nephrotoxicity
	Erythromycin	↓ Erythromycin
	Neuromuscular blocking agents	↑ Neuromuscular blockade
Ciprofloxacin	1A2 Substrates (Table 82.1)	↑ Substrate
(1A2 inhibitor)	Cyclosporine	↓ Ciprofloxacin
	Sucralfate	↓ Ciprofloxacin
	Calcium, iron, antacids	↓ oral Ciprofloxacin
Clarithromycin	1A2, 3A4 Substrates (Table 82.1)	↑ Substrate
(1A2, 3A4 inhibitor)	Digoxin	↑ Digoxin
Colistin	Neuromuscular blocking agents	↑ Neuromuscular blockade
Linezolid	SSRIs	↑ Serotonin
	Tramadol	concentrations
	Tricyclic antidepressants	↑ Linezolid
		↑ Linezolid
Piperacillin-tazobactam	Methotrexate	↑ Methotrexate

(continued)

TABLE 82.2	Frequent Drug-Drug Interactions in Critically Ill Patients (*continued*)

Medication	Interacting drug	Effect [a]
Quinupristin-dalfopristin (3A4 inhibitor)	3A4 Substrates (Table 82.1)	↑ Substrate
Vancomycin	NSAIDs	↑ Vancomycin
Antifungals		
Caspofungin	Carbamazepine	↓ Caspofungin
	Cyclosporine	↑ Caspofungin
	Dexamethasone	↓ Caspofungin
	Phenytoin	↓ Caspofungin
	Rifampin	↓ Caspofungin
	Tacrolimus	↓ Tacrolimus
Fluconazole, voriconazole (2C9, 3A4 inhibitor)	2C9, 3A4 Substrates (Table 82.1)	↑ Substrate
Itraconazole Ketoconazole (3A4 inhibitor)	3A4 Substrates (Table 82.1) Acid suppressants	↑ Substrate ↓ Oral capsule form itra/ketoconazole
Posaconazole	3A4 Substrates (Table 82.1) Cimetidine Phenytoin Rifabutin	↑ Substrate ↓ Posaconazole (avoid concomitant use) ↓ Posaconazole (avoid concomitant use) ↓ Posaconazole (avoid concomitant use)
Antivirals		
Foscarnet	Ciprofloxacin	↑ Seizures

SSRIs, selective serotonin reuptake inhibitors; NSAIDs, nonsteroidal anti-inflammatory drugs.
[a]↑, increase serum/tissue concentration; ↓, decrease serum/tissue concentration.

| TABLE 82.3 | Drugs Associated with QT-Interval Prolongation[a] |

Antiarrhythmic agents

Amiodarone	Procainamide
Disopyramide	Propafenone
Dofetilide	Quinidine
Flecainide	Sotalol
Ibutilide	

Antimicrobials

Azithromycin	Ciprofloxacin
Clarithromycin	Levofloxacin
Erythromycin	Moxifloxacin
Telithromycin	Pentamidine
Foscarnet	Azole antifungals

Antidepressants

Amitriptyline	Fluoxetine
Desipramine	Fluoxetine
Imipramine	Sertraline
Doxepin	Venlafaxine

Antipsychotics

Droperidol	Thioridazine
Haloperidol	Chlorpromazine
Quetiapine	Ziprasidone
Risperidone	

Other Agents

Dolasetron	Octreotide
Indapamide	Tacrolimus
Methadone	Tizanidine

[a]The combination of these agents may increase the risk for adverse arrhythmic event including torsades de pointes.
From Owens RC, Nolin TD. Antimicrobial-associated QT interval prolongation: pointes of interest. *Clin Infect Dis.* 2006;43:1603–1611; Olsen KM. Pharmacologic agents associated with QT interval prolongation. *J Fam Pract.* 2005;S8–14; and *N Engl J Med. Roden DM. Drug-induced prolongation of the QT interval.* 2004;350:1013–1022, with permission.

TABLE 82.4	Drugs with Serotonergic Properties[a]

Increased release of serotonin

Amphetamines and derivatives	MAOIs
Cocaine	Mirtazapine
Levodopa	

Inhibition of serotonin metabolism

Linezolid	Selegiline
MAOIs	St. John's wort

Impaired presynaptic reuptake

Amphetamines and derivatives	SSRIs
Bupropion	St. John's wort
Cocaine	Tramadol
Dextromethorphan	Trazadone
Fentanyl	Tricyclic antidepressants
Meperidine	Venlafaxine
Propoxyphene	

Direct serotonin receptor agonism

5-HT1 receptor agonists (i.e., sumatriptan)	Buspirone
Lithium	Carbamazepine

MAOIs, monoamine oxidase inhibitors; SSRIs, selective serotonin reuptake inhibitors.
[a]The combination of these agents may increase the risk for serotonin toxicity manifested by a triad of symptoms including: 1) cognitive changes, 2) autonomic instability, and 3) neuromuscular excitability.
From Taylor JJ, Wilson JW, Estes LL. Linezolid and serotonergic frug interactions: a retrospective survey. *Clin Infect Dis.* 2006;43:180–187, with permission.

COMMON DRUG DOSAGES AND SIDE EFFECTS

83

Lee P. Skrupky and Scott T. Micek

TABLE 83.1 **Shock**

Drug class/ prototypes	Dosing	Rare toxicities	Common toxicities
Norepinephrine	0.02–3 mcg/kg/ min	Tissue hypoxia, tachycardia, arrhythmias, myocardial ischemia, extravasation-associated tissue necrosis	Hyperglycemia
Epinephrine	0.01–0.1 mcg/kg/ min	Tachycardia, arrhythmias, myocardial ischemia, splanchnic and renal hypoxia, extravasation-associated tissue necrosis	Tachycardia, hyperglycemia
Phenylephrine	0.5–10 mcg/kg/ min	Tachycardia, reduced cardiac output, myocardial ischemia, extravasation-associated tissue necrosis	—
Dopamine	5–20 mcg/kg/min	Tachycardia, arrhythmias, myocardial ischemia, tissue hypoxia, extravasation-associated tissue necrosis	—
Vasopressin	0.01–0.04 U/min	Reduced cardiac output, myocardial ischemia, hepatosplanchnic hypoperfusion, thrombocytopenia, hyponatremia, ischemic skin lesions	—
Dobutamine	2.5–20 mcg/kg/min	Arrhythmias	Tachycardia
Milrinone	50 mcg/kg bolus, then 0.25–0.75 mcg/kg/min	Thrombocytopenia, arrhythmias	Hypotension
Corticosteroids Hydrocortisone	Septic Shock: 200–300 mg/day in 3–4 divided doses	—	Short-term: hyperglycemia, mood changes, insomnia, gastrointestinal irritation, increased appetite

(continued)

TABLE 83.1	Shock[a]		
Drug class/ prototypes	**Dosing**	**Rare toxicities**	**Common toxicities**
			Long-term: osteoporosis, acne, thin skin, fat redistribution, muscle wasting, cataracts HPA axis suppression, increased blood pressure, infection
Mineralocorticoids Fludrocortisone	Septic shock: 50–100 mcg PO q24h	—	Increased blood pressure, edema, hypernatremia, hypokalemia
Drotrecogin alfa	24 mcg/kg/hr × 96 hours	—	Bleeding
Alteplase	Pulmonary embolism: 100 mg IV over 2 hr	—	Bleeding

HPA, hypothalamic-pituitary-adrenal; PO, by mouth; IV, intravenous.
[a]Toxicities were classified as "rare" and "common" in a relative fashion for each agent. This table does not include an exhaustive list of possible adverse effects.

TABLE 83.2	Respiratory Disorders

Drug class/ prototypes	Dosing	Rare toxicities	Common toxicities
ARDS, status asthmaticus, COPD exacerbation			
Corticosteroids Methylprednisolone	2 mg/kg/day in 3–4 divided doses, tapering schedule dependant on disease process	—	Short-term: hyperglycemia, mood changes, insomnia, gastrointestinal irritation, increased appetite Long-term: osteoporosis, acne, thin skin, fat redistribution, muscle wasting, cataracts, HPA axis suppression, increased blood pressure, infection
Beta-agonists Albuterol Levalbuterol	2–4 puffs BID to QID 0.63–0.125 mg TID	Tachycardia, insomnia, irritability/ nervousness, tremor, hyperglycemia, hypokalemia	—
Anticholinergics Ipratropium	2–4 puffs BID to QID	Dry mucous membranes, tachycardia	—
Pulmonary hypertension			
Calcium channel blockers Diltiazem Nifedipine[a]	up to 720 mg/day up to 240 mg/day both in divided doses	Gingival hyperplasia, increased cardiovascular events	Peripheral edema flushing, headache, dizziness, hypotension
Warfarin	Target goal INR	Skin necrosis, purple-toe syndrome	Bleeding
Prostacyclins Epoprostenol	2–50 ng/kg/minute IV 5,000–20,000 ng/mL continuous nebulization	—	Jaw pain, nausea, headache, flushing, hypotension, infusion-site pain*
Treprostinil* Iloprost	10–150 ng/kg/min SC 2.5–5 mcg inhaled 6–9 times daily		
Endothelin antagonists Bosentan	62.5 mg PO bid × 1 month, then 125 mg PO BID, as tolerated	Hepatotoxicity, anemia	Headache, hypotension, flushing
PDE-5 inhibitors Sildenafil	20 mg PO TID	Vision changes	Headache, hypotension, flushing, dyspepsia
Nitric oxide	5–40 parts per million	Methemoglobinemia, elevated nitrogen dioxide	Hypotension

HPA, hypothalamic-pituitary-adrenal; BID, twice daily; QID, four times a day; INR, international normalized ratio; IV, intravenous; SC, subcutaneously; PO, by mouth.
[a]Immediate-release form.

TABLE 83.3	Cardiac Disorders		

Drug class/ prototypes	Dosing	Rare toxicities	Common toxicities
	Acute myocardial infarction		
Aspirin	160–325 mg PO daily	Tinnitus, anaphylaxis, gastritis	Bleeding, dyspepsia
Beta-blockers		Heart block,	Bradycardia,
Metoprolol	5 mg IV q5min × 3 dose 50–200 mg PO q12h	bronchospasm, depression, nightmares, altered	hypotension, fatigue, malaise, cold extremities
Esmolol	500 mcg/kg bolus, then 50–300 mcg/kg/min	glucose metabolism, dyslipidemia, sexual dysfunction	
Nitrates		—	Headache, flushing,
Nitroglycerin	10–200 mcg/min		dizziness,
Isosorbide dinitrate	5–40 mg PO TID		hypotension,
Isosorbide mononitrate	30–120 mg PO daily		tachycardia
Morphine	2–4 mg IV q5min	Respiratory depression, hypotension, pruritis	Constipation, dyspepsia, nausea, drowsiness, dizziness
Fibrinolytics	STEMI	—	Bleeding
Alteplase	15 mg bolus, then 0.75 mg/kg (up to 50 mg) × 30 min, then 0.5 mg/kg (up to 35 mg) × 60 min (max, 100 mg over 90 min		
Reteplase	10 mg IV, then 10 mg IV 30 min after first dose		
Tenecteplase	One time bolus: ≤60 kg = 30 mg 61–70 kg = 35 mg 71–80 kg = 40 mg 81–90 = 45 mg ≥90 kg = 50 mg		
Streptokinase	1.5 million units over 2 hr		
Unfractionated heparin	60 U/kg bolus, then 12 U/kg/hr, adjust to aPTT 1.5–2.5 × control	Type II heparin-induced thrombocytopenia, hyperkalemia	Bleeding, type I heparin-induced thrombocytopenia bleeding
Low-molecular-weight Heparins		—	
Enoxaparin	1 mg/kg SC q12h		
Dalteparin	120 U/kg SC q12h		

(*continued*)

| TABLE 83.3 | Cardiac Disorders (*continued*) |

Drug class/ prototypes	Dosing	Rare toxicities	Common toxicities
Direct thrombin inhibitors	PCI	Hypersensitivity reactions*	Bleeding
Argatroban	350 mcg/kg bolus, then 25 mcg/ kg/min		
Bivalirudin	1 mg/kg bolus, then 2.5 mg/kg/hr		
GPIIb/IIIa inhibitors	PCI:	Thrombocytopenia	Bleeding
Abciximab	0.25 mg/kg bolus, then 0.125 mcg/ kg/min		
Eptifibitide	180 mcg/kg bolus, then 2 mcg/kg/min		
Tirofiban	0.4 mcg/kg/min × 30 minutes, then 0.1 mcg/kg/min		
Clopidogrel	75 mg PO daily	Thrombotic thrombocytopenic purpura	Nausea, vomiting, diarrhea, bleeding
Arrhythmias and conduction abnormalities			
Atropine	1 mg IV q3–5 min	—	Dry eyes, dry mouth, urinary retention, tachycardia
Epinephrine	1 mg IV q3–5min	—	Tachycardia, hypertension
Vasopressin	40 units IV		
Procainamide	15–18 mg/kg bolus then 1–6 mg/min	Torsade de pointes	Diarrhea, nausea, vomiting
Lidocaine	1–1.5 mg/kg bolus (may repeat doses 0.5–0.75 mg/kg in 5–10 min up to max 3 mg/kg), then 1–4 mg/min	Confusion, drowsiness, slurred speech, psychosis, paresthesias, muscle twitching, seizures, bradycardia	—
Amiodarone	300 mg bolus, then 1 mg/min for 6 hr, then 0.5 mg/min for ≥18 hr	Heart block, pulmonary fibrosis, hypo/ hyperthyroidism, blue-gray skin discoloration, torsade de pointes, corneal microdeposits, optic neuropathy	Bradycardia, hypotension, nausea
Calcium channel blockers Diltiazem	0.25 mg/kg bolus (may repeat 0.35 mg/kg bolus after 15 min), then 5–15 mg/hr	Heart block, heart failure, exacerbation	Bradycardia, hypotension, constipation (verapamil > diltiazem) headache, flushing, edema

(continued)

TABLE 83.3	Cardiac Disorders (*continued*)		

Drug class/ prototypes	Dosing	Rare toxicities	Common toxicities
Verapamil	5 mg bolus (may repeat up to total 20 mg), then 5–15 mg/hr		
Adenosine	6 mg IV, if not effective in 1–2 min can give 12 mg, may repeat 12 mg	—	Flushing, lightheadedness, headache, nervousness/anxiety
Congestive heart failure			
Nesiritide	2 mcg/kg bolus, then 0.01–0.03 mcg/ kg/min	—	Hypotension, increased serum creatinine
Digoxin	Load: 10–15 mcg/kg; give 50% of load in initial dose, then 25% at 6–12 hr intervals × 2 Maintenance: 0.125–0.5 mg/day (Dose should be reduced by 20%–25% when changing from oral to IV)	Arrhythmias, heart block, visual disturbances (blurred or yellow vision), mental disturbances	Bradycardia
ACE inhibitors		Anaphylaxis, angioedema	Cough, hyperkalemia, hypotension, renal insufficiency
Captopril	6.25–50 mg PO TID		
Lisinopril	2.5–40 mg PO BID		
Enalapril	2.5–10 mg PO BID		
Ramipril	1.25–5 mg PO BID		
Aldosterone receptor Antagonists		Gynecomastia (spironolactone > eplerenone), hyponatremia	Hyperkalemia
Spironolactone	12.5–50 mg PO daily		
Eplerenone	25–50 mg PO daily		
Loop diuretics[a]		Ototoxicity	Hypokalemia, hypomagnesemia, hypocalcemia, orthostatic hypotension, azotemia
Furosemide	20–80 mg/day IV/PO in 2–3 divided doses		
Torsemide	10–20 mg IV/PO daily		
Bumetanide	0.5–2 mg/day in 1–2 doses		
Hypertensive emergencies			
Nitroprusside	Usual, 0.25–3 mcg/ kg/min Max, 10 mcg/kg/min	Muscle spasm	Nausea, vomiting, hypotension, tachycardia, thiocyanate and cyanide toxicity

(*continued*)

TABLE 83.3	Cardiac Disorders (*continued*)

Drug class/ prototypes	Dosing	Rare toxicities	Common toxicities
Nicardipine	3–15 mg/hr	—	Hypotension, tachycardia, headache, flushing, peripheral edema
Labetalol	20–40 mg (max, 80 mg) as IV bolus at 10–20 min intervals, then 0.5–2 mg/min if needed	Heart block, bronchoconstriction	Hypotension, bradycardia, nausea, vomiting
Clonidine	0.1–0.3 mg PO BID–TID	—	Drowsiness, dizziness, hypotension, bradycardia, dry mouth
Hydralazine	10–40 mg IV q4–6h or 10–75 mg PO TID-QID	Drug-induced lupuslike syndrome, rash peripheral neuropathy	Hypotension, tachycardia, flushing, headache
Enalaprilat	1.25–5 mg IV q6h	Anaphylaxis, angioedema	Hypotension, hyperkalemia, renal insufficiency

PO, by mouth; IV, intravenous; TID, three times a day; STEMI, ST-segment elevation myocardial infarction; aPTT, activated partial thromboplastin time; PCI, percutaneous coronary intervention; BID, twice daily.
[a]Usual starting doses are listed for furosemide and torsemide; dosing is highly variable and much larger doses are often used.

TABLE 83.4	Electrolyte Abnormalities

Drug class/ prototypes	Dosing	Rare toxicities	Common toxicities
Hyponatremia			
Conivaptan	20 mg IV bolus, then 0.8– 1.6 mg/hr IV continuous infusion	—	Diarrhea, hypokalemia
Hyperkalemia			
Regular Humulin insulin	10–20 units IV (given with dextrose, every ~1 unit for 4–5 g dextrose)	Local skin reactions	Hypoglycemia, hypokalemia, weight gain
Sodium bicarbonate	1 mEq/kg IV	Extravasation-associated tissue necrosis	Metabolic alkalosis, hypernatremia, hypokalemia
Albuterol	10–20 mg nebulized over 30–60 min	Tachycardia, insomnia, irritability/ nervousness tremor, hyperglycemia, hypokalemia	—
Calcium gluconate	1 gm IV over 2 min	Arrhythmias, phlebitis (chloride > gluconate)	Hypercalcemia, constipation (oral)
Hypercalcemia			
Bisphosphonates Pamidronate Zoledronic acid	60–90 mg IV bolus 4 mg IV bolus	Thrombophlebitis; bone, joint, muscle pain	Fever, fatigue
Calcitonin	Initial 4 U/kg IM q12h, up to 8 U/kg IM q6h	Allergic reaction	Facial flushing, nausea, vomiting
Hypophosphatemia			
Phosphate salts Potassium phosphate* Sodium phosphate†	0.08–0.16 mmol/kg IV over 6 hr	—	Hyperphosphatemia. Hypocalcemia. Hypomagnesemia. hyperkalemia* hypernatremia† diarrhea (oral)

IV, intravenously; IM, intramuscularly.

| TABLE 83.5 | Endocrine Disorders | | |

Drug class/ prototypes	Dosing	Rare toxicities	Common toxicities
	Hypothyroid		
Thyroid hormones Levothyroxine	Myxedema coma: 50–100 mcg IV q6–8h × 24 hr, then 100 mcg IV q24h	Signs and symptoms of hyperthyroidism with excessive doses (tachycardia, angina pectoris, arrhythmias, myocardial infarction, heat intolerance, diaphoresis, hyperactivity)	—
	Hyperthyroid		
Thiourea drugs Propylthiouracil*	Initial 300–600 mg/day in 3 divided doses q8h, maintenance 50–300 mg per day	Agranulocytosis, aplastic anemia, hepatotoxicity, lupuslike syndrome, hypoprothombinemia, polymyositis*	Rash, arthralgias, fever, leukopenia, nausea, vomiting
Methimazole	Initial 30–60 mg/day in 3 divided doses q8h, Maintenance 5–30 mg per day		
Beta-blockers Propranolol	10–40 mg PO q6h	Heart block, bronchospasm, depression, nightmares, altered glucose metabolism, dyslipidemia, sexual dysfunction	Bradycardia, hypotension, fatigue, malaise, cold extremities
SS potassium iodide	1–2 drops PO q12h	Hypersensitivity reactions	Metallic taste, nausea, stomach upset, diarrhea, salivary gland swelling
	Adrenal insufficiency		
Corticosteroids Hydrocortisone Dexamethasone	100 mg IV q8h 10 mg IV prior to ACTH stimulation test	—	Short-term: hyperglycemia, mood changes, insomnia, gastrointestinal irritation, increased appetite Long-term: osteoporosis, acne, thin skin, fat redistribution, muscle wasting, cataracts HPA axis suppression, increased blood pressure, infection

(continued)

TABLE 83.5	Endocrine Disorders (*continued*)

Drug class/ prototypes	Dosing	Rare toxicities	Common toxicities
Mineralocorticoids Fludrocortisone	50–200 mcg PO q24h	—	Increased blood pressure, edema, hypernatremia, hypokalemia
Insulin	—	Local skin reactions	Hypoglycemia, hypokalemia, weight gain

IV, intravenous; PO, by mouth; ACTH, adrenocorticotropin hormone; HPA, hypothalamic-pituitary-adrenal; PRN, as needed; NSAIDs, nonsteroidal anti-inflammatory drugs; TID, three times a day.

TABLE 83.6	Oncologic Emergencies

Drug class/ prototypes	Dosing	Rare toxicities	Common toxicities
Allopurinol	600–800 mg/day in 2–3 divided doses	Nausea, vomiting	Rash
Rasburicase	0.2 mg/kg/day	Hypersensitivity reactions, methemoglobinemia, hemolysis	Nausea, vomiting, fever, headache, rash, diarrhea, constipation

IV, intravenous; PO, by mouth; ACTH, adrenocorticotropin hormone; HPA, hypothalamic-pituitary-adrenal; PRN, as needed; NSAIDs, nonsteroidal anti-inflammatory drugs; TID, three times a day.

TABLE 83.7	Temperature Regulation

Drug class/ prototypes	Dosing	Rare toxicities	Common toxicities
Acetaminophen	325–1,000 mg PO q4–6h PRN	Hepatotoxicity	—
NSAIDs Ibuprofen	200–800 mg PO q3–6h PRN	Gastric ulceration, bleeding, acute renal failure, increased risk of cardiovascular events	Gastric irritation, nausea
Ketorolac	15–30 mg IM or 10 mg PO PRN		
Dantrolene	1–2.5 mg/kg IV; may repeat q5–10min to max cumulative dose 10 mg/kg	Hepatotoxicity, muscle weakness	Drowsiness, dizziness, diarrhea, nausea, vomiting
Bromocriptine	2.5–5 mg PO TID	—	Headache, dizziness, nausea, diarrhea, hypotension, nasal congestion

IV, intravenous; PO, by mouth; ACTH, adrenocorticotropin hormone; HPA, hypothalamic-pituitary-adrenal; PRN, as needed; NSAIDs, nonsteroidal anti-inflammatory drugs; TID, three times a day.

| TABLE 83.8 | Toxicology | | |

Drug class/ prototypes	Dosing	Rare toxicities	Common toxicities
Activated charcoal	25–100 g	Bowel obstruction	Vomiting, constipation, fecal discoloration (black)
Naloxone	0.4–2 mg IV q2min, up to 10 mg	Abrupt reversal may cause withdrawal symptoms (sweating, agitation, hypertension, tachycardia, nausea, vomiting, cardiovascular events, seizures) pulmonary edema	—
Flumazenil	0.2–0.5 mg IV q1min, up to 5 mg	Abrupt reversal may cause withdrawal symptoms (sweating, agitation, hypertension, tachycardia, nausea, vomiting, cardiovascular events, seizures)	—
N-Acetylcysteine	Oral 140 mg/kg loading dose, then 70 mg/kg q4h × 17 doses IV 150 mg/kg bolus, then 12.5 mg/kg/hr × 4 hr, then 6.25 mg/kg/hr × 16 hr	Anaphylactic reactions	Nausea, vomiting (oral), unpleasant odor (oral)
Deferoxamine	1 g IV bolus, then 500 mg IV q4h × 2 doses	Infusion-related reactions (hypotension, tachycardia, erythema, urticaria) anaphylactic reactions acute respiratory distress syndrome	Urine discoloration (orange-red)
Fomepizole	15 mg/kg IV bolus, then 10 mg/kg IV q12h × 4 doses, then 15 mg/kg IV q12h until ethylene glycol or methanol level <20	—	—

IV, intravenous.

TABLE 83.9	Infectious Diseases

Drug class/ prototypes	Dosing	Rare toxicities	Common toxicities
Antibacterial agents			
Penicillins		Anaphylaxis, seizures, hemolytic anemia, neutropenia, thrombocytopenia, drug fever	Diarrhea, nausea, vomiting, rash
Ampicillin	2–3 g IV q4–6h		
Aqueous penicillin G	2–4 million U IV q4h		
Antistaphylococcal Penicillins		Anaphylaxis, neutropenia, thrombocytopenia, acute interstitial nephritis, hepatotoxicity	Diarrhea, nausea, vomiting, rash
Nafcillin	2 g IV q4–6h		
Oxacillin	2 g IV q4–6h		
B-lactam/ B-lactamase Inhibitors		Anaphylaxis, seizures, hemolytic anemia, neutropenia, thrombocytopenia, *Clostridium difficile* colitis, cholestatic jaundice,* drug fever	Diarrhea, nausea, vomiting, rash
Amoxicillin/ clavulanate	875 mg PO BID		
Ampicillin/ sulbactam	1.5–3 g IV q6h		
Piperacillin/ Tazobactam*	3.375–4.5 g IV q6h		
Ticarcillin/ clavulanate	3.1 g IV q4–6h		
Cephalosporins		Anaphylaxis, seizures, neutropenia, thrombocytopenia, drug fever	Diarrhea, nausea, vomiting, rash
Cefazolin	1–2 g IV q8h		
Cefoxitin	1–2 g IV q4–8h		
Ceftriaxone	1–2 g IV q12–24h		
Cefepime	500 mg–2 g IV q8–12h		
Carbapenems		Anaphylaxis, seizures (imipenem> meropenem> ertapenem), C. .difficile colitis, drug fever	Diarrhea, nausea, vomiting
Imipenem	500 mg–1 g IV q6–8h		
Meropenem	1 g IV q8h		
Ertapenem	1 g IV q24h		
Glycopeptides		Ototoxicity, nephrotoxicity (unlikely without concomitant nephrotoxins), thrombocytopenia	Red-man syndrome
Vancomycin	15 mg/kg IV q12h		
Oxazolidinones		More common with long-term use: peripheral and optic neuropathy, myelosuppression Possible with short-term use: lactic acidosis	Diarrhea
Linezolid	600 mg IV/PO q12h		
Lipopeptides		Myopathy, anemia	Diarrhea, constipation, vomiting
Daptomycin	4–6 mg/kg IV q24h		
Streptogramin		—	Arthralgia, myalgia, inflammation, pain, edema at infusion site, hyperbilirubinemia
Quinupristin/ dalfopristin	7.5 mg/kg IV q8h		

(*continued*)

TABLE 83.9	Infectious Diseases (*continued*)		

Drug class/ prototypes	Dosing	Rare toxicities	Common toxicities
Aminoglycosides	—	—	Nephrotoxicity
Amikacin	8 mg/kg IV q12h or 15 mg/kg extended interval	—	Ototoxicity
Gentamicin	3 mg/kg bolus, then 2 mg/kg IV q8h or 5–7 mg/kg extended interval		
Tobramycin	See gentamicin		
Fluoroquinolones		Anaphylaxis, QTc	Nausea, vomiting,
Ciprofloxacin	500–750 mg PO BID or 400 mg IV q8–12h	prolongation, joint toxicity in children, tendon rupture	diarrhea, photosensitivity, rash,
Levofloxacin	500–750 mg IV/PO q24h		CNS stimulation, dizziness, somnolence
Moxifloxacin	400 mg IV/PO q24h		
Gemifloxacin	320 mg PO q24h		
Macrolides		QTc prolongation	Nausea, vomiting,
Erythromycin*	250–500 mg PO qid or 0.5–1 g IV q6h	(erythromycin > clarithromycin >	diarrhea, abnormal taste
Azithromycin	250–500 mg IV/PO daily	azithromycin), cholestasis*	
Clarithromycin	250–500 mg PO BID		
Ketolides		Acute hepatic failure,	Nausea, vomiting,
Telithromycin	800 mg PO q24h	QTc prolongation	diarrhea
Clindamycin	600–900 mg IV q8h	*C. difficile* colitis	Nausea, vomiting, diarrhea, abdominal pain, rash
Tetracyclines		Tooth discoloration and	Photosensitivity,
Tetracycline*	250–500 mg PO q6h	retardation of bone	diarrhea
Doxycycline	100 mg IV/PO q12h	growth (in children),	
Minocycline[†]	200 mg PO, then 100 mg PO q12h	renal tubular necrosis,* dizziness,[†] vertigo,[†] pseudotumor cerebri	
Glyclcyclines		—	Nausea, vomiting,
Tigecycline	100 mg bolus, then 50 mg IV q12h		diarrhea
Trimethoprim/ sulfamethox- azole	5 mg/kg IV q8h (based on the trimethoprim component)	Myelosuppression, Stevens-Johnson syndrome, hyperkalemia, aseptic meningitis, hepatic necrosis	Rash, nausea, vomiting, diarrhea
Metronidazole	500 mg IV/PO q8h	Seizures, peripheral neuropathy	Nausea, vomiting, metallic taste, disulfiramlike reaction

(*continued*)

| TABLE 83.9 | Infectious Diseases (*continued*) |

Drug class/ prototypes	Dosing	Rare toxicities	Common toxicities
Antifungal agents			
Azoles		Hepatic failure, increased AST/ALT, cardiovascular toxicity,* hypertension,* edema*	Nausea, vomiting, diarrhea rash, visual disturbances,[†] phototoxicity[†]
Fluconazole	100–800 mg PO/IV daily		
Itraconazole*	200 mg IV/PO q24h		
Voriconazole[†]	4 mg/kg IV q12h or 200 mg PO BID		
Amphotericin B products		Nephrotoxicity (less common with lipid formulations), acute liver failure, myelosuppression	Acute infusion-related reactions, hypokalemia, hypomagnesemia
Amphotericin B deoxycholate	0.3–1.5 mg/kg q24h		
ABLC	5 mg/kg IV q24h		
ABCD	3–4 mg/kg IV q24h		
Liposomal amphotericin B	3–5 mg/kg IV q24h		
Echinocandins		Hepatotoxicity, infusion-related rash, flushing, itching	—
Caspofungin	70 mg IV bolus, then 50 mg IV q24h		
Micafungin	50–150mg IV q24h		
Anidulafungin	200 mg IV bolus, then 100 mg IV q24h		
Flucytosine	25–37.5 mg/kg PO q6h	Myelosuppression, hepatotoxicity, confusion, hallucinations, sedation	Nausea, vomiting, diarrhea, rash
Antiviral agents			
Nucleoside analogs		Nephrotoxicity, rash, encephalopathy, inflammation at injection site phlebitis	Bone marrow suppression,[†] headache, nausea, vomiting, diarrhea (with oral forms)
Acyclovir	400 mg PO TID or 5 mg/kg IV q8h		
Valacyclovir[†]	1,000 mg PO q8h		
Ganciclovir[†]	5 mg/kg IV q12hr		
Valganciclovir	900 mg PO daily–BID		
Amantadine	100 mg PO BID	CNS disturbances (amantadine > rimantadine)	Nausea, vomiting, anorexia, xerostomia
Rimantadine	100 mg PO BID		
Neuraminidase inhibitors		Anaphylaxis,* bronchospasm,[†]	Nausea, vomiting,* cough,[†] local discomfort[†]
Oseltamivir*	75 mg PO BID		
Zanamivir[†]	10 mg inhaled q12h		
Cidofovir	5 mg/kg IV weekly plus probenecid 2 g PO 3 hr before the infusion and then 1 g at 2 and 8 hr after the infusion	Anemia, neutropenia, fever, rash	Nephrotoxicity, uveitis/iritis, nausea, vomiting

(*continued*)

| TABLE 83.9 | Infectious Diseases (*continued*) | | |

Drug class/ prototypes	Dosing	Rare toxicities	Common toxicities
Foscarnet	60 mg/kg IV q8h or 90 mg/kg IV q12h	Seizures, anemia, fever	Nephrotoxicity, electrolyte abnormalities (hypocalcemia, hypomagnesemia, hypokalemia, hypophosphatemia), nausea, vomiting, diarrhea, headache

IV, intravenous; PO, by mouth; BID, two times a day; AST/ALT, alanine aminotransferase/aspartate aminotransferase; TID, three times a day.

TABLE 83.10	Hepatic Disorders

Drug class/ prototypes	Dosing	Rare toxicities	Common toxicities
Lactulose	20–30 g (30–45 mL) PO q2h until initial stool, then adjust to maintain 2–3 soft stools/day	—	Diarrhea, flatulence, nausea
Neomycin	500–2,000 mg PO q6–12h	Nephrotoxicity, neurotoxicity	Nausea, vomiting, diarrhea, irritation or soreness of mouth or rectal area
Rifaximin	400 mg PO TID		Headache
Nonspecific Beta-Blockers Propranolol Nadolol	20–80 mg PO q12h 20–80 mg PO q24h	Heart block, bronchospasm, depression, nightmares, altered glucose metabolism, dyslipidemia, sexual dysfunction	Bradycardia, hypotension, fatigue, malaise, cold extremities
Spironolactone	12.5–100 mg PO q24h	Gynecomastia, hyponatremia	Hyperkalemia

PO, by mouth.

TABLE 83.11	Gastrointestinal Disorders

Drug class/ prototypes	Dosing	Rare toxicities	Common toxicities
Proton pump inhibitors Pantoprazole	20–40 mg PO q12–24h 80 mg IV bolus, then 8 mg/hr × 72 hr	Headache, dizziness, somnolence, diarrhea, constipation, nausea	—
Omeprazole Lansoprazole Esomeprazole	20–40 mg PO q12–24h 30–60 mg PO q12–24h 20–40 mg PO q24h		
Octreotide	25–50 mcg IV bolus, then 25–50 mcg/hr infusion	Arrhythmias, conduction abnormalities, hypothyroidism, cholelithiasis (long-term use)	Diarrhea, flatulence, nausea, abdominal cramps, bradycardia, dysglycemia

PO, by mouth; IV, intravenous.

TABLE 83.12	Neurologic Disorders

Drug class/ prototypes	Dosing	Rare toxicities	Common toxicities
	Status epilepticus		
Benzodiazepines Lorazepam	0.1mg/kg at 2 mg/min up to 8 mg	Paradoxical excitation, hypotension, respiratory depression (high doses)	CNS depression
Midazolam	0.2 mg/kg bolus, then 0.75–10 mcg/kg/min		
Phenytoin	20 mg/kg IV bolus, then 5–7 mg/kg day	Idiosyncratic: rash, fever, bone marrow suppression, Steven-Johnson syndrome, hepatitis	Concentration-dependent: nystagmus, diplopia, ataxia, sedation, lethargy, mood/ behavior changes, coma, seizures
Fosphenytoin	20 mg phenytoin equivalents/kg IV/IM bolus	Associated with chronic use: gingival hyperplasia, folic acid deficiency, hirsutism, acne, vitamin D deficiency, osteomalacia	IV form: hypotension, bradycardia, phlebitis
Phenobarbital	20 mg/kg IV bolus	Rash, bone marrow suppression	Sedation, nystagmus, ataxia, nausea, vomiting IV form: hypotension, bradycardia, respiratory depression
Propofol	30–250 mcg/kg/min	Pancreatitis, propofol infusion syndrome	Hypotension, bradycardia, CNS depression, hypertriglyceridemia
Levetiracetam	500–1,000 mg IV/PO q12h	Behavioral disturbances	Somnolence, nausea, vomiting
Valproate	1,000–2,500 mg/day IV/PO in 2–4 divided doses	Hepatotoxicity, pancreatitis, thrombocytopenia, hyperammonemia, rash	Somnolence, diplopia nausea, vomiting, diarrhea
	Intracranial pressure elevation		
Hypertonic saline (23.4% NaCl)	For mannitol-refractory patients: 30–50 mL q3–6h as needed (central line only) 0.686 mL of 23.4% saline is equiosmolar to 1 g of mannitol	—	Hypernatremia, hyperchloremia
Mannitol	1–1.5 g/kg IV bolus, then 0.25–1 g/kg q3–6h as needed	—	Hypotension, acute renal failure, fluid and electrolyte imbalances

(*continued*)

| TABLE 83.12 | Neurologic Disorders (*continued*) |

Drug class/ prototypes	Dosing	Rare toxicities	Common toxicities
		Stroke	
Alteplase	Ischemic stroke: 0.9 mg/kg IV (NOT to exceed 90 mg), infused over 60 min with 10% of the dose given as an initial bolus over 1 min	—	Bleeding
Factor VII	Hemorrhagic stroke: 1.2–4.8 mg IV	Thrombosis	Hypertension
		ICU delirium	
Haloperidol	2–80 mg IV/PO q6h	QTc prolongation, extrapyramidal side effects (dystonia, akathisia, pseudoparkinsonism, tardive dyskinesia), neuroleptic malignant syndrome	CNS depression, orthostatic hypotension
		ICU sedation	
Benzodiazepines Lorazepam Midazolam	2–4 mg bolus, 0.5–4 mg/hr 1–5 mg bolus, 1–10 mg/hr	Paradoxical excitation, hypotension, respiratory depression (high doses)	CNS depression
Propofol	25–100 mcg/kg/min	Pancreatitis, propofol infusion syndrome	Hypotension, bradycardia, CNS depression, hypertriglyceridemia
Dexmedetomidine	0.2–0.7 mcg/kg/hr	—	Hypotension, bradycardia

IV, intravenous; IM, intramuscular; PO, by mouth; ICU, intensive care unit.

TABLE 83.13   **Hematopoeitic Disorders**

Drug class/ prototypes	Dosing	Rare toxicities	Common toxicities
Direct thrombin inhibitors Lepirudin*	Initial 0.1–0.15 mg/kg/hr infusion, adjust based on aPTT measurements	Allergic reactions*	Bleeding
Argatroban	Initial 2 mcg/kg/min, adjust based on aPTT measurements		
DDAVP	0.3 mcg/kg slow IV	Hyponatremia, hypotension, tachycardia, thrombosis	Facial flushing
Phytonadione (vitamin K)	1–10 mg q24h Can be given PO, SQ, or IV	IV form: anaphylaxis, hypotension	—
Warfarin	Initial 1–5 mg/day, adjust based on INR measurements	Skin necrosis, purple-toe syndrome	Bleeding

aPTT, activated partial thromboplastin time; IV, intravenous; PO, by mouth; SQ, subcutaneous; INR, international normalized ratio.

TABLE 83.14	Pregnancy[a]		

Drug class/ prototypes	Dosing	Rare toxicities	Common toxicities
Magnesium	4–6 g IV over 15–20 min, then 2 g/hr infusion	—	Hypermagnesemia, diarrhea (oral)
Phenytoin	20 mg/kg IV bolus, then 5–7 mg/kg day	Idiosyncratic: rash, fever, bone marrow suppression, Steven-Johnson syndrome, hepatitis Associated with chronic use: gingival hyperplasia. folic acid deficiency. hirsutism, acne. vitamin D deficiency. osteomalacia	Concentration-dependent: nystagmus, diplopia, ataxia. sedation, lethargy. mood/behavior changes. coma, seizures IV form: hypotension, bradycardia, phlebitis
Labetalol	100–800 mg PO q8–12h, max 2.4 g/day	Heart block, bronchoconstriction, drug-induced lupuslike syndrome, rash, peripheral neuropathy	Hypotension, bradycardia. nausea, vomiting.
Hydralazine	10–40 mg IV q4–6h or 10–75 mg PO TID–QID		hypotension, tachycardia. flushing, headache

IV, intravenous; PO, by mouth; TID, three times a day; QID, four times a day.